RADIATION ONCOLOGY
A Question-Based Review
SECOND EDITION

Editors:

Boris Hristov, MD
Chief, Radiation Oncology
Tumor Board Chairman
88th Medical Group
Wright-Patterson AFB, Ohio

Steven H. Lin, MD, PhD
Assistant Professor
Department of Radiation Oncology
The University of Texas MD Anderson Cancer Center
Houston, Texas

John P. Christodouleas, MD, MPH
Department of Radiation Oncology
Hospital of the University of Pennsylvania
Philadelphia, Pennsylvania

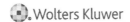

Wolters Kluwer

Philadelphia • Baltimore • New York • London
Buenos Aires • Hong Kong • Sydney • Tokyo

Senior Executive Editor: Jonathan W. Pine, Jr.
Acquisitions Editor: Julie Goolsby
Senior Product Development Editor: Emilie Moyer
Production Product Manager: Priscilla Crater
Manufacturing Manager: Beth Welsh
Strategic Marketing Manager: Stephanie Manzo
Senior Designer: Joan Wendt
Production Service: Aptara, Inc.

Copyright 2015 by Wolters Kluwer Health
Two Commerce Square
2001 Market Street
Philadelphia, PA 19103 USA
First Edition © 2011 by LIPPINCOTT WILLIAMS & WILKINS, a WOLTERS KLUWER
business

All rights reserved. This book is protected by copyright. No part of this book may be reproduced in
any form by any means, including photocopying, or utilized by any information storage and retrieval
system without written permission from the copyright owner, except for brief quotations embodied in
critical articles and reviews. Materials appearing in this book prepared by individuals as part of their
official duties as U.S. government employees are not covered by the above-mentioned copyright.
Printed in USA.

Library of Congress Cataloging-in-Publication Data
Radiation oncology (Hristov)
   Radiation oncology : a question-based review / edited by Boris Hristov, Steven H. Lin,
John P. Christodouleas. – Second edition.
      p. ; cm.
   Includes bibliographical references and index.
   ISBN 978-1-4511-9199-8 (paperback : alk. paper)
   I. Hristov, Boris, editor. II. Lin, Steven H., editor. III. Christodouleas, John P., editor. IV. Title.
   [DNLM: 1. Neoplasms–radiography–Examination Questions. QZ 18.2]
   RC271.R3
   616.99′40642–dc23

                                                                              2014009259

Care has been taken to confirm the accuracy of the information presented and to describe generally
accepted practices. However, the authors, editors, and publisher are not responsible for errors or omis-
sions or for any consequences from application of the information in this book and make no warranty,
expressed or implied, with respect to the currency, completeness, or accuracy of the contents of the
publication. Application of the information in a particular situation remains the professional responsibility of the practitioner.

   The authors, editors, and publisher have exerted every effort to ensure that drug selection and
dosage set forth in this text are in accordance with current recommendations and practice at the time
of publication. However, in view of ongoing research, changes in government regulations, and the
constant flow of information relating to drug therapy and drug reactions, the reader is urged to check
the package insert for each drug for any change in indications and dosage and for added warnings and
precautions. This is particularly important when the recommended agent is a new or infrequently
employed drug.

   Some drugs and medical devices presented in the publication have Food and Drug Administration
(FDA) clearance for limited use in restricted research settings. It is the responsibility of the health care
provider to ascertain the FDA status of each drug or device planned for use in their clinical practice.

To purchase additional copies of this book, call our customer service department at (800) 638-3030 or
fax orders to (301) 223-2320. International customers should call (301) 223-2300.

Visit Lippincott Williams & Wilkins on the Internet at LWW.com. Lippincott Williams & Wilkins
customer service representatives are available from 8:30 am to 6 pm, EST.
10 9 8 7 6 5 4 3

QBV0717

In memory of our Senior Executive Editor and friend, Jonathan W. Pine, Jr.

Section Editors

Ida Ackerman, MD, FRCP(C)
Associate Professor
Department of Radiation Oncology
University of Toronto
Associate Director Postgraduate Radiation
  Oncology Program
Odette Cancer Centre
Sunnybrook Health Science Centre
Toronto, Ontario, Canada
Gynecology

John P. Christodouleas, MD, MPH
Assistant Professor
Department of Radiation Oncology
Hospital of the University of Pennsylvania
Philadelphia, Pennsylvania
Genitourinary

Clifton David Fuller, MD, PhD
Assistant Professor
Department of Radiation Oncology
The University of Texas MD Anderson
  Cancer Center
Houston, Texas
Eye and Ear; Skin

Eli Glatstein, MD
Professor of Radiation Oncology
University of Pennsylvania
Philadelphia, Pennsylvania
Bone and Soft Tissue Sarcoma

Salma K. Jabbour, MD
Associate Professor
Department of Radiation Oncology
Rutgers Cancer Institute of New Jersey,
  Robert Wood Johnson Medical School
Rutgers, The State University of New
  Jersey
New Brunswick, New Jersey
Gastrointestinal

Joshua A. Jones, MD, MA
Assistant Professor of Radiation
  Oncology
Hospital of the University of
  Pennsylvania
Perelman Center for Advanced
  Medicine
Philadelphia, Pennsylvania
Palliative and Benign

Alexander Lin, MD
Assistant Professor
Department of Radiation Oncology
University of Pennsylvania
Philadelphia, Pennsylvania
Head and Neck

Steven H. Lin, MD, PhD
Assistant Professor
Department of Radiation Oncology
The University of Texas MD Anderson
  Cancer Center
Houston, Texas
Thoracic

Anita Mahajan, MD
Professor
Department of Radiation Oncology
The University of Texas MD Anderson
  Cancer Center
Houston, Texas
Pediatrics

Amit Maity, MD
Professor of Radiation Oncology
Hospital of the University of
  Pennsylvania
Philadelphia, Pennsylvania
Hematology

Susan L. McGovern, MD, PhD
Department of Radiation Oncology
The University of Texas MD Anderson
  Cancer Center
Houston, Texas
Central Nervous System

Welela Tereffe, MD, MPH
Associate Professor
Department of Radiation Oncology
The University of Texas MD Anderson
  Cancer Center
Houston, Texas
Breast

Michelle Alonso-Basanta, MD, PhD
Helene Blum Assistant Professor
Department of Radiation Oncology
University of Pennsylvania
Philadelphia, Pennsylvania

Brian C. Baumann, MD
Resident
Department of Radiation Oncology
Hospital of the University of Pennsylvania
Philadelphia, Pennsylvania

Abigail T. Berman, MD
Resident
Department of Radiation Oncology
Hospital of the University of Pennsylvania
Philadelphia, Pennsylvania

Andrew J. Bishop, MD
Resident
Department of Radiation Oncology
The University of Texas MD Anderson
    Cancer Center
Houston, Texas

Katherine Osusky Castle, MD
Resident
Department of Radiation Oncology
The University of Texas MD Anderson
    Cancer Center
Houston, Texas

Kevin Camphausen, MD
Head, Imaging and Molecular
    Therapeutics Section Branch Chief
Center for Cancer Research
National Cancer Institute
Bethesda, Maryland

Eva N. Christensen, MD, PhD
Resident
Department of Radiation Oncology
The University of Texas MD Anderson
    Cancer Center
Houston, Texas

Deborah E. Citrin, MD
Investigator
Head, Section of Translational Radiation
    Oncology
Radiation Oncology Branch
National Cancer Institute
Bethesda, Maryland

David V. Eastham, MD, MPH
Radiation Oncologist
David Grant Medical Center
Travis AFB, California

Mark Edson, MD, PhD
Resident
Department of Radiation Oncology
The University of Texas MD Anderson
    Cancer Center
Houston, Texas

Delnora L. Erickson, MD
Chief Resident
National Capital Consortium
Bethesda, Maryland

Annemarie Fernandes, MD
Resident
Department of Radiation Oncology
University of Pennsylvania
Philadelphia, Pennsylvania

Deborah A. Frassica, MD
Associate Professor
Johns Hopkins Department of Radiation
  Oncology and the University of
  Maryland Department of Radiation
  Oncology
Central Maryland Radiation Oncology
Columbia, Maryland

Eli Glatstein, MD
Professor of Radiation Oncology
University of Pennsylvania
Philadelphia, Pennsylvania

Phillip J. Gray, MD
Instructor
Radiation Oncology
Massachusetts General Hospital
Harvard Medical School
Boston, Massachusetts

Surbhi Grover, MD, MPH
Resident
Department of Radiation Oncology
University of Pennsylvania
Philadelphia, Pennsylvania

Thomas J. Guzzo, MD, MPH
Vice-Chief, Division of Urology
Associate Program Director, Urology
Assistant Professor of Urology
The Hospital of the University of
  Pennsylvania
Philadelphia, Pennsylvania

Lauren M. Hertan, MD, MS
Resident
Department of Radiation Oncology
University of Pennsylvania
Philadelphia, Pennsylvania

Emma B. Holliday, MD
Resident
Department of Radiation Oncology
The University of Texas MD Anderson
  Cancer Center
Houston, Texas

Boris Hristov, MD
Chief, Radiation Oncology
Tumor Board Chairman
88th Medical Group
Wright-Patterson AFB, Ohio

Salma K. Jabbour, MD
Associate Professor
Department of Radiation Oncology
Rutgers Cancer Institute of New Jersey,
  Robert Wood Johnson Medical School
Rutgers, The State University of New Jersey
New Brunswick, New Jersey

Anusha Kalbasi, MD
Resident
Department of Radiation Oncology
Hospital of the University of Pennsylvania
Philadelphia, Pennsylvania

Jason D. Kehrer, DO
Resident
Department of Radiation Oncology
National Cancer Institute
Bethesda, Maryland

György Kovács, MD, PhD
Professor of Radiation Therapy
Head of Interdisciplinary Brachytherapy
  Unit
University of Lübeck
Lübeck, Germany

Vincent J. Lee, MD
Associate Staff
Radiation Oncology
The Permanente Medical Group
Sacramento, California

Anna O. Likhacheva, MD, MPH
Attending Physician
Department of Radiation Oncology
Banner MD Anderson Cancer Center
Gilbert, Arizona

Adjunct Professor
The University of Texas MD Anderson
  Cancer Center
Houston, Texas

Sarah McAvoy, MD
Resident
Department of Radiation Oncology
The University of Texas M.D. Anderson
  Cancer Center
Houston, Texas

Robert G. Prosnitz, MD, MPH
Vice Chair, Department of Radiation
    Oncology
Lehigh Valley Health Network
Allentown, Pennsylvania

Anand Shah, MD, MPH
Postdoctoral Residency Fellow
Department of Radiation Oncology
Columbia University Medical Center
New York, New York

Shervin Shirvani, MD, MPH
Banner Thunderbird Medical Center
Glendale, Arizona

**William K. J. Skinner, Lt Col, USAF, MC,
FS (MD)**
Assistant Professor, Department of
    Radiation Biology
Assistant Program Director,
National Capital Consortium (NCC)
    Radiation Oncology Residency Program
Walter Reed National Military Medical
    Center
Bethesda, Maryland

Bronwyn R. Stall, MD
Staff Physician
Radiation Oncology
San Antonio Military Medical Center
Fort Sam Houston, Texas

Michael J. Swartz, MD
Attending Radiation Oncologist
Department of Radiation Oncology
John T. Vucurevich Cancer Care Institute
Rapid City, South Dakota

Vinita Takiar, MD, PhD
Resident
Department of Radiation Oncology
The University of Texas M.D. Anderson
    Cancer Center
Houston, Texas

Randa Tao, MD
Resident
Department of Radiation Oncology
The University of Texas MD Anderson
    Cancer Center
Houston, Texas

Nikhil G. Thaker, MD
Resident
Department of Radiation Oncology
The University of Texas MD Anderson
    Cancer Center
Houston, Texas

Reid F. Thompson, MD, PhD
Resident
Department of Radiation Oncology
The Hospital of the University of
    Pennsylvania
Philadelphia, Pennsylvania

Richard Tuli, MD
Assistant Professor
Department of Radiation Oncology
Samuel Oschin Comprehensive Cancer
    Institute
Cedars-Sinai Medical Center
Los Angeles, California

Gary V. Walker, MD, MPH
Resident
Department of Radiation Oncology
The University of Texas MD Anderson
    Cancer Center
Houston, Texas

Jingya Wang, MD
Resident
Department of Radiation Oncology
The University of Texas MD Anderson
    Cancer Center
Houston, Texas

Jing Zeng, MD
Assistant Professor
Department of Radiation Oncology
University of Washington
Seattle, Washington

Acknowledgments

The Editors wish to acknowledge the contributions of the following people who submitted chapters for the first edition.

Michelle Alonso-Basanta, MD, PhD

Fariba Asrari, MD

Gopal K. Bajaj, MD

Justin E. Bekelman, MD

M. Kara Bucci, MD

Kevin Camphausen, MD

Timothy A. Chan, MD, PhD

Joe Y. Chang, MD, PhD

John P. Christodouleas, MD, MPH

Deborah E. Citrin, MD

Theodore L. DeWeese, MD

Roland Engel, MD

Deborah A. Frassica, MD

Eli Glatstein, MD

Thomas J. Guzzo, MD

Naomi B. Haas, MD

Russell K. Hales, MD

Joseph M. Herman, MD, MSC

Boris Hristov, MD

Salma Jabbour, MD

Melenda D. Jeter, MD, MPH

Atif Khan, MD

Ritsuko Komaki, MD

Vincent J. Lee, MD

Zhongxing Liao, MD

Alexander Lin, MD

Lilie Lin, MD

Steven H. Lin, MD, PhD

Robert A. Lustig, MD, FACR

Anita Mahajan, MD

Charles H. Matthews, MD, MBA

William P. O'Meara, MD

Daniel G. Petereit, MD

John P. Plastaras, MD, PhD

Robert Prosnitz, MD

Kristin Janson Redmond, MD, MPH

Ramesh Rengan, MD, PhD

Daniele Rigamonti, MD, FACS

Howard M. Sandler, MD, MS

Giuseppe Sanguineti, MD

Ori Shokek, MD

Benjamin D. Smith, MD

Danny Y. Song, MD

Bronwyn R. Stall, MD

Robert C. Susil, MD, PhD

Michael J. Swartz, MD

Owen C. Thomas, MD, PhD

Brent A. Tinnel, MD

Richard Tuli, MD, PhD

Neha Vapiwala, MD

James Welsh, MD

Moody D. Wharam, Jr., MD

Shiao Y. Woo, MD, FACR

Tse-Kuan Yu, MD, PhD

Richard C. Zellars, MD

Jing Zeng, MD

Preface

It is with great pleasure that we introduce the second edition of *Radiation Oncology: A Question-Based Review*. Based on the favorable response to the first edition, we believe that this text will continue to serve as an important reference for trainees as well as practicing radiation oncologists. While this second edition has been completely reviewed and updated, the book's core format and objectives have essentially remained the same.

The handbook's question-based approach is designed to provide medical students, residents, and radiation oncologists with a quick primer on the clinical management of all the major cancer types and conditions that are currently treated with radiation. One enduring goal of this edition is to serve as a user-friendly means for self-assessment and to help both practicing and aspiring radiation oncologists build more intuitively upon their existing knowledge of the field. With this in mind, we include various memory aids and incorporate many useful facts from other relevant disciplines such as radiology, anatomy, and medical oncology. We also emphasize providing the clinician with the best evidence and rationale for modern radiation oncology practice by continuing to highlight practice-changing developments, major randomized trials, and the best retrospective data available for various cancer types. Finally, each section of the book (e.g., Pediatrics, GI, Breast, etc.) has been meticulously reviewed in its entirety by a single experienced faculty physician specializing in that particular area of radiation oncology.

We hope that our second edition of *Radiation Oncology: A Question-Based Review* continues to serve as an invaluable and high-yield learning tool and that clinicians and students of radiation oncology alike continue to benefit from its unique approach and format.

The Editors

Abbreviation Key

Abbrev	Full Spell-Out
2D	two-dimensional
3D	three-dimensional
3D-CRT	three-dimensional conformal radiation therapy
5-FU	5-fluoro uracil
ABMT	autologous bone marrow transplant
APBI	accelerated partial breast irradiation
abnl	abnormal
ACTH	adrenocorticotropic hormone
ADH	antidiuretic hormone
adj	adjuvant
Adr	Adriamycin
AFP	alpha-feto protein
AIDS	acquired immune deficiency syndrome
AJCC	American Joint Committee on Cancer
aka	also known as
alk phos	alkaline phosphatase
Alt	alternated with
am	morning (ante meridian)
ANC	absolute neutrophil count (lab)
ant	anterior
anterolat	anterolateral
AP	anterior-posterior
APC	adenomatous polyposis coli (gene mutation)
appx	approximately
APR	abdomino-perineal resection
ARUBA	A Randomized Trial of Unruptured Brain Arteriovenous Malformations
ASCUS	atypical squamous cells of unknown significance
ASTRO	American Society for Therapeutic Radiation and Oncology
AUC	area under the curve
avg	average
BAT	B-mode acquisition and targeting
b/c	because
b/t	between
bFFP	biochemical freedom from progression
β-HCG	beta-human chorionic gonadotropin
bid	twice daily
bilat	bilateral
BM	bone marrow

Abbrev	*Full Spell-Out*
BMI	body mass index
BMP	basic metabolic panel
BMT	bone marrow transplant
BTSG	Brain Tumor Study Group
BWS	Beckwith-Wiedemann Syndrome
Bx	biopsy/biopsies
C	cervical (spine level)
c/w	Compared with
CA 19-9	cancer antigen 19-9
CA 125	cancer antigen 125
CALGB	Cancer and Leukemia Group B
C/A/P	chest/abdomen/pelvis
CBC	complete blood count (lab)
CCCG	Colorectal Cancer Collaborative Group
cCR	clinical complete response
CD	cone-down
CD4	cluster of differentiation 4 (for immune cells)
CEA	carcinoembryonic antigen
CESS	Cooperative Ewing Sarcoma Study
CHART	Continuous Hyperfractionated Accelerated Radiotherapy Trial
chemo	chemotherapy
CHF	congestive heart failure
CIN	cervical intraepithelial neoplasia
CIS	carcinoma in situ
cm	centimeter/centimeters
CMP	complete metabolic panel (lab)
c-myc	(gene)
cN0	clinically node-negative
CN	cranial nerve
CNS	central nervous system
Co-60	cobalt-60
COG	Children's Oncology Group
contralat	contralateral
CPT	common procedural terminology
Cr	creatinine
CR	complete response
CRT	chemoradiation
CSF	cerebrospinal fluid
CSI	craniospinal irradiation
CSM	cancer-specific mortality
CSS	cause-specific survival
CT	computed tomography
cT	clinical T-stage
CTV	clinical target volume
Cx	Cervical (spine level)
CXR	chest x-ray
D/C	discontinue/discontinued

(Continued)

Abbrev	Full Spell-Out
D&C	dilation and curettage
DCC	deleted in colorectal cancer (gene)
DDx	differential diagnosis
DFS	diseasefree survival
DI	diabetes insipidus
DLBCL	diffuse large-B cell lymphoma
DLCO	lung diffusion capacity testing
DM	distant metastasis
DMFS	distant metastasisfree survival
DOI	depth of invasion
DRE	digital rectal examination
DSS	disease-specific survival
d/t	due to
DVH	dose volume histogram
DVT	deep venous thrombosis
Dx	diagnosis/diagnoses
Dz	disease/diseases
EB	external beam
EBRT	external beam radiation therapy
EBUS	endobronchial ultrasound
EBV	Epstein-Barr virus
ECE	extracapsular extension
ECOG	Eastern Cooperative Oncology Group
EFRT	Extended field ratiotherapy
EFS	eventfree survival
e.g.	for example
EGFR	epidermal growth factor receptor
EM	electron microscopy
ENI	elective nodal irradiation
EORTC	European Organisation for Research and Treatment of Cancer
Epo	erythropoetin
ESR	erythrocyte sedimentation rate (lab)
et al.	and others
EUA	exam under anesthesia
EUS	endoscopic ultrasound
EWS	Ewing sarcoma
exam	examination
f/b	followed by
FAP	familial adenomatous polyposis
FDA	Food and Drug Administration
FDG	fluorine-18 2-fluoro-2-deoxy-D-glucose
FEV	forced expiratory volume
FFS	failurefree survival
FFTF	freedom from treatment failure
FIGO	International Federation of Gynecology and Obstetrics
FH	Favorable histology
FHIT	fragile histidine triad

Abbrev	Full Spell-Out
FISH	fluorescence in situ hybridization
FKHR	Forkhead (drosophilia) homolog 1 (rhabdomyosarcoma) (gene)
FLAIR	fluid attenuation inversion recovery
F:M	female to male ratio
FN rate	false-negative rate
FNA	fine needle aspiration
FOLFOX	5-FU/leukovorin/oxaliplatin
FPR	false-positive rate
FSH	follicle-stimulating hormone
FSR	fractionated stereotactic radiotherapy
fx	fraction/fractions
GBM	glioblastoma multiforme
GH	growth hormone
GI	gastrointestinal
GN-CSF	granulocyte-macrophage colony-stimulating factor
GnRH	gonadotropin-releasing hormone
GTR	gross total resection
GTV	gross target volume
GU	genitourinary
Gy	Gray
gyn	gynecologic
H&N	head and neck
H&P	history and physical
HA	headache
HAART	highly active antiretroviral therapy
HCG	human chorionic gonadotropin (lab test)
HDC+SCT	high-dose chemotherapy with stem cell transplant
HDR	high dose rate
Hgb	hemoglobin
HGG	High-grade glioma
HGSIL	High-grad squamous intraepithelial lesion
HIV	human immunodeficiency virus
HNPCC	hereditary nonpolyposis colon cancer
HPV	human papilloma virus
hr/hrs	hour/hours
HR	hazard ratio
HRT	hormone replacement therapy
HSV	herpes simplex virus
HTN	hypertension
HVA	homovanillic acid
Hx	history/histories
Hyperfx	Hyperfractionation
IBCSG	International Breast Cancer Study Group
IC	Internal carotid
ICP	intracranial pressure
IDL	isodose line
i.e.	that is
IELCAP	International Early Lung Cancer Action Project

(Continued)

Abbrev	Full Spell-Out
IFN	interferon
IgA	immunoglobulin A
IGF	insulinlike growth factor
IgG	immunoglobulin G
IGRT	image-guided radiation therapy
IJROBP	*International Journal of Radiation Oncology, Biology, and Physics*
IMA	inferior mesenteric artery
IMRT	intensity-modulated radiation therapy
inf	inferior
INR	international normalized ratio
intraop	intraoperative
IORT	intraoperative radiation therapy
ipsi	ipsilateral
IQ	intelligence quotient
ITV	internal target volume
IVC	inferior vena cava
JAMA	*Journal of the American Medical Association*
JCO	*Journal of Clinical Oncology*
JCOG	Japan Clinical Oncology Group
JCRT	Joint Center for Radiation Therapy
JHH	Johns Hopkins Hospital
JNCI	*Journal of the National Cancer Institute*
JPA	juvenile pilocytic astrocytoma
KPS	Karnofsky performance status
L	lumbar (spine level)
LA	lymphadenopathy
lab	laboratory/laboratory test
LAD	lymphadenopathy
LAMP	Locally Advanced Multimodality Protocol
LAO	left anterior oblique
lat	lateral
LC	local control
LDH	lactate dehydrogenase
LDR	low dose rate
LE	lower extremity
LEEP	loop electrosurgical excision procedure
LF	local failure
LFT	liver function test
LGSIL	low-grade squamous intraepithelial lesion
LH	luteinizing hormone
LINAC	linear accelerator
LLL	left lower lobe
LML	left middle lobe
LN	lymph node
LND	lymph node dissection
LOH	loss of heterozygosity
LP	lumbar puncture
LPO	left posterior oblique

Abbrev	Full Spell-Out
LR	local recurrence
LRC	locoregional control
LRF	locoregional failure
LRFS	local recurrencefree survival
LRR	locoregional recurrence
LUL	left upper lobe
LVI	lymphovascular invasion
LVSI	lymphovascular stromal invasion
MALT	mucosa-associated lymphoid tissue
max	maximal/maximum
MB	medulloblastoma
MDACC	MD Anderson Cancer Center
med	medication
MEN	multiple endocrine neoplasia
mets	metastasis/metastases
M:F	male to female ratio
MFS	metastasesfree survival
MGMT	O^6-methylguanine DNA-methyltransferase
MI	myocardial infarction
MIBG	metaiodobenzylguanidine
min	minimal/minimum
MLD	mean lung dose
MN	mediastinal node
mo/mos	month/months
MRC	Medical Research Council
MRI	magnetic resonance imaging
MS	median survival
MSKCC	Memorial Sloan Kettering Cancer Center
MTD	maximum tolerated/tolerable dose
Mtx	Methotrexate
MVA	multivariate analysis
NB	neuroblastoma
N/C	nuclear to cytoplasm ratio
NCCN	National Comprehensive Cancer Network
NCCTG	North Central Cancer Treatment Group
NCI	National Cancer Institute
NCIC	National Cancer Institute of Canada
NED	no evidence of disease
NEJM	*New England Journal of Medicine*
neoadj	neoadjuvant
NF	neurofibromatosis
NF	neurofibromatosis
NGGCT	non-germinomatous germ cell tumor
NHL	non-Hodgkin lymphoma
NPCR	National Program of Cancer Registries
NPV	negative predictive value
NPX	nasopharynx
NR	no response

(Continued)

Abbrev	Full Spell-Out
NSABP	National Surgical Adjuvant Breast and Bowel Project
NSAID	nonsteroidal anti-inflammatory drug
NSE	neuron-specific enolase
NSS	not statistically significant
NTR	near-total resection
n/v	nausea/vomiting
NWTS	National Wilms Tumor Study
NZ	New Zealand
OPX	oropharynx
OR	odds ratio
ORN	Osteoradionecrosis
ORR	overall response rate
OS	overall survival
PA	posterior-anterior
PAP	Papanicolau
PCI	prophylactic cranial irradiation
PCNSL	primary CNS lymphoma
PCP	pneumocystic pneumonia
PCR	polymerase chain reaction
pCR	pathologic complete response
PDGFR	platelet-derived growth factor receptor
PEG (tube)	percutanous endoscopic gastrostomy tube
periop	perioperative
PET	positron emission tomography
PF	posterior fossa
PFS	progressionfree survival
PFT	pulmonary function test
Plt	platelets
pm	afternoon (post meridian)
PM	para-meningeal (for rhabdomyosarcoma)
PMH	Princess Margaret Hospital
pN0	pathologically node negative
PNET	primitive neuroectodermal tumor
PNI	perineural invasion
PNS	paranasal sinuses
PORT	postoperative radiation therapy
post	posterior
posterolat	posterolateral
postop	postoperative
PPV	positive predictive value
PR	partial response
PrA	para-aortic (for lymph nodes)
PrT	paratesticular (for rhabdomyosarcoma)
preop	preoperative
PS	performance status
PSA	prostate-specific antigen
pt/pts	patient/patients
PTHrP	parathyroid hormone–related peptide

Abbrev	Full Spell-Out
PT	prothrombin time
pT	pathologic tumor stage
PTV	planning target volume
PUVA	psoralen and long-wave ultraviolet radiation
q	every
qd	daily
QOL	quality of life
QUANTEC	quantitative analysis of normal tissue effect in the clinic
RAO	right anterior oblique
RASSFIA	Ras Association (RalGDS/AF-6) domain family member 1A
RB	restinoblastoma
RBE	relative biologic effectiveness
RCC	renal cell carcinoma
RCT	randomized controlled trial
rcv	receive/received
RFS	relapsefree survival
RLL	right lower lobe
RML	right middle lobe
RMS	rhabdomyosarcoma
r/o	rule out
ROM	range of motion
RPO	right posterior oblique
RR	relative risk
RT	radiation or radiation therapy
RTOG	Radiation Therapy Oncology Group
RUL	right upper lobe
RUQ	right upper quadrant
Rx	prescription/prescriptions
S	sacral (spine level)
SBO	small bowel obstruction
SC	sSpinal cord
SCC	squamous cell carcinoma
SCCa	squamous cell carcinoma
SCV	supraclavicular
Sg	Surgery
SEER	Surveillance Epidemiology and End Results (data)
SFOP	French Society of Pediatric Oncology
Sg	surgery
SIADH	syndrome of inappropriate secretion of antidiuretic hormone
SIL	squamous intraepithelial lesion
SQ	subcutaneous
s/p	status post
SPECT	single photon emission computed tomography
SRS	stereotactic radiosurgery
SS	statistically significant
SSD	source to skin distance
ST	Soft tissue (as in sarcoma)
STD	sexually transmitted disease

(Continued)

Abbrev	*Full Spell-Out*
STR	subtotal resection
STS	soft-tissue sarcoma
sup	superior
SVC	superior vena cava
Sx	symptom/symptoms
T	thoracic (spine level)
TD	tolerance dose
TFT	thyroid function test
tid	three times a day
TMZ	temozolomide
TNM	Tumor/Node/Metastasis
trilat	trilateral
TRUS	transrectal ultrasound
TSH	thyroid-stimulating hormone
Tx	treatment/treatments
UA	urinalysis
UCSF	University of California at San Francisco
UE	upper extremity
UH	unfavorable histology
UK	United Kingdom
unilat	unilateral
US	ultrasound
U.S.	United States
UV	ultraviolet
VALCSG	Veterans Administration Lung Cancer Study Group
VCE	vincristine, carboplatin, etoposide (chemo regimen)
VMA	vanillylmandelic acid
vs.	versus
WBC	white blood cell
WBRT	whole brain radiation therapy
WHO	World Health Organization
wk/wks	week/weeks
WLE	wide local excision
yo	year old/years old
yr/yrs	year/years

Symbols	
+	meaning *with or and* (as in Surgery + RT)
→	meaning *followed by*
↑	meaning *increasing, high(er),* or *elevated*
↓	meaning *decreasing or low(er)*

Contents

Section Editors … *v*
Updating Authors … *vii*
Acknowledgments … *x*
Preface … *xi*
Abbreviation Key … *xii*

PART I   Pediatrics … 1

1   Rhabdomyosarcoma … 1
Updated by Vinita Takiar

2   Ewing Sarcoma … 13
Updated by Randa Tao

3   Wilms Tumor … 20
Updated by Eva N. Christensen

4   Neuroblastoma … 31
Updated by Jingya Wang

5   Retinoblastoma … 39
Updated by Vinita Takiar

6   Langerhans Cell Histiocytosis … 44
Updated by Mark Edson

7   Medulloblastoma … 47
Updated by Nikhil G. Thaker

8   Ependymoma … 57
Steven H. Lin, Ori Shokek, and
Updated by Mark Edson

9   Intracranial Germ Cell and Pineal Tumors … 62
Updated by Nikhil G. Thaker

10   Craniopharyngioma … 67
Updated by Andrew J. Bishop

11   Hemangioblastoma … 71
Updated by Sarah McAvoy

12   Brainstem Glioma … 74
Updated by Andrew J. Bishop

PART II		**Central Nervous System**	**77**
	13	General Central Nervous System *Updated by Jingya Wang*	77
	14	Low-Grade Glioma *Updated by Andrew J. Bishop*	81
	15	High-Grade Glioma *Updated by Sarah McAvoy*	87
	16	Optic Pathway Glioma *Updated by Andrew J. Bishop*	94
	17	Primary Central Nervous System Lymphoma *Updated by Gary V. Walker*	96
	18	Meningioma *Updated by Mark Edson*	104
	19	Pituitary Tumor *Updated by Emma B. Holliday*	107
	20	Primary Spinal Cord Tumor *Boris Hristov, Timothy A. Chan, and Updated by Eva N. Christensen*	113
	21	Choroid Plexus Carcinoma and Papilloma *Updated by Jingya Wang*	117
	22	Arteriovenous Malformation *Updated by Sarah McAvoy*	120
	23	Vestibular Schwannoma/Acoustic Neuroma *Updated by Sarah McAvoy*	124
PART III		**Eye**	**129**
	24	Ocular Melanoma *Updated by Vinita Takiar*	129
	25	Orbital and Intraocular Primary Eye Lymphomas *Updated by Randa Tao*	135
	26	Thyroid Ophthalmopathy *Updated by Randa Tao*	139
	27	Orbital Pseudotumor *Updated by Randa Tao*	142
PART IV		**Head and Neck**	**145**
	28	Nasopharyngeal Cancer *Updated by Eva N. Christensen*	145
	29	Sinonasal Tract Tumors *Updated by Vinita Takiar and Gopal K. Bajaj*	151

30	Oral Cavity Cancer	156
	Updated by Anna O. Likhacheva and Gopal K. Bajaj	
31	Oropharyngeal Cancer	164
	Updated by Gary V. Walker	
32	Salivary Gland Cancer	173
	Updated by Vinita Takiar	
33	Laryngeal and Hypopharyngeal Cancers	179
	Updated by Anna O. Likhacheva and Gopal K. Bajaj	
34	Thyroid Cancer	190
	John P. Christodouleas and Updated by Mark Edson	
35	Head and Neck Cancer of Unknown Primary	197
	Boris Hristov, Giuseppe Sanguineti, and Updated by Gary V. Walker	
36	Neck Management and Postoperative Radiation Therapy for Head and Neck Cancers	202
	Updated by Gary V. Walker	

PART V   Thorax   **207**

37	Early-Stage (I–II) Non–Small Cell Lung Cancer	207
	Updated by Nikhil G. Thaker and Steven H. Lin	
38	Advanced-Stage (III–IV) Non–Small Cell Lung Cancer	220
	Updated by Steven H. Lin	
39	Small Cell Lung Cancer and Bronchial Neuroendocrine Tumor	233
	Updated by Shervin M. Shirvani and Ritsuko Komaki	
40	Thymoma and Thymic Carcinoma	243
	Updated by Shervin M. Shirvani and Melenda D. Jeter	
41	Pleural Mesothelioma	250
	Updated by Nikhil G. Thaker and Steven H. Lin	

PART VI   Breast   **257**

42	General Breast Cancer	257
	Updated by Katherine Osusky Castle	
43	Ductal and Lobular Carcinoma In Situ	264
	Updated by Emma B. Holliday	
44	Early-Stage (I–II) Breast Cancer	272
	Updated by Emma B. Holliday	
45	Locally Advanced Breast Cancer	283
	Updated by Jingya Wang	

PART VII	**Gastrointestinal**	**297**
46	**Esophageal Cancer** *Updated by Sonny Batra*	297
47	**Gastric Cancer** *Updated by Boris Hristov*	307
48	**Pancreatic and Periampullary Adenocarcinoma** *Updated by Anusha Kalbasi*	316
49	**Hepatocellular Carcinoma** *Updated by Richard Tuli*	328
50	**Biliary Tree and Gallbladder Cancer** *Updated by Anusha Kalbasi*	334
51	**Colorectal and Small Bowel Cancer** *Updated by Richard Tuli*	341
52	**Anal Cancer** *Updated by Richard Tuli*	353
PART VIII	**Genitourinary**	**363**
53	**Low-Risk Prostate Cancer** *Updated by Anand Shah*	363
54	**Intermediate- and High-Risk Prostate Cancer** *Updated by Abigail T. Berman and John P. Christodouleas*	374
55	**Adjuvant and Salvage Treatment for Prostate Cancer** *Updated by Jing Zeng*	385
56	**Metastatic Prostate Cancer** *Updated by Phillip J. Gray*	390
57	**Brachytherapy for Prostate Cancer** *Updated by Anand Shah and György Kovács*	395
58	**Bladder Cancer** *Updated by Brian C. Baumann and John P. Christodouleas*	400
59	**Seminoma** *Updated by Reid F. Thompson*	408
60	**Testicular Nonseminomatous Germ Cell Tumor** *Updated by Reid F. Thompson and Thomas J. Guzzo*	414
61	**Penile Cancer** *Updated by Jing Zeng*	419
62	**Urethral Cancer** *Updated by Reid F. Thompson*	425
63	**Renal Cell Carcinoma** *Updated by Phillip J. Gray and Thomas J. Guzzo*	429

PART IX   **Gynecology**   **435**

     64   Cervical Cancer   **435**
           Updated by Jing Zeng

     65   Ovarian Cancer   **445**
           Updated by Surbhi Grover

     66   Endometrial Cancer   **451**
           Updated by Surbhi Grover

     67   Uterine Sarcoma   **461**
           Updated by Surbhi Grover

     68   Vulvar Cancer   **464**
           Updated by Surbhi Grover

     69   Vaginal Cancer   **470**
           Updated by Surbhi Grover

PART X   **Hematology**   **475**

     70   Hodgkin Lymphoma   **475**
           Updated by Annemarie Fernandes

     71   Non-Hodgkin Lymphoma   **483**
           Updated by Annemarie Fernandes

     72   MALT Lymphoma (Gastric and Ocular
           Adnexa and Other Sites)   **491**
           Updated by Annemarie Fernandes

     73   Plasmacytoma/Multiple Myeloma   **497**
           Updated by Robert Prosnitz

     74   Mycosis Fungoides   **502**
           Updated by Lauren M. Hertan

     75   Transplant/Total Body Irradiation   **508**
           Updated by Delnora L. Erickson and Deborah E. Citrin

PART XI   **Bone**   **513**

     76   Osteosarcoma   **513**
           Updated by David V. Eastham and Deborah A. Frassica

     77   Chondrosarcoma   **517**
           Updated by Vincent J. Lee and Deborah A. Frassica

     78   Chordoma   **520**
           Updated by Vincent J. Lee and Michelle Alonso-Basanta

PART XII   **Soft Tissue Sarcoma**   **525**

     79   General and Extremity Soft Tissue Sarcoma   **525**
           Updated by Abigail T. Berman and Deborah A. Frassica

80 Hemangiopericytoma and Solitary
Fibrous Tumors 534
Updated by Boris Hristov

81 Desmoid Tumors 536
Updated by William K. J. Skinner and Deborah A. Frassica

82 Retroperitoneal Soft Tissue Sarcoma 540
Updated by David V. Eastham and Deborah A. Frassica

PART XIII Skin 545

83 Melanoma 545
Updated by Anna O. Likhacheva

84 Squamous Cell and Basal Cell Carcinomas
(Nonmelanoma Skin Cancers) 553
Updated by Anna O. Likhacheva

85 Merkel Cell Carcinoma 559
Updated by Anna O. Likhacheva

86 Nonmelanoma Cutaneous Ear Cancer 563
Updated by Eva N. Christensen

PART XIV Palliative 567

87 Brain Metastases 567
Updated by Jason D. Kehrer and Bronwyn R. Stall

88 Bone Metastases 577
Updated by Delnora L. Erickson and Bronwyn R. Stall

89 Cord Compression 584
Updated by Jason D. Kehrer and Bronwyn R. Stall

90 Superior Vena Cava Syndrome 588
Updated by Delnora L. Erickson and Bronwyn R. Stall

PART XV Benign Disease 593

91 Heterotopic Ossification Prophylaxis 593
Updated by Jing Zeng and Michael J. Swartz

92 Keloids 596
Updated by Jing Zeng and Michael J. Swartz

Appendix
Normal Tissue Constraint Guidelines 599
INDEX 605

Part I Pediatrics

1 Rhabdomyosarcoma

Updated by Vinita Takiar

▶ BACKGROUND

What are the 3 most commonly tested rhabdomyosarcoma (RMS) cases on the radiation oncology oral boards?

Bladder (trigone), parameningeal (PM), and orbit

What are the 2 incidence age peaks of RMS and their associated histologies?

2–6 yo (embryonal) and 15–19 yo (alveolar)

What is the estimated overall annual incidence of RMS in the U.S.?

350 cases/yr of RMS in the U.S., 3% of all childhood cancers (#1 soft tissue sarcoma)

What are the most common sites of RMS? List them in order of approximate frequency in %.

Most common sites of RMS:
1. H&N 40% (PM 25%, orbit 9%, non-PM 6%)
2. GU 30%
3. Extremity 15%
4. Trunk 15%

What are the most common sites of mets?

Bone, BM, and lung

What % of pts present with mets? What types are prone to have hematogenous mets?

15% of pts present with mets. The prostate, trunk, and extremities are prone to hematogenous mets.

What is the most common origin of RMS?

Mesenchymal stem cells. Sporadic RMS is the most common.

What genetic syndromes are associated with RMS?

Genetic syndromes: Beckwith-Wiedemann syndrome (BWS), Li Fraumeni, NF-1, Costello syndrome, and Noonan syndrome

What are the 4 major histologies of RMS and their associated subtypes (if any)? Which is most common?

Major histologies of RMS and subtypes:
1. Embryonal (classic, spindle cell, and botryoid) (Most common: 60%)
2. Alveolar
3. Pleomorphic
4. Undifferentiated

What genetic change is associated with embryonal RMS?

LOH 11p15.5 (embryonal) is associated with *IGF2* **gene deletion,** seen in BWS; also, abnormalities in chromosomes 2, 8, 12, and 13 are associated with MYCN, MDM2, CDK4, CDKN2A (p16), CDKN2B, and TP53 genes.

What translocations are associated with alveolar RMS? What are the genes involved in the fusion?

Alveolar RMS is associated with **t(2;13)** (70%) and **t(1;13)** (20%). Genes involved are **PAX3 or PAX7 with FOX01 (also known as FKHR).**

Which is the most common histology of RMS in infants? Young children? Adolescents? Adults?

Most common RMS histology **(by age group):**
Infants: botryoid
Young children: embryonal
Adolescents: alveolar
Adults: pleomorphic

Which histologies are most commonly associated with each organ site (H&N, GU, extremities/trunk)?

Most common RMS histologies **(by site):**
H&N: embryonal
GU: botryoid
Extremities/Trunk: alveolar

What is the most important cytogenetic tumor marker for RMS?

MyoD (and other myogenic proteins: actin, myosin, desmin, myoglobin)

What is the DDx for small round blue cell tumors of childhood?

Medulloblastoma, rhabdomyosarcoma, leukemia/lymphoma, Ewing sarcoma, retinoblastoma, neuroblastoma, Wilms tumor

List the histologies of RMS in terms of prognosis from best to worst.

1. Spindle cell and botryoid
2. Classic embryonal
3. Alveolar
4. Undifferentiated

What are the ~5-yr OS rates for each of the histologic subtypes?

~5-yr OS **(by histology):**
Botryoid: 95%
Spindle cell: 88%
Embryonal: 66%
Alveolar: 54%
Undifferentiated: 40%

Which sites require LND b/c of a high propensity for LN mets? What is the risk of LN mets for these sites?

The following sites are associated with >**20%** LN mets rate and thus require LND:

    <u>Paratesticular</u> (PrT): (only if >10 yo)

    <u>Bladder:</u> pelvic

    <u>H&N:</u> nasopharynx (NPX), LND typically not done for NPX

    <u>Extremities:</u> upper extremity (UE) (axillary) and lower extremity (LE) (inguinal/femoral) (*La TH et al., IJROBP 2011*)

Which International Rhabdomyosarcoma Study (IRS) called for routine LN sampling in RMS of the extremity?

IRS-IV (*Neville HL et al., J Pediatr Surg 2000*): 139 extremity pts, 76 patients had surgical LN evaluation; of the 10% who were cN+, 50% were pN+; **of those cN0, 17% were pN+.**

What are considered nonregional mets/LNs for various sites (UE, LE, pelvic organs [PrT, vagina, uterus])?

Non regional LN stations by primary site:

    <u>UE:</u> scalene node

    <u>Pelvic (PrT/vagina/uterus):</u> inguinal

    <u>Retroperitoneal (RP):</u> para-aortic (PrA) (except if immediately adjacent)

    <u>LE:</u> iliacs/PrA

What are the 4 favorable organ sites and their ~3-yr OS rate?

Favorable organ sites:

1. Orbit
2. Non-PM H&N
3. Nonprostate/bladder GU
4. Biliary

The ~3-yr OS is **94%**.

What is the estimated 3-yr OS for RMS arising from unfavorable sites (PM H&N, prostate, bladder, extremities/trunk)?

For unfavorable sites, overall ~3-yr OS is **70%**.

What are the PM H&N sites?

PM H&N sites:

    Middle ear

    Mastoid

    Nasal cavity

    Nasopharynx

    Infratemporal f**O**ssa

    Pterygopalatine f**O**ssa

    Paranasal sinuses

    Parapharyngeal space

(Mnemonic: **MMNNOOPP**)

What are the non-PM H&N sites?

Scalp, cheek, parotid, oral cavity, oropharynx, and larynx

► **WORKUP/STAGING**

List the general workup for RMS.	RMS workup: H&P, basic labs (CMP, CBC, lactate dehydrogenase [LDH]), EUA, CT/MRI primary, CT chest/abdomen, bone scan, BM Bx, and primary site core Bx/incisional Bx; PET/CT may be useful in determining extent of Dz
What specific workup studies are needed for PM RMS?	PM RMS workup: MRI brain, CSF cytology (neuroaxial MRI if +)
What specific workup studies are needed for bladder RMS?	Bladder RMS workup: EUA and cystoscopy
Summarize the TNM criteria for RMS.	**T1:** confined to anatomic site of origin **T1a:** ≤5 cm **T1b:** >5 cm **T2:** extension or fixed to adjacent tissue **T2a:** ≤5 cm **T2b:** >5 cm **N1:** regional node involvement **M1:** DM
Summarize the preop staging of RMS.	**Stage I:** favorable site (any T, any N, M0) **Stage II:** unfavorable site, T1a or T2a (≤5 cm), N0, M0 **Stage III:** unfavorable site, T1b or T2b (>5 cm), and/or N1, M0 **Stage IV:** M1
Summarize the postop grouping for RMS.	**Group I:** R0 resection, localized Dz **Group II:** R1 resection and/or resected +LN **Group III:** R2 (both primary and +LN) or Bx only **Group IV:** DM
Most RMS pts present with what group of Dz?	Most (~50%) present with **group III** Dz.
Define the risk groups for RMS (based on IRS-VI).	**Low risk** (5-yr OS 90%–95%): nonmetastatic, embryonal, *and* a. favorable site all groups *or* b. unfavorable site groups I–II **Intermediate risk:** a. nonmetastatic, group III embryonal, unfavorable site (5-yr OS 70%–85%) *or* b. nonmetastatic unfavorable histology (UH), any site (5-yr OS 55%–60%) **High risk: all metastatic Dz,** including 2–10 yo embryonal (5-yr OS 25%–35%)

▶ **TREATMENT/PROGNOSIS**

What is the Tx paradigm for RMS?

The Tx for RMS in the IRS studies varies based on site, histology, and tumor size.

RMS Tx paradigm: **generally, max safe resection (or Bx alone) → chemo +/– RT (timing of CRT depends on risk groupings)**

What chemo regimens are commonly used in RMS?

Vincristine/Actinomycin D/Cytoxan (VAC) and vincristine/actinomycin D (VA) are commonly used.

Ifosfamide/etoposide (IE) is also used in subsets of RMS.

How does age factor into the prognosis of metastatic embryonal RMS?

>10 yo is worse than <10 yo (EFS 14% vs. 47%).

What factors make PM RMS high risk?

Subarachnoid space involvement with skull base erosion, CN palsy, intracranial extension; DFS 51% vs. 81% (without risk factors)

What is the seminal trial that 1st supported the use of chemo for RMS?

Heyn RM et al. (Cancer 1974): VA chemo vs. nothing after surgery improved OS.

IRS-I: What did it answer?

Group I: favorable histology (FH); **RT not needed**

Group II: RT + VA × 1 yr (no need for Cytoxan)

Groups III–IV: RT + VAC × 2 yr (no Adriamycin [Adr] needed)

DM is more common than LF.

No dose response for RT; no difference in RT field size (large = involved field):

PM RMS ↑ CNS relapse if certain high-risk features are present.

IRS-II: What did it answer?

Group I: VA × 1 yr same as VAC × 2 yrs (except in UH)

Group II: RT + VA × 1 yr same as RT + VAC + 1 yr (except in UH, use VAC + RT).

Groups III–IV: no benefit adding Adr to VAC + RT (except in UH).

Better PM outcomes than **IRS-I** with prophylactic WBRT for high-risk pts.

Chemo alone for special pelvic sites with VAC is not adequate (bladder preservation only 22% b/c of inadequate response).

According to IRS I–II analysis, which RMS site was shown to carry the highest risk for LN mets?

The **prostate** (~40% with LN+ Dz) was shown to have the highest risk for LN mets.

IRS-III: What did it answer?

Groups I–II UH: better with vincristine/Adriamycin/cyclophosphamide (VAdrC) alternating with VAC + RT, than RT + VA or VAC.

Groups II–III favorable site: VA + RT adequate

Groups II–III unfavorable site and group IV FH/UH: VAC + RT; no benefit adding Adr

WBRT prophylaxis did not reduce CNS relapse.

There was an improved bladder preservation rate and OS in the multimodality Tx of special pelvic sites.

Who did not get RT in IRS-III?

Group I FH and group III special pelvic sites (if CR after chemo) did not get RT.

In IRS-III, the OS was mainly driven by what groups of pts?

Groups I–II UH getting VAdrC alternating with VAC and group III FH special pelvic sites

What did IRS-III demonstrate about the Tx of special pelvic sites?

Pelvic site I (bladder dome, vagina, uterus): VAdrC alternating with VAC × 2 yrs → second-look surgery (SLS) at 20 wks → if PR, then RT at wk 20 + Adriamycin/etoposide × 2 cycles; if CR, no RT and continue chemo.

Pelvic site II (bladder neck/trigone, prostate): VAdrC alternating with VAC × 2 yrs → RT (wk 6) → SLS at 20 wks.

Bladder preservation rate 60% vs. 25% (IRS-I–II) and better OS rate (83% vs. 72%).

IRS-IV: What did it answer?

IRS-IV focused on improving outcome for group III: utility of adding IE to VAC, and bid RT (1.1 Gy bid to 59.4 Gy) vs. conventional RT (1.8–50.4 Gy).

Conventional once daily RT remains standard.

VAC remains standard, even for the alveolar type.

However, **for group IV, VAC + IE is standard** (IE vs. vincristine/melphalan).

What trial utilized WBRT prophylaxis for high-risk PM RMS, and how did it differ from other IRS trials?

IRS-II–III, with whole brain to 30 Gy with intrathecal chemo, all started day 0. IRS-IV started day 0 but did not treat the whole brain—just to tumor + 2-cm margin on day 0.

For **IRS-IV,** RT started week 9 except at day 0 for spinal cord compression and week 1 for high-risk PM (direct intracranial extension, base of skull invasion, CN palsy).

What did *Wolden et al.* data show about the importance of RT in clinical group (CG)-I UH RMS?

Wolden et al. (*JCO 1999*) analyzed **IRS-I–III,** RT vs. no RT in **CG-I** pts: showed only a trend to improved FFS and no OS with RT in FH; however, **in CG-I UH, RT improved FFS and OS.**

What was the purpose of COG-D9602?

To determine whether the lowest risk patients from IRS-III and IRS-IV (localized, grossly resected, or gross residual [orbit only]) embryonal RMS could be treated with reduced toxicity by reducing RT dose and eliminating cyclophosphamide. (*Raney RB et al., JCO 2011*)

What are the 2 subsets of low-risk pts on COG-D9602?

Subsets of low-risk pts on COG-D9602:
 Subset A (treated with VA + RT on **IRS-III–IV**): stage 1, CG-I–II, orbit CG-III, stage 2, CG-I–II. Now treated with VAC × 4 cycles **(reduced chemo) → 4 cycles VA + RT.**
 Subset B (treated with VAC + RT on **IRS-III–IV**): stage 1, CG-III (nonorbit), stage 3 CG-I–II. Now treated with VAC × 4 cycles **(reduced chemo) → 12 cycles VA + RT.**

What did the results of COG-D9602 demonstrate?

5-yr FFS rate (88%) and OS rate (97%) were similar to comparable IRS-III pts, even with lower RT doses but were worse than comparable IRS-IV pts receiving VA + cyclophosphamide. (*Raney RB et al., JCO 2011*)

What radiation doses were used in COG-D9602?

Dose depended on clinical group (extent of surgery) and LN positivity. After resection, pts with microscopic residual and uninvolved LN received 36 Gy. Involved LN: **41.4–50.4 Gy.** Orbital primary: **45 Gy.** (*Breneman J et al., IJROBP, 2012*)

What are the major study questions for intermediate-risk pts in COG-ARST0531?

VAC vs. VAC alternating with vincristine/irinotecan (VI); timing of RT (wk 4 vs. wk 10, **IRS-IV**)

What are the major study questions for high-risk pts in COG-ARST0431?

VAC alternating with IE using interval dose compression; ability to improve LC in metastatic RMS by using VI with RT.

What is the timing of RT in IRS-V?

 Low risk: **wk 3**
 Intermediate risk: **wk 12**
 High risk: **wk 15**

What is the timing of RT in COG-D9602?

 Low risk: **wk 13**
 Intermediate risk: **wk 4**
 High risk: **wk 20**

What were the secondary objective questions for RT in COG-D9602?	Whether 36 Gy is adequate for N0, R1 and if 45 Gy is adequate for orbital RMS.
What is the dose for CG-I with FH?	**0 Gy. No RT is required** for CG-I with FH.
What study provided the rationale for reduced RT doses of 36 Gy in IRS-V– COG-D9602?	MSKCC retrospective review (*Mandell L et al., JCO 1990*): in only 32 CG-II pts, no difference in LC between <40 Gy vs. >40 Gy.
All pts with initial nodal involvement, regardless of response to induction therapy or SLS, must get what?	RT to **41.4 Gy if R0-R1** resected; all gross or suspected **gross Dz** treated to **50.4 Gy.** **RT is NEVER omitted for node+ Dz.**
Under what circumstances should RT be interrupted?	ANC <750 µL or Plt <75 K, and if uncontrolled infection or Hgb <10. RT is restarted after these are normalized; if a low blood count is a problem, chemo should be withheld or modified until RT is completed.
How do you treat PA nodes (if +)?	AP/PA to 36 Gy → boost to 50.4 Gy with off-cord technique, IMRT, or protons (allowed on COG studies).
What is defined as a minor deviation of an RT plan?	95% IDL covers <90% PTV but between 90% and 100% CTV, or >110% PTV
What is defined as a major deviation of an RT plan?	95% IDL covering <90% of CTV
What % of CG-III pts get a GTR at SLS?	**25%** of **CG-III** pts get a GTR at SLS.
PT RMS arises from where?	PT RMS arises from the **distal spermatic duct**.
Which RMS tumors have a better prognosis: hyperdiploid or diploid?	**Hyperdiploid** (found in embryonal histologies) vs. diploid (in alveolar histologies)
Based on a review of IRS-III data, where do failures mostly occur after Tx? What is the #1 prognostic factor for LF?	**LF > DM. LN positivity** is the biggest predictor for LF.

What evidence supports the use of ≤40 Gy in the management of CG-II RMS (and therefore the rationale for a test dose of 36 Gy in COG-D9602)?

St. Jude data (*Regine WF et al., IJROBP 1995*) suggest that for the 24 CG-II pts in this study, the LC rate with <40 Gy (89%) was not statistically different from ≥40 Gy (100%).

MSKCC data (*Mandell L et al., JCO 1990*): 32 CG-II pts treated with various doses also found that the LC for doses <40 Gy was equivalent to doses ≥40 Gy.

What evidence is there to support IMRT for H&N RMS (as endorsed by IRS-VI)?

Wolden et al. reviewed 28 pts (21 PM) treated with IMRT. A 1.5-cm margin was used, with a median dose of 50.4 Gy. There was excellent LC (95%) despite reduced margins used, min late toxicity, and comparable acute toxicity. (*IJROBP 2005*)

In IRS-V, what additional dose must be given if Tx is delayed by 2–3 wks? How about >3 wks? If <2 wks?

2–3 wks: **1.8 Gy**
>3 wks: **3.6 Gy**
<2 wks: no change in dose

What 3 issues must be considered when treating an extremity site?

Considerations when treating an extremity site:
1. Evaluate the need to radiate regional nodes.
2. Include scars/drains in the field.
3. Try to spare a strip of skin or portion of the joint/epiphyses.

If a CR is obtained after induction chemo with a group III, N0 embryonal tumor of the vagina, cervix, and uterus, what RT dose would you use?

No RT if CR! These are "special sites."

What dose of RT would you give for a pt with stage III, group I embryonal RMS? How about alveolar RMS?

No RT for ALL embryonal group I pts (stages I–III). For UH group I pts, **36 Gy** RT is given.

If a pt is high risk (i.e., metastatic), should the mets be treated as well as the primary with RT?

At the discretion of the radiation oncologist. At the Johns Hopkins Hospital, the preference is to treat the primary and let the pt finish chemo; if the pt responds to chemo, then mets are treated with RT. Consider treating the mets concurrently with the primary if not too large a BM volume is irradiated.

For what 2 sites of the H&N would you *not* recommend primary resection?

The **orbit and PM** sites are not recommended for primary resection.

For what RMS tumor sites would LND be recommended?

LND is recommended for the following RMS tumor sites:
1. GU (PrT/bladder) (pelvic and PA)
2. Extremities/Trunk (axillary, inguinal)

What are 2 favorable prognostic factors in pts with CG-IV RMS?

Per **IRS-IV, ≤2 metastatic sites and embryonal histology** were associated with better OS. (*Breneman JC et al., JCO 2003*)

▶ TOXICITY

Per COG-D9602, what is the dose constraint for the whole kidney?

The dose constraint for the whole kidney is **19.8 Gy.**

What is the max allowed dose to the whole liver?

The max dose to the whole liver is **23.4 Gy.**

Per COG-D9602, what is the dose limit to the chiasm?

The dose limit to the chiasm is **46.8 Gy.**

What is the max allowed dose to the whole heart? Whole abdomen/pelvis?

The max dose to the whole heart is **30.6 Gy.** The max dose to the whole abdomen/pelvis is **24 Gy (at 1.5 Gy/fx).**

What is the dose limit to the lungs, if less than half of the combined lung volume is in the PTV?

In this situation, the dose limit to the lung is **15 Gy (in 1.5 Gy/fx).**

What is a major side effect of VAC besides myelosuppression?

Veno-occlusive Dz of the liver

Table 1.1	Radiation Doses for Favorable Histology Tumors (per COG-ARST0331, closed)
Stage 1, clinical group I	No radiotherapy
Stage 1, clinical group II, N0	Conventional RT: 36 Gy
Stage 1, clinical group II, N1	Conventional RT: 41.4 Gy
Stage 1, clinical group III	Conventional RT: 45 Gy (orbit only)
Stage 1, clinical group III	Conventional RT: 50.4 Gy (nonorbit)
Stage 2, clinical group I	No radiotherapy
Stage 2, clinical group II, N0	Conventional RT: 36 Gy
Stage 3, clinical group I	No radiotherapy
Stage 3, clinical group II, N0	Conventional RT: 36 Gy
Stage 3, clinical group II, N1	Conventional RT: 41.4 Gy

RT, radiation therapy.

For certain clinical group III pts, the radiotherapy dose may be modified by the use of 2nd-look surgery.

Source: http://members.childrensoncologygroup.org (ARST0331).

Table 1.2	Radiation Doses for Unfavorable Histology Tumors (per COG-ARST0531, completed)
Clinical Group	**Dose**
Group I, alveolar only	36 Gy
Group II, node negative	36 Gy
Group II, node positive	41.4 Gy
Group III, alveolar, orbit only	45 Gy
Group III, all others	50.4 Gy

Table 1.3 Principles of Radiation Therapy (per COG-D9602, completed)

Low risk: Surgery 1st, then chemo. If group I → chemo only, no RT. All pts with initial +node must get RT regardless of response to induction chemo or SLS (at least 41.4 Gy, 50.4 Gy to gross Dz). Vincristine is given with RT and dactinomycin is given at wk 13 prior to RT, but they are not given concurrently.

Target volume: GTV—pre-Tx volume + involved LN; CTV = GTV + 1 cm; PTV = CTV + 0.5 cm. For CG-III to 50.4 Gy, CD at 36 Gy to pre-Tx GTV + 0.5 cm (CTV), with PTV = CTV + 0.5 cm. The planning organ-at-risk volume is based on organs at risk; GTV can be defined by exam, CT, MRI, or PET.

Timing: RT begins wk 13 after postop chemo. The exceptions are those who get SLS and those with vaginal primaries. For those who get SLS, RT starts after surgery at wk 13 (to allow time for healing).

All pts with initial CG-III in a favorable site (stage I, except orbit and paratesticular sites) should be considered for SLS at wk 13.

Intermediate risk: RT given at wk 4 (compare with data from wk 10 on IRS-IV). IMRT/proton/brachytherapy/electron and PET imaging are all allowed. CRT = VC or VI concurrently. Simulation occurs before wk 4 to begin on time.

Margins: CD after 36 Gy for tumors with "pushing" rather than invasive (lung, intestine, bladder). Boost to 50.4 Gy with new GTV representing response + 1 cm (CTV) and 0.5 cm (PTV). If 36 or 41.4 Gy, there is no volume reduction. GTV is pre-Tx volume + margin, except intrathoracic or intra-abdominal tumors (GTV as pre-Tx volume excluding intrathoracic or intra-abdominal/pelvic tumor from which it was debulked, since these are "pushing" borders).

Timing: All at wk 4. Emergency RT for *symptomatic cord compression* and high-risk PM (intracranial extension) can be given on wk 1 (day 1). Management of BOS erosion and CN palsy was not specified in the protocol, so it can be managed according to the discretion of the radiation oncologist.

High risk: RT given on wk 20 to primary and metastatic sites (except high-risk PM sites with IC extension and emergency RT).

High-risk PM sites with only BOS and/or CN palsy will get RT at wk 20. PM sites with intracranial extension will rcv RT at wk 1 (day 0) (but within 2 wks of the 1st cycle of chemo to start RT) and Tx to the metastatic site at wk 20 (unless the metastatic site is within the same Tx port as the primary). Emergency RT for cord compression is on day 0.

(continued)

Table 1.3	Principles of Radiation Therapy (per COG-D9602, completed) *(Continued)*

CRT: VI is given concurrently with RT, starting on wk 19 (day 0 if an emergency or PM with IC). *Alternative:* VC, if VI is not tolerable.

Margins: CD after 36 Gy for tumors with "pushing" rather than invasive (lung, intestine, bladder). Boost to 50.4 Gy with new GTV representing response + 1 cm (CTV) and 0.5 cm (PTV). If 36 or 41.4 Gy, GTV is pre-Tx volume + margin.

Bilat whole lung 15 Gy (10 fx) for pulmonary mets or pleural effusion (can boost to gross Dz) to 50.4 Gy.

IRS, International Rhabdomyosarcoma Study; chemo, chemotherapy; RT, radiation therapy; pt, patient; +node, positive node; SLS, second-look surgery; Gy, gray; Dz, disease; wk, week; GTV, gross target volume; Tx, treatment; LN, lymph node; CTV, clinical target volume; cm, centimeter; PTV, planning target volume; CG, clinical group; CD, cone down; exam, examination; CT, computed tomography; MRI, magnetic resonance imaging; PET, positron emission tomography; postop, postoperative; IMRT, intensity modulated radiation therapy; CRT, chemoradiation; VC, vincristine/ Cytoxan; VI, vincristine/irinotecan; PM, parameningeal; BOS, base of skull; CN, cranial nerve; IC, internal carotid; rcv, receive; bilat, bilateral; fx, fraction; met, metastasis.

Table 1.4	Principles of Surgery (per COG-D9602, completed)

1. WLE with margin preferred, no amputation for group IV setting. The rest get incisional or core Bx (orbit, PM H&N).
2. Sentinel LN Bx should be done for extremity sites.
3. Needle Bx or open Bx can be done; an aggressive LN sample is most appropriate.
4. Definitive surgery can be carried out after initial Bx or noncancer surgery. This subsequent PRE is followed by local adj therapy based on pathology from the definitive PRE.
5. A subsequent delayed resection can be done after chemo and RT (for initial Bx only) if the tumor has diminished enough to make resection feasible. SLS takes place on wk 13 (except orbit, PT).
6. If residual tumor persists after SLS, subsequent-look procedures can be done after further therapy, if the tumor appears resectable. SLS should be done to max extent if it is cosmetically and functionally feasible.
7. H&N sites: no neck dissection unless there is clinical involvement.
8. PrT: Only ipsi RP LN dissection should be done. Do not do radical bilat regional node dissection. Regional LNs are ipsi iliac and RP nodes up to the hilum of the ipsi kidney. Orchiectomy and resection of the entire spermatic cord is via inguinal excision. Bx can take place prior to excision (but must ensure there is no spillage).
9. GU (bladder/prostate): if laparotomy is preformed, then iliac/para-aortic node sample should be done, and any other clinically involved site(s) should be biopsied. Bladder preservation rate is 50%–60%. Partial cystectomy should be done for bladder dome tumors.
10. Elective LND is not indicated except for extremities and PT lesions. Open Bx or LN sampling should be done for any gross enlarged nodes.

WLE, wide local excision; Bx, biopsy; PM, parameningeal; H&N, head and neck; LN, lymph node; PRE, pretreatment re-excision; adj, adjuvant; chemo, chemotherapy; RT, radiation therapy; SLS, second-look surgery; wk, week; PrT, paratesticular; max, maximum; ipsi, ipsilateral; RP, retroperitoneal; bilat, bilateral; GU, genitourinary; LND, lymph node dissection.

2 Ewing Sarcoma

Updated by Randa Tao

 BACKGROUND

What is the annual incidence of Ewing sarcoma (EWS) in the U.S.? How common is it relative to other bone tumors?	**200 cases/yr** of EWS in the U.S.; **2nd most common bone tumor** (osteosarcoma #1)
What is the median age of presentation of EWS?	The median age of EWS is **14–15 yrs**.
Is EWS associated with congenital Dz?	**No.** However, it can occur as a 2nd malignant neoplasm secondary to chemotherapy (i.e., VP16) or radiation.
What is the racial and gender predilection?	EWS is more common in **whites** (>90% of cases) and among **males** (1.5:1).
What is the embryologic tissue and cell of origin in EWS?	**Neuroectodermal tissue** is the embryonic tissue of origin for EWS and it is derived from a primordial bone marrow mesenchymal stem cell.
What is the most common genetic change seen in EWS?	1. **t(11;22)** in 90%, FLI1(11): EWS(22). Other minor translocations include 2. t(21;22) in 10% of cases and 3. t(7;22).
What other neoplasms are associated with the EWS translocation?	PNET, malignant melanoma of soft parts, and desmoplastic small round cell tumor (DSRCT)
Which exon fusion in t(11;22) is most common, and why is this important?	The most common fusion is **exon 7** of EWS and **exon 6** of FLI1 in 60% of cases. It is **associated with a lower proliferative rate and better prognosis.**
What type of cell morphology is expected to be seen in EWS?	**Small round blue cells** should be seen in EWS.
What constitutes the Ewing family of tumors?	**EWS** (osseous and extraosseous), **PNET, DSRCT,** and **Askin tumor**

What other tumors also have small round blue cells?

Lymphoma
Ewing
Acute lymphoblastic leukemia
Rhabdomyosarcoma
Neuroblastoma (NB)
Neuroepithelioma
Medulloblastoma
Retinoblastoma

(Mnemonic: **LEARN NMR**)

What markers help differentiate EWS from other small round blue tumors?

Markers that differentiate EWS:
1. Vimentin
2. HBA-71
3. β_2-microglobulin
4. ↑c-myc (vs. n-myc in NB)

How is PNET similar to and different from EWS histologically?

PNET and EWS have similar translocations and are both CD99 (MIC2)+ and vimentin+. However, **PNET is neuron-specific enolase (NSE)+**, S100+, more differentiated, and has more neuroendocrine features. **EWS is NSE−** and S100 variable.

What major factors have been classically associated with a poor prognosis in EWS?

Male gender
Age >15 yrs (>17 yrs in some)
Pelvic/axial **S**ite or rib origin
Size (>8 cm per St. Jude or >100 cc per **CESS-81** [Cooperative Ewing Sarcoma Studies])
Stage (presence/absence of metastatic Dz is strongest prognostic factor)
↑**LDH**
Poor **response** to chemo (>10% viable tumor)

(Mnemonic: **MASSSive LDH response**) (*Jürgens H et al., Klin Padiatr 1988*)

What is Askin tumor?

Askin tumor is **nonosseous PNET of the chest wall** (worse prognosis than other sites).

What % of EWS pts present with mets?

25% of EWS pts present with mets. Mets typically occur in the **lung** (40%–50%) > bone.

Where do mets typically occur?

(25%–40%) ≥ **BM** (~25%) and LNs (<10%).

What % of pts with localized Dz vs. lung mets have BM micromets?

25% (localized) vs. 40% (lung mets)

▶ WORKUP/STAGING

What is the typical clinical presentation with EWS?

Pain (96% of cases) and swelling (63% of cases) are most common → fever (21%) and fractures (16%).

What Sx at presentation portends a particularly poor prognosis in EWS?

Pts who present with **fever** (21% of cases) tend to have a poor prognosis.

What is the most commonly involved site in EWS at presentation?

Extremities (53%) > **axial skeleton** (47%). The **lower extremity** is the most common region (41%), and the **femur** is most common site (~20% of cases) followed by the pelvis (26%), chest wall (16%), upper extremity (9%), spine (6%), and skull (2%).

If an EWS tumor presents centrally, what is the most common site?

The **pelvis** (26% of cases) is more common than the axial skeleton (12% of cases).

List the general workup for a pt who presents with an extremity mass.

Extremity mass workup: H&P, plain x-ray, MRI/CT primary, and core needle Bx or incisional Bx. Once a Dx of a sarcoma (EWS) is confirmed, complete the workup with CBC, BMP, LDH, ESR, LFTs, CXR, CT chest, bone scan, or PET/CT (preferred), and bilateral BM Bx.

What are the characteristic findings on plain x-ray in EWS? How does this compare to osteosarcoma?

Classically, EWS shows an **"onion skin"** reaction on plain films, whereas osteosarcoma is associated with a "sunburst" appearance. The **Codman triangle,** an area of new subperiosteal bone as a result of periosteal lifting by underlying tumor, can be seen in both EWS and osteosarcoma.

How is EWS staged?

No standard staging system exists. Tumors are either localized or metastatic.

In EWS, what is meant by expendable bones? Name 3.

Expendable bones are ones that can be resected with minimal morbidity, such as:
1. Proximal fibula
2. Ribs
3. Distal four fifths of clavicle
4. Body of scapula
5. Iliac wings

▶ **TREATMENT/PROGNOSIS**

Summarize the current Tx paradigm for EWS.

EWS Tx paradigm: **induction VAdriaC** (vincristine, doxorubicin, and cyclophosphamide **alternating with ifosfamide/etoposide (IE)** → **local therapy at wk 12** (surgery ± RT or definitive RT with non-Adria chemo given during RT, usually 2 cycles) → **further adj chemo to wk 48.** Surgery when possible, give PORT when necessary, and whole lung irradiation (WLI) for lung mets.

Estimate the 5-yr OS for localized and metastatic EWS.

5-yr OS for localized EWS is **60%–80% (60% for pelvic, 80% extremities) and 20% for metastatic EWS (bone mets 5 yrs 30%; lung mets 5 yrs 50%).**

What are the RT doses given for EWS in the definitive vs. the postop setting?

Definitive: 55.8 Gy (45 Gy to prechemo volume with 1.5–2-cm margin with boost to postchemo volume to 55.8 Gy).

Postop: **50.4 Gy for microscopic**/tumor spill and **55.8 Gy for gross** residual; **45 Gy for vertebral body** involvement because of spinal cord tolerance.

What is the LF rate for EWS after definitive RT?

Overall, 5%–25%; worse with pelvic sites (LF 15%–70%); worse with large (>8 cm) lesions (LF 20%)

What are considered adequate surgical margins in EWS?

Per COG protocol **AEWS0031,** adequate margins are >1 cm for bone, >0.5 cm for soft tissue, and >0.20 cm for fascia. (*Womer RB et al., JCO 2012*)

What are 3 indications for adj RT after surgery in EWS?

+Margin, tumor spill, and >10% viable tumor after induction chemo (poor chemo response)

Is there a difference in LC between EWS pts who rcv preop RT vs. postop RT vs. definitive RT?

Yes. *Schuck et al.* performed a secondary analysis of 1,085 pts in **CESS-81 and -86** and **EICESS 92** (European Intergroup CESS) and found no difference in LF between preop and postop RT (5.3% vs. 7.5%), but LF was significantly worse in the definitive RT arm (26%). However, there was a strong negative selection bias against the definitive RT cohort. There was no difference in LF between RT alone and surgery + post-RT if only partial resection was achieved. Preop RT may improve LC if STR is deemed likely. (*IJROBP 2003*)

When is surgery preferred to RT as a local therapy in EWS?

Surgery is preferred when expendable bones are involved, if there is a pathologic fracture, and when there is a lower extremity lesion in a child (<10 yo).

What Tx were compared in IESS-1? Summarize the study's major results (OS, RFS, and LR).

IESS-1 compared induction vincristine/actinomycin D/Cytoxan (VAC) alone vs. vincristine/actinomycin D/Cytoxan/doxorubicin (VACAdr) vs. VAC + prophylactic WLI. 5-yr OS was significantly worse in the VAC alone arm (28%) compared to VACAdr (65%) or VAC + whole-lung irradiation (WLI) (53%). 5-yr OS was not significantly different between VACAdr and VAC + WLI. However, the VACAdr arm had an improved 5-yr RFS (60%) compared to VAC + WLI (44%). 5-yr LR was not significantly different between arms (~15%). (*Nesbit ME et al., JCO 1990*)

In IESS-1, which site had the worst prognosis?

In **IESS-1,** pts with pelvic primaries had significantly worse 5-yr OS (pelvic 34% vs. nonpelvic 57%). (*Nesbit ME et al., JCO 1990*)

What Tx were compared in IESS-2? Summarize the study's major results (OS).

IESS-2 randomized 214 patients between induction high-dose intermittent (HDI) VACAdr to moderate-dose continuous (MDC) VACAdr in nonpelvic localized tumors. HDI given q3wks vs. MDC given weekly. **5-yr OS favored the HDI arm** (77% vs. 63%). (*Burgert EO et al., JCO 1990*)

What Tx were compared in INT-0091 (IESS-3)? Summarize the study's major results (OS and LR).

INT-0091 randomized patients to induction **VACAdr vs. VACAdr alternating with IE.** The study enrolled 518 pts with EWS, PNET of bone and primitive sarcoma of bone, and pts with both localized and metastatic Dz. In pts with nonmetastatic Dz, induction VACAdr alternating with IE improved 5-yr OS (72% vs. 61%) and 5-yr LR **(5% vs. 15%).** There was no 5-yr OS advantage with adding IE for pts with metastatic Dz at presentation (~34%). (*Grier HE et al., NEJM 2003*)

When was local therapy given in INT-0091?

In **INT-0091,** local therapy (surgery +/– PORT or RT alone) was given at **wk 12.**

How was RT given in INT-0091 compared to IESS-1–2?

> **INT-0091:** definitive RT was given with IE to **GTV + 3-cm** margin to 45 Gy → CD to postchemo volume to 55.8 Gy. For PORT: if R0, then no PORT; if R1, then 45 Gy (initial GTV + 1 cm); if R2, then 55.8 Gy.
>
> **IESS-1–2:** definitive RT to **whole bone** to 45–50 Gy → CD to 55–60 Gy

In INT-0091, what pt characteristics were associated with the largest benefit from the addition of alternating IE?

In **INT-0092,** benefit from the addition of alternating IE was associated with **pelvic tumors, large tumors, and age <17 yrs.**

In INT-0091, for pts with pelvic primaries, did LR differ between surgery alone, surgery + PORT, and definitive RT?

LR did not differ by local therapy for pts with pelvic primaries (~**15%**). (*Yock TI et al., JCO 2006*)

What RT Tx techniques were compared in POG-8346? Summarize the study's major results.

In **POG-8346,** osseous EWS pts who rcv definitive RT for local therapy after induction chemo were randomized to **whole bone RT (39.6 Gy → 55.8 Gy boost to GTV +2 cm) vs. involved-field RT (GTV +2 cm to 55.8 Gy).** All pts then rcv maintenance chemo. The RT Tx techniques had similar 5-yr EFS (~41%) and LC (~53%). (*Donaldson SS et al., IJROBP 1998*)

What are 2 Tx options in EWS pts with lung mets?

In addition to chemo, **consider WLI or surgical resection (if <5 mets)** in EWS pts with lung mets.

What 2 key retrospective studies support the use of WLI in pts with metastatic EWS?

EICESS secondary analyses: *Paulussen et al.* reviewed the outcomes of EWS pts with (a) isolated pulmonary mets or (b) combined lung + bone/BM mets who were treated +/– WLI as part of a series of protocols from the EICESS. WLI was associated with improved EFS in both subgroups. (*Ann Oncol 1998*)

St. Jude's retrospective study: *Rodriguez-Galindo et al.* reviewed outcomes in EWS pts with isolated pulmonary recurrence. Pts who rcv WLI had improved 5-yr postrecurrence survival (30% vs. 17%). (*Cancer 2002*)

What doses and technique are used for WLI in EWS?

The WLI dose in EWS depends on age: if <14 yo, then **15 Gy (1.5 Gy/fx); if ≥14 yo, then 18 Gy (mostly in European protocols, but U.S. protocols still use 15 Gy).**

Describe the field borders used in WLI for EWS.

Superior-Inferior: 1 cm above 1st rib to L2
Lateral: 1 cm lat rib cage

Block PA kidney at 7.5 Gy.

Is there a difference in prognosis for metastatic EWS pts who present with isolated lung mets, bone-only mets, or both?

Yes. Metastatic EWS pts who present with either isolated pulmonary mets or skeletal mets have a similar EFS. However, EFS is significantly worse in pts with both.

5-yr OS for metastatic EWS:
Lung mets: ~35%
Bone/BM mets: ~25%
Lung 1 bone/BM mets: ~15%

(*Paulussen M et al., Ann Oncol 2009*)

What evidence supports the use of hemithorax RT in chest wall EWS?

Schuck A et al. retrospectively reviewed 138 pts with localized chest wall EWS treated in **CESS-86** and **EICESS 92.** 42 pts rcv hemithorax RT. If <14 yo, then 15 Gy; otherwise, 20 Gy at 1.5 Gy/fx or 1.25 Gy bid. All RT pts rcv a boost to the primary site of 45–60 Gy. Despite worse baseline prognostic factors in the hemithorax RT cohort, 7-yr EFS trended in its favor (63% vs. 46%). Improvements in EFS appeared to be due to reductions in pulmonary mets. A major criticism of this study is that the RT group had superior chemo. (*IJROBP 2002*)

Does hyperfractionation improve outcomes in EWS?

No. **CESS-86** randomized localized osseous EWS pts being treated with definitive RT to conventional fractionation (60 Gy in 1.8–2.0 Gy/fx) during a chemo break or split-course hyperfractionated RT concurrently with chemo. Hyperfractionated RT was 1.6 Gy bid to 60 Gy with a 12-day break after the initial 22.4 Gy and 44.8 Gy. LC was somewhat higher in the hyperfractionation arm (86% vs. 76%), but the difference was not SS. Benefits of this altered fractionation may have been lost due to the Tx breaks. (*Dunst J et al., IJROBP 1995*)

In EWS, how are the Tx volumes defined, and what are the margins used for the following scenarios?
1. **Bone-only lesion**
2. **Bone lesion with soft tissue extension**
3. **Postop setting**

In EWS, **RT volumes depend on the chemo response**.
1. **Bone only:** treat prechemo GTV + 2 cm to block margin (1-cm CTV, 0.5-cm PTV) to 55.8 Gy.
2. **Bone with soft tissue extension:** treat prechemo GTV + 2 cm to 45 Gy, then CD to initial/prechemo bone and postchemo soft tissue extent + 2 cm to 55.8 Gy.
3. **Postop setting:** treat preop, prechemo volume (except pushing borders in areas of lung or intestines) + 2 cm to 45 Gy, then CD to postop residual + 2 cm to 55.8 Gy.

In EWS pts with resected node + Dz, what RT dose is used to treat the nodal bed?

In EWS pts with resected node+ Dz, treat the nodal bed to **50.4 Gy**.

Based on the SFOP (France) metastatic EWS protocol, what was the 5-yr EFS with the addition of high-dose busulfan and melphalan as consolidation?

High-dose oral busulfan and melphalan were used → stem cell rescue as consolidation after 5 cycles Cytoxan/Adr and 2 cycles IE → local therapy (surgery and/or RT). 5-yr EFS was 52% for lung-only mets and 36% for bone-only mets (no BM involvement). With BM involvement, survival was **4%**. (*Oberlin O et al., JCO 2006*)

Based on the SFOP (France) metastatic EWS protocol, how was local therapy delivered?

Local therapy was delivered either before or after consolidative high-dose chemo. RT was given alone or after incomplete resection (55–60 Gy).

RT after R0 resection was given if >5% viable cells were seen (40 Gy). If <5% viable cells were seen, no RT was given. (*Oberlin O et al., JCO 2006*)

► TOXICITY

What is the 20-yr cumulative risk of 2nd malignancies in pts treated for EWS?	*Kuttesch et al.* retrospectively reviewed 266 EWS pts treated at St. Jude's Hospital. 20-yr cumulative incidence was 9.2% for any malignancy and 6.5% for sarcoma. There appeared to be a RT dose–response relationship with a 2nd malignancy **RR of 40** if RT was >60 Gy. (*JCO 1996*)
What GU side effect is of particular concern when treating pelvic EWS tumors?	Since EWS pts are typically treated with ifosfamide and cyclophosphamide, **RT cystitis** is of particular concern.
What dose causes premature epiphyseal closure?	**>20 Gy** causes premature epiphyseal closure. Decreased bone growth can occur at ~10 Gy.
How can lymphedema be minimized in the extremities when treating with RT?	Attempt to spare a 1–2-cm strip of skin on the extremity or minimize the circumferential RT dose to 20–30 Gy.
What are some factors that influence fracture risk?	Total dose, extent of cortical disruption at Dx, younger age, and 2nd bone malignancy in the RT field.

3   Wilms Tumor

Updated by Eva N. Christensen

► BACKGROUND

What is the estimated annual incidence of Wilms tumor (WT) in the U.S.?	**~500 cases/yr** of WT are diagnosed in the U.S.
What is the median age at Dx?	Median age at Dx is **3–4 yrs** (95% <10 yrs) for WT.
Is there a sex predilection?	**Yes. Females** are more commonly affected than males.

How does the age of presentation differ with Wilms when compared to neuroblastoma (NB)?	NB often presents at **<2 yrs. Unilateral WT** presents at **3.5–4 yrs.**
What is the age of presentation for hereditary/bilat tumors?	Hereditary/bilat tumors often present at **2.5 yrs** (younger than sporadic cases).
Name 3 genetic syndromes associated with Wilms.	1. WAGR 2. Denys-Drash 3. Beckwith-Wiedemann
What is WAGR syndrome, and what is the associated genetic change?	**Mnemonic: WAGR:** **W**ilms **A**niridia **G**U anomalies Mental **R**etardation <u>Associated genetic change</u>: **del 11q13** (WT1 deletion)
What is Denys-Drash syndrome, and what is the associated genetic change?	**Denys-Drash:** Wilms, renal Dz (proteinuria during infancy, nephritic syndrome, progressive renal failure), male pseudohermaphroditism <u>Associated genetic change</u>: point mutation of WT1 gene
What is Beckwith-Wiedemann syndrome, and what is the associated genetic change?	**Beckwith-Wiedemann:** macrosomia, macroglossia, omphalocele, hemihypertrophy <u>Associated genetic change</u>: **11p15.5,** duplication of WT2 locus
What transcription factor is important for normal kidney/gonadal development and is associated with Wilms?	**WT1** (a zinc finger protein) is associated with Wilms and is important for normal kidney/gonadal development.
What is the function of WT2?	Function of WT2 is **unknown.** It affects IGF2, the H19 tumor suppressor, and p57 cell cycle protein.
What are the other genetic defects seen in Wilms?	LOH 1p + 16q, FWT1 (17q), and FWT2 (19q)
Name 1 paternal and 1 maternal environmental risk factor for WT.	Fathers who are welders/machinists (RR 5.3); mothers who use hair dyes (RR 3.6)
What are some poor prognostic factors seen in Wilms?	**Unfavorable histology** (UH), advanced **tumor stage, molecular** (+telomerase) and **genetic** (LOH 1p + 16q) markers, **age >24 mos**

What histology has the worst outcome in Wilms?	**Diffuse anaplasia** (DA), followed by rhabdoid and clear cell sarcoma. A review of NWTS-1 and -2 studies involving ~1,200 children, DA had the shortest survival time compared to non-anaplastic histologies (*Bonadio F et al., JCO 1985*). In another study, DA was seen in 10% of cases, but accounted for 60% of the deaths (*Faria P et al., Am J Surg Pathol 1996*).
What study demonstrated the prognostic importance of LOH 1p + 16q for Wilms?	**NWTS**-5 analysis (*Grundy PE et al., JCO 2005*). For favorable histology (FH), LOH 1p or 16q is associated with ↑ (RR) of relapse. LOH of both ↑ RR of relapse + death.
What are the UH subtypes in Wilms?	Anaplastic: focal or diffuse
How is focal anaplasia defined?	Focal anaplasia is sharply localized within the primary tumor, without atypia in the rest of the tumor.
What renal tumors are not Wilms tumor but are treated similarly to Wilms tumors?	Malignant rhabdoid tumor and clear cell sarcoma of the kidney
What are the 4 sets of criteria used to define DA?	Criteria to define DA: 1. Nonlocalized 2. Localized with severe nuclear unrest elsewhere in the tumor 3. Anaplasia outside the tumor capsule or mets 4. Anaplasia revealed by random Bx
What is the stage-by-stage 4-yr OS for anaplastic/UH WT?	4-yr OS for anaplastic/UH Wilms: Stage I: 83% Stage II: 83% Stage III: 65% Stage IV: 33% (*Dome JS et al., JCO 2006*)
How does the 4-yr OS compare between focal and diffuse anaplasia?	Overall: 97% vs. 50% Stage I: 100% Stage II: 93% vs. 55% Stage III: 90% vs. 45% Stage IV: 80% vs. 4%
What are the typical presenting Sx in Wilms? How does this compare to NB?	Asymptomatic abdominal mass (83%) → abdominal pain (37%), HTN (25%, due to ↑ renin), hematuria (25%), fever, anemia (due to ↓ erythropoietin) NB most commonly presents with systemic Sx. (Mnemonic: **WWNN**—**W**ilms are **W**ell, **N**euroblastomas are **N**ot well)

▶ **WORKUP/STAGING**

What is the typical workup for an abdominal mass of unclear etiology in a child?

Abdominal mass workup: H&P (focusing on congenital defects), labs, UA (including urinary catecholamines), abdominal US, CXR, and CT C/A/P

What is the recommended 1st-line imaging modality for an abdominal mass?

US is the recommended 1st-line study for imaging the abdomen.

Pts with what histologic subtype(s) require bone scan?

Clear cell

With a Dx of Wilms, what 2 chest imaging modalities can be employed for staging purposes?

Both **CXR and CT** are used for chest imaging. Lesions seen on CT but not visible on CXR may be treated more conservatively than lung mets visible on CXR.

Pediatric pts with what renal tumors need BM Bx?

Pts with **clear cell and rhabdoid** require BM Bx.

Pediatric pts with what renal tumors require MRI of the head as part of their workup?

Rhabdoid: 10%–15% will have PNET in brain (atypical teratoid rhabdoid tumors)
Clear cell: to r/o brain mets

What is the typical appearance of WT on CT?

Large round mass with pseudocapsule usually without calcifications.

Under what circumstances should Bx be performed?

Do not Bx unless the tumor is **unresectable** or **bilat** Dz. If Bx is necessary, use a **posterior approach** to avoid contaminating the abdomen.

On what issues should the surgeon comment at the time of surgery?

Involvement of regional nodes, opposite kidney, peritoneum, liver, renal vein/IVC. Also, if there is tumor spillage and if it is confined to the ipsi flank.

What% of patients present with each of the features summarized in this table?

Presenting Features	Patients (%)
Bilat Dz	7
Multifocal Dz	12
Renal vein invasion	10
LN involvement	20
Mets	10

What are some common sites of mets?

Lung (80%) → liver → bone, brain (clear cell), LN (outside abdomen and pelvis)

How commonly is calcification seen in Wilms?

Calcification is seen in 10%–15% of cases but is seen in 85% of NB cases.

How many stages are there in Wilms?

There are **5 stages** in Wilms.

Summarize the staging of WT.

I (40% of pts): limited to kidney

II (20%): extension to outside capsule, vessel involvement >2 mm

III (20%): R1-R2 resection, +LN, local spillage or diffuse peritoneal spillage, Bx (including FNA), +implants, +margin, transected tumor thrombus, piecemeal resection, unresectable tumor

IV (10%): hematogenous mets or LN+ outside the abdomen/pelvis

V (4%–8%): bilat Dz; each side staged independently

Is adrenal involvement considered a met?

No. Adrenal involvement is considered local extension.

▶ TREATMENT/PROGNOSIS

What is the Tx paradigm for WT in the U.S.?

WT Tx paradigm: initial surgical resection → risk-adapted adj chemo +/– RT

What is the major difference between the International Society of Pediatric Oncology (SIOP) Tx paradigm (European Cooperative Group) and the National Wilms Tumor Study (NWTS) paradigm (American Cooperative Group)?

SIOP trials incorporate **preop therapy** (CRT), whereas the NWTS/COG trials do not.

Under what circumstance is the SIOP paradigm favored in the U.S.?

In **unresectable or bilat Wilms,** preop chemo is used.

What are the indications for postop RT in the current COG protocols (AREN0532,533)?

Indications for postop RT depend on **histology and stage:**
    Favorable histology: stages III–IV
    Unfavorable histology: stages I–IV

What chemotherapeutic agents are typically used in Wilms?

Vincristine, actinomycin D (Adr/VP-16/Cytoxan/carboplatin added in UH)

What did the early NWTS-1 and NWTS-2 studies show?	1. Vincristine and actinomycin D (VA) are better together than either alone. 2. RT is not needed for stage I FH pts, but when given it should preferably start within 9 days of surgery (but no later than postop day 14). 3. There was no RT dose response from 10–40 Gy.
Which study demonstrated that whole abdomen irradiation (WAI) is not needed for local spillage?	**NWTS-1;** flank fields suffice if spillage is local.
Which study demonstrated that adding Adr to VA benefited group 2–4 pts?	**NWTS-2;** adding Adr benefited group 2–4 FH, especially group 2–4 UH pts (OS 38% vs. 78%).
Which study demonstrated that 10 wks was equal to 6 mos of chemo for stage I pts?	**NWTS-3;** 4-yr OS was 96%–97%.
Which study showed that stage II FH pts do not need RT as long as VA is given?	**NWTS-3** (4-arm: vincristine/Actinomycin D/ Adriamycin [VAAdr] vs. VA vs. +/– RT → 4-yr OS ~90%–95%, no difference)
Which study eliminated Adr from stage II FH?	**NWTS-3.** VA alone was sufficient.
Which study demonstrated that 10 Gy was equal to 20 Gy if Adr was added to stage III pts?	**NWTS-3** demonstrated the noninferiority of lower RT doses with Adr.
Which study addressed the addition of Cytoxan to VAAdr for high-risk pts?	**NWTS-3.** Cytoxan improved outcome in UH stage II–IV but not FH stage IV.
Which study addressed pulse-intense (PI) chemo?	**NWTS-4.** 6 mos of PI was equal to 15 mos of conventional chemo.
What are the main advantages of PI chemo?	With PI chemo, there is ↓ **hematologic toxicity** and ↓ **total cost** b/c fewer drugs are used.
Which study found that local spillage (old stage II) without RT results in a ↑ LR?	**NWTS-4;** ↑ LR, but no difference in OS; so, moved to stage III for FH (need adj RT)
What question does NWTS-5 address? (*Dome JS et al., JCO 2006*)	Nonrandomized, assesses prognostic importance of LOH 1p + 16q

For which pts did NWTS-5 show ↑ (13.5%) rates of relapse with nephrectomy alone and without adj chemo?

Stage I FH, pts <2 yo, **and tumors** <550 g. Most (>70%) were salvaged successfully, however.

What chemo regimen in NWTS-5 improved outcomes for stages II–IV with DA?

Vincristine/Adr/cyclophosphamide/etoposide

Did stage I anaplastic tumors qualify for RT in NWTS-5?

No. Anaplastic tumors did not qualify for RT in **NWTS-5.**

What do the current protocols (COG AREN0532, 0533) address?

Tx intensification based on LOH 1p16q status; stage I anaplastic pts get RT + Adr (with VA).

What were the factors that determine risk groups in the COG AREN0532/0533?

Age (>2 yo worse), tumor weight (550 g), stage, LOH 1p + 16q, and chemo response

What subset of pts on the current COG protocol could get surgery alone without adj Tx?

Very low risk group **(stage I FH, pts <2 yo, and tumors <550 g)** and if there is central pathology review and LN sampling

What are the RT doses to the postop bed for Wilms pts ≥16 yo and/or those with rhabdoid and/or DA? How about for other pts?

19.8 Gy to flank for stage III DA or rhabdoid stages I–III (+10.8 Gy boost to mets/gross Dz = 30.6 Gy), **10.8 Gy** for the rest (stage III FH, stages I–III FA, stages I–II DA, stages I–III clear cell, age <16 yrs, infants with DA or rhabdoid histology)

What are the indications and the RT doses for WAI?

Seeding/rupture/diffuse spill; **10.5 Gy (1.5 Gy/fx),** boost to 21 if bulky (but 19.8 Gy for DA or rhabdoid)

What are the indications for flank RT?

Stage III FH, localized spill, stages I–III UH, and recurrent Wilms (also done for certain stage IV pts)

What is the standard flank RT dose?

The standard flank RT dose is **10.8 Gy in 6 fractions.**

What is the dose to unresected +LNs?

19.8 Gy to entire chain → boost with optional 5.4–10.8 Gy; 30.6 Gy if >16 yo

What is the preferred Tx for localized liver mets? Diffuse liver mets?

Surgery is preferred for localized liver mets. For diffuse liver mets, **19.8 Gy** to the entire liver (with optional boost of 5.4–10.8 Gy) is an option.

What dose is given to resected +LNs?

Resected +LNs get a dose of **10.8 Gy.**

At what age can pts rcv greater flank doses and greater doses to mets?

≥**16 yo** (19.8 Gy to flank or WAI and 30.6 Gy to mets in bone, LNs, and brain)

When is whole lung irradiation (WLI) not required in a Wilms pt with lung mets?

WLI is not required in these pts **if mets are seen only on CT and not on CXR** or **if a CR is seen after VAAdr at wk 6.**

When is WLI indicated? What are the doses?

WLI is indicated when there is no CR seen on CT at wk 6 after 3-drug chemo (per current protocol); it is not based on # of mets, size, or detectability on CT or CXR. The dose for WLI is **12 Gy (>1 yo)** or **10.5 Gy (<1 yo)** in **1.5 Gy/fx.** If there is persistent Dz after WLI, consider a **7.5 Gy boost.**

What med should pts take when treated with WLI?

Trimethoprim/sulfamethoxazole (Bactrim) for PCP prophylaxis

How is bilat Wilms treated?

Initial surgery or Bx to **stage each side** → **chemo** → **2nd-look surgery at 6 wks** for a max safe resection (spare two-thirds of 1 kidney if possible) → continuation of chemo. **RT is given after surgery based on the final local stage.**

RT should preferably start by which day and should begin no later than which day after surgery?

RT should preferably start by **day 9** and should begin no later than **day 14.** Secondary analyses of **NWTS-1** and **NWTS-2** showed worse outcomes when RT was delayed >10 days.

How long is the chemo regimen for stages I–II and III–IV FH?

18 wks (VA); **24 wks** (VAAdr)

What is the medial border of a flank field?

1 cm from the contralat vertebral body edge. Be aware of the intact kidney location.

What are the preferred RT margins/techniques for a flank field?

Preop GTV + 1 cm; AP/PA for flank; conformal for boost (residual + 2 cm)

What is the dose for brain mets?

The dose for brain mets is WBRT to 21.6 Gy if <16 yo (+ 10.8 Gy boost = 32.4 Gy) or 30.6 Gy (–boost) if >16 yo.

What is the dose for bone mets?

The dose for bone mets is **25.2 Gy** (30.6 Gy if >16 yo).

How do you manage a pt who presents with mets and a resectable tumor?

These pts are treated the same way as nonmetastatic pts, except mets are treated at the same time as abdominal RT, if needed.

What is the outcome for relapsed Wilms treated with VA only for stage I or II Dz?	4-yr EFS/OS: 71% (stage I) vs. 82% (stage II). Pt salvaged with surgery, RT, and chemo with vincristine/Adr/Cytoxan/etoposide. Lung mets only, 4-yr EFS/OS: 68% (stage I) vs. 81% (stage II).
What about relapsed stages III–IV Dz?	Relapse after stages III–IV Tx is worse (4-yr EFS/OS: 42% vs. 48%, respectively), lung only mets: 4-yr EFS/OS: 49% vs. 53%, respectively. (*Green DM et al., Ped Blood Cancer 2007; Malogolowkin M et al., Ped Blood Cancer 2008*)

▶ TOXICITY

What is the dose constraint for the kidney?	One-third of contralat kidney <14.4 Gy
What is the dose constraint for the liver?	One-half of uninvolved liver <19.8 Gy; with liver mets, 75% of liver ≤30.6 Gy
Pts are at risk for what late effects with flank RT? WLI?	Scoliosis of the spine, muscular hypoplasia, kyphosis, iliac wing hypoplasia, SBO, veno-occlusive Dz of the liver;
	Breast hypoplasia (four-fifths of females who get WLI will have underdeveloped breasts), pneumonitis, CHF, 2nd malignancy, and renal failure
What is the risk of SBO at 15 yrs after flank/abdominal RT?	15%.
What is the risk of a 2nd malignancy at 15 yrs?	1.6%–2%.
The reirradiation tolerance of which organ decreases with time after initial RT?	Reirradiation tolerance of the **kidney** decreases with time.
What is the TD 5/5 for an entire kidney?	The TD 5/5 is **23 Gy.**
What is the cumulative maximal total dose (including prior RT) for WT pts?	30.6 Gy (if <3 yrs) or 39.5 Gy (if >3 yrs)

Table 3.1	Current Children's Oncology Group Wilms Protocol (AREN0532/533)

Goals: Reduce Tx-related toxicity in low-risk tumors and improve outcome for high-risk tumors with chemo intensification.

Tumor Risk Classification	Multimodality Treatment
Very low risk FH WT >2 yrs, stage I FH, <550 g	Surgery, *no* therapy if central pathology review and LN sampling
Low-risk FH WT	Surgery, no RT, regimen EE4A
≥2 yrs, stage I FH, ≥550 g	
Standard-risk FH WT	Surgery, regimen DD4A
Stages I–II FH with LOH	Surgery, RT, regimen DD4A
Stage III FH without LOH	
Stages III–IV FH with LOH	Surgery, RT, regimen M, WLI
Stage IV FH (slow/incomplete responders)	
Stage IV FH: CR of lung mets at wk 6/ DD4A (rapid early responders)	Surgery, RT, regimen DD4A; no WLI
Stages I–III FA	Surgery, RT, regimen DD4A
Stage I DA	
Stage IV FA	Surgery, RT, regimen UH1
Stages II–IV DA	
Stage IV CCSK	
Stage IV RTK	
Stages I–III CCSK	Surgery, RT, regimen 1

FH, favorable histology; WT, Wilms tumor; LN, lymph node; RT, radiation therapy; LOH, loss of heterozygosity; WLI, whole lung irradiation; CR, complete response; FA, focal anaplasia; DA, diffuse anaplasia; CCSK, clear cell sarcoma of the kidney; RTK, rhabdoid tumor of the kidney.

Table 3.2	Chemotherapy Regimens on AREN0532/533 Protocols

Regimen	Agents
EE4A	VCR/AMD
DD4A	VCR/AMD/ADR
M	VCR/AMD/ADR; CY/ETOP
I	VCR/DOX/CY; CY/ETOP
UH1	CY/CARBO/ETOP; VCR/DOX/CY

VCR, vincristine; AMD, dactinomycin; ADR, Adriamycin; CY, Cytoxan; ETOP, etoposide; DOX, doxorubicin; CARBO, carboplatin.

Table 3.3 Radiation Planning and Doses on Protocols AREN0532/533

RT timing: Concurrent with VCR, surgery day 1, RT ≤day 10 (max day 14).

Exception: Medical contraindication or delay in central pathology review.

RT field design:

I. Flank RT: GTV = preop CT/MRI (tumor and involved kidney).

$$CTV + PTV = \leq 1 \text{ cm}$$

Medial border across midline to include vertebral bodies + 1-cm margin but sparing contralat kidney. Other field borders placed at edge of PTV. Use AP/PA.
If + PA and surgically removed, then treat entire PA chain to 10.8 Gy.
If + residual Dz, then boost with 10.8 Gy after initial 10.8 Gy (3D-CRT, GTV = postop volume).

Dose limits: Two-thirds contralat kidney to 14.4 Gy, one-half of undiseased liver to 19.8 Gy.

II. WAI: CTV = entire peritoneal cavity from diaphragm to pelvic diaphragm.

Superior border: 1 cm above dome of diaphragm.

Inferior border: Bottom of obturator foramen.

Laterally: 1 cm beyond lat abdominal wall; block femoral heads.

Dose 10.5 Gy (1.5 Gy/fx) except for diffuse anaplasia or rhabdoid tumors (dose is 19.8 Gy, shield kidney to keep <14.4 Gy).

III. WLI: CTV includes lungs, mediastinum, and pleural recesses. PTV = CTV + 1 cm.

Inf border at L1, sup border 1 cm above 1st rib, block humeral heads.
Can boost after 12 Gy (1.5 Gy/fx) (10.5 Gy for <12 mos) for persistent Dz after 2 wks → +7.5 Gy (19.5 Gy) to residual with conformal fields.

IV. Liver mets: Surgery for solitary mets, excised to –margins. Whole liver RT for diffuse liver mets to 19.8 Gy (with additional 5.4–10.8 Gy at discretion).

V. Brain: WBRT to 21.6 Gy (30.6 Gy if >16 yo). If 21.6 Gy → conformal RT boost with additional 10.8 Gy.

VI. Bone: GTV + 3-cm margin, AP/PA to 25.2 Gy (30.6 Gy if >16 yo).

VII. Unresected nodes: Cover entire LN chain to 19.8 Gy (30.6 Gy if >16 yo), with optional 5.4–10.8 Gy boost. If removed +PA LN, use 10.8 Gy to cover.

RT, radiation therapy; VCR, vincristine; max, maximum; GTV, gross target volume; preop, preoperative; CT/MRI, computed tomography/magnetic resonance imaging; CTV, clinical target volume; PTV, planning target volume; cm, centimeter; contralat, contralateral; AP/PA, anterior-posterior/posterior-anterior; +, positive; Gy, gray; Dz, disease; 3D-CRT, three-dimensional conformal radiation therapy; postop, postoperative; WAI, whole abdomen irradiation; lat, lateral; fx, fractions; WLI, whole lung irradiation; inf, inferior; sup, superior; mos, months; wks, weeks; mets, metastasis; –, negative; WBRT, whole brain radiation therapy; yo, years old; LN, lymph node.

4 Neuroblastoma

Updated by Jingya Wang

What are the 3 types of neuroblastic tumors?

3 types of neuroblastic tumors:
1. Neuroblastoma (NB)
2. Ganglioneuroblastoma
3. Ganglioneuroma

These tumors differ in the degree of cellular maturation.

What are the 4 most common malignancies of childhood?

4 most common malignancies of childhood:
1. Leukemia
2. Brain tumors
3. Lymphoma
4. NB

What is the most common malignancy in infants?

NB is the most common malignancy in infants.

Estimate the annual incidence of NB in the U.S.

There are ~**650 cases/yr** of NB in the U.S.

What is the median age at Dx for NB?

The median age at Dx is **17 mos,** with a range between birth and 15 yrs. NBs in adults are rare and tend to have slower growth rate than in children.

Name 3 genetic syndromes associated with NB.

3 genetic syndromes associated with NB:
1. NF
2. Hirschsprung Dz
3. Fetal hydantoin syndrome

What tests have been used to screen infants for NB?

Historically, infants were screened for NB using **urinary catecholamines (vanillylmandelic acid/ homovanillic acid).**

Does screening improve survival in NB?

This is **controversial.** Screening infants for NB with urinary catecholamines has been evaluated in multiple studies; however, the value of catecholamine-based screening is limited by its false+ rate and b/c a significant % of infant NBs spontaneously regress.

What markers distinguish NB from other small round blue tumors?

NB-specific markers:
1. Neuron-specific enolase
2. Synaptophysin
3. Neurofilament

What is the cell of origin for NB?	NB arises from **neural crest cells of the sympathetic ganglion.**
What % of NB pts have detectable urinary catecholamines?	**90%**
What genetic changes are associated with n-myc amplification?	**Double-minute chromatin bodies and homogeneously staining regions** are associated with n-myc amplification.
What are the genetic/ chromatin changes that portend a poor prognosis in NB?	Genetic/chromatin changes with a poor prognosis in NB: 1. **n-myc amplification** 2. LOH 1p + 11q 3. diploid DNA 4. ↑ telomerase activity
In which pts does DNA content _not_ have prognostic importance?	DNA content does not have prognostic importance in **metastatic pts.**
What % of NB pts present with n-myc amplification?	**30%–40%** of pts present with n-myc amplification. An n-myc amplification is associated with poor prognosis.
What % of NB pts present with 1p deletions?	70% of pts present with 1p deletions.
What is the genetic variation on 6p22 that is associated with clinically aggressive NB?	Homozygosity for 3 single nucleotide polymorphisms on 6p22 is associated with stage IV Dz, n-myc amplification, and Dz relapse. (_Maris JM et al., NEJM 2008_)
What are the most common sites of presentation for NB?	Adrenal medulla > paraspinal > postmediastinum
In what age group is thoracic presentation of NB more common?	Thoracic NB is more common in **infants.**
What are some presenting Sx of NB?	Along with the presentation of a mass, NB may be associated with **constitutional Sx** (fever, malaise, pain, weight loss), periorbital ecchymosis (**"raccoon eyes"**), **"blueberry muffin" sign** (nontender blue skin mets), scalp nodules, bone pain, irritable/ill appearance, diarrhea (↑ vasoactive intestinal peptide), Horner syndrome, opsomyoclonus truncal ataxia (rare paraneoplastic syndrome of ataxia, random eye movement, and myoclonic jerking associated with early stage but persists after cure), and Kerner-Morrison syndrome (diarrhea, low K).

What % of NB pts present with mets overall? How does this differ by age?

75% of all NB pts present with mets overall. 60% of pts <1 yr present with localized disease, while 70% of patients >1 yr present with mets.

What are the most common sites of mets for NB?

NB commonly metastasizes to **bone (~50%), LNs (35%),** BM, liver, skin, and orbits. **Lung mets are rare.**

What are the most common bony sites of metastatic Dz in NB?

Bones of the skull and orbit (proptosis, ecchymosis, scalp mass)

What features distinguish NB from Wilms tumor?

(1) **NB (85%)** is more likely to exhibit calcifications vs. 5%–10%, in Wilms, (2) median age of presentation for **NB** is 1 yr vs. 3.5 yrs for Wilms, (3) Wilms is more common in African Americans, (4) Wilms patients appear healthy vs. **NB** patients appear sick, (5) Wilms arises from and destroys the kidney vs. **NB** displaces the kidney, (6) **NB** can cross midline (Wilms does not), (7) **NB** rarely metastasizes to the lungs (Wilms can metastasize to the lungs).

What are the classic histologic findings seen in NB?

Homer-Wright pseudorosettes, hemorrhage, and calcification

Does screening change the mortality rate of NB?

No. The **Quebec project** increased the detection rate of NBs but failed to have an impact on mortality in the screened populations. The high spontaneous regression rate led to overdiagnosis of clinically insignificant Dz.

▶ WORKUP/STAGING

Outline the workup for pts with suspected NB.

Suspected NB workup:
1. H&P
2. Labs (CBC, BUN/Cr, LFTs, serum markers, UA, urine catechol)
3. Imaging of primary: CT C/A/P, abdominal US, or MRI abdomen/liver/spine)
4. Workup of mets (bone scan, I-131 metaiodobenzylguanidine [MIBG] scan, BM Bx, CT/MRI as needed)
5. Pathology (DNA content, n-myc amplification, and cytogenetics)

Why is a BM Bx important in the workup of NB?

BM Bx may obviate the need for primary site surgery if the testing is positive and the clinical picture is clear.

What % of NB pts have uptake on an I-131 MIBG scan?

~90% of NB pts have uptake on an I-131 MIBG scan.

What are the currently used NB staging systems?

As of 2010, most cooperative group trials use the **International Neuroblastoma Staging System (INSS),** which involves the extent of surgical resection. However, a new staging system that uses only pre-Tx factors has been developed: the **International Neuroblastoma Risk Group (INRG).** These 2 staging systems will likely be used concurrently to allow for comparisons between trials. (*Monclair T et al., JCO 2009*)

Summarize the INSS staging system.

Stage 1: unilat localized tumor s/p GTR +/– microscopic residual Dz; ipsi LN–, though LNs attached and removed with the primary may be involved

Stage 2A: unilat localized tumor s/p STR only; ipsi LN–, though LNs attached and removed with the primary may be involved

Stage 2B: unilat localized tumor s/p GTR or STR with involved non-adherent ipsi LNs; enlarged contralat LN–.

Stage 3: unresectable localized tumor extending across the midline +/– regional LN involvement; unilat localized tumor with contralat regional LN involvement

Stage 4: distant Dz except as defined by stage 4S

Stage 4S: localized unilat primary as defined by stage 1, 2A, or 2B; distant Dz limited to the liver, skin, and/or <10% of BM in infants <1 yo

What are the prognostic factors in NB per INRG?

Age, stage, histologic category, grade, n-myc amplification, 11q aberration, DNA ploidy

Summarize the INRG staging system.

In the **INRG system,** locoregional tumors are staged **L1** or **L2** based on the absence or presence of 1 or more of 20 image-defined radiographic findings (IDRFs). These IDRFs generally affect whether or not a tumor is surgically resectable and to what degree. The authors of the INRG system avoided the terms resectable and unresectable since that may depend more on the surgeon's style and subjective judgment. **Metastatic tumors** are defined as stage **M,** except for stage **MS,** in which mets are confined to the skin, liver, and/or BM in pts <18 mos old. (*Monclair T et al., JCO 2009*)

What is the INRG stage of an 8-mo-old pt with metastatic Dz to bone only?

An 8-mo-old pt with metastatic Dz to bone only is INRG **stage M** (only BM, liver, and skin mets qualify for stage MS).

What is the INSS stage of a 14-mo-old pt with metastatic Dz to BM only?

A 14-mo-old pt with metastatic Dz to bone marrow only is INSS **stage 4** (only pts <12 mos old qualify for stage 4S).

What 2 clinical factors are most predictive of cure in NB?

The 2 clinical factors most predictive of cure are **age** and **stage at Dx.**

In children with metastatic Dz, what is the most important prognostic factor?

In children with metastatic Dz, **age (<1 yo best)** is the strongest prognostic factor, even more so than n-myc.

The Shimada classification system divides NB into what 2 categories? What 5 features are used to classify pts in this system?

The Shimada classification system divides NB into **favorable histology** (FH) and **unfavorable histology** (UH). Favorable factors:
  Stroma-rich (Schwann cell stroma)
  Age (young)
  Differentiation (well differentiated)
  Mitotic/karyorrhectic index (low)
  Nodularity (nonnodular)

(Mnemonic: Dr. Shimada has a **SAD MiNd**)

What 5 factors are used to classify NB pts into low-, intermediate-, and high-risk groups per the COG?

5 factors used to classify NB in COG low-, intermediate-, and high-risk groups:
  1. **S**tage, INSS
  2. **A**ge
  3. **N**-myc status
  4. **D**NA ploidy
  5. **S**himada classification

(Mnemonic: **SANDS**)

An NB pt with stage I Dz and n-myc amplification is in what risk group?

All stage I NB pts are **low risk.**

Can a pt with n-myc amplification be classified as intermediate risk?

No. All NB pts with n-myc are either low risk or high risk.

What makes a stage 2 or stage 3 pt high risk?

Stage 2 patients are high risk if they have all 3 risk factors: (1) n-myc amplification, (2) unfavorable histology, and (3) >1 yo.

Stage 3 patients need 1 risk factor to be high risk: either (1) n-myc amplification, or (2) both unfavorable histology ≥1 yo.

What feature makes NB pts with stage 4S Dz high risk?

NB stage 4S pts are high risk if tumors are **n-myc amplified.**

What features make NB pts with stage 4S Dz intermediate risk?

NB stage 4S pts are intermediate risk if tumors are **not n-myc amplified** and are **either Shimada UH or have diploid DNA.**

In which COG risk group do NB pts most commonly present?

NB pts are most commonly **high risk (55%)** → low risk (30%).

▶ TREATMENT/PROGNOSIS

Estimate the 3-yr OS for low-, intermediate-, and high-risk NB.

NB 3-yr OS by risk group:
Low risk: 95%–100%
Intermediate risk: 75%–98%
High risk: <30%

What percentage of stage 4S patients experience spontaneous regression?

Up to 85% of patients with stage 4S NB experience spontaneous regression. Thus, low-risk stage 4S patients can be observed.

What is the Tx paradigm for low-risk NB?

Low-risk NB Tx paradigm: surgery alone with chemo reserved for persistent or recurrent Dz

What is the Tx paradigm for low-risk stage 4S NB, and which study supports this approach?

Low-risk stage 4S NB Tx paradigm: Bx → supportive care. Chemo and/or RT are reserved for rapidly growing or symptomatic Dz. A subgroup analysis of **CCG 3881** showed that supportive care is sufficient for 57% of pts. The protocol resulted in a 5-yr EFS of 86% and an OS of 92%. (*Nickerson HJ et al., JCO 2000*)

Which studies support the use of observation (without resection) in infants with localized NB without n-myc amplification?

The use of observation (without resection) in infants with localized NB without n-myc amplification was evaluated in the German GPOH trials **NB95-S and NB97.** Of 93 pts with gross Dz, 44 had spontaneous regression. OS and DM-free survival were no different from outcomes of pts treated with surgery or chemo in these trials (3-yr OS 99%, DM-free survival 94%). (*Hero B et al., JCO 2008*)

What is the role of RT in the Tx of intermediate-risk NB?

In intermediate-risk pts, RT is typically reserved for those who are symptomatic due to tumor bulk and are not responding to initial chemo, such as pts with respiratory distress due to hepatomegaly or with neurologic compromise due to cord compression. RT is not indicated as a consolidative therapy even with persistent Dz. Indications for RT based on **A3961:** Symptomatic palliation, viable residual Dz in Tx-refractory pts, and recurrent Dz.

What is the Tx for unfavorable stage 4S (intermediate-risk) Dz?

The Tx is **chemo × 8 cycles.**

What is the Tx paradigm for high-risk NB?

High-risk NB Tx paradigm: induction chemo, then resection, then high-dose chemo and stem cell transplant → **consolidation RT,** then oral cis-retinoic acid and immunotherapy (anti-GD2 + IL2/GM-CSF).

Which targeted agent has recently been demonstrated as promising new adj therapy for high-risk NB?

Promising results have been observed **with immunotherapy targeting the surface glycolipid molecule disialoganglioside (GD2).** A recent phase III randomized trial showed a significant improvement in event-free survival and OS for children with high-risk NB receiving chimeric anti-GD2 (ch14.18) combined with cytokines (IL2 and GM-CSF) and isotretinoin after myeloablative consolidation therapy. (*Yu AL et al., NEJM 2010*)

In low-risk and intermediate-risk NB, what dose of radiation is generally used?

In low-risk NB, radiation to 21 Gy at 1.5 Gy/fx can be used for Sx that do not respond to chemo. In intermediate-risk NB, if PR to chemo and viable residual disease after second-look surgery, then RT can be given locally to the primary + 2-cm margin to 24 Gy at 1.5 Gy/fx.

In high-risk NB, what tissues are targeted during RT and to what dose?

Per current **COG0532,** high-risk NB pts are treated with RT to their **postchemo, preop tumor bed** to a total dose of **21.6 Gy in 1.8 Gy/fx if GTR** and 36.0 Gy (21.6 Gy to preop GTV → 14.4 Gy boost) **if gross residual.**

In high-risk NB, should elective nodal RT be given?

No. In high-risk NB, only clinically+ or pathologically+ LN regions are covered in the RT volumes.

What study indirectly demonstrated an RT dose response in high-risk NB?

Haas-Kogan et al. performed a secondary analysis of **CCG 3891** and found that high-risk NB pts who rcvd 10 Gy local EBRT + 10 Gy total body irradiation (TBI) as part of a transplant preparation regimen had better LC than pts who did not get TBI (or a transplant) (5-yr LR rate was 22% vs. 52%). (*IJROBP 2003*)

These results support the current use of 21.6 Gy in high-risk protocols.

What study demonstrated the benefits of high-dose chemo → BMT as well as adj cis-retinoic acid in high-risk NB?

In **CCG 3891,** 379 high-risk NB pts were treated with induction chemo → surgery and 10 Gy to gross residual. Pts were then randomized to 3 cycles of nonmyeloablative chemo vs. myeloablative chemo, TBI, and BM T. Pts underwent secondary randomization to observation vs. cis-retinoic acid × 6 mos. Both the myeloablative chemo and cis-retinoic acid improved OS. 5-yr OS for pts who rcvd both was 59%. (*Matthay KK et al., JCO 2009*)

What is the appropriate Tx for NB pts with cord compression?

Consider chemo initially for NB-related cord compression. Unresponsive Dz can be treated with surgery or RT.

What is the RT dose and dose/fx used for NB pts being treated for symptomatic cord compression?

For symptomatic cord compression:
1. If pt is <3 yo, treat to **9 Gy** (1.8 Gy/fx).
2. If pt is ≥3 yo, treat to **21.6 Gy** (1.8 Gy/fx).

What is the RT dose and dose/fx used for NB pts being treated for symptomatic hepatomegaly?

Symptomatic hepatomegaly is treated to **4.5 Gy** (1.5 Gy × 3).

Can the vertebral body be split during radiation planning?

No. It is necessary to always cover the full width of the vertebrae to avoid scoliosis.

What chemo drugs are typically used in NB?

Chemo drugs typically used in NB:
1. Cytoxan
2. Doxorubicin
3. Etoposide
4. Carboplatin
5. Ifosfamide

What is the role of I-131 MIBG in NB?

I-131 MIBG can be used for refractory NB, based on a promising phase II study showing a 36% response rate. (*Matthay KK et al., JCO 2007*)

▶ TOXICITY

In NB, what dose constraint is used for the contralat kidney?

Limit the dose to the entire contralat kidney to **<15 Gy.**

In NB, what dose constraint is used for the liver?

Limit liver V15 to **66%.**

In NB, what dose constraint is used for the lung?

Limit lung V15 to **<66%.**

What are some complications of radiation treatment in NB?

Disturbances of growth, infertility, neuropsychologic sequelae, endocrinopathies, cardiac effects, pulmonary effects, bladder dysfunction, secondary malignancy

Table 4.1	Children's Oncology Group Risk Groupings				
Risk Group	**INSS Stage**	**Age (yrs)**	**N-myc**	**Shimada**	**DNA Index**
Low	1	0–21	Any	Any	Any
	2	<1	Any	Any	Any
	2	>1	Normal	Any	Any
	2	>1	Amplified	Fav	Any
	4S	<1	Normal	Fav	>1
Intermediate	3	<1	Normal	Any	Any
	3	1–21	Normal	Fav	Any
	4	<1	Normal	Any	Any
	4S	<1	Normal	Any	=1
	4S	<1	Normal	Unfav	Any
High	2	1–21	Amplified	Unfav	Any
	3	<1	Amplified	Any	Any
	3	1–21	Normal	Unfav	Any
	3	1–21	Amplified	Any	Any
	4	<1	Amplified	Any	Any
	4	1–21	Any	Any	Any
	4S	<1	Amplified	Any	Any

INSS, International Neuroblastoma Staging System; Fav, favorable; Unfav, unfavorable.

5 Retinoblastoma

Updated by Vinita Takiar

▶ BACKGROUND

What is the incidence and median age for presentation of retinoblastoma (RB)?

250–300 cases/yr of RB; **95% <5 yo** (1 yo for familial, 2 yo for sporadic)

What is the most common eye tumor in infants?

Metastatic leukemia (1,000 cases/yr). RB is the #1 primary tumor.

What are the 3 most common ocular tumors (considering all age groups)?

Metastatic carcinoma, melanoma, and RB

What % of multifocal RB is inherited vs. from de novo germline mutations?

40% are heritable (only 10% have a positive family Hx ["familial"]), and **60% are from new germline mutations;** 93% have a negative family Hx.

What % of RBs are bilat/ multifocal vs. unilat at presentation?

25% bilat/multifocal vs. 70%–80% unilat. Bilat tumors are typically multifocal (~5 tumors on avg) and present younger (~15 mos).

To what other malignancy are RB pts particularly prone?

RB pts are prone to **osteosarcoma.**

What gene is mutated in RB?

The **RB1 tumor suppressor gene** is mutated in RB.

On what chromosome is the RB tumor suppressor gene located?

The RB tumor suppressor gene is located on **chromosome 13.**

What cell cycle checkpoint does RB1 affect?

RB1 affects the **G1/S** checkpoint.

What is the cell of origin for RB?

RB arises from **neuroepithelial cells** (from the nucleated photoreceptor layer of the inner retina).

How do the 1st hit vs. the 2nd hit differ in terms of mechanisms?

1st hit: germline deletion
2nd hit: somatic loss of heterozygosity due to mitotic recombination error, allelic loss, or loss of ch13

What pathway is involved in the 3rd hit that leads to tumor formation?

3rd hit: p53 suppression with MDM2 amplification (two-thirds of tumors)

Are there mutational hot spots on the RB gene?

No. Various mutations are seen in each of the 20 exons involved, but there are no mutational hot spots on the RB gene.

What is the unique histologic feature/pattern associated with RB?

Flexner-Wintersteiner rosettes (also small round blue cells, $+Ca^{2+}$, necrosis)

What are the 5 patterns of spread for RB?

Patterns of spread for RB:
1. Local extension
2. Optic nerve to brain
3. CSF to leptomeninges/subarachnoid
4. Heme mets
5. LN from conjunctiva, ciliary body, iris

What are the most common sites of hematogenous spread in RB? What % of pts present with DMs?

Bone, liver, and spleen. **10%–15%** of pts present with DMs.

What are 2 tumor-related factors that correlate with an increased risk for mets?	**Thickness** (relates to invasion of optic nerve, uvea, orbit, choroid) and **size** of lesion
What is trilat RB? How common is it? What is the prognosis?	Trilat RB is **bilat RB + CNS midline PNET** (pineal or suprasellar), representing **3%–9% of hereditary RB** (rare). It is almost **uniformly fatal.**
How does RB present grossly?	Endophytic mass (projects into vitreous) and less frequently exophytic
How do pts present with RB in the U.S. vs. in developing countries?	In the U.S.: **leukocoria** > strabismus > painful glaucoma, and irritability. Leukocoria refers to an abnl white reflection from the retina. In developing countries: proptosis, orbital mass, and mets (more advanced)
What are the major negative prognostic factors in RB?	Delay in Dx of >6 mos, Hx of intraocular surgery leading to seeding, cataracts, thick tumors, and Hx of RT (because of high risk for secondary cancers), extraocular extension

▶ WORKUP/STAGING

What is the DDx for pts who present with leukocoria?	Toxocariasis, hyperplastic primary vitreous, Coat's Dz, retrolental fibrodysplasia, congenital cataracts, and toxoplasmosis
Is Bx done for RB?	**Generally not.** Because of the fear of seeding, the Dx is established clinically.
What is the typical workup for pts with an intraocular mass?	Intraocular mass workup: H&P (EUA, max dilated pupil, scleral indentation, ocular US), labs, US/CT, MRI (most sensitive to evaluate extraocular extension)
When are bone scan, BM Bx, and LP indicated?	If the tumor is not confined to the globe (with deep invasion), BM Bx, LP, and bone scan are indicated.
What % of RBs are calcified?	**90%** of RBs are calcified.
What is the most commonly used staging system for RB? For what does this system predict?	**Reese-Ellsworth grouping system;** used to predict for **visual preservation after EBRT** (does *not* predict for survival)
What staging system is used in ongoing COG protocols?	The **International Classification for Intraocular Retinoblastoma** is used for staging in ongoing COG protocols.
Summarize the International Classification for Intraocular Retinoblastoma.	**Group A:** all tumors ≤3 mm in thickness, confined to retina, and ≥3 mm from foveola and ≥1.5 mm from optic disc

Group B: all tumors confined to retina, clear subretinal fluid ≤3 mm from tumor with no subretinal seeding

Group C: discrete tumors, subretinal fluid without seeding involving up to one-fourth of retina, local fine vitreous seeding close to discrete tumor, local subretinal seeding <3 mm from tumor

Group D: massive or diffuse tumors; subretinal fluid or diffuse vitreous seeding; retinal detachment; diffuse or massive Dz including greasy seeds or avascular tumor masses; subretinal seeding may include subretinal plaques or tumor nodules

Group E: presence of any of the following features: tumor touching lens, tumor ant to ant vitreous surface involving ciliary body or ant segment, diffuse infiltrating RB, neovascular glaucoma, opaque media from hemorrhage, tumor necrosis with aseptic orbital cellulites, phthisis bulbi (shrunken, nonfunctional eye)

▶ TREATMENT/PROGNOSIS

What is the Tx paradigm for unilat intraocular RB?

Unilat intraocular RB Tx paradigm: preserve eye with chemoreduction × 6 cycles (vincristine/carboplatin/etoposide [VCE]) → focal therapy

What are some focal therapies used for RB?

Enucleation, EBRT or brachytherapy (plaque), cryotherapy, photocoagulation (laser), thermochemo (thermal + carboplatin), sub-Tenon injection of carboplatin, intra-arterial chemotherapy.

When can cryotherapy/laser be used in RB?

Small lesions, at least 4 disc diameters from the fovea/optic disc

What is the generally accepted Tx breakdown based on the international RB groupings?

UCSF (*Lin P et al., Am J Ophthalmol 2009*):
  Group A: focal therapy only (laser, cryotherapy, hyperthermia, brachytherapy)
  Group B: vincristine + carboplatin × 6 cycles; focal therapy after 2–6 cycles
  Group C: VCE × 6 cycles; focal therapy
  Group D: same as group C; EBRT
  Group E: enucleation; 3-agent chemo

When is EBRT typically used in the management of RB without enucleation?

Dz persistence or progression with chemo; extraocular extension, small intraocular tumor in the macula, diffuse vitreous seeding, or subretinal implants; used **only if visual preservation is possible**

What evidence supports the addition of consolidative local therapy after chemoreduction in RB pts with seeding at Dx?

Per *Shields et al.* (retrospective): chemo vs. chemo + local Tx: in eyes with seeding before Tx, the addition of local Tx to chemo × 6 cycles decreased the vitreous and subretinal seeding recurrences from 75% to 0% (*p* = 0.04) and 67% to 0% (*p* = 0.003), respectively. (*Ophthalmology 1997*)

What are commonly used EBRT doses?

36–45 Gy with progressive Dz

How is bilat RB managed?

Individualize the Tx for each eye (bilat eye preservation, if possible).

How is extraocular Dz managed?

Orbital EBRT, chemo +/– RT for palliation; intrathecal chemo, high-dose chemo with stem cell transplant

What is the eye preservation rate in most RB series?

60%–90% (95% for Reese-Ellsworth groups I–III)

How is EBRT given, and what are the volumes irradiated?

4–6 MV IMRT/3D, proton therapy, electron therapy if available to entire globe + 5–8 mm of optic nerve (spare lens and iris for lower stages), 0.5-cm bolus if needed

What RT fields/setups are used for unilat vs. bilat RB?

Old standard for unilateral Dz is 4 ant oblique fields **and for bilateral** Dz opposed lat + ant oblique fields. Currently, with advanced techniques, there are no specific beam arrangement, but do tend to be anterior or anterior obliques.

What chemo agents are employed in RB?

Vincristine and carboplatin. If there is advanced Dz, add topoisomerase inhibitors.

What are the indications for enucleation? How much optic nerve needs to be removed?

Group E tumors, occupying >50% of the globe, no vision, painful eyes, extension to optic nerve; need to remove 10–15 mm of optic nerve with globe.

When is CRT indicated after enucleation for RB?

Adj CRT is indicated for RB whenever there is a +**margin or +LN** post-enucleation

What are the indications for episcleral brachytherapy? What is the dose used?

Solitary lesion **6–15 mm base diameter, ≤10 mm thick, >3 mm from disc/fovea; 40–45 Gy** to apex, **100–120 Gy** to base

What isotopes and plaque sizes are used in episcleral brachytherapy for RB?

I-125 or Ru-106 (more uniform loading, lower energy [beta] and less dose to anterior ocular structures), diameter of tumor + 4 mm (**2-mm margin** around the tumor)

What are the main advantages of proton RT in the Tx of RB?

Better orbital bone sparing (*Lee CT et al., IJROBP 2005*) and **better lens sparing** when the whole eye does not need to be treated (*Krengli M et al., IJROBP 2005*)

▶ TOXICITY

What is the 2ⁿᵈ malignancy rate in familial cases of RB treated with RT vs. no RT?	<u>With RT</u>: 4% at 10 yrs, 18% at 35 yrs, **50% at 50 yrs** <u>Without RT</u>: **15%–35% rate at 50 yrs,** mainly sarcomas (soft tissue and osteosarcoma) and melanomas
Is the risk of 2ⁿᵈ malignancy also increased in sporadic forms treated with RT?	**Yes,** but minimally—**5% at 50 yrs** (*Wong FL, JAMA 1997*)
What are some complications from RT?	Midfacial/orbital hypoplasia, 2ⁿᵈ malignancy (sarcoma), and cataracts
What are the complications from episcleral plaque therapy?	Retinopathy, maculopathy, glaucoma, and papillopathy
In what manner and how often should pts with bilat RB be screened for trilat RB?	With **biannual MRIs** of the brain for at least 5 yrs

6   Langerhans Cell Histiocytosis

Updated by Mark Edson

▶ BACKGROUND

What is the estimated annual incidence of Langerhans cell histiocytosis (LCH) in the U.S.?	**~1,200 cases/yr** of LCH in the U.S. It is likely underdiagnosed in the general population and is most common in children 1–3 yrs.
Is there a sex predilection in LCH?	**Yes. Males** are more commonly affected than females (3:2).

What is the cell of origin of LCH?

LCH results from dysregulation of the **mononuclear** cell line (not the skin Langerhans cell)

What are the diagnostic histopathologic characteristics of LCH?

Birbeck granules on electron microscopy and **CD1a, S100, and CD207 (Langerin)** positivity are typical for LCH.

What is the normal function of Langerhans cells? Where are they normally found?

Langerhans cells serve as **antigen presenting cells to lymphocytes** and are typically found in **skin, mucosa, spleen, and lymphatics.**

What organs are typically involved in LCH?

Bones (children) and lungs (adults), but LCH can present in any organ (e.g., liver, skin, etc.).

What defines low-risk groups vs. high-risk groups?

Low risk: unifocal lesion in bone, LN, GI tract, CNS

High risk: <2 yo with organ dysfunction (hepatosplenomegaly, pancytopenia); liver, spleen, BM involvement

How does LCH relate to other histiocytosis entities like eosinophilic granuloma, Letterer-Siwe Dz, Hand-Schuller-Christian Dz, and histiocytosis X?

Eosinophilic granuloma is an older term for focal LCH, while the eponyms represent multifocal Dz. Histiocytosis X is the older term for LCH. All are antiquated terms.

What is Hand-Schuller-Christian Dz?

Hand-Schuller-Christian Dz refers to the proliferation of histiocytes that results in **exophthalmos, skull lesions, diabetes insipidus** (DI), **and hemangiomas** (poor prognosis).

In what age group are widespread seborrheic rashes in the scalp/groin, +LAD, and liver involvement seen with LCH?

These Sx are seen in LCH pts **<2 yo.**

For what age group is DI a common presentation of LCH?

>2 yo (20%–50%). In this group, bone (pain +/– soft tissue mass), lung, oral mucous membrane, and cerebral involvement by LCH can be seen.

▶ WORKUP/STAGING

Is bone scan useful for LCH? Why?

No. LCH bone lesions are usually purely lytic.

What type of workup is necessary?

LCH workup: H&P, labs, skeletal survey (lucency in the medullary cavity), and **Bx**

What is the appearance of LCH lesions on plain radiograph?

LCH lesions appear **lytic** or **"punched-out"** on plain radiograph.

What staging system is used for LCH?	There is no staging system. LCH is described as **single-system** (unifocal or multifocal involvement of an organ/body system) or **multisystem** (≥2 organ or body systems).

▶ **TREATMENT**

What are the indications for RT in LCH?	No signs of local healing, relapse after surgery, if other local therapy (i.e., curettage) is not appropriate, potential compromise of critical structures from expansile bone lesions, pain relief, and DI
What is the largest series supporting RT for DI from LCH?	**Mayo data** (*Kilpatrick SE et al., Cancer 1995*): 45 pts. There was a 36% rate of DI improvement with RT.
Within how many days after Dx should RT be given for DI?	RT should be administered within **14 days** of DI Dx. (*Kilpatrick SE et al., Cancer 1995*)
When is RT not indicated in LCH?	RT is not indicated for **sclerotic LCH lesions and collapsed vertebral lesions** (only indicated if such lesions are painful).
What data support the use of RT for localized osseous LCH lesions?	**German meta-analysis** (*Olschwski T et al., Strahlenther Onkol 2006*): LC was 96% and CR was 93% for single-system Dz with RT.
What are the commonly used doses and volumes for LCH?	DI: **15 Gy** to pituitary/hypothalamus Bone (small margin): **5–10 Gy** Adults: **15–24 Gy** (in 2 Gy/fx)
When is chemo used in LCH?	**Multisystem Dz** (e.g., if fever, pain, severe skin involvement, failure to thrive, and organ dysfunction)
What systemic agents are used for LCH?	**Prednisone (1ˢᵗ-line), then vinblastine.** Single-agent chemo is as good as multiagent chemo. Vincristine can also be used.
How are asymptomatic, organ-confined LCH lesions managed?	Asymptomatic LCH lesions are typically **observed.**
How is a symptomatic bony LCH lesion managed?	A symptomatic bony LCH lesion is typically managed by surgery **(curettage, excision) and/or local injection of steroids.**
How are symptomatic LCH skin lesions managed?	Symptomatic LCH skin lesions are managed by **topical therapy with nitrogen mustard, steroids, or systemic therapy.**
How is LCH of the eye, ear, spine, or weight-bearing bones managed?	LCH of these areas is managed by **systemic steroids or local RT.**

How is asymptomatic multifocal LCH Dz with organ dysfunction managed?	Such asymptomatic LCH Dz is typically **observed.**
How is symptomatic multifocal LCH Dz with organ dysfunction managed?	Symptomatic multifocal LCH Dz with organ dysfunction is managed by **systemic therapy** (as described above). If the pt is symptomatic due to organ failure, consider transplant (liver, lung).
What is the long-term OS for solitary LCH lesions?	The OS for solitary LCH lesions is ~**100%.**
What is the long-term OS for multisystem LCH with organ dysfunction?	The long-term OS for multisystem LCH with organ dysfunction is **33%–54%.**
What is the long-term OS for multisystem LCH without organ dysfunction?	The long-term OS for multisystem LCH without organ dysfunction is **82%–96%.**

▶ **TOXICITY**

What is the RT TD 5/5 dose threshold for developing hypopituitarism?	The TD 5/5 for hypopituitarism is **40–45 Gy** (GH levels decrease first with doses as low as 18 Gy, then LH/FSH, then TSH/ACTH)

7 Medulloblastoma
Updated by Nikhil G. Thaker

 BACKGROUND

Estimate the annual incidence of medulloblastoma (MB) in the U.S. What is its frequency relative to other CNS tumors in children?	~**500 cases/yr** of MB in the U.S. It is the **2nd most common** pediatric CNS tumor (20% of cases; #1 is low-grade glioma at 35%–50%). It is the most common malignant brain tumor in the posterior fossa (PF) in children and adolescents, comprising 40% of all PF tumors.

What is the median age of MB at Dx?

MB has a bimodal age distribution, with a median age of ~7 yrs in children (**peak incidence between 5 and 9 yrs**) and ~25 yrs in adults.

Is there a sex predilection to MB?

Yes. Males are more commonly affected than females (2:1).

What is the cell of origin?

Neuroectodermal cells from the superior medullary velum (germinal matrix of cerebellum) or cerebellar vermis

MB is a subtype of what class of tumors?

MB is a subtype of **embryonal tumors** (along with PNET and atypical teratoid rhabdoid tumor [ATRT]).

Mutation of which gene distinguishes ATRT from MB?

Loss of *INI1* distinguishes ATRT from MB. *INI1* is found on chromosome 22 and functions as a tumor suppressor gene.

What % of pts present with CSF spread at Dx?

30%–40% of MB cases present with CSF spread at Dx.

For what MB age group is CSF spread more common?

This is more common in **younger pts.**

Does extra-axial spread occur in MB? If so, where?

Extra-axial spread is **rare,** but when it does occur it is typically to **bone.**

What are the characteristic histologic features and markers for MB?

MB appears as **small round blue cells.** 40% have **Homer-Wright rosettes,** and most stain + for neuron-specific enolase, synaptophysin, and nestin.

What are some other types of small round blue cell tumors?

Other small round blue cell tumors include:
1. **L**ymphoma
2. **E**wing
3. **A**cute lymphoblastic leukemia
4. **R**habdomyosarcoma
5. **N**euroblastoma
6. **N**euroepithelioma
7. **M**edulloblastoma
8. **R**etinoblastoma

(Mnemonic: **LEARN NMR**)

What are the 3 histologic variants of MB?

Histologic variants of MB:
1. Classic
2. Nodular/Desmoplastic (better prognosis)
3. Large cell/Anaplastic (worse prognosis)

The desmoplastic histologic variant of MB is associated with what clinical features?

The desmoplastic variant is associated with:
1. LOH 9q
2. Older age at Dx
3. Better prognosis

What is the most aggressive histologic variant that also has a particularly high rate of CSF dissemination?

Large cell/Anaplastic is the most aggressive MB variant.

What % of MBs are familial, and what are some associated genetic syndromes?

2%–5% of MBs are familial. Associated genetic syndromes include **Gorlin** (*PTCH1* mutation leading to nevoid basal cell carcinoma syndrome) and **Turcot** (APC mutation, also seen in colorectal cancer or familial adenomatous polyposis).

What are the common cytogenetic abnormalities in MB?

Common cytogenetic abnormalities in MB include:
1. **Deletion of 17p** (40%–50%)
2. **Isochromosome 17q**
3. **Deletion of 16q**

Where does MB most commonly arise?

Midline cerebellar vermis (75%), with the rest in cerebellar hemispheres

What is the DDx for a PF mass?

DDx for a PF mass includes:
1. **MB**
2. Ependymoma
3. ATRT
4. Astrocytoma
5. Brainstem glioma
6. Juvenile pilocytic astrocytoma
7. Hemangioblastoma
8. Mets

What are the 4 genetic MB subgroups and what mutations tend to occur in each subgroup?

1. WNT group: *CTNNB1* mutation. Associated with Turcot. Least common (10%) subgroup.
2. SHH group: *PTCH1, GLI3, MYCN*. 30% of MB, often desmoplastic. Overrepresented in infants and adults (bimodal).
3. Group 3: *MYC* amplification, GABAergic expression. Enrich for large cell histology and are frequent mets at Dx.
4. Group 4: *MYCN, CDK6* amplification

(*Northcott PA et al., JCO 2011*)

Describe the prognosis for each subgroup.

Good prognosis: WNT group and **infants** in SHH group
Intermediate prognosis: Group 4 and SHH group
Poor prognosis: Group 3

▶ WORKUP/STAGING

What are some common presenting Sx for MB?

HA (nocturnal or morning), n/v, altered mentation due to hydrocephalus, truncal ataxia, head bob, and diplopia (CN VI)

To what are the common presenting Sx in MB?

Obstructive hydrocephalus/↑ICP (HA and vomiting) and cerebellar dysfunction

What symptoms would be expected with midline vs. lateral cerebellar tumors?	Midline tumors may cause gait ataxia or truncal instability (i.e., broad-based gate, difficulty with heel-to-toe), whereas tumors in the lateral hemispheres (more common in adults) may cause limb ataxia (i.e., dysmetria, intention tremor, difficulty with heel-to-shin). ATRT more likely to involve lateral hemispheres.
What is the "setting-sun" sign?	Downward deviation of gaze from $\uparrow$ ICP (CNs III, IV, and VI)
List the general workup for a PF mass at presentation.	PF mass workup: H&P (funduscopic exam, CN exam), CBC/CMP, MRI brain/spine, CSF cytology (may not be possible due to herniation risk), and baseline ancillary tests. Consider bone scan and CXR depending on presentation and risk factors.
What are some important ancillary tests to obtain prior to starting Tx?	Baseline audiometry, IQ testing, TSH, and growth measures
Is a tumor Bx necessary for Dx? Is a BM Bx necessary?	Per current COG MB protocol **ACNS0331**, a **tumor Bx is unnecessary; pts often go straight to surgery. BM Bx is not part of the standard workup.**
Is there any risk of CSF dissemination with shunt placement for MB?	**No.** There is no risk of CSF dissemination.
What tests should be obtained on days 10–14 postop?	MRI spine, CSF cytology. (Delay until day 10 to avoid a false+ result from surgical debris.)
When is MRI of the brain done? Of the spine?	MRI brain: preop and 24–48 hrs postop MRI spine: preop or 10–14 days postop
What can be done before Tx to reduce ICP?	Ventricular drain or shunt, steroids, acetazolamide (Diamox)
List the T staging according to the modified Chang staging system for MB.	**T1:** <3 cm, confined **T2:** ≥3 cm **T3a:** >3 cm, with extension into aqueduct of Sylvius or foramen of Luschka **T3b:** >3 cm, with unequivocal extension into brainstem **T4:** >3 cm, extends beyond aqueduct of Sylvius or foramen magnum to involve 3rd ventricle/midbrain/upper cervical cord
List the M staging according to the modified Chang staging system for MB.	**M0:** no subarachnoid or hematogenous mets **M1:** +CSF **M2:** nodular intracranial seeding **M3:** nodular seeding in spinal subarachnoid space **M4:** extraneural spread (esp BM, bone)

Define standard-risk and high-risk MB.	**Standard risk (two-thirds):** >3 yo, GTR/NTR <1.5 cm^2 residual, and M0 **High risk (one-third):** <3 yo or STR >1.5 cm^2 residual, or M+
What may contribute to the poor prognosis of <3 yo?	Reduction in volume and/or dose or elimination of RT in very young children due to concerns of toxicity may contribute to the poor prognosis in this age group.

▶ TREATMENT/PROGNOSIS

What is the most important prognostic factor at Dx for MB? What are other poor prognostic factors for MB?	**M stage** is the most important prognostic factor. Other poor prognostic factors include male sex, age <3 yrs, and unresectable Dz/STR.
What is the management paradigm for standard-risk MB?	COG approach: Standard-risk MB management: max safe resection → RT with concurrent weekly vincristine → adj chemo (8 6-wk cycles of cisplatin/CCNU/vincristine). **RT is CSI to 23.4 Gy → cone down 1 (CD1) to PF to 36 Gy, then cone down 2 (CD2) to cavity/residual; or PF to 54–55.8 Gy; or cavity/residual to 54–55.8 Gy (MDACC).**
What chemo regimens are typically used for MB?	Initial studies that established the efficacy of reduced-dose CSI (23.4 Gy) with chemo in standard-risk MB used **concurrent vincristine with RT → adj cisplatin/CCNU/vincristine.** The **CCG A9961** trial recently found similar outcomes when cyclophosphamide was substituted for CCNU. (*Packer R et al., JCO 2006*)
What is the management paradigm for high-risk MB?	High-risk MB management paradigm for pts >3 yo: same as standard risk, but the **CSI dose is 36 Gy;** also, nodular intracranial or spinal mets may to be boosted to 45–50.4 Gy depending on location (whether lesion is above or below spinal cord terminus).
For high-risk MB pts, what is the total boost dose for pts with intracranial (M2) vs. spinal (M3) mets?	Per COG **ACNS0332,** boost intracranial mets to 50.4 Gy, focal spinal mets below the cord terminus to 50.4 Gy, focal spinal mets above the cord terminus to 45 Gy, and diffuse spinal Dz to 39.6 Gy.
Estimate the 5-yr EFS for standard- and high-risk MB.	The 5-yr EFS for standard risk is **~80%** and for high risk **~50%–60%.**

What is the management paradigm for MB pts <3 yo?

MB pts <3 yo management paradigm: max safe resection → chemo until pt reaches 3 yo. At 3 yo, consider standard therapy with CSI → more chemo. If desmoplastic histology, consider omitting RT altogether. New protocols use surgical bed RT alone after induction chemotherapy in 18- to 36-mo patients.

What are the potential risks of aggressive surgery in the PF?

The major risk of aggressive surgery in the PF is **PF syndrome (10%–15% of cases):** mutism, ataxia, dysphagia, hypotonia, respiratory failure, and mood lability caused by disruption of the dentatorubrothalamic pathway to the supplemental motor cortex. PF syndrome typically presents 12–24 hrs postop and improves over several mos. Other potential complications include aseptic meningitis and CSF leakage.

In MB, how are NTR, STR, and "Bx only" defined?

NTR: <1.5 cm^2 residual on postop MRI
STR: 51%–90% resection
Bx only:

In MB, is there a difference between NTR vs. GTR in terms of EFS? How about STR and GTR?

Retrospective studies suggest that pts who obtain an **NTR and GTR have similar outcomes** (*Gajjar A et al., Ped Neurosurg 1996*). However, 5-yr EFS is worse in STR pts (54%) compared to GTR/NTR pts (78%). (*Zeltzer PM et al., JCO 1999*)

What chemo agent improved DFS and OS according to MB studies in the 1990s?

Cisplatin. Prior to the introduction of cisplatin, several studies (**SIOP I** and **CCG 942**) failed to show improved OS with the addition of adj chemo.

What 2 studies demonstrated the need for chemo with reduced-dose CSI (23.4 Gy) for standard-risk MB?

There has been no RCT comparing reduced-dose CSI +/– cisplatin-based chemo. The need for cisplatin-based chemo is inferred from the following 2 studies:

1. **POG 8631/CCG 923:** randomized standard-risk MB to 36 Gy vs. 23.4 Gy CSI alone (no chemo). There was a trend toward ↓ EFS and OS in the 23.4-Gy arm. (*Thomas PR et al., JCO 2000*)
2. **CCG 9892 (phase II):** standard-risk MB treated with 23.4 CSI with concurrent weekly vincristine → 55.8-Gy boost to PF → adj cisplatin/CCNU/vincristine. 5-yr PFS was 79%, which was similar to historical controls treated with 36 Gy CSI and similar chemo. (*Packer R et al., JCO 1999*) Basis for POG A9961 reduced dose CSI.

Can RT be delayed for MB pts <3 yo by using chemo alone? What studies support this?

Yes. Given the toxicity of RT in pts <3 yo, it is reasonable to delay RT until 3 yo, **especially with desmoplastic histology.**

Baby POG (*Duffner PK et al., Neurooncol 1999, NEJM 1993*): <3 yo, 206 pts, high-/low-risk MB + other PNET, chemo alone (Cytoxan + Vincristine (VCR) × 2–> cisplatin + etoposide) × 2 yrs if <2 yo, × 1 yr if 2–3 yo. 5-yr OS was 40%, and PFS was 32%.

German BTSG data (*Rutkowski S et al., NEJM 2005*): <3 yo, 43 pts, high-/low-risk MB, chemo (Cytoxan, vincristine, methotrexate, carboplatin, VP-16, intrathecal methotrexate). 5-yr PFS was 58%, and OS was 66%. The majority of pts had a desmoplastic variant histology. The benefit was best in M0 pts (5-yr PFS of 68% and OS of 77%)

SFOP data (*Grill J et al., Lancet Oncol 2005*): <5 yo, 79 pts. 5-yr OS was best in R0M0 (73%) vs. 13% with M+.

What was the Tx regimen on COG A9934 for MB pts <3 yo?

Initial surgery → induction chemo × 4 mos with Cytoxan, vincristine, cisplatin, etoposide → 2nd surgery for identifiable or residual Dz → age/risk group/response-adapted conformal RT to PF + primary site (*no* CSI) → maintenance chemo × 8 mos. Enrolled children were older than 8 mos but younger than 3 yrs, all M0 MB.

Age/risk/response-adapted RT:
If <24 mos and CR: 18 Gy to PF → tumor bed boost to 50.4 Gy, or 54 Gy if PR/SD/+ residual
If >24 mos and CR or PR: 23.4 Gy to PF → tumor bed boost to 54 Gy

(*Ashlet DM et al., JCO 2012*)

What evidence supports the use of >50 Gy total doses in MB?

Retrospective data suggest that LC in the PF varies with dose above and below 50 Gy. In 60 MB cases, if the PF dose was >50 Gy, the LC was 79%. However, if the PF dose was <50 Gy, the LC was 33%. (*Hughes EN et al., Cancer 1988*)

In MB pts, does the entire PF need to be boosted to >50 Gy?

Retrospective evidence suggests that **few failures occur in the PF outside the tumor bed (<5%).**

Fukunaga-Johnson et al. reviewed 114 pts treated with CSI → boost to the entire PF. The solitary site of the 1st failure within the PF but outside the tumor bed occurred in 1 of 27 failures. (*IJROBP 1998*)

Wolden et al. reviewed 32 pts treated with tumor bed boost only. There were 6 total failures: 5 outside the PF and 1 within the PF but outside the boost volume. (*JCO 2003*)

Merchant et al. conducted a prospective phase II trial of 23.4 Gy CSI + PF boost to 36 Gy and primary site to 55.8 Gy with dose-intensive chemo. 5-yr EFS was 83%, and PF failure was 5%. Reduced doses to temporal lobes, cochlea, hypothalamus. (*IJROBP 2008*)

What are the RT technique questions being addressed in COG ACNS0331?

In **ACNS0331, standard-risk pts 3–7 yo** are randomized to **CSI to 18 Gy vs. 23.4 Gy.** For the **18 Gy arm, all pts got a PF boost to 23.4 Gy.** All standard-risk pts 3–7 yo underwent a 2nd randomization: CD to **54 Gy to whole PF vs. tumor bed only.** Standard-risk pts 8–22 yo: 23.4 Gy CSI → randomization to CD to 54 Gy to PF vs. tumor bed only.

What was the rationale for 18-Gy CSI in ACNS0331?

CSI doses in excess of 20 Gy still pose a significant risk for cognitive and growth outcomes, particularly in young children. Pilot study in 10 children with PNET of the PF showed comparable outcomes to higher doses. (*Goldwein J et al., IJROBP 1996*)

What question does ACNS0334 attempt to address?

Phase III trial in children **<3 yrs with high-risk MB or PNET.** Trial addresses the addition of high-dose MTX to the 4-drug induction chemo regimen of VCR, etoposide, cytoxan, cisplatin → 2nd surgery, consolidation, and peripheral blood stem cell rescue. RT is at the discretion of the institution.

Is there a role for pre-RT chemo in MB pts >3 yo?

No. In MB pts >3 yo, intensive chemo prior to RT (vs. RT then chemo) is associated with ↑ RT toxicity, RT Tx delays, and worsened RFS. (German **HIT 91:** *Kortmann RD et al., IJROBP 2000*)

What benefit does proton therapy have in the Tx of MB?

Retrospective data suggest that proton plans have ↓ **dose to the cochlea/temporal lobe compared to IMRT** (0.1%–2% vs. 20%–30%), and virtually no exit dose to the abdomen, chest, heart, pelvis. Recent study suggests less morbidity, including GI and heme toxicity (although this is in adults). (*Brown AP et al., IJROBP 2013*)

Is there a role for hyperfractionated RT to reduce cognitive sequelae of MB Tx?

MSFOP 98, a phase II trial, evaluated hyperfractionated RT in MB and showed promising results. 48 standard-risk pts were treated with CSI 1 Gy bid to 36 Gy → tumor bed boost 1 Gy bid to 68 Gy. **6-yr OS was 78%, and EFS was 75%. Decline in IQ appeared less pronounced than in historical controls.** (*Carrie C et al., JCO 2009*)

How are MB pts simulated?

MB simulation: supine or **prone, neck extended** (so PA spine field does not exit through the mouth), head mask, **shoulders positioned inferiorly** (to allow for lat cranial fields). Depending on institutional experience, can simulate supine, which allows better airway access during anesthesia, most places are now doing supine technique.

What modalities of RT have been used for CSI?

Photons, electrons (at MDACC in years past), and protons are the more commonly used RT modalities for CSI therapy.

In CSI, which fields are placed 1st?

Spinal fields are placed 1st (to allow calculation of collimator angle for the cranial field based on spinal field beam divergence).

Cranial fields are placed 2nd (down to C5-6 or as low as possible but need to ensure laterals do not go through shoulder).

By what angle are the cranial field collimators rotated?

Arctan (one-half length of sup spine field/SSD), which matches the cranial field to the spine field divergence

What are the borders of the spine field(s)?

Superior: matched to cranial field
Inferior: end of thecal sac (near S2-3, check on sagittal spine MRI)
Lateral: 1 cm past pedicles (some centers plan with wider margins in sacrum to cover neural foramina)

By what angle is the couch kicked and in which direction?

Couch kick for CSI: **arctan (one-half length of cranial field/source axis distance);** couch kicked **toward** side treated to match cranial field divergence (for breast, kick is **away**)

What is a potential problem with a couch kick?

Couch could be rotated in the opposite direction than intended. At MDACC, treatments are usually planned without a couch kick to eliminate moving table in wrong direction. A small amount of overlap occurs lat to cord, but doses used are relatively low and amount of overlap is decreased by feathering the junction.

If multiple spinal fields are used, what is the skin gap? At what depth is the match?

With multiple spine fields, the **skin gap = ([0.5 × Length 1 × d]/SSD1) + ([0.5 × Length 2 × d]/SSD2)** where d is the depth of the match, which is typically at the ant cord edge.

How is "feathering" done? Why is it used?

There are several techniques, and feathering is dependent upon institutional experience. Feathering helps reduce hot and cold spots in plan. At MDACC, several techniques are used, including inter- and intrafractional junctioning for photons, electron junction technique, and proton junction technique.

Interfractional junctioning may be modulated with field-in-field technique and consists of moving junction superiorly 0.5 cm on 7th and 13th fraction. This creates 12 fields with junctions.

Intrafractional junctioning may be modulated with step-and-shoot technology. 3 junction control points at 1-cm gaps (i.e., 0, 1, and 2 cm with the use of multileaf collimators [MLCs]) are created, and each control point delivers one-third of the fractional dose. MLC leaves remain outside the field to ensure minimal interleaf leakage.

Where should the isocenter be placed in the cranial field for CSI? What cranial structure should be assessed for adequate coverage?

For the half-beam block technique, the isocenter should be placed **behind the lenses** to minimize divergence of beams into the opposite lens; the **cribriform plate** is not optimally visualized on conventional simulation films. A generous margin must be given in this area, or CT contours of the cribriform plate can be outlined to ensure coverage.

What CSI techniques can be employed if the entire spine cannot be included in 1 field?

The practitioner can **increase the SSD (i.e., 100 cm → 120 cm) or rotate the collimator** using a single field, but if the length is >36–38 cm, then **2 spinal fields** are needed, with the inf field's isocenter placed at the junction (using half-beam block to minimize the cold spot). Match at L1-2, as this is the area where the depth of cord changes the most.

▶ TOXICITY

What is Collins' law as it pertains to the max length of follow-up needed for pediatric tumors?

Defines period of risk for recurrence (**age at Dx + 9 mos** [gestational period]). If tumor was present in utero, then **age at Dx + 9 mos** determines rate of growth for it to become clinically evident. Residual Dz should become evident in same timeframe. (*Sure U, Clin Neurol Neurosurg 1997*)

What factors predict for greater decline in IQ after CSI?

Factors for decline in IQ after CSI:
  Age <7 yrs (most important)
  Higher dose (36 Gy vs. 23.4 Gy)
  Higher IQ at baseline
  Female sex

(*Ris MD et al., JCO 2001*)

For how long can the pt's IQ decline after CSI?

>**5 yrs.** *Hoppe-Hirsch et al.* reviewed 120 MB pts treated with CSI to 36 Gy. At 5 yrs, 58% had an IQ >80. At 10 yrs, only 1% had an IQ >80. (*Childs Nerv Syst 1990*)

What are some important factors influencing IQ scores/neurotoxicity after RT?

Age at Tx with RT (most important), volume and dose of RT, and sex (female > male)

What is the dose constraint to the cochlea?

V30 <50% is the dose constraint to the cochlea (max is 35 Gy with chemo).

What is the most common hormone deficiency after RT to the brain? What is the dose threshold?

GH. The threshold dose for GH deficiency is ~10 Gy.

What is the annual IQ drop after full PF boost in MB pts younger and older than 7 yrs? What structure is most important?

IQ drop of **5 points/yr if <7 yo and 1 point/yr if >7 yo.** The dose to the **supratentorial brain** (temporal lobes) is most important.

8   Ependymoma

Steven H. Lin, Ori Shokek, and
Updated by Mark Edson

▶ **BACKGROUND**

In children and adults, what % of brain tumors are ependymomas?

<u>Children:</u> 5% (3rd most common childhood CNS tumor)
<u>Adults:</u> 2%

What is the median age of Dx for ependymomas?

Bimodal peak distribution, with peaks at **5 yrs** and **35 yrs**

What % of ependymomas arise intracranially, and how does this differ in children vs. adults? What are the most common locations?

Children: 90% intracranial (10% cord). If intracranial, the posterior fossa is the most common site (60% infratentorial [floor of 4th ventricle], 40% supratentorial [lat ventricle]).
Adults: 75% arise in spinal canal. Of intracranial tumors, two-thirds are supratentorial and one-third are infratentorial.

What is the cell of origin for ependymomas?

Ependymomas arise from the **ependymal cells lining the ventricles.**

What % of primary spinal tumors is ependymoma?

~20% (meningiomas comprise 33%, spinal nerve tumors 27%)

What genetic syndrome is associated with spinal cord ependymoma?

Spinal cord ependymoma is associated with **NF-2.**

What % of ependymoma pts present with CSF seeding? What features predispose to seeding?

5%–10%; infratentorial location, high-grade tumors, and LF predispose to CSF seeding.

What is the WHO classification of ependymoma?

Grade I: myxopapillary and subependymoma
Grade II: classic ependymoma
Grade III: anaplastic
Grade IV: ependymoblastoma

Where do grade IV ependymomas generally arise?

Grade IV ependymomas usually arise in the **supratentorium.**

What is the classical pathologic feature of ependymomas?

Perivascular pseudorosettes are a classical pathologic feature of ependymomas.

What defines malignant ependymomas on pathology?	Greater number of mitoses, cellular atypia, and more necrosis
Which histopathologic subtype is most commonly found in the lumbosacral spinal cord?	**Myxopapillary ependymomas** usually arise in the conus/filum region of the spinal cord.
What is the typical presentation of ependymomas?	**Depends on location.** *If infratentorial:* CN deficits, ↑ ICP; *if supratentorial:* seizures, focal deficits
With what neurologic deficits are spinal cord ependymoma pts likely to present?	Sensory deficits (vs. cord astrocytomas, which present with pain/motor deficits)

 WORKUP/STAGING

What is the workup for ependymoma?	Ependymoma workup: H&P, basic labs, CSF cytology/sampling, and MRI brain/spinal cord
When is LP contraindicated?	LP is contraindicated with a **posterior fossa tumor with surrounding mass effect.**
When should spinal MRI or CSF cytology be obtained after resection?	**2 wks (10–14 days) postop** to avoid false+.

▶ **TREATMENT/PROGNOSIS**

What is the Tx paradigm for ependymoma?	Traditional ependymoma Tx paradigm: max safe resection with adj RT for children >3 yo (adj chemo if <3 yo)
Under what circumstances should CSI be done for ependymomas?	CSI should be done if **+CSF, +MRI neuroaxis, and ependymoblastoma** histology. For all others, local RT is sufficient.
What evidence supports the omission of CSI for anaplastic ependymomas after resection if there is no evidence of neuroaxial involvement?	Multiple retrospective reviews reveal the following: LR is the primary pattern of failure (>90%) regardless of field size; spinal seeding is uncommon without LR; and prophylaxis with CSI or WBRT does not affect survival when compared to local RT.

What is the role of chemo in ependymoma? What is the response rate?	Traditionally, chemo is utilized for <3 yo to delay RT and for salvage (cisplatin, VP-16, temozolomide, nitrosoureas). The response rate typically is 5%–15%. However, a new prospective study from St. Jude's Children's Hospital (*Merchant TE et al., Lancet Oncol 2009*), which included many pts <3 yo (78%) treated with maximal safe resection and postoperative conformal RT to 59.4 Gy with 10-mm margin around postop bed, suggests that RT can be given safely and effectively for pts <3 yo. The 7-yr OS was 81%, EFS was 69%, and LC rate was 87.3% (cumulative LF rate is 16.3%). Therefore, young age should not preclude pts from receiving high-dose RT after surgery, except for infants <1 yo. Current protocols require postop RT in completely resected infratentorial ependymoma starting at age 18 mos. If STR, chemo may be used to see if GTR is possible with 2nd-look surgery after 2 cycles of chemo.
What is the single most important favorable prognostic factor in ependymoma?	**Completeness of surgical resection** (correlates closely with LC for ependymomas)
What is the difference in 5-yr OS between GTR and STR for ependymomas?	**75% vs. 35%** (similar for low-grade vs. high-grade ependymomas)
What ependymoma locations are most amenable to GTR? Least?	**Spinal** (GTR ~100%) > supratentorial (80%) > infratentorial
What is given to children <3 yo after STR for ependymoma?	2 cycles of chemo can be used as a bridge Tx to see if GTR can be achieved. RT can be deferred with chemo until >18 mos, based on the St. Jude's trial (*Merchant TE et al., Lancet Oncol 2009*) and SEER analysis (*Koshy M et al., J Neurooncol 2011*). Both suggest that postop RT in children <3 yo improves survival.
What types of chemo are typically used for ependymoma?	**Cisplatin, cyclophosphamide, and etoposide** are typical chemo agents for ependymoma.
What is the dose and volume of RT to be used if no CSI is given for ependymomas?	Preop GTV + 1–2-cm margin to **54–59.4 Gy** (54 Gy for children <18 mos and >18 mos with GTR)

How is ependymoblastoma treated? What is the total dose to spine lesions vs. cranial lesions?

Treat like high-risk medulloblastoma/PNET: **CSI 36 Gy + vincristine** +/– carboplatin, boost to cavity/gross Dz. 45–50.4 Gy if spine and 54–59.4 Gy if cranial → vincristine/Cytoxan/prednisolone 6 wks after RT.

How is infratentorial ependymoma managed?

Max safe resection followed by **involved field postop RT** to a dose of **54–59.4 Gy.**

How is supratentorial ependymoma managed?

If not anaplastic (i.e., if grades I–II), observation after max GTR is acceptable.

How is recurrent ependymoma managed?

If no prior RT: surgery → RT
If prior RT: surgery → stereotactic RT or chemo

Which phase II study showed min neurocognitive decrement with conformal/small RT fields?

St. Jude's study ACNS0121 (*Merchant TE et al., JCO 2004*): 88 pts, 33 pts with grade 3. 3-yr PFS was 74%. IQ testing was stable after 2 yrs.

What is a major reason infratentorial lesions should get adj RT, regardless of histologic grade?

Difficulty with complete resection due to proximity to floor of 4th ventricle, or laterally protrusion through foramen of Luschka and involvement of CN nerves or CNS vessels → higher LR if infratentorial without RT

Which recent studies showed a benefit with adj RT after GTR for posterior fossa ependymomas?

Rogers L et al.: 10-yr LC GTR/RT 100% vs. 50% GTR alone. Nonsignificant benefit in 10-yr OS GTR (67%), GTR/RT (83%). (*J Neurosurg 2005*)

Merchant TE et al.: 5.3-yr median follow-up update from the phase II study **ACNS0121**. All rcvd conformal RT to 59.4 Gy for NTR/all sites and grade, and for R0 infratentorial lesions of all histologies. Well-differentiated lesions after GTR were observed. Chemo for STR, then evaluated for surgery and RT. 7-yr OS was 81%, LC was 87.3%, and EFS was 69.1%. Median age 2.9 yrs, with 78% of the pts <3 yo. (*Lancet Oncol 2009*)

When is RT used in spinal ependymomas?

When resection is incomplete or anaplastic histology (Kaiser data: *Volpp PB et al., IJROBP 2007*)

What fields/doses are used for spinal ependymomas?

Include 2 vertebral bodies/sacral nerve roots above and below tumor to 45 Gy (boost if below cord to 50.4–59.4 Gy)

What molecular profile is associated with poor outcomes in ependymoma?

Overexpression of erbB-2/erbB-4 is associated with poor outcomes in ependymoma.

Do young children or young adults with ependymoma have a worse prognosis?

Children. Age <4 yrs is a poor prognostic factor.

Which ependymoma lesions have a poorer prognosis: supratentorial or infratentorial?

Supratentorial (↑ high grade and more STR) (*Mansur DB et al., IJROBP 2005*)

What are the 5- and 10-yr OS rates for pts with grades II–III ependymomas?

70% and 55%, respectively (*Mansur DB et al., IJROBP 2005*); no difference between grade II and grade III tumors ($p = 0.71$)

What % of ependymoma pts eventually die of their Dz?

50% of ependymoma pts eventually die of their Dz.

▶ **TOXICITY**

How long of a follow-up is required for pts with ependymoma?

At least **10 yrs,** because late recurrences of >12 yrs after surgery can occur.

What imaging is required during the follow-up for ependymoma pts?

Craniospinal MRI q3–4mos for yr 1, then q4–6mos for another yr, then q6–12mos.

What is a commonly used dose constraint for the spinal cord?

45 Gy is the usual dose constraint for the spinal cord.

What is a commonly used dose constraint for the chiasm?

50.4–54 Gy is the usual max point dose constraint for the chiasm.

9 Intracranial Germ Cell and Pineal Tumors

Updated by Nikhil G. Thaker

▶ BACKGROUND

What are the 2 broad categories of germ cell tumors?

Gonadal and extragonadal

Pineal tumors represent what % of adult and children's tumors?

<u>Pediatric:</u> 5%
<u>Adult:</u> 1%

Germ cell tumors represent what % of pediatric and adult brain tumors?

<u>Pediatric:</u> 3%–11% (more frequent in Japan and Asia)
<u>Adult:</u> 1%

What would a "germinoma" of the testicles or ovaries be referred to?

Germinoma is referred to as seminoma in the testicles and dysgerminoma in the ovaries.

What are the 3 subtypes of extragonadal germ cell tumors? Which are more common in adults vs. children?

Sacrococcygeal, retroperitoneal, and intracranial. In adults, most common sites are ant mediastinum, retroperitoneum, pineal/suprasellar areas. In infants or children, intracranial and sacrococcygeal teratomas are more common.

What are the 2 subtypes of intracranial germ cell tumors? Which has a more favorable prognosis? Which is more common?

Germinoma and nongerminomatous germ cell tumor (NGGCT). Germinoma has a more favorable prognosis and requires less-intensive therapy. **Germinomas are more common** (two-thirds of all intracranial germ cell tumors).

What are 4 subtypes of intracranial NGGCTs?

Endodermal sinus tumor (yolk sac, elevated AFP), choriocarcinoma (elevated β-HCG), teratoma (immature and mature), embryonal (elevated β-HCG and AFP), and mixed (25% of NGGCT).

What are the median age at Dx and the sex/race predilection for germinomas?

10–12 yrs, males > females (2–3:1), **Asian** > white (4% vs. 1% pediatric CNS tumors in Asia vs. the U.S.)

Where do the majority of intracranial germinomas and NGGCTs arise?

Midline proximal 3rd ventricular structures: two-thirds pineal and one-third suprasellar. Other sites include basal ganglia, thalamus, cerebral hemisphere, and cerebellum. 5%–10% present with both pineal and suprasellar tumors, may be bifocal rather than metastatic, and are usually pure germinomas.

What % of germinomas have CSF dissemination at Dx?

10%–15% (50% of pineoblastomas have leptomeningeal dissemination)

What is the probability of spinal failure in pts with various types of pineal-based tumors without evidence of spinal seeding at Dx?

Mature and immature teratoma: 0% (0 of 16)
Mixed NGGCT: 4% (1 of 24)
Other NGGCT: 39% (3 of 9) (teratomas with malignant transformation and yolk sac tumors)
Germinoma: 17% (8 of 46)
Pineocytoma: 0% (0 of 7)
Pineal parenchymal tumor (PPT), pineoblastoma, or PPT of intermediate differentiation: 8 of 14 (57%)
Pineoblastoma and NGGCT have the highest propensity for CSF dissemination.
(*Schild SE et al., Cancer 1996*)

What is the typical presentation of a tumor in the pineal region?

↑ ICP (due to obstructive hydrocephalus, causing, n/v, papilledema, lethargy, somnolence); Parinaud syndrome (decreased upward gaze, accommodates but abnl light response); endocrinopathies rare but diabetes insipidus (DI) sometimes observed.

Pressure/mass effect on what anatomic structure causes Parinaud syndrome?

Pressure/mass effect on the **superior colliculus** causes Parinaud syndrome.

How do pts with suprasellar masses present?

Triad of **visual** difficulties (bitemporal hemianopsia), **DI,** and precocious or delayed/**abnl sexual development.** Other aspects of hypothalamic/pituitary dysfunction possible, including GH deficiency, hypothyroidism, and adrenal insufficiency.

▶ WORKUP/STAGING

What is the DDx for a pediatric brain tumor in the pineal region?

Pineoblastoma, pineocytoma, PPT of intermediate differentiation, germinoma, NGGCT, glioma, meningioma, lymphoma, benign cyst, Langerhans cell histiocytosis, hamartoma; most are germ cell tumors.

What is the DDx for a pediatric brain tumor in the suprasellar region?

Germinoma, NGGCT, craniopharyngioma, pituitary adenoma, meningioma, glioma, aneurysm, infection, metastases

What is the workup for a suspected germ cell tumor?	Suspected germ cell tumor workup: H&P (esp CNs, funduscopic exam), MRI brain/spine, basic labs, serum AFP/β-HCG, CSF AFP/β-HCG (more sensitive than serum), and CSF cytology
What AFP levels exclude the Dx of a germinoma?	An **AFP >10 ng/mL** excludes the Dx of pure germinoma.
What β-HCG levels exclude the Dx of germinoma?	None are truly exclusive, but if the β-HCG is >50 ng/mL, then it probably is not a germinoma. Very high levels are consistent with choriocarcinoma.
What stain definitively confirms the Dx of a germinoma?	**Placental alkaline phosphatase** staining confirms the Dx of germinoma.
What is the role of surgery in Dx of GCT?	If AFP and β-HCG are normal, surgery can distinguish pure germinoma or mature teratoma from other benign or malignant lesions. If β-HCG is elevated but normal AFP, surgery can distinguish β-HCG secreting germinoma from immature teratoma or choriocarcinoma (i.e., NGGCT).
What are the typical MRI findings of pure germinoma? Are there any distinctions on imaging from NGGCTs?	Homogeneous or heterogeneous pattern, hypointense T1, hyperintense T2, +Ca, cysts. These are indistinguishable from NGGCTs on imaging.
Historically, how was RT used in the Dx of intracranial germinomas?	**Tumors were irradiated with a diagnostic dose of 10–20 Gy.** If there was a response, then the Dx was germinoma and RT was continued to a definitive dose of 40–56 Gy. *This is no longer done.*
What staging system is used for intracranial GCTs M staging?	The **medulloblastoma staging** (modified Chang) system is used for staging of intracranial GCTs M staging, but usually M0 or M+ (disseminated) is adequate.

▶ TREATMENT/PROGNOSIS

What is the most important prognostic factor in germ cell tumors?	**Histology** is the most important prognostic factor in germ cell tumors.
What is the prognosis of pure germinomas vs. NGGCTs?	The prognosis is **better for germinomas** (5-yr PFS >90% vs. 40%–70%, respectively).
Describe 2 Tx paradigms for localized pure germinomas.	Tx paradigms for localized germinoma: 1. Definitive RT *or* 2. Neoadj chemo → lower dose RT (experimental protocol)

Describe the definitive RT technique for localized germinoma.

Whole ventricular radiation therapy (WVRT) to **21–24 Gy,** boost to primary tumor to 40–45 Gy

For which pineal tumor type is surgery generally *not* done?

Surgery is generally not done for **germinomas,** since they are radiosensitive tumors and can lead to morbidity. However, extent of resection is important for NGGCT.

What is the RT technique for disseminated germinoma/CSF spread?

CSI to 24 Gy, gross Dz **boost to 45 Gy**

Can chemo replace RT in the Tx of pure germinomas?

No. In a large CNS GCT study (*Balmaceda C et al., JCO 1996*), 45 germinomas were treated with carboplatin/etoposide/bleomycin. 84% had CR, but 48% recurred in 13 mos and 10% of pts died due to Tx toxicity. >90% were salvaged by RT (ifosfamide/carboplatin/etoposide [ICE] × 3 → involved-field radiation therapy [IFRT] of 24 Gy).

What hypothesis is being tested in the current germinoma study ACNS1123?

ACNS1123 is attempting to determine **if neoadj chemo can help reduce RT doses in *localized* germinoma and NGGCT.**

Describe the RT technique with neoadj chemo for localized germinoma.

Reduced RT doses: CR to chemo: WVRT to **18 Gy;** boost to **30 Gy in 1.5 Gy/day in patients who achieve a CR on chemo on current COG protocol. PR/stable Dz to chemo WVRT to 24Gy +12 Gy boost**

In germinoma protocols, what does "occult multifocal germinoma" refer to? What is the boost volume?

Pineal-region tumor and DI. Boost volume is the enhancing tumor (pineal region), infundibular region, and the 3rd ventricle after WVRT.

In ACNS1123, what chemo agents are being tested?

Carboplatin and etoposide are being tested in **ACNS1123.**

With pre-RT chemo, what are the RT doses in the experimental arm of ACNS1123 for germinoma?

In **ACNS1123,** the RT doses depend on the chemo response.
Induction chemo, carbo/etoposide × 4 cycles.
If CR, WVRT to 18 Gy + boost to 30 Gy with IFRT alone.
If <CR, 24 Gy whole ventricular irradiation + 12-Gy boost.

What studies showed that even with CR to chemo, IFRT (without WVRT) may not be sufficient?

SIOP CNS GCT96 (*Calaminus G et al., Neurooncol, 2013*): M0 pts treated with CSI 24 Gy + 16-Gy boost vs. 2 × ICE → IFRT 40 Gy. CRT 5-yr EFS was 85% vs. 91% with RT alone; 5-yr OS was 92% vs. 94%. All CRT failures were within the ventricular system. Conclusion: Suggest inclusion of ventricles in RT fields. Reduced-dose CSI to 24 Gy effective in M+ Dz.

What other evidence demonstrates that involved-field RT may not be sufficient for germinomas?

Rogers SJ et al.: literature review of 788 pts. There was a greater failure rate in focal RT vs. WBRT or WVRT + boost or CSI + boost (23% vs. 4%–8%). The pattern of relapse was mostly isolated spinal (11%), but there was no difference in WVRT vs. CSI in spinal relapse (3% vs. 1%). Conclusion: WVRT + boost should replace CSI. (*Lancet Oncol* 2005) Similar findings were found in a **Seoul study.** (*Eom KY et al., IJROBP 2008*)

What early studies established the feasibility of RT dose reduction?

German MAKEI 83/86/89 studies (from 50 Gy to 34 Gy)

Describe 2 Tx paradigms for NGGCT.

NGGCT Tx paradigms:

1. **Induction** platinum-based **chemo** 4–6 cycles → **CSI RT 30–36 Gy** (lower dose for CR) → **boost primary to 50.4–54 Gy;** surgery for residual or recurrent Dz
2. Max surgical resection → adj platinum-based chemo; restage; if no neuroaxial involvement, consolidate with IFRT; if +neuroaxial Dz, CSI to 30–36 Gy, boost to 50.4 Gy

When is chemo indicated in the Tx of NGGCTs?

Chemo is **always** indicated for NGGCTs (influences survival).

What is the Tx paradigm for pineoblastoma?

Pineoblastoma Tx paradigm: treat as **high-risk** medulloblastoma (CSI 36 Gy + local boost to 54 Gy)

What is the Tx paradigm for pineocytoma?

Pineocytoma Tx paradigm: treat like a low-grade glioma (GTR → observation; STR → consideration of adj RT or observation with Tx at the time of progression [50–54 Gy])

Which study showed that bifocal germinoma can be treated as localized Dz?

Canadian data (*Lafay-Cousin L et al., IJROBP 2006*): chemo and then limited-field RT (WVRT + boost) resulted in a CR.

▶ **TOXICITY**

Which recent study showed better QOL with CRT (dose/field reduction) than with RT alone?	**Seoul study** (*Eom KY et al., IJROBP 2008*), need for hormonal therapy: RT alone 69% vs. CRT 38% (however, all RT alone pts rcvd CSI)
What is the long-term rate of RT-induced 2nd CNS malignancies? What type is most common?	5%–10%; usually **glioblastoma multiforme**
What chemo agent should be avoided with brain RT? Why?	**6-mercaptopurine.** It is associated with **high rates of secondary high-grade gliomas.**

10 Craniopharyngioma
Updated by Andrew J. Bishop

▶ **BACKGROUND**

What is the origin of craniopharyngioma?	Epithelial tumor derived from **Rathke's pouch,** the embryonic precursor to the anterior pituitary
In what region of the brain does it usually arise?	**Suprasellar region (most common),** sella proper (less common)
Are craniopharyngiomas malignant?	**No.** They are histologically benign but behave aggressively with frequent local recurrences and morbidity due to the location of Dz.
Approximately how many cases of craniopharyngioma occur annually in the U.S.?	**~300–350 cases/yr** of craniopharyngioma in the U.S., accounting for 1%–3% of all pediatric brain tumors.

At what ages does craniopharyngioma occur?

Commonly occur between ages 5–10 yrs. There is a bimodal distribution (5–15 yrs and 45–60 yrs); one-third of cases occur in pts aged 0–14 yrs.

What are the 2 histologic subtypes of craniopharyngioma?

Adamantinomatous and squamous; thought of as WHO grade 1 tumors

Which subtype is characterized by a solid and cystic pattern?

Adamantinomatous craniopharyngioma has a solid and cystic pattern. A recent study suggests this histology has more frequent LR. (*Pekmezci et al., Neurosurgery 2010*)

Historically, how has the cyst fluid consistency been described?

"Crankcase (machine) oil"–like (very proteinaceous fluid with cholesterol crystals)

What structures do cysts usually abut superiorly?

Tumors/cysts usually abut the **3rd ventricle and the hypothalamus** superiorly.

Name the most common presenting signs/Sx of craniopharyngioma.

1. HA, n/v (i.e., ↑ ICP)
2. Visual change (bitemporal hemianopsia)
3. Endocrinopathies (TSH, GH, LH/FSH)

What is the most common hormone deficiency at presentation?

At presentation, **GH** is the most common hormone deficiency.

Do craniopharyngioma tumors respond rapidly or slowly to RT?

Craniopharyngioma tumors respond **slowly** to RT.

▶ **WORKUP/STAGING**

What is the workup for a craniopharyngioma?

H&P, basic labs, endocrine/pituitary panel, and MRI of brain

What ancillary studies need to be done before Tx?

Endocrine, audiology, vision, and neuropsychiatric studies

What is the classic appearance of craniopharyngiomas on CT/MRI?

Heterogenous partially calcified nodular suprasellar masses with associated cysts on CT/MRI

Is histology absolutely necessary for the Dx of craniopharyngioma?

No. If necessary, a Dx can be made based on radiographic appearance and cyst fluid analysis.

What is the staging of craniopharyngioma?

There is **no formal staging.**

► TREATMENT/PROGNOSIS

What is the Tx paradigm for craniopharyngioma?

Tx paradigm: max *safe* resection. Consider EBRT or intracystic chemo adjuvantly or at recurrence

While controversial, what is the favored treatment approach?

STR + RT. The morbidity of a GTR can be detrimental. An STR spares some morbidity and has better QOL (e.g., St. Jude's data [2002] showed that the surgery group lost an avg of 9.8 IQ points; the more limited surgery + RT group lost an avg of 1.25 points).

What surgical approach is typically employed for craniopharyngioma resection?

Lat pterional approach (temporal craniotomy). Approach depends on location of tumor relative to 3rd ventricle and optic nerves.

What is the rate of GTR?

Large referral centers report GTR rates in **50%–79%** of patients.

What % of attempted craniopharyngioma GTRs result in STR?

Depends on location, but overall, **20%–30%.** (*Tomita T et al., Childs Nerv Syst 2005*)

Is observation ever appropriate after incomplete resection for craniopharyngioma?

Yes. Observation is especially appropriate in young pts. Adj and salvage therapy may have similar LC in closely followed pts. However, more surgical procedures often lead to higher morbidity.

What are the RT doses used for craniopharyngioma?

50.4–54 Gy with EBRT in 1.8 Gy/fx, **12–14 Gy** with SRS (limited by nearby critical structures)

What volumes are typically irradiated for craniopharyngioma?

GTV is decompressed/postop volume = tumor + cyst wall (cysts decompressed before Tx); PTV is GTV + 0.5–1 cm; **no CTV** because no microscopic invasion. **Be aware of cyst(s) and monitor during RT.**

Estimate the 10-yr LC with surgery alone vs. surgery + postop RT for craniopharyngioma.

Surgery (GTR + STR) alone ~**42%;** surgery + RT ~**84%** (*Stripp DC et al., IJROBP 2004*)

Estimate the 10-yr LC with adj RT vs. salvage RT.

Similar rates. **Both ~83%–84%.** (*Stripp DC et al., IJROBP 2004*) RT can be deferred for children <5–7 yo after surgery.

In what 3 ways can craniopharyngioma cysts be managed?

Aspiration, radioactive isotope injection, and bleomycin injection, also using intracystic interferon now. (*Cavalheiro S et al., Neurosurg Focus 2010*)

What isotopes have been used for intracystic RT and what do they deliver?

β-emitting isotopes (yttrium-90, P-32, Rh-186); **200–250 Gy** to the cyst wall, be aware of location of chiasm relative to cyst wall.

What is the energy and half-life of P-32 and to what depth is it effective?

0.7 MeV, 2 wks. The effective depth is **3–4 mm.**

What are the indications for intralesional cyst management (vs. cyst aspiration)?

Intralesional Tx is an option if the cyst is >50% of total tumor bulk *and* the number of cysts is ≤3 (ideal if there is a **solitary cyst**) or for those with **recurrent cysts** after prior resection

What intracystic chemo has been used?

Bleomycin typically has been used for intralesional cyst management.

What is the typical response rate to intralesional bleomycin?

Limited data, **~65% ORR** (29% CR). Median PFS is 1.8 yrs. (*Hukin J et al., Cancer 2007*)

If a pt has worsening visual Sx while getting adj RT, is this likely due to an acute side effect from RT?

No. Acute Sx during RT are likely due to a rapidly enlarging cystic component; therefore, urgent surgical intervention for decompression is indicated. Radiographic cyst monitoring during RT is recommended to allow for smaller PTV. 15% of cysts increase in size during RT.

Is there a dosimetric advantage to protons vs. photon therapy?

Yes. Compared to IMRT, proton therapy has been shown to reduce dose to the brain and body. (*Beltran C et al., IJROBP 2012; Boehling NS, IJROBP 2012*) Meaningful clinical differences are uncertain.

What important treatment consideration is needed when treating with protons for craniopharyngioma?

Cyst dynamics. Frequent imaging or resimulations are necessary when treating with protons (or any conformal techniques) to ensure adequate coverage of the cysts (*Winkfield KM et al., IJROBP 2009*).

What factors have been shown to correlate with inferior LC in craniopharyngioma?

Size >5 cm (Joint Center data: *Hetelekidis S et al., IJROBP 1993*) and **RT dose <55 Gy** (Pittsburgh data: *Varlotto JM et al., IJROBP 2002*)

What is the significance of cyst regrowth after RT?

Cyst regrowth may occur after definitive Tx (does not mean failure, as RT can take a long time to exert its ablative effects). Repeat aspirations are in order if the pt is symptomatic.

What study proposed a risk-stratification scheme to guide the aggressiveness/extent of surgery for craniopharyngioma?

A **French study by *Puget et al.*** showed significant reductions in endocrine and hypothalamic dysfunction if pts were stratified prospectively before surgery based on the degree of hypothalamic involvement: grades 0–1, attempt GTR; grade 2, STR (+ RT if >5 yo, observe if <5 yo). (*J Neurosurg 2007*)

What is the 10-yr OS of pts with craniopharyngioma?

10-yr OS is **70%–92%**

What is the long-term survival for pts with craniopharyngioma?

The 20-yr OS is **76%.**

▶ **TOXICITY**

What is the mortality and morbidity rate from surgery for craniopharyngioma?	In modern series, mortality is **<4%.** Morbidity ranges between **8% and 14%.**
What are the most common/serious side effects of surgery?	**Diabetes insipidus, hypothalamic obesity, vision loss (<2%), and other hypothalamic injury** (defective short-term memory, sleep disturbances)
What are the potential long-term side effects of RT?	**Hypopituitarism,** cognitive dysfunction or ↓IQ (10%), 2nd malignancy, and vasculopathy
The hypothalamus should be kept at or below what total RT dose?	If possible, the hypothalamus should not exceed **45 Gy.**
How long does it usually take for tumors to regrow? What follow-up is needed?	**2 yrs on avg.** However, there is a big range, and regrowth can take up to 9 yrs. Thus, the pt requires **long-term follow-up** with serial MRIs and neuro-ophthalmology or endocrinology exams.

11 Hemangioblastoma
Updated by Sarah McAvoy

▶ **BACKGROUND**

What is the typical age of presentation for hemangioblastoma?	**20–50 yrs** is the typical age of presentation for hemangioblastoma (primarily in young adults).
Where do most hemangioblastomas arise anatomically?	Hemangioblastomas arise in the **cerebellum.** They account for 7%–10% of tumors arising in the posterior fossa in adults.
What genetic disorder is associated with hemangioblastomas?	**Von Hippel-Lindau** (VHL; hemangioblastomas, pancreatic/renal cysts, renal cell carcinoma)
Are hemangioblastomas benign/low grade or malignant/high grade?	**Benign/low grade** (WHO grade I)

What is the cell of origin or hemangioblastomas, and what is the associated pathology?

Endothelial stem cells; closely packed vascular lesions with a stroma of large oval "foamy" cells that result in a "clear cell" morphology.

The # of lesions seen in hemangioblastomas correlates with what in terms of etiology?

Single lesion (sporadic, older pts) **vs. multiple lesions** (familial, younger pts)

What characteristics are common in hemangioblastomas associated with VHL?

Diagnosed at **younger age,** mean of 29 yrs. Distribution is 50% in spinal cord, 40% in cerebellum, and 10% brainstem. Usually, multiple lesions.

What hematologic abnormality is present in pts with hemangioblastomas? Why?

Polycythemia is present because of erythropoietin production by the tumor.

How do hemangioblastomas cause morbidity if not treated?

Local compression and hemorrhage

What are common Sx of hemangioblastoma at presentation?

HA, hydrocephalus, and imbalance

▶ WORKUP/STAGING

What steps are critical during the workup of a hemangioblastoma?

Thorough **neurologic exam and MRI** (craniospinal); **angiography** to aid in embolization before surgery

What is the typical radiographic appearance of a hemangioblastoma?

Eccentric/peripheral cystic mass (70%) in the posterior fossa.

How do hemangioblastomas appear on MRI?

On MRI, hemangioblastomas are **intensely enhancing.**

▶ TREATMENT/PROGNOSIS

What are the 2 main Tx approaches for hemangioblastoma?

Surgery (max safe resection is curative and preferred) **and SRS**

What are the LC rates of surgery vs. SRS for hemangioblastomas?

Surgery: 50%–80%
SRS: 82%–92% at 2 yrs, 75% at 5 yrs

What is the SRS dose range used for the Tx of hemangioblastomas?

15–21 Gy to 50% IDL (dose ranged from 15–40 Gy with median dose of 22 Gy in *Moss JM et al., Neurosurgery 2009*).

What does the older dose-response data show for fractionated EBRT for the Tx of hemangioblastomas?	It showed **better results with higher doses.** (*Smalley SR et al., IJROBP 1990:* better OS with dose >50 Gy; *Sung DI et al., Cancer 1982:* better survival with 40–55 Gy vs. 20–36 Gy)
What are the traditionally employed EBRT doses for hemangioblastomas?	**50–55 Gy** at 1.8 or 2 Gy/fx
For cystic hemangioblastoma lesions, what component does *not* have to be removed during surgery?	If there is a negative margin, there is no need to remove the **entire cyst.** In this case, only the mural nodule/tumor should be removed.
When has RT (either SRS or EBRT) been traditionally used in the management of hemangioblastomas?	**After recurrence** (i.e., after definitive surgery or after STR for recurrence), for surgically inaccessible locations, or for patients with multiple lesions (i.e., VHL disease).
For what type of hemangioblastoma lesions is fractionated EBRT a better choice than SRS?	Multiple tumors, larger lesions (>3 cm), and lesions in eloquent regions of the brain
Which hemangioblastoma pts have a better prognosis after EBRT: VHL+ or VHL−pts?	**VHL**+ pts have a better prognosis after EBRT. (Princess Margaret Hospital data: *Koh ES et al., IJROBP 2007*)
What is the prognostic significance of a cyst component after SRS for hemangioblastoma?	**LC is worse if the tumor is cystic.** (Japan data: *Matsunaga S et al., Acta Neurochir 2007*)
What is the median time to recurrence after EBRT or SRS for hemangioblastoma?	Hemangioblastomas tend to recur **2–4 yrs** after radiation.
What is the pattern of failure after EBRT for pts with hemangioblastoma?	Failure is **predominantly local.**

▶ **TOXICITY**

What is the surgical mortality rate of pts treated for hemangioblastoma?	The surgical mortality rate is **10%–20%** in pts treated for hemangioblastoma.

12 Brainstem Glioma

Updated by Andrew J. Bishop

▶ BACKGROUND

What is the prevalence of brainstem gliomas (BSGs) in relation to pediatric CNS tumors overall?

BSGs comprise up to **20% of pediatric primary CNS tumors** (<2% of adult CNS tumors).

What is the peak age of presentation for BSGs? What is the sex predilection?

The peak age of BSG presentation is **5–9 yrs. Males** are more commonly affected than females.

What are the 2 classes of BSGs? Where are they most commonly located, and what is the prognosis?

The 2 classes of BSGs are **focal and diffuse:**

Focal (20%): in the **upper midbrain/lower medulla;** best prognosis

Diffuse (80%): in the **pons and upper medulla;** infiltrative and worst prognosis

What are the anatomical subdivisions of BSGs?

Diffuse intrinsic pontine glioma (DIPG), exophytic medullary glioma, and midbrain or tectal glioma

What BSG histology most commonly involves the medulla? The pons? The midbrain?

BSG that arise from midbrain, medulla, and cervicomedullary junction are typically low grade (grade 1 or 2) and are focal, discrete, well-circumscribed tumors without local invasive growth or edema. Pontine gliomas are predominantly diffuse, high-grade, and locally infiltrative.

Why does adult BSG tend to have a better prognosis?

Lesions in adults tend to be **mostly low grade.**

What is the median OS of BSG in adults vs. children vs. the elderly?

Adults: 7.3 yrs
Children: 1 yr
The elderly: 11 mos

Overall, the Dz is fatal in >90% of pts.

▶ WORKUP/STAGING

What are some typical clinical findings with diffuse pontine glioma?

Typical findings with diffuse pontine glioma:

1. CN palsy (CNs VI–VII)
2. Ataxia
3. Long tract signs (hyperreflexia, etc.)

What is the typical workup for a child with a suspected BSG?	Suspected BSG workup for a child: H&P, labs, MRI, typically *no* Bx
When should Bx be done for BSG?	When mass lesions have an **unusual MRI appearance** or there is an **atypical clinical course** (either possible benign tumors or an infectious/inflammatory etiology)
How is BSG staged?	There is **no formal staging** of BSG.

▶ TREATMENT/PROGNOSIS

What is the typical Tx paradigm for BSG?	BSG Tx paradigm: steroids/shunts → RT
Is there a role for temozolomide (TMZ) after RT?	**No** (*Broniscer A et al., Cancer 2005*). MS is 12 mos.
Is there a role for concurrent TMZ in DIPG?	**No.** Despite glioblastoma multiforme being the most common histology of DIPG, a COG study did not find a benefit of concurrent/adj TMZ. (*Cohen KJ et al., Neuro Oncol 2011*)
Is there any benefit with other chemos in BSG?	**No.** There is minimal response with single and combination. Concurrent gefitinib has minimal benefit in a subset of pts in phase II. (*Pollack IF et al., Neuro Oncol 2011*) There are ongoing studies with systemic therapies.
What type of BSG is amenable to surgical resection +/– adj RT?	**Dorsally exophytic BSGs** have a 75% 10-yr OS with surgery +/– RT. These are usually juvenile pilocytic astrocytomas (JPAs) with a good prognosis.
What is the typical RT dose for BSGs?	The typical RT dose for BSGs is **54 Gy** in 1.8–2 Gy/fx.
What proportion of BSG pts will have stabilization or improvement of Sx after RT?	After RT, **two-thirds** of pts will have stabilization or improvement of Sx.
Is there a role for hyperfractionation or dose escalation in BSG?	**No.** Both did not improve survival in multiple POG/CCG trials (only better radiographic response at higher doses with greater radionecrosis and steroid dependence).
Is there a role for hypofractionation in BSG?	**Yes.** For pts with DIPG, RT over 3–4 wks offers equal OS and PFS as conventional RT with less Tx burden. (*Janssens GO et al., IJROBP 2013*)
Is there a role for brachytherapy or Gamma Knife boost after RT in BSG?	**No.** There is no role for brachytherapy or Gamma Knife boost after RT.

How are midbrain tectal plate tumors managed? What is their histology?	Tectal plate tumors are typically managed with **observation and a ventriculoperitoneal shunt** for obstruction. They are typically **JPAs** (indolent).
What are the major prognostic factors dictating outcome in pts with BSGs?	1. Diffuse vs. focal 2. Adult vs. child 3. Histology
What is the survival of pts with diffuse vs. focal BSG lesions?	<u>Diffuse</u>: 12 mos (median) <u>Focal</u>: 10-yr OS 50%–70%
What usually causes death in pts with BSGs?	**Local expansion** usually causes death in pts with BSGs.

 TOXICITY

What is the RT dose tolerance of the brainstem?	The dose tolerance of the brainstem is **54 Gy** (if fractionated EBRT) and **12 Gy** (if SRS).

13

General Central Nervous System

Updated by Jingya Wang

▶ **BACKGROUND**

What is the estimated annual incidence of primary CNS tumors in the U.S.?	**~50,000–55,000 cases/yr** of CNS tumors (per the National Program of Cancer Registries database)
What is the most common intracranial tumor?	**Brain mets** (20%–40% of all cancer pts develop brain mets)
What are the most common primary histologies associated with brain metastases?	Most common: lung, breast, melanoma
Which primary histologies are associated with hemorrhagic metastases?	Renal cell carcinoma, melanoma, and choriocarcinoma are associated with hemorrhagic mets.
Which primaries tend to metastasize to the posterior fossa?	GU/Pelvic primaries tend to go to the posterior fossa, where they are more likely to have a mass effect
What is the most common type of primary CNS tumor?	**Glioma (~40%) > meningioma** (15%–20%)
What % of CNS tumors are metastases vs. glioma vs. other?	Of all CNS tumors, roughly one-third are mets, one-third are gliomas, and one-third are other (meningioma, schwannoma, pituitary, lymphoma, etc.)
What % of adult astrocytomas are low grade vs. high grade?	25% low grade vs. 75% high grade

What is the most common histologic type of malignant CNS tumor in children? In adults?

<u>Children</u>: juvenile pilocytic astrocytoma (JPA)
    (20% <14 yo vs. 12% >14 yo)
<u>Adults</u>: glioblastoma

What is the most common benign intracranial tumor in adults?

Meningioma

What is the strongest risk factor for developing CNS tumors?

Ionizing RT in children (no threshold—glioma, meningioma, nerve sheath)

What CNS tumors are linked to the following?

1. **NF-1**
2. **NF-2**
3. **Tuberous sclerosis**

4. **Von Hippel-Lindau**
5. **Li-Fraumeni**
6. **Cowden**
7. **Gorlin**
8. **Turcot**
9. **Retinoblastoma (RB)**
10. **Ataxia telangiectasia**
11. **MEN-1**

1. Optic glioma, JPA
2. Bilat acoustic neuroma, spinal ependymoma
3. Subependymal giant cell astrocytoma, retinal hamartoma
4. Hemangioblastoma

5. Glioma
6. Meningioma
7. Medulloblastoma
8. Medulloblastoma, glioblastoma
9. Pineoblastoma

10. CNS lymphoma

11. Pituitary adenoma

What are the 4 factors used for grading in the WHO brain tumor grading system?

Nuclear **A**typia
Cellularity and **M**itosis
Endothelial proliferation
Necrosis

(Mnemonic: **AMEN**)
WHO grade I = no factors present
WHO grade II = atypia
WHO grade III = atypia, mitoses
WHO grade IV = endothelial proliferation or necrosis

Which CNS structures cross midline?

Glioblastoma multiforme (GBM), radiation necrosis, meningioma (extra-axial can spread along meninges to contralateral side), epidermoid cyst, multiple sclerosis

What CNS tumors tend to have CSF spread?

Medulloblastomas and other blastomas (except astroblastoma/GBM), CNS lymphoma, choroid plexus carcinomas, germ cell tumors, and mets

What is the pathway in which CSF flows?	CSF is produced by the choroid plexus → lateral ventricles → foramen of Monroe → third ventricle → cerebral aqueduct of Sylvius → fourth ventricle → foramen of Magendie, and 2 lateral foramina of Lushka
What CNS tumors have Flexner-Wintersteiner rosettes?	Pineoblastoma and RB (any PNET)
What CNS tumors have psammoma bodies?	Meningioma and pituitary tumors (uncommon)
What CNS tumor type exhibits Verocay bodies? Schiller-Duval bodies?	**Schwannomas** exhibit Verocay bodies, and **yolk sac tumors** exhibit Schiller-Duval bodies.
Which CNS tumors have Homer-Wright rosettes?	**Neuroblastoma, medulloblastoma, pinealoblastoma, and PNET**
What CNS tumor has pseudorosettes?	**Ependymoma**
What receptors are commonly overexpressed in gliomas?	**EGFR** (30%–50% in GBM tumors) **and PDGFR** (non-GBM tumors)
Neural stem cells express which marker? Why are they important?	**CD133.** Neural stem cells are thought to be **precursors for astrocytomas.**
What gene on chromosome 17 is frequently lost in both low-grade and high-grade gliomas?	The **p53** gene is frequently lost in low- and high-grade gliomas.
What is the genetic mutation in NF-1, and for which sites does it predispose to gliomas?	In NF-1, the genetic mutation is **17q11.2/ neurofibromin.** It predisposes to **optic/intracranial gliomas.**

▶ **WORKUP/STAGING**

Which structures enhance on the MRI sequences, T_1, T_2, and FLAIR?	T_1 enhances fat and soft tissue, does not enhance fluid. T_1 **with contrast** is generally the best way to visualize intracranial tumors. T_2 enhances fluid (CSF, edema) and does not enhance fat. **FLAIR** removes the increased CSF signal on T_2 and shows abnormal fluid (masses and edema).
Which structures enhance with contrast?	**M**ets, **A**bscess, **G**BM, **L**ymphoma, +/– **A**A or **A**O [anaplastic astrocytoma/anaplastic oligodendroglioma]) (Mnemonic: **MAGLA**), meningioma, pilocytic astrocytoma, gliosis, cerebritis

Which structures do not enhance with contrast?	Grade 2 low-grade gliomas, +/− AA or AO, rare for GBM to not enhance.
Which gyri contain the sensory and motor area?	The precentral gyrus contains the motor area, and the postcentral gyrus contains the somatosensory area. Medial = body, lower extremities, feet. Lateral = trunk, arms, head.
What brain region is associated with expressive aphasia?	The **Broca motor area** (dominant/left frontal lobe) is associated with expressive aphasia.
What brain region is associated with receptive aphasia?	The dominant/left temporal lobe at the post end of the lateral sulcus (**Wernicke area**) is associated with receptive aphasia.
Which CN exits on the dorsal side of the brain (midbrain)?	**CN IV** exits on the dorsal side of the brain.
What structures are in the cavernous sinus?	CNs III, IV, VI, V1, and V2; internal carotid artery
What common defect does tumor involving the cavernous sinus produce?	**CN VI palsy** (no abduction of the lateral rectus)
What components traverse the superior orbital fissure?	CNs III, IV, VI, and V1
What nerve passes through the foramen rotundum?	**V2** passes through the foramen rotundum.
What nerve passes through the foramen ovale?	**V3** passes through the foramen ovale.
What structures pass through the foramen spinosum?	The **middle meningeal artery and vein** as well as the **nervus spinosus** (branch of CN V3), pass through the foramen spinosum.
Through what structure do CNs VII–VIII traverse?	CNs VII–VIII traverse through the **internal auditory meatus.**
Through which foramen does CN VII traverse the skull base?	CN VII emerges through the **stylomastoid foramen.**
What passes through the jugular foramen?	**CNs IX–XI** pass through the jugular foramen.
How many spinal nerves are there in the spinal cord?	There are **31 spinal nerves** in the spinal cord (8 cervical, 12 thoracic, 5 lumbar, 5 sacral, and 1 coccygeal).

Where does the cord end? Where does the thecal sac end?	The cord ends at **L3–4 in children** and **L1–2 in adults.** The thecal sac ends at **S2–3 in both children and adults.**
What tumors present with a dural tail sign?	**Meningioma** (60%), also chloroma, lymphoma, and sarcoidosis

▶ TOXICITY

Name some acute RT complications in pts receiving RT for CNS tumors.	Alopecia, dermatitis, fatigue, transient worsening of neurologic Sx, n/v, otitis externa, seizures, and edema
What is the timing and mechanism of somnolence syndrome?	**6–12 wks post-RT,** due to transient **demyelination** of axons
What are some late complications of RT to the CNS? What is the timing for these?	Radionecrosis, leukoencephalopathy, retinopathy, cataracts, endocrine deficits, memory loss, learning deficits, and hearing loss; **3 mos to 3 yrs**

14 Low-Grade Glioma

Updated by Andrew J. Bishop

▶ BACKGROUND

Low-grade gliomas (LGGs) account for what % of all primary brain tumors?	~10% of all primary brain tumors are LGGs.
Is there a racial predilection for LGG?	**Yes. Whites** are more commonly affected than blacks (2:1).
What are the histologic subtypes of LGGs?	Histologic subtypes of LGG: Grade I: pilocytic astrocytoma, subependymal giant cell tumor Grade II: (fibrillary, protoplasmic, gemistocytic), astrocytoma, oligodendroglioma, and oligoastrocytoma

What 4 pathologic features determine glioma grading?	**N**ecrosis **A**typia **M**itotic figures **E**ndothelial proliferation (Mnemonic: **NAME** or AMEN)
Which subtype of grade II glioma has the worst prognosis?	The **gemistocytic subtype** tends to de-differentiate and has the worst prognosis. Some prefer to treat it like a high-grade glioma.
Where does pilocytic astrocytoma most commonly present?	Most commonly presents in the **posterior fossa** (80% cerebellar, 20% supratentorial).
What pathologic feature is characteristic of pilocytic astrocytoma?	**Rosenthal fibers** are characteristic of pilocytic astrocytoma.
Where do grade II LGGs most commonly present?	Grade II LGGs most commonly present in the **supratentorium.**
What is the median age of Dx for pilocytic astrocytoma vs. other LGG?	The median age for **pilocytic astrocytoma is 10–20 yrs** and for grade II **LGG is 30–40 yrs.**
What genetic changes are important prognostic factors in LGG?	In LGG, **LOH 1p19q and isocitrate dehydrogenase (IDH) mutations** portend a better survival. **p53 mutation** indicates poorer survival and time to malignant transformation.
What genetic change is prognostic in oligodendroglioma?	**LOH 1p19q** (50%–70%) is prognostic in oligodendroglioma. Associated with superior OS and PFS. (*Jenkins RB et al., Cancer Res 2006*)
What is the characteristic pathologic appearance of oligodendroglioma?	**"Fried egg"** appearance (round cells with nuclear halo) is characteristic of oligodendroglioma.
Where do most oligodendrogliomas occur in the brain?	Most oligodendrogliomas occur in the **hemispheres** (80%).
Anaplastic transformation from LGG to HGG occurs in what % of pts?	**~70%–80%** of pts with LGG will undergo anaplastic transformation (based on **EORTC 22845**).
What is the genetic mutation in NF-1, and with what type of gliomas is it associated?	NF-1 is a result of a mutation on the long arm of **chromosome 17** and is associated with **optic/ intracranial gliomas.**
What is the genetic mutation in tuberous sclerosis, and with what glioma is it associated?	Tuberous sclerosis is a result of a mutation on **chromosome 9** and is associated with **subependymal giant cell astrocytoma.**

What syndrome is associated with gliomas and GI polyposis?	**Turcot syndrome** is associated with gliomas and polyposis.
With what Sx do LGGs most commonly present?	**Seizures** (60%–70%, better prognosis) > HA, focal neurologic Sx
What is the 5-year OS of LGG?	The 5-yr OS is **60%–70%.**

▶ **WORKUP/STAGING**

What is the workup for suspected glioma?	Suspected glioma workup: H&P, basic labs, and MRI brain
How should tissue be acquired for Dx?	Tissue should be acquired by **maximal safe resection** (per the NCCN), otherwise by stereotactic Bx.
What is the typical MRI characteristic seen in LGG?	On MRI, LGGs appear hypointense on T_1, are **nonenhancing with gadolinium,** and show T_2 prolongation.
What is the typical MRI appearance of pilocytic astrocytoma?	Well-circumscribed, cystic mass, intensely enhancing solid mural nodule
What % of nonenhancing lesions are grade III gliomas?	**~30%** are grade III gliomas (65% are LGG).
What feature has been associated with oligodendrogliomas on imaging?	**Calcifications** are a prominent feature on imaging of oligodendrogliomas.
What is suggestive of a malignant tumor on MR spectroscopy?	**Increased choline** (cell membrane marker), **low creatine** (energy metabolite), and **low N-acetyl-aspartate** (a neuronal marker) are suggestive of malignancy on MR spectroscopy.
What is the staging of LGG?	There is **no formal staging** for LGG.

▶ **TREATMENT/PROGNOSIS**

What are the 5 negative prognostic factors for LGG as determined by EORTC 22844 and 22845?	Negative prognostic factors per the EORTC index: 1. Age >40 yrs 2. Astrocytoma histology 3. Tumors >6 cm 4. Tumors crossing midline 5. Preop neurologic deficits *(Pignatti F et al., JCO 2002)*

What is the general Tx paradigm used for LGGs?

LGG Tx paradigm: max safe resection → observation for GTR or STR with stable Dz; reserving RT or chemo for progression/recurrence.

What prospective data support initial observation over adj RT in LGG (early vs. delayed)?

EORTC 22845 ("Non-Believers Trial") randomized 314 LGG pts to early RT vs. delayed RT until time of progression. Concluded early RT lengthens PFS (5.3 yrs vs. 3.4 yrs) and seizure control (25% vs. 41%) but does not impact OS. (*Van den Bent MJ et al., Lancet 2005*)

What adj and salvage chemo regimens are typically used in LGG?

Chemos used in LGG:

1. Temozolomide (TMZ)
2. BCNU/CCNU (carmustine/lomustine)
3. PCV (procarbazine/CCNU/vincristine)

What RT dose is typically used for LGG?

LGG is commonly treated to **50.4–54 Gy (1.8 Gy/fx)**

A complete resection can be achieved in what proportion of pts with LGGs?

Approximately one-third of pts with LGGs have a GTR.

Within what timeframe should postop MRI be obtained for pts with LGGs? Why is it needed?

Postop MRI should be done within 48–72 hrs of surgery to assess for residual Dz/extent of resection.

In LGG, how are the RT Tx volumes defined, and what margins are typically used?

Per RTOG1072/ECOG E3F05:

GTV = cavity + T_2/FLAIR + enhancement
CTV = GTV + 1 cm; PTV = CTV + 0.5 cm

In what 2 clinical circumstances can adj RT be considered for LGGs?

1. For pts s/p STR/Bx only and with Sx
2. For pts with 3 of 5 high-risk features per the EORTC index (above). No LOH 1p19q or IDH mutation are also adverse features that may be considered.

What % of LGG pts undergoing initial observation in EORTC 22845 eventually required salvage RT?

In **EORTC 22845, 65% of pts** in the observation arm received subsequent salvage RT.

What proportion of pts do not need salvage RT when observed after surgical resection for LGG?

Per EORTC 22845, approx one-third of patients will not require salvage RT.

In EORTC 22845, how did the OS after progression compare in the adj vs. observation arms?

Survival after progression was better in initially observed pts, most of whom received salvage RT. OS after 1st recurrence was **3.4 yrs vs. 1 yr** (SS).

Is there prospective evidence to support dose escalation with adj RT for LGG?

No. Dose escalation in LGG has been evaluated in 2 RCTs, neither of which showed a benefit:

1. **EORTC 22844** randomized 343 pts to adj RT 45 Gy vs. 59.4 Gy. **There was no difference in 5-yr OS (58%–59%) or PFS (47%–50%).** (*Karim AB et al., IJROBP 1996*)
2. **INT/NCCTG** randomized 203 pts to adj RT 50.4 Gy vs. 64.8 Gy. **There was no difference in 5-yr OS (65%–72%). 92% of failures were in-field.** (*Shaw EG et al., JCO 2002*)

Is adjuvant therapy needed after GTR or STR for pilocytic astrocytoma in adults?

No. *Brown et al.* prospectively followed 20 adult pilocytic astrocytoma pts s/p GTR, STR (6 pts), or Bx (3 pts). **5-yr PFS was 95%.** (*IJROBP 2004*)

Is there a benefit of chemo with RT for LGGs with high-risk features?

This is **controversial. RTOG 9802** stratified pts into low risk (age <40 yrs s/p GTR) and high risk (age >40 yrs or STR/Bx only). Low-risk pts were observed. **High-risk pts were randomized to adj RT alone (54 Gy) vs. RT + PCV.** Outcomes were better in the chemo arm but did not reach SS (5-yr OS: 63% vs. 72%; PFS: 46% vs. 63%). For pts living 2 years, the probability of an additional 5-yr survival favored RT + PCV (74% vs. 59%, *p* = 0.02), suggesting a possible delayed benefit. (*Shaw EG et al., JCO 2012*)

In RTOG 9802, what were the 5-yr OS and PFS for low-risk pts observed after GTR?

In **RTOG 9802,** low-risk pts (<40 yo s/p GTR) were observed and had **5-yr OS of 94% and PFS of 50%.** (*Shaw EG et al., ASCO 2006*)

Is there a role for TMZ in the initial Tx of LGG?

Results of 2 trials are **preliminary:**

1. **EORTC 22033** randomized high-risk LGG pts (3 of 5 EORTC features) to adj RT vs. adj TMZ. No clear benefit of TMZ in PFS or OS. RT remains standard of care. Results need further maturation. (*Baumert BG et al., ASCO 2013*)

2. **RTOG 0424** is a phase II study that enrolled high-risk LGG pts (3 of 5 EORTC features) and treated with RT (54 Gy) + concurrent TMZ then adjuvant TMZ. Preliminary results show a 3-yr OS rate of 73%, which is higher than historic controls (*Fisher BJ et al., ASCO 2013*)

For pilocytic astrocytoma, what is the estimated 10-yr RFS in pts treated with GTR alone?

10-yr RFS is **~95%** in pilocytic astrocytoma pts treated with GTR alone. (*Watson GA et al., Semin Radiat Oncol 2001*)

In pts with oligodendroglioma/mixed oligodendroglioma, what is the median OS for those +/−LOH for 1p19q?

With LOH 1p19q: median OS ~13 yrs
Without LOH 1p19p: median OS ~9 yrs
(*Jenkins RB et al., Cancer Res 2006*)

▶ TOXICITY

How does RT affect QOL in the Tx of LGG?

QOL in LGG is impacted by **surgery, RT, chemo, and seizure meds.** Based on the **EORTC 22844** dose escalation study, higher-dose RT was significantly associated with fatigue/malaise and insomnia and ↓ emotional functioning. (*Kiebert GM et al., Eur J Cancer 1998*)

Does RT predispose LGG lesions to malignant transformation?

No. RT is not associated with an ↑ rate of malignant transformation. In **EORTC 22845,** there was a 70% transformation rate in both the adj and observation arms.

What is the commonly used RT dose constraint for the chiasm with fractionated RT vs. SRS?

The chiasm is commonly constrained to **54 Gy** in 1.8–2 Gy/fx and **8 Gy** in a single fx.

What is the commonly used RT dose constraint for the cochlea?

The cochlea is commonly constrained to a **mean dose of 30–35 Gy** in 1.8–2 Gy/fx.

What is the commonly used RT dose constraint for the brainstem with SRS?

The brainstem is commonly constrained to **12 Gy** in a single fx.

What is the cause of somnolence syndrome after brain RT?

Somnolence syndrome is thought to be caused by **demyelination.**

15 High-Grade Glioma

Updated by Sarah McAvoy

► BACKGROUND

What % of primary CNS tumors are malignant?
~40% of primary brain tumors are considered malignant.

In adults, what is the most common malignant CNS neoplasm?
~80% of CNS neoplasms in adults are **glioblastoma** (GBM), which constitutes 20% of all primary tumors. ~22,000 new malignant primary brain tumors are diagnosed annually in the U.S.

What are the WHO classifications for high-grade CNS tumors?
WHO III: anaplastic astrocytoma (AA)/anaplastic oligodendroglioma (AO)/anaplastic oligoastrocytoma (AOA)
WHO IV: GBM

What are some common genetic changes seen in malignant brain tumors?
↑ EGFR (50%) and phosphatase and tensin homolog (PTEN) mutation (30%–40%)

What are the initial genetic changes associated with primary vs. secondary GBM?
Primary: ↑ EGFR/MDM2 amplification/LOH 10/ p16 loss
Secondary: p53 mutation → low-grade glioma (LGG) → LOH 19q/p16 loss → AA → LOH 10, DCC → 2nd GBM

What % of GBMs are multicentric?
<5% of GBMs are multicentric.

What are the 4 pathologic characteristics used for astrocytoma grading?
Nuclear **A**typia, **M**itoses, **E**ndothelial proliferation, and **N**ecrosis
(Mnemonic: **AMEN**)

What is the defining pathologic characteristic of GBM?
Necrosis

► WORKUP/STAGING

What is the Cushing triad, and what does it represent in brain tumors?
HTN, bradycardia, respiratory irregularity. It represents ↑ ICP.

With what Sx do high-grade gliomas (HGGs) most commonly present?
HA (especially in the morning, 50%), seizures (20%), focal neurologic dysfunction, and mental status change

What are the common imaging characteristics of HGGs on MRI?	Hypodense on T_1, **gadolinium enhancing,** T_2 enhancing, and + T_2 FLAIR (edema)

▶ TREATMENT/PROGNOSIS

What is the MS for LGG vs. HGG?	<u>Low grade</u>: pure oligodendroglioma: 10 yrs; oligoastrocytoma: 7 yrs; anaplastic oligodendroglioma (AO): 5 yrs <u>High grade</u>: AA: 3 yrs; GBM: 14 mos
What are the most important factors used for the RTOG recursive partitioning analysis (RPA) stratification?	Age 50 yrs, histology (AA or GBM), Karnofsky performance status (KPS) of 70, MS changes, and Sx ≥3 mos (*Curran WJ et al., J Natl Cancer Inst 1993*)
What is the MS of a pt with RPA classes I–II, III–IV vs. V–VI?	MS by RPA class: **Classes I–II:** 40–60 mos (3–5 yrs) **Classes III–IV:** 11–18 mos (1–1.5 yrs) **Classes V–VI:** 5–9 mos
Under what RPA classes can GBM fall?	GBMs fall under **classes III–VI:** **Class III:** <50 yo, KPS 90–100 **Class IV:** <50 yo, KPS <90 or >50 yo, good KPS **Class V:** >50 yo, KPS <70 but no change in MS **Class VI:** KPS <70 and MS change
On what is the current modified RPA based?	**Outcomes with temozolomide** (TMZ) (*Mirimanoff RO, JCO 2006*)
What is the 4-yr OS and MS for RT + TMZ vs. RT alone for the adapted RPA groups for malignant gliomas (per *Mirimanoff RO, ASTRO 2007 update*)?	<u>Overall survival</u>: <u>class III</u> (<50 yo, performance status [PS] 0): **28.4%** vs. 6.4%; <u>class IV</u>: **11.3%** vs. 3.3%; <u>class V</u> (>50 yo, Mini-Mental State Examination <27, Bx only): **6%** vs. 1% <u>Median survival</u>: <u>class III</u>: 21 mos vs. 15 mos; <u>class IV</u>: 16 mos vs. 13 mos; <u>class V</u>: 10 mos vs. 9 mos
What additional factors did the European Nomogram (European GBM Calculator) investigate for stratification purposes?	**MGMT methylation status** and extent of resection; only MGMT, age, PS, and MS were prognostic (*Gorlia T et al., Lancet Oncol 2008*)
What is MGMT, and why is it important?	MGMT is a **DNA repair enzyme that removes alkyl groups from the O^6 position of guanine.** When methylated the MGMT gene is inactive and therefore, there is no ability to repair the damage caused by TMZ = chemosensitive. Methylated MGMT leads to increased OS regardless of the type of treatment.

What is the mechanism of action of TMZ?

Oral agent that cross links DNA (alkylating)

When should anticonvulsants be started?

Anticonvulsants should be started **only if the pt is symptomatic or has a Hx of seizures.**

What is the impact of resection extent in HGGs?

Data suggest that the extent of resection correlates with **improved outcomes.** (*Sanai N et al., Neurosurgery 2008; Stummer W, Lancet Oncol 2006*)

What is the Tx paradigm for AA and GBM?

AA Tx paradigm: surgery → RT to 57–59.4 Gy +/– TMZ or PCV
GBM Tx paradigm: surgery → RT to 60 Gy + TMZ → TMZ × 6 months

What is the dose of TMZ, and how is it administered/scheduled?

Oral pill; 7 days/wk at **75 mg/m²** concurrent with RT → 1-mo break → 6 cycles of adj TMZ at **150–200 mg/m²** given 5 days of every 28 days

With the current Tx paradigm, what additional pharmacologic therapies are often necessary?

Steroids, proton pump inhibitors, and PCP prophylaxis

Which early GBM studies demonstrated significant (doubled) survival with RT vs. supportive care and helped RT become a standard component of Tx?

GBM studies showing significant survival:
BTSG 69–01 (*Walker MD et al.*): randomized to observation, BCNU (carmustine), WBRT, and BCNU + WBRT. There was no difference between WBRT vs. WBRT + BCNU, but RT was better than no RT. (*J Neurosurg 1978*)
BTSG 72–01 (*Walker MD et al.*): Randomized to MeCCNU (semustine), *RT* alone, BCNU + RT, and semustine +RT. MS 3–6 mos without RT, 9–12 mos with RT. (*NEJM 1980*)
Scandinavian Glioblastoma Study Group (SGSG) (*Kristiansen K et al.*): 45 Gy + bleomycin vs. 45 Gy vs. observation: MS 10.8 mos vs. 10.8 mos vs. 5.2 mos (SS). (*Cancer 1981*)

Which randomized study supports the use of RT vs. best supportive care for the elderly with GBM?

French data (*Keime-Guibert F et al.*): pts >70 yo, KPS ≥70, to 50.4 Gy vs. observation. **MS improved with RT:** 6.7 mos vs. 3.9 mos. There was no difference in QOL or cognition. (*NEJM 2007*)

What studies support the use of hypofractionation in elderly GBM pts with a poor KPS?

Roa W et al. (*JCO 2004*), *Bauman GS et al.* (*IJROBP 1994*), *and Malmström A et al.* (*Lancet Oncol 2012*) suggest feasibility of hypofractionation. All 3 trials looked at hypofractionated courses vs. standard fractionation in patients >60–65 yrs or with poor KPS and showed hypofractionation was as good or better than standard fractionation in terms of OS. Dose fractionation schemes included 40 Gy in 15 fx (Roa), 30 Gy in 10 fx (Bauman), and 34 Gy in 10 fx (Malmström).

Which study suggested that WBRT is not required (i.e., that limited-field RT is sufficient) in the Tx of HGGs?

BTCG 80–01 (*Shapiro WR et al., J Neurosurg 1989*): prospective RCT, 510 pts, WBRT to 60 Gy vs. WBRT to 43 Gy → CD to 60 Gy. There was no difference in survival in the RT arms. This study also demonstrates that BCNU single agent is equivalent to a multiagent regimen.

What evidence supports current RT volumes being used in the Tx of HGGs?

Hochberg FH: CT correlation with postmortem tissue, CT abnl + 2-cm margin encompassed tumor extent by 83%. Recurrence by imaging also occurred within 2 cm of the margin in primary Dz in 90% of cases. (*Neurology 1980*)
Kelly PJ: correlated imaging (MRI + CT) with stereotactic Bx in untreated gliomas. The study found that isolated tumor cells extended at least as far as T2, suggesting that T1 enhancement is equivalent to GTV and a +T2 is equivalent to subclinical Dz. (*J Neurosurg 1987*)

What evidence supports the current RT dose of 60 Gy used for HGGs?

Combined analysis of 3 BTSG trials (*Walker MD, IJROBP 1979*): 4 doses (<45 Gy, 50 Gy, 55 Gy, and 60 Gy). MS was 4 mos, 7 mos, 9 mos, and 10 mos, respectively. MRC data (*Bleehen NM et al., Br J Cancer 1991*): RCT, 474 pts, 45 Gy vs. 60 Gy (no chemo). MS was 9 mos vs. 12 mos.

Is there evidence for a dose escalation benefit beyond 60 Gy in HGGs?

No. There is no evidence for a dose escalation benefit. In **RTOG 7401,** there was no benefit for 70 Gy vs. 60 Gy in >600 pts. (*Chang CH, Cancer 1983*)
Chan JL et al. escalated the dose to 90 Gy without survival benefit. Of those who failed at 90 Gy, 91% failed in-field. (*JCO 2002*)

Is there evidence supporting RT hyperfractionation for GBM?

No. RTOG 8302: >700 pts, randomized phase I, 64.8 vs. 81 Gy bid. There was no benefit. **RTOG 9006** also showed no benefit.

Is there a benefit to radiosurgery boost for HGGs?

No. RTOG 9305 showed no benefit and higher toxicity. (*Souhami L et al., IJROBP 2004*)

Before the TMZ data, was there any benefit to CRT for HGGs?

Yes. This was shown by evidence from 2 large meta-analyses: The *MRC Glioma Meta-analysis Trialist Group* showed a small improved median PFS (7.5 mos vs. 6 mos) with chemo, reduced risk of death by 15%, and ↑ 1-yr OS by 6%. There was no RT dose response with less or more than 60 Gy. (*Stewart LA et al., Lancet 2002*)

What is the evidence that supports the current gold standard in GBM Tx with TMZ?

EORTC/NCIC data (*Stupp R et al., NEJM 2005* and 5-yr update *Stupp R et al., Lancet Oncol 2009*): 5-yr OS 10% (+ TMZ) vs. 2% (– TMZ), **MS 14.6 mos (+ TMZ) vs. 12 mos (– TMZ).** Benefit in all groups including ages 60–70. In pts with methylated MGMT there is a PFS benefit to TMZ + RT vs. RT alone.

Which modified RPA class did TMZ + RT not benefit significantly (per *Mirimanoff RO et al., JCO 2006*)?

Class V. MS per RPA: class III, 17 mos; class IV, 15 mos; and class V, 10 mos. The only significant benefit of TMZ + RT vs. RT alone was in classes III–IV.

What is the role of MGMT methylation in terms of response to Tx with HGGs?

Greater response to TMZ + RT in those with methylated MGMT (*Hegi ME et al., NEJM 2005; Mirimanoff RO, ASTRO 2007*): 4-yr OS <u>unmethylated</u> (RT alone vs. RT + TMZ): **0% vs. 11%** and <u>methylated</u> **5% vs. 22%,** all SS

What are the options for recurrent GBM?

TMZ, bevacizumab, reirradiation to ~36 Gy (*Combs SE et al., BMC Cancer 2007*), radiosurgery, brachytherapy (GliaSite), Gliadel, or clinical trial

What is the dose used for GliaSite in GBM? What is the radioisotope used?

60 Gy to 5–10 mm at a dose rate of 0.5 Gy/hr (*Chan TA, IJROBP 2005*); **I-125**

What are the approved uses of Gliadel?

<u>FDA approval</u>: recurrent dz with re-resection improved survival advantage 31 vs. 23 wks. (*Brem H et al., Lancet 1995*)
<u>In newly diagnosed adj setting</u>: MS was 13.9 mos vs. 11.6 mos. (*Westphal M, Neurooncol 2003*)

What are the general guidelines for RT target volume delineation in GBMs?

RTOG:
<u>Initial volume (46 Gy)</u>: GTV1 = T_1/tumor bed + T_2/FLAIR, CTV1 = GTV1 + 2 cm
<u>Boost volume (14 Gy)</u>: GTV2 = T_1/tumor bed, CTV2 = GTV2 + 2 cm. PTV adds 0.5 cm to all CTVs. Postop imaging (with MRI fusion) should be used for target delineation.

Alternative MDACC technique with simultaneous integrated boost (*Chang et al., IRJOBP 2007*): GTV = T_1/tumor bed, CTV = GTV + 2 cm. PTV 50 = CTV + 5-mm dose to 50 Gy in 30 fractions, PTV 60 = GTV + 5-mm dose 60 Gy in 30 fx

Which recent study showed similar survival outcomes with adj RT vs. adj chemo with procarbazine/lomustine/ vincristine (PCV) or TMZ in WHO III gliomas (AA)?

German **NOA-04** study (*Wick W et al., JCO 2009*): same PFS/OS for all arms (RT alone or 2 chemo agents alone). Good predictors: extent of resection, oligo component (oligodendroglioma or oligoastrocytoma), IDH1 mutation, MGMT promoter hypermethylation, 1p19q codeletion. Toxicity: grades 3–4 hematologic toxicity was significantly higher for PCV than for TMZ.

Which study investigated sequential PCV → RT vs. RT alone in oligodendroglial tumors?

RTOG 9402/INT-0149 (*Cairncross G et al., JCO 2006 and Cairncross G et al., JCO 2013*): AO or AOA s/p resection randomized to PCV × 4 → RT 59.4 Gy vs. RT alone. No median OS benefit. There was improved median PFS (8.4 yrs vs. 2.9 yrs) with chemo. Pt with 1p19q co-deletion (unplanned subgroup analysis) had improved median OS with PCV vs. RT alone (14.7 vs. 7.3 yrs). PCV increased toxicity.

Which recent study investigated sequential RT → BCNU vs. RT alone in AA? What did it find?

EORTC 26882 (*Hildebrand J et al., Eur J Cancer 2008*): no OS or PFS difference

What study tested the role of adj PCV after RT in oligodendroglial tumors?

EORTC 26951 (*Van den Bent MJ et al., JCO 2006 and JCO 2013*): With long-term follow-up OS better with RT + PCV (24.3 mos vs. 13.2 mos). 1p19q deleted pts did better. There was no long-term difference in QOL after PCV.

What phase III study investigated the efficacy of combining RT with either TMZ or nitrosourea in anaplastic gliomas?

RTOG 9813 (*Chang S, Neurooncol 2008*): Study closed early with 201 pts enrolled. Showed increased toxicity with BCNU vs. TMZ.

What studies are investigating the role of TMZ in AO/AOA?

NCCTG N0577: pts **with** 1p19q codeletion randomized to RT + PCV vs. RT + TMZ → TMZ vs. TMZ × 12 cycles.
EORTC 26053: anaplastic gliomas **without** 1p19q del 2 × 2 randomization RT vs. RT + TMZ then observation vs. adj TMZ.

What is the Tx paradigm for gliosarcoma?

Gliosarcoma Tx paradigm: treat like GBM (surgery → RT + TMZ → TMZ)

Which study tested dose-intensified TMZ after TMZ + RT?

RTOG 0525 (*Gilbert M et al., ASCO 2011*). This study randomized pts after TMZ + RT (after a 1-mo break) to TMZ on days 1–21 vs. standard days 1–5 for up to 12 cycles (max) depending on the response. Prelim results showed more toxicity in dose-dense arm and no difference in OS or PFS. Final data are pending as are neurocognitive and QOL results.

What ongoing phase III studies looked at bevacizumab in the upfront setting for GBM?

RTOG 0825 (*Gilbert M et al., ASCO 2013*): all treated with RT + TMZ then randomized to concurrent bevacizumab vs. placebo. Preliminary results show no OS or PFS benefit, but bevacizumab arm had worse QOL, cognitive function, and Sx burden.

AVAglio (*ASCO 2013*): all treated with RT + TMZ then randomized to bevacizumab vs. placebo. Early results suggest PFS benefit.

▶ TOXICITY

What is the radiographic appearance of radionecrosis?

Central hypodensity, ring enhancement, edema, and low PET avidity (occurs >6 mos post-RT)

What was the grade 3–4 toxicity rate from the Stupp R et al. trial (NEJM 2005) for the RT + TMZ arm? What main toxicity was noted?

7%; mostly hematologic from TMZ (thrombocytopenia and lymphocytopenia)

What does the follow-up entail after RT for HGGs?

MRI 1-mo post-RT, then q3mo; weekly labs (blood counts) while on TMZ

What % of HGG recurrences are local?

80%–90% of HGG recurrences are local.

What % of pts may show pseudoprogression after RT + TMZ?

Up to **50%** (*Taal W et al., Cancer 2008*)

Does MGMT promoter methylation status influence the incidence of pseudoprogression in HGGs?

Yes. MGMT methylation status increases the incidence of pseudoprogression after TMZ + RT. (*Brandes AA et al., JCO 2008*)

16 Optic Pathway Glioma

Updated by Andrew J. Bishop

▶ BACKGROUND

What is the typical age distribution of patients diagnosed with optic pathway gliomas (OPGs)?

OPGs have a bimodal distribution with **peaks at 5 yrs and 52 yrs of age.** 75% of all OPGs occur in **children** <10 yo.

OPG represents what % of all CNS tumors in children?

OPG represents **5%** of all CNS tumors in children.

What histologic grade is typical of OPG?

OPGs are typically **low grade.** Pilocytic astrocytoma (grade I) is the predominant histology. However, grade II has been reported.

Is there a sex predilection in OPG?

Yes. In children, girls are more commonly affected than boys. **In adults, males** are more commonly affected than females.

What genetic syndrome is associated with OPG?

OPG is strongly associated with **NF-1.** Most patients with OPGs have NF-1 (typically diagnosed before age 6 yrs due to screening), while ~15%–20% of NF-1 pts have OPG. (NF-2 is associated with acoustic neuromas.)

What are the subtypes of OPGs?

OPGs are organized by location:
1. Ant/prechiasmal
2. Chiasmatic
3. Hypothalamic

Which OPG subtype is more common in children vs. adults?

Ant OPG is more common in younger children (and in pts with NF-1). Chiasmatic and hypothalamic gliomas are more common in adults.

Which subtype has the worst prognosis?

Hypothalamic OPG has the worst prognosis (OS **50%–80%**/LC **40%–60%**) vs. other types (OS **90%–100%**/LC **60%–90%**).

How do pts with OPGs typically present?

A common presenting Sx is **painless proptosis.** Other Sx include ↓ visual acuity, visual field defects, changes in appetite or sleep/precocious puberty (hypothalamic), and new-onset HA and n/v (obstructive hydrocephalus).

▶ **WORKUP/STAGING**

What is the workup for pts with suspected OPG?	Suspected OPG workup: H&P (including a neuro-ophthalmic exam with a quantitative visual acuity assessment), MRI brain and orbits, genetic evaluation, and baseline endocrinology
What is the DDx of an optic nerve mass?	Optic neuritis, retinoblastoma, optic nerve meningioma, and lymphoma, hamartomas
How do OPGs appear on MRI?	On MRI, OPGs appear as **well-circumscribed, homogeneously enhancing lesions** (isointense on T_1 and iso- to hyperintense on T_2). Contrast enhancement and presence of cysts are more common in sporadic OPGs than in NF-1 associated.
Is Bx necessary for Dx?	**No.** Imaging and the clinical exam are sufficient for OPG Dx.

▶ **TREATMENT/PROGNOSIS**

What is the preferred initial Tx for pts with OPGs?	OPG Tx (controversial): Initial management most commonly is **observation.** Tx is typically reserved for pts with **documented progression or declining visual acuity.**
What is the Tx paradigm once pt progresses?	1. Chemo: first step due to risks of local therapy, especially if pt <10 yo 2. RT: good tumor control but typically delayed as long as possible due to long-term toxicity 3. Debulking surgery: reserved for refractory or symptomatic
What chemo agents are generally used for OPG?	**Carboplatin + vincristine** or etoposide
What data support prolonged chemo as a way of avoiding/delaying RT without compromising OS or visual function?	*Laithier V et al.* prospectively evaluated prolonged chemo (alternating procarbazine/carboplatin, etoposide/cisplatin, and vincristine/cyclophosphamide q3wks). 2nd-line chemo was given at relapse before RT. The objective response rate was 42%, 5-yr OS was 89%, and 5-yr freedom from RT was 61%. (*JCO 2003*)
What data support initial RT instead of initial chemo?	*Awdeh RM et al.* from St. Jude's prospectively followed 20 pts (*IJROBP 2012*). Visual acuity was better in patients treated with upfront RT compared to those treated with chemotherapy and RT as salvage therapy.
What is the ongoing Children's Cancer Group (CCG) protocol (A9952) comparing?	**CCG A9952** compares **chemo regimens** (carboplatin/ vincristine vs. thioguanine/procarbazine/lomustine/ vincristine)

When is RT indicated in OPG?	RT is typically used after **chemo options are exhausted,** when there are **progressive Sx,** or when there is **intracranial extension.**
OPGs are typically treated using what RT dose, fractionation, and technique?	OPGs are typically treated to **45–54 Gy in 1.8Gy/fx.** Proton therapy may have dosimetric advantages, especially in children. Fractionated stereotactically guided RT has good outcomes (5-yr PFS 72%) (*Combs SE et al., IJROBP 2005*).
What is the estimated 5-yr OS in OPG?	The estimated 5-yr OS is **89%.** (*Laithier V et al., JCO 2003*)

▶ TOXICITY

What is the main risk of surgery for OPGs?	**Visual morbidity** is the main surgical risk.
What are the more common late complications of RT in the Tx of OPGs?	Late complications of RT include **endocrine dysfunction, vasculopathy, and possible decline in visual acuity.**
What is a major disadvantage of RT in NF-1 pts?	**High incidence of 2nd CNS tumors** (RR 5.3: *Sharif S et al., JCO 2006*)
What is the RT TD 5/5 dose threshold for developing hypopituitarism?	The hypopituitarism TD 5/5 is **40–45 Gy** (GH levels ↓ 1st, then LH/FSH, followed by TSH/ACTH.)

17 Primary Central Nervous System Lymphoma

Updated by Gary V. Walker

▶ BACKGROUND

What are the incidence and median age at Dx of primary central nervous system lymphoma (PCNSL)?	**1,000 cases/yr** of PCNSL; median age **55 yrs (immunocompetent)** vs. **35 yrs (immunocompromised)**

What % of primary brain tumors are PCNSL?

~4%

What is the sex predilection, and how does it relate to immunocompetency?

Immunocompetent pts: males > females (2:1)
AIDS pts: 95% males

What risk factors are often associated with CNS lymphoma?

Immunodeficiency (congenital or acquired) and EBV infection

What type of non-Hodgkin lymphoma (NHL) is most often associated with PCNSL?

Diffuse large B-cell lymphoma is most often associated with PCNSL.

What % of PCNSL has ocular involvement?

15% of PCNSL has ocular involvement (vitreous, retina, choroid > optic nerve) that is typically bilat.

What is the most common genetic alteration seen in PCNSL?

The most common genetic alteration in PCNSL is the **gain of chromosome 12** (12p12–14), which corresponds to the amplification of MDM2 to enhance p53 suppression

If the pt presents with ocular lymphoma, what % later develop CNS involvement?

75% of pts who present with ocular lymphoma develop CNS involvement.

With what is orbital lymphoma often associated?

Systemic NHL is often associated with orbital lymphoma.

What % of pts present with isolated spinal cord/ meningeal involvement?

<5% of pts present with isolated spinal cord/ meningeal involvement.

What proportion of pts present with CSF involvement?

One-third of pts present with CSF involvement.

What % of pts present with PCNSL but have a negative systemic lymphoma workup?

Nearly all pts (>95%) who present with PCNSL have a negative lymphoma workup, so if lymphoma is found outside the CNS, it is NHL with involvement of the CNS.

What are the high-risk features of systemic NHL that increase the risk of CNS mets?

Burkitt, lymphoblastic lymphoma, immunocompromised pt, BM+, parameningeal presentation (nasopharynx, paranasal sinuses), and testicular relapse

What % of pts present with multifocal Dz?

Immunocompetent pts: 50%
AIDS pts: 100%

What % of pts with grossly unifocal Dz are actually microscopically multifocal?	**>90%** of pts with grossly unifocal Dz are microscopically multifocal.
What % of AIDS pts develop CNS lymphoma?	**2%–13%** of AIDS pts develop CNS lymphoma. Invariably all are EBV+.
What has happened to the incidence of PCNSL over the past 30 yrs?	There has been a dramatic **increase** (3-fold) in immunocompetent and immunocompromised PCNSL pts.
In what regions of the CNS does PCNSL arise?	Brain, spinal cord, leptomeninges, and globe (retina, vitreous)
What virus has been associated with PCNSL?	**EBV** has been associated with PCNSL (60% of immunocompromised cases).
Are B cells normally found in the CNS?	**No.** They develop as part of the pathologic process.
What is the more radioresistant NHL: intracranial or extracranial?	**Intracranial.** Per RTOG 8315, pts received 40 Gy WBRT + 20 Gy boost and 25 of 41 pts (61%) failed in the brain.
What % of PCNSLs are supratentorial?	The majority of PCNSLs **(75%)** are supratentorial.

▶ WORKUP/STAGING

With which CNS symptoms do patients present?	Focal neurologic deficits (70%), neuropsychiatric/personality change (frontal lobe involvement [43%]), ↑ ICP ([33%] HA, n/v, CN VI deficit, blurred vision), seizures, leg weakness, urinary incontinence/retention, and ocular Sx (blurry vision)
With which systemic symptoms do patients present?	Fever, night sweats, and weight loss (80%)
All PCNSLs are what stage? What type of NHL?	All PCNSLs are **stage IE.** PCNSL is considered an **extranodal NHL.**
What brain location and specific structures are commonly involved?	The #1 location is the **frontal lobe, often the deep white matter and frequently periventricular** (↑CSF spread).
What are considered deep structures of the brain according to the International Extranodal Lymphoma Study Group (IELSG)?	Corpus callosum, basal ganglia, brainstem, and cerebellum

How is the Dx of ocular lymphoma made?	The Dx of ocular lymphoma is made by **vitrectomy.**
What infectious etiology is often confused with CNS lymphoma?	**Toxoplasmosis** is the infectious etiology often confused with CNS lymphoma.
What is the DDx?	Secondary metastatic lymphoma, other primary brain tumors, metastasis, abscess, hemorrhage, multiple sclerosis, sarcoidosis, and toxoplasmosis in AIDS
What is the workup of a pt suspected of having CNS lymphoma (per NCCN)?	Suspected CNS lymphoma workup: H&P (ophthalmic slit lamp exam to r/o ocular involvement), CBC, CMP, LDH, EBV titer, HIV status, CSF cytology (if safe), MRI, and tissue Bx, consider BM Bx, testicular US (men >60 yo)
What imaging studies should be performed?	MRI brain (MRI spine if Sx or CSF+), CT C/A/P, and SPECT (if immunocompromised)
What clinical scenario and testing results obviate the need for Bx for a definitive Dx?	**In an AIDS pt, +EBV and +SPECT** lead to a sensitivity/specificity of 90%–100%. If both are negative, treat empirically for toxoplasmosis. If only 1 is positive, perform a tissue Bx.
How does CNS lymphoma appear on MRI?	Indistinct fluffy borders, periventricular location common, T_1 enhancement with gadolinium, and ring enhancement (due to central necrosis, often seen in AIDS)
When is PCNSL more likely to be multifocal?	PCNSL is more likely to be multifocal when the **pt is immunocompromised** (50%–80% of such pts).
What chemical abnormalities are seen in the CSF of pts with CNS lymphoma?	↑ Protein (85%), ↓ glucose (33%), ↑ LDH, ↑ β_2-microglobulin
What additional tests are necessary for AIDS pts with a possible Dx of CNS lymphoma?	Toxoplasmosis titer (r/o this and other opportunistic infections) and BM Bx
How can the Dx of PCNSL be most definitively established?	Bx brain/globe or CSF sampling
What additional workup is done for pts with suspected PCNSL?	Additional PCNSL workup: H&P with neurology emphasis (include visual/spinal Sx), MRI brain +/– spine, and ocular slit lamp exam. Consider PET/CT and/or testicular US for elderly men (per NCCN), labs (basic, LDH, HIV, toxoplasmosis, +/– BM Bx), and LP with cytology if such testing would be safe.

What are the 5 poor prognostic factors for PCNSL according to the IELSG?	Poor prognostic factors for PCNSL: 1. Age >60 yrs 2. ECOG performance status >1 3. Elevated LDH 4. Elevated CSF protein 5. Deep brain involvement (*Fererri AJ et al., JCO 2003*)
What is the 2-yr OS for pts with 0–1, 2–3, and 4–5 factors?	2-yr OS for these pts is **80%, 50%, and 15%, respectively.** (*Fererri AJ et al., JCO 2003*)
What are other prognostic factors for PCNSL?	Poor response to chemo, AIDS, and multifocality
Who are considered "good-risk" immunocompromised pts with PCNSL?	Non-HIV immunosuppression and HIV+ with CD4 >200

▶ TREATMENT/PROGNOSIS

What is the management paradigm for a immunocompetent pt with PCNSL and KPS ≥40?	PCNSL management paradigm: high-dose methotrexate (Mtx) (good CNS penetration) or multiagent chemo. If there is a CR, observe (particularly >60 yrs). Use RT for recurrence.
What is the management paradigm for a KPS <40?	Give steroids. If KPS improves, chemo, otherwise WBRT (per NCCN).
What is the 1st intervention in a symptomatic pt after Bx?	The use of **high-dose steroids** is the 1st intervention in a symptomatic pt after Bx.
If a pt is suspected of harboring PCNSL, why should steroids *not* be started right away before obtaining a Bx?	**Tumor regression (in 90%) with subsequent Bx yielding nondiagnostic results;** Bx 1st → start of steroids (upfront steroids only for unstable pts)
How does the RT response differ between PCNSL and other types of extranodal NHL?	PCNSL is **very radioresistant** (5-yr OS is 4%). Extranodal NHL response is 90%.
How did the IELSG determine the prognostic groups that may predict for better survival?	*Fererri AJ et al.:* 378 pts from 1980–1999, **HIV–** with CNS lymphoma. All were treated with various regimens (+/– chemo, +/– RT). (*JCO 2003*)

How do survival outcomes differ between CRT and RT alone?

MS is 40 mos (CRT) vs. 12 mos (RT alone). 5-yr OS is 30% (CRT) vs. 5% (RT alone).

What is the outcome of pts with ocular lymphoma?

The outcome of pts with ocular lymphoma is **uniformly fatal.** MS is only 6–18 mos.

Is cyclophosphamide HCl/doxorubicin/ Oncovin/prednisone (CHOP) effective against PCNSL? Is cyclophosphamide HCl/ doxorubicin/Oncovin/ dexamethasone (CHOD) effective?

No. There is ineffective blood–brain barrier penetration. 3 RCTs, including **RTOG 8806** (*Schultz C et al., JCO 1996*), demonstrated no benefit of CHOP or CHOD.

Which study demonstrated that an RT boost is not beneficial for PCNSL?

RTOG 8315 (phase II): WBRT 40 Gy → CD to 60 Gy. MS was 11.5 mos. 80% failed in the boost field.

What does the Memorial Sloan Kettering Cancer Center (MSKCC) data demonstrate on the use of high-dose Mtx + WBRT and the relation of age to developing neurotoxicity?

MSKCC data: phase II, 52 pts. MS was 60 mos. High-dose Mtx × 5 cycles (3.5 g/m^2) was alternated with intrathecal Mtx (12 mg) → procarbazine/ vincristine + WBRT 45 Gy → high-dose cytosine arabinoside (Ara-C) (intravenous 3 mg × 2). Of those aged >60 yrs, some did not rcv RT. Survival was the same between no RT vs. RT, but DFS was worse if there was no RT. Those >60 yrs who rcvd RT had ↑ risk of neurotoxicity (83%) vs. age <60 yrs (6%). With chemo alone, only 1 pt developed neurotoxicity. (*Abrey LE et al., JCO 2000*)

In the Abrey study, what was the response rate to pre-RT chemo?

CR 56% and PR 33% **(ORR 89%).** (*Abrey LE et al., JCO 2000*)

In RTOG 9310, did 36 Gy (1.2 Gy bid) benefit PCNSL pts when compared to 45 Gy (conventional qd) WBRT?

RTOG 9310 (*Fisher B et al., J Neurooncol 2005*): no difference in control and survival, but worse neurotoxicity (23% vs. 4%); prospective study of Abrey chemo regimen → **45 Gy vs. 36 Gy bid** (if CR to chemo) (63 pts rcvd 45 Gy, and 16 pts rcvd 36 Gy. MS was 37 mos).

What study examined the feasibility of observation after CR to high-dose Mtx?

NABTT 96–07, phase II study (*Batchlor T et al., JCO 2003*): intravenous high-dose Mtx (8 g/m^2) was given every 2 wks until CR or until 8 cycles. Once there was a CR, the pt rcvd 2 → high-dose Mtx q2wks and 11 cycles of high-dose Mtx q28d. MS was not reached at 22.8 mos. There was no neurotoxicity. CR was 52%, and PR was 22%.

In pts with failure after high-dose Mtx, what salvage RT regimens/ doses are used?	**45 Gy.** Recent Massachusetts General Hospital data suggests **36 Gy WBRT** (*Nguyen PL et al., JCO 2005*). MS s/p RT was 10.9 mos, and overall MS was 30 mos. There was neurotoxicity in 3 pts >60 yrs and in those who rcvd >36 Gy (31% vs. 0%).
What is the typical response rate to salvage WBRT for pts failing initial chemo?	CR 37% and PR 37% (*Nguyen PL et al., JCO 2005*)
What critical volumes need to be covered with WBRT?	The **post retina and CNS down to C2** need to be covered.
What volumes are treated with RT if the pt presents with an ocular primary?	WBRT to C2, + bilat orbits with opposed lats to 36 Gy → CD to WBRT + post retina to 45 Gy
How should AIDS+ PCNSL be treated?	**Trial of toxoplasmosis antibiotics.** If there is no response, consider Bx. Chemo is not well tolerated. Consider intrathecal Mtx. Consider palliative WBRT alone (30–45 Gy). If the pt is severely immunocompromised, consider HAART 1st.
Why is chemo not preferred in AIDS-related PCNSL?	Chemo is not preferred in AIDS-related PCNSL b/c **CD4 counts are already low** (usually <50).
What is the Tx paradigm in such severely immunocompromised HIV pts?	Immunocompromised HIV pt Tx paradigm: **WBRT to 36–45 Gy with concurrent HAART**
What was the Tx regimen in RTOG 93–10? What was the MS?	Intravenous/intrathecal Mtx/vincristine/procarbazine → WBRT to 45 Gy → intravenous cytarabine. MS was **3 yrs.** (*DeAngelis LM et al., JCO 2002*)
What options are there for leptomeningeal PCNSL?	Intrathecal Mtx or CSI to 36 Gy with a boost to 45–50 Gy
What is the Tx paradigm for ocular lymphoma?	Ocular lymphoma Tx paradigm: **RT to 36 Gy or intraocular chemo**
What is the rationale for omitting WBRT in the elderly with PCNSL?	**Neurotoxicity** in older pts (*Abrey LE et al., JCO 2000*): 80% of pts >60 yo had neurocognitive defects after 45 Gy; 6% if <60 yo. Some pts >60 yo did not get WBRT and had similar OS (worse DFS with no WBRT, however).
What is the WBRT dose for PCNSL after CR to chemo?	**24–36 Gy.** Consider omitting RT altogether if the pt is >60 yo.

What is the WBRT dose for PCNSL after PR to chemo?

36–45 Gy WBRT; focal CD to gross Dz to 45 Gy

What prospective data support RT omission/ deferral after high-dose chemo (Mtx/Ara-C)?

German data support RT omission/deferral following high-dose chemo. (*Pels H et al., JCO 2003, Jahnke K et al., Ann Oncol 2005*)

What is 1 additional option after RT, especially after PR to initial chemo?

Consolidation Ara-C is an additional option after RT.

What is the role of rituximab (Rituxan) in PCNSL? How can it be incorporated, and what studies support its use?

Can be used with Mtx/procarbazine/vincristine) as induction regimen → dose-reduced WBRT to 23.4 Gy if CR (45 Gy if PR) → Ara-C consolidation. MSKCC data (*Shah GD et al., JCO 2007*): 2-yr OS was 67% and two-thirds of pts had a CR (these pts were able to rcv reduced-dose RT).

What did RTOG 8315 investigate? What did it show?

RTOG 8315: RT alone/dose escalation (40 Gy + 20 Gy boost). There was high LR in the brain at 61% and significant neurotoxicity with higher doses. (*Nelson DF et al., IJROBP 1992*)

Which recent randomized international phase II study investigated the use of induction cytarabine for PCNSL? What did it find?

IELSG (*Ferreri AJ et al., Lancet 2009*): randomized to 4 cycles of Mtx vs. Mtx/cytarabine → WBRT. CR rates were 18% vs. 46% and ORR 40% and 69%, respectively.

What regimen was used in CALGB 50202 and what were the results?

Mtx, temozolomide, and rituximab (MT-R) followed by etoposide/cytarabine consolidation (EA), with no WBRT. CR is 66% with 2-yr PFS of 57%—comparable to previous regimens with WBRT. (*Rubenstein JL et al., JCO 2013*)

▶ **TOXICITY**

What is the dose tolerance of the lacrimal gland?

The dose tolerance of the lacrimal gland is **36 Gy.**

What was the toxicity rate in the RTOG 93–10 study?

RTOG 93–10: 15% had severe delayed neurotoxicity (especially if >60 yo). (*DeAngelis LM et al., JCO 2002*)

What was the Tx-related mortality for pts treated with chemo alone in the German trials?

In German trials, Tx-related mortality with chemo alone was **9%.**

Primary central nervous system lymphoma: results of a pilot and phase II study of systemic and intraventricular chemotherapy with deferred radiotherapy. (*Pels H et al., JCO 2003*)

18 Meningioma

Updated by Mark Edson

BACKGROUND

What % of all primary CNS tumors do meningiomas account for in adults?

34%. Meningioma is the most common benign 1st-degree CNS tumor. (*Central Brain Tumor Registry of the United States, 2012 update*). Autopsy studies suggest prevalence of subclinical meningiomas in up to 3% of the general population.

What are the age and sex predilection for meningiomas?

Meningiomas appear **late in life** (mean age at Dx 62, incidence peaks in the 8th decade). **Females** are more commonly affected than males (2:1).

What are some risk factors for meningiomas?

Prior RT (RR 10, median interval to development 20 yrs), **NF-2,** and **HRT** in women (RR 2).

Which protein is defective in NF-2, and to what else does NF-2 predispose?

Merlin; bilat acoustic neuromas/ependymomas and juvenile subcapsular cataracts

What histologic features can be seen in meningiomas?

Psammoma bodies and calcifications

List 5 negative prognostic factors for meningiomas.

Negative prognostic factors for meningiomas:
1. High grade
2. Young age
3. Chromosome alterations
4. Poor performance status
5. STR

What is the grade classification of meningiomas?

WHO **grade I** (benign), **grade II** (atypical), **and grade III** (anaplastic/malignant).

According to the 2007 WHO classification, what criterion upgrades an otherwise grade I meningioma to grade II?

Brain invasion.

What is the prevalence of grades II–III meningiomas? Name the histologies associated with WHO grades II–III meningiomas.

6% and 4%, respectively. **90% are grade I.**

Grade II: atypical, clear cell, chordoid
Grade III: anaplastic, rhabdoid, papillary

Of grade I meningiomas, which histologic subtype is most aggressive?

The **angioblastic** subtype is the most aggressive grade I meningioma.

What is the OS difference between atypical and anaplastic meningiomas?

Atypical 12 yrs vs. anaplastic 3.3 yrs (*Yang SY et al., J Neurol Neurosurg Psychiatry 2008*)

What are some prognostic factors identified for anaplastic meningiomas?

Brain invasion, adj RT, extent of resection, and p53 overexpression (*Yang SY et al., J Neurol Neurosurg Psychiatry 2008*)

▶ WORKUP/STAGING

What is the most common Sx at presentation for meningiomas?

HA is the most common presenting Sx.

What is the appearance of meningiomas on CT/MRI?

Homogeneously and intensely enhancing mass, +/– dural tail

What % of meningiomas exhibit a dural tail? In what other tumors/lesions can dural tails be seen?

60%. Dural tails can also be seen in **chloroma, lymphoma, and sarcoidosis.**

What proportion of incidentally found meningiomas remain stable on imaging?

Two-thirds. The majority remain stable on imaging.

For meningiomas, with what are slower growth rates associated?

Slower growth rates are associated with **older pts and calcifications.**

What surgical grading system is used in meningiomas? For what does it predict?

Simpson grade (I/GTR–V/decompression) predicts the **likelihood of LR.**

In what anatomic regions is GTR more difficult to achieve for meningioma resection?

Cavernous sinus, petroclival region, postsagittal sinus, and optic nerve.

How is optic sheath meningioma diagnosed?

Optic sheath meningioma is diagnosed clinically/radiographically by a neuro-ophthalmologist/MRI (*no* Bx).

▶ TREATMENT/PROGNOSIS

What are the Tx paradigms for meningiomas?

Meningioma Tx paradigms:
  If incidental/asymptomatic: observation
  If grade I and symptomatic/progressive: surgery +/– RT
  If grade II or III: surgery + RT

For which types of meningioma is RT the primary Tx modality?

Optic nerve sheath and cavernous sinus (inaccessible regions)

When should observation be considered?

Observation should be considered with **incidental/asymptomatic and stable lesions.** Consider surgery for large (≥30 mm) lesions, if accessible.

When is RT utilized after surgery for meningiomas?

RT should be utilized after surgery if there is **recurrent Dz or STR** or if there is **anaplastic histology or brain invasion.**

What is the avg time to recurrence after surgery for meningiomas?

4 yrs is the avg time to recurrence after surgery.

What are the 10-yr recurrence rates with surgery alone after either GTR or STR?

10-yr recurrence rates with surgery alone are **~10% after GTR** and **60% after STR.**

Is there a benefit to upfront RT after STR for grade I meningioma?

This is **controversial** (upfront control rates are considered equivalent to salvage rates). RTOG 0539 will attempt to address this question in its low-risk cohort.

What are the RT doses employed for meningiomas?

RT doses are **54 Gy for benign** and **60 Gy for malignant** tumors (PTV = GTV + 1–2 cm).

Is there any RT dose-response data for meningiomas?

Yes. *Goldsmith BJ et al.* showed improved PFS with doses >52 Gy. (*J Neurosurg 1994*)

What are typical SRS doses used for meningiomas?

Typical SRS doses range from **12–16 Gy** to 50% IDL at the tumor margin (depending on location/size).

What is the 5-yr LC rate for meningiomas after SRS?

The 5-yr LC rate is **~95% for grade I tumors.** For grades II–III, it is 68% and 0%, respectively. (*Stafford SL et al., Neurosurgery 2001*)

What poor prognostic factors have been identified in pts receiving SRS for meningiomas?

Male sex, previous surgery, tumors located in parasagittal/falx/convexity regions (*Pollock BE et al., Neurosurgery 2012*)

Should the dural tail be covered in the RT field?

In general, no; however this is controversial. Some studies have shown improved 5-yr DFS when the dural tail was included in SRS prescription isodose. (*DiBiase SJ et al., IJROBP 2004*)

▶ TOXICITY

What is the surgical complication rate after resection for meningiomas?

After resection, the surgical complication rate is **2%–30%** depending on the location/type; 1%–14% mortality (worse in the elderly).

If observed, pts should get MRIs at what intervals?

At **3 mos, 6 mos, and 12 mos, then every 6–12 mos for 5 yrs,** then every 1–3 yrs if stable

What is the toxicity rate for SRS if doses >16 Gy are used?	There is **temporary toxicity in 10%** of pts and **permanent toxicity in 6%** of pts. Perilesional edema is observed in 15%. (*Kullova A et al., J Neurosurg 2007*)
What is the RT dose limitation to the chiasm when SRS is used?	The chiasm should be limited to **8 Gy** with SRS.
How are optic nerve sheath/cavernous sinus meningioma pts followed?	These pts should be followed with **serial MRIs, neuro-ophthalmology exams, and regular endocrinology exams.**

19 Pituitary Tumor

Updated by Emma B. Holliday

▶ BACKGROUND

What is the % of pituitary tumors in relation to all primary brain tumors?	~10%–15% of all diagnosed primary brain tumors are of pituitary origin with up to 25% seen on autopsy series.
What % of pituitary tumors are functional vs. nonfunctional?	75% of pituitary tumors are functional, while **25%** are nonfunctional.
What are the sex and age predilection for pituitary tumors with symptomatic presentations?	Symptomatic pituitary tumors occur mostly in **females.** 70% occur from **30–50 yrs.**
What are some heritable syndromes that predispose to pituitary tumors, and what is the inheritance pattern?	**MEN-1** (3 "Ps": pituitary, parathyroid, pancreas), 11q13 mutant/menin. Autosomal dominant inheritance.
What is Nelson syndrome?	Nelson syndrome is **ACTH-secreting adenoma that develops after adrenalectomy** (pts can develop hyperpigmentation of the skin due to a melanocyte-stimulating hormone).

What are the embryonic derivatives of the ant pituitary vs. post pituitary?

Anterior: Rathke pouch (oral ectoderm)
Posterior: extension of the 3rd ventricle (neuroectoderm)

What is the name for the bony structure that houses the pituitary?

The **sella turcica** houses the pituitary.

What are the boundaries of the sella?

Tuberculum sellae anteriorly, dorsum sellae posteriorly, sphenoid sinus inferiorly, dural folds superiorly, and posterior clinoid processes laterally.

What CN deficit is most commonly caused by pituitary adenoma?

CN II. Pituitary adenomas are the most common cause of optic chiasm compression. Less commonly, CN III, CN IV, and CN VI deficits can cause ocular motility symptoms.

What hormones are secreted by lobes of the pituitary?

Anterior: prolactin (PL), GH, ACTH, TSH, LH, FSH
Intermediate: melanocyte-stimulating hormone (MSH)
Posterior: ADH, oxytocin

What is the histopathologic description of the cells of nonfunctional tumors?

Histopathologically, the cells of nonfunctional tumors are **chromophobic.**

What hormones are secreted by basophilic cells? Acidophilic cells?

Basophilic: ACTH, TSH, LH, FSH
Acidophilic: GH, PL

What is the most common functional pituitary tumor? 2nd most common? 3rd most common?

Prolactinoma (30%) > GH (25%) > ACTH (~15%)

Which pituitary tumors are more common in males and the elderly? Which are more common in females?

Males and the elderly: nonfunctioning or GH
Females: PL and ACTH secreting

Which are the more common pituitary tumors: micro- or macroadenomas?

Macroadenomas (≥1 cm) are the more common pituitary tumors.

Which are the most common pituitary tumors in females?

Microadenomas (<1 cm) are the most common pituitary tumors in females, particularly those that are PL secreting.

What is the most common cause of pituitary dysfunction in adults? Children?	<u>Adults</u>: pituitary adenoma <u>Children</u>: craniopharyngioma
What histologic features are prominent in prolactinomas?	**Calcifications and amyloid deposits** are prominent in prolactinomas.
What immunohistochemical stains are positive in pituitary adenomas?	Synaptophysin, chromogranin, and hormone-specific stains

▶ WORKUP/STAGING

With what signs/Sx do pts with a nonsecretory pituitary tumors present?	Bitemporal hemianopsia (optic chiasm compression), HA (↑ICP), oculomotor deficits: CNs III–IV, VI, V1–V2 (cavernous sinus compression), hydrocephalus (3rd ventricle compression), hyperprolactinemia (disruption of PL suppression from hypothalamus due to compression of pituitary stalk), or panhypopituitarism (from general glandular disruption).
With what signs/Sx do pts with secretory pituitary tumors present?	<u>PL secreting (50%)</u>: galactorrhea, amenorrhea, infertility, and vaginal dryness for women, loss of libido, erectile dysfunction and infertility for men <u>GH secreting (25%)</u>: acromegaly <u>ACTH secreting (20%)</u>: Cushing disease <u>TSH secreting (≤1%)</u>: hyperthyroid symptoms
What is the DDx of a pt with a pituitary mass?	Pituitary tumor, craniopharyngioma, meningioma, glioma, suprasellar germ cell, mets, and benign lesions (cyst, aneurysm, empty sella syndrome)
What is the workup of a pt with a pituitary tumor?	Pituitary tumor workup: H&P (physical: CNs, visual field, endocrinopathy), labs, including hormone levels, thin-slice MRI through the base of skull, and tissue Dx (transsphenoidal resection)
What lab findings are suggestive of a prolactinoma?	**Normal prolactin is ~2–25. If >100–200, prolactinoma is suspected, particularly in the setting of a pituitary mass.**
What are other causes of elevated PL?	**Pregnancy, lactation,** polycystic ovary syndrome, **hypothyroidism** (thyroid-releasing hormone from hypothalamus stimulates PL secretion), **seizures, and cirrhosis.**
What lab findings are suggestive of a GH adenoma?	**GH >10 (not suppressed by glucose) and elevated IGF-1** are findings that suggest GH adenoma.

What lab abnormalities are noted in Cushing Dz?	High cortisol not suppressed by low-dose dexamethasone and normal or ↑ACTH
What is Cushing syndrome?	Cushing syndrome is **elevated cortisol due to a variety of causes** (e.g., adrenal production, exogenous use). Pts have low ACTH, unlike in Cushing Dz.
What primary malignancies most commonly metastasize to the pituitary?	Breast and lung cancer. Usually in the setting of diffuse metastatic disease with >4 other sites.

▶ TREATMENT/PROGNOSIS

What are the Tx paradigms of choice for the management of pituitary adenomas?	1. Observation if small, nonsecreting microadenomas or prolactinomas 2. Medical management with bromocriptine or cabergoline for a microadenoma prolactinoma not causing local symptoms. However, 30% cannot tolerate bromocriptine due to nausea, HA, and fatigue. 3. Surgical resection if hypersecreting or symptomatic (due to mass effect for nonsecreting tumors) → observation or postop radiation if fail to suppress biochemically. Can also consider external radiation therapy alone for definitive local treatment with either stereotactic radiosurgery or fractionated radiation.
How long does it take for normalization of the PL level to occur after initiating pharmacologic suppression?	Normalization of the PL level takes **1–2 mos** following the initiation of pharmacologic suppression.
What pharmacologic agents are used for GH-secreting pituitary adenomas?	Somatostatin, octreotide, and pegvisomant (GH receptor antagonist)
What pharmacologic agents are used for ACTH-secreting pituitary adenomas?	Ketoconazole (best), cyproheptadine (inhibits ACTH secretion), mitotane (↓ cortisol synthesis), RU-486 (blocks glucocorticoid receptor), and metyrapone
What is the hormone normalization rate after surgery for a hyperfunctioning pituitary tumor?	Hormone levels normalize in 80%–90% of those with microadenoma and ~65% of those with macroadenoma.
What types of surgical resection are used for pituitary tumors, and what are the indications?	<u>Transsphenoidal microsurgery</u>: for microadenomas, decompression, debulking of large tumors, reducing hyperfunctioning tumors <u>Frontal craniotomy</u>: for large tumors with invasion into cavernous sinus, frontal/temporal lobes

Where is the scar located after transsphenoidal resection?

There is **no visible scar.** Transsphenoidal resection is done through the nose or alternatively from behind the upper lip.

What are the LC rates after transsphenoidal resection? Are they better for macroadenomas or microadenomas?

95%. LC rates are better for **microadenomas** after surgical resection.

What are some poor prognostic factors after transsphenoidal resection of prolactinoma?

Size >2 cm, high preop PL level, ↑age, and longer duration of amenorrhea

What are some poor prognostic factors after surgical resection of GH-secreting tumors?

High preop GH and somatomedin-C levels, tumors >1 cm, and extrasellar extension

Which pituitary tumors have a high recurrence rate after resection?

TSH-secreting tumors (risk factors: Hx of thyroid ablation, Hashimoto thyroiditis, prior RT/surgery)

What are the indications for radiotherapy in the Tx of pituitary tumors?

Pituitary tumor indications for radiotherapy:

1. Medically inoperable or otherwise not felt to be good surgical candidate due to proximity to vessels or cavernous sinus.
2. Persistence of hormone defect after surgery
3. Macroadenoma with STR or decompression
4. Recurrent tumor after surgery

What are the long-term control rates for hormone-secreting tumors after RT?

Best outcomes with RT for GH-secreting tumors (80%) > ACTH (50%–80%) > PL (30%–40%)

What should be done with medical/pharmacologic Tx before initiating RT for pituitary adenomas?

Medical Tx **needs to be D/C** b/c of lower RT sensitivity with concurrent medical Tx. (*Landolt AM et al., J Clin Endocrinol Metab 2000*)

What is the typical LC rate with RT for pituitary tumors?

The LC after RT is >**90%** for most pituitary tumors (*Loeffler JS et al., J Clin Endocrinol Metab 2011*).

What are the typical RT volumes and doses used for pituitary tumors?

With IMRT or proton beam therapy: Treat operative bed + gross disease + 0.3 – 0.5 cm PTV; **45–50.4 Gy in 1.8 Gy/fx if postop with no gross Dz, 54 Gy for gross Dz.**

How long does it typically take for hormone stabilization to occur after Tx with RT?

It takes **yrs** for hormone stabilization after Tx with RT (GH: 50% normalize at 2–5 yrs, 70% after 10 yrs).

What evidence supports at least 45 Gy as the min effective RT dose for pituitary tumor control?

Older Florida data (*McCollough WM et al., IJROBP 1991*): 10-yr LC was 95%.

What are the indications for and the benefits of SRS in the Tx of pituitary adenomas?

SRS is used for **microadenomas** and yields **better control of hormone secretion** (same LC as fractionated and is more convenient).

What are the typical SRS doses used for functional vs. nonfunctional tumors?

Functional SRS dose: ~20 Gy
Nonfunctional SRS dose: ~14–18 Gy

What are the differences between LINAC-based and Gamma Knife (GK)-based SRS for pituitary tumors?

With GK, there is **less homogeneous dose to the tumor, more precise setup, and slightly less normal tissue treated** (similar outcomes/conformality can be achieved with LINAC-based SRS, however).

When is FSR preferred instead of SRS for pituitary adenomas?

FSR is preferred **when the pituitary lesion is >3 cm and/or the lesion is <2 mm from the chiasm.**

What RT doses are used with fractionated EBRT? When is EBRT typically used?

45–50 Gy (nonfunctioning), 50–54 Gy (functioning). Fractionated EBRT is typically **used for large adenomas and/or lesion is < 2 mm from chiasm or optic nerves.**

What form of radiation can be used to reduce dose to normal tissues with fractionated EBRT?

Proton therapy. The Loma Linda experience showed it to be effective (*Ronson BB et al., IJROBP 2006*). However, long-term results needed to determine clinical results from normal tissue sparing.

▶ **TOXICITY**

What is the most common toxicity of pituitary irradiation?

Hypopituitarism. Risk is ~20% at 10 yrs posttreatment (*Brada et al., Clin Endocrinol 2002*) with fractionated radiation or SRS (*Sheehan et al., J Neurosurg 2013*).

What is the RT TD 5/5 tolerance dose threshold for developing hypopituitarism?

The TD 5/5 is **40–45 Gy.** GH levels ↓ 1st, then LH/FSH → TSH/ACTH.

What is the tolerance of the optic nerves/chiasm with the use of conventional RT?

With conventional RT, **50–54 Gy** is the tolerance of the optic nerves/chiasm.

What is the TD of the optic nerve to single-fx SRS?

8 Gy is the TD of the optic nerve with single-fx SRS.

What are the main benefits of using SRS for pituitary adenomas?

Benefits of SRS include ↓ **neurocognitive sequelae and possible preservation of normal pituitary function** by reducing the dose to the hypothalamus (↑ risk of damage to the optic nerve/chiasm).

What is the best way to assess the response to RT in GH-secreting tumors?

The response to RT can be assessed by **monitoring IGF-1 levels.**

What hormone is the 1ˢᵗ to respond/decrease after RT?

GH is the 1ˢᵗ hormone to respond/decrease after RT.

What is the operative mortality/complication rate after surgery?

Mortality: 1%–2%
Complication rate: 15%–20%

What are the most common surgical complications after resection of pituitary tumors?

Diabetes insipidus (6%) → hyponatremia and CSF leak

Which pituitary pts/ tumor types are prone to increased rates of 2ⁿᵈ malignancies after Tx with RT?

Men with **GH-secreting pituitary adenomas** have increased rates of 2ⁿᵈ malignancies after RT. (*Norberg L et al., Clin Endocrinol 2007*)

20 Primary Spinal Cord Tumor

*Boris Hristov, Timothy A. Chan,
and Updated by Eva N. Christensen*

▶ BACKGROUND

At what level does the spinal cord (SC) end in adults? Newborns?

Adults: L1–2
Newborns: L3–4

What is the filum terminale?

A **filamentous process that anchors the dural sac inferiorly to the coccyx.**

What is the conus medullaris?

The **inf/tapering portion of the SC.**

What % of all primary CNS malignancies arise in the SC?	2%–4%
How are spinal tumors classified?	By their anatomic location relative to the **(1) dura mater** (lining around the cord) **and (2) spinal cord** (medullary)
What % of primary spinal tumors are extramedullary vs. intramedullary?	**67% extramedullary and 33% intramedullary**
What are the most common intramedullary spinal tumors?	Gliomas (ependymomas, astrocytomas, and less commonly, oligodendrogliomas); intramedullary mets are much less common.
What grade is most common for primary SC astrocytomas?	~90% are **low grade**/WHO grades I–II (pilocytic/fibrillary).
What is the most common intramedullary tumor in adults, and at what age does presentation peak?	Ependymoma, peaking between 30 and 40 yrs
What is myxopapillary ependymoma and why is it considered to be a special case of ependymoma?	Ependymoma typically arising from the filum terminale, a **filamentous process that anchors the dural sac inferiorly to the coccyx.** These tumors are biologically different from other ependymomas.
In what part of the spine are ependymomas most commonly located?	Lumbar/sacral spine
In what part of the spine are astrocytomas most commonly located, and with what are they associated?	Cervical/thoracic spine; associated with cysts
What are the most common intradural-extramedullary spinal tumors?	Nerve sheath tumors (schwannomas and neurofibromas) and meningiomas
From what anatomic portion of the meninges do meningiomas arise?	Arachnoid
What are the most common extradural spinal tumors?	Mets, often arising in vertebral bodies
What are primary extradural spinal tumors?	Chordomas, sarcomas, lymphomas, plasmacytoma, multiple myeloma, Langerhans cell histiocytosis

▶ WORKUP/STAGING

What is the most common presenting Sx of primary SC tumors, and over what timeframe do Sx present?

Pain (75%), with Sx presenting over **mos to yrs** (long prodrome).

What is particularly important as part of the workup for a SC tumor?

Detailed neurologic exam and SC imaging (MRI or CT myelogram)

What is the difference between astrocytomas and ependymomas on MRI (location/appearance)?

Astrocytoma: eccentric/asymmetric expansion of SC
Ependymoma: central/symmetric expansion of SC

What is the MRI appearance of SC lipomas?

Bright on T_1 without contrast, and signal disappears on fat suppression.

Which primary SC tumors require imaging of the entire craniospinal axis?

Ependymomas, glioblastoma multiforme, and anaplastic astrocytomas

▶ TREATMENT/PROGNOSIS

What is the Tx paradigm for primary SC tumors?

Primary SC tumor Tx paradigm: max resection +/– RT or definitive RT alone

What are the 2 main advantages of upfront surgical resection?

Histologic confirmation and decompression of the cord

After GTR, which meningiomas—spinal or intracranial—have higher rates of recurrence?

Intracranial meningiomas have a 10%–20% recurrence rate, while spinal meningiomas have ~5% recurrence rate.

What is the most important predictor of recurrence for meningiomas/ependymomas?

Extent of resection. There are few recurrences after GTR.

In what % of SC meningioma/ependymoma pts is GTR achievable?

>90% of pts. (Retrospective series: *Gezen F et al., Spine 1976, Peker S et al., J Neurosurg Sci 2005*)

In what proportion of SC astrocytoma pts is GTR possible?

<33% of pts

Why is RT controversial for most SC tumors, even after STR?

Most SC tumors are indolent (slow growing), and there is **potential for SC toxicity** with RT.

What RT options are available after STR for meningioma/ ependymoma?

At MDACC, the practice is fractionated EBRT with protons to 45–54 Gy (*Amsbaugh MJ et al., IJROBP 2012*). It is also possible to use photons or stereotactic techniques depending on the histology and volume of Dz.

Does WHO grade I or grade II spinal ependymoma carry a worse prognosis?

WHO grade I (*Tarapore PE et al., Neurosurg 2013*)

What Tx options are available for SC astrocytomas?

Low grade: observe after GTR/45–50.4 Gy after STR
High grade: 45–54 Gy

What retrospective series support RT in pediatric pts with low-grade SC astrocytomas?

Johns Hopkins Hospital: After surgical resection, 12 of 20 pts rcvd radiation to a median dose of 47.5 Gy. Acute radiation toxicity was low grade, and long-term side effects were uncommon and manageable. In 7 of 8 pts with low-grade tumors who rcvd adj or salvage RT, there was no Dz progression or recurrence. (*Guss ZD et al., IJROBP 2013*)

What retrospective studies support use of RT in SC astrocytomas?

Princess Margaret Hospital: PFS was significantly influenced by RT in low- and intermediate-grade tumors; however, the RT group had fewer complete resections as compared with the surgery alone group (13% vs. 53%; $p = 0.01$). (*Rodrigues GB et al., IJROBP 2000; Abdel-Wahab M et al., IJROBP 2006*)

What data support the RT dose response for SC ependymomas?

Garcia DM: <40 Gy, 23% OS; >40 Gy, 83% OS (*IJROBP 1985*)
Mayo Clinic data: 35% LF for <50 Gy vs. 20% for >50 Gy (*Shaw EG et al., IJROBP 1986*)

For what type of SC tumor has adj RT been shown to be beneficial, regardless of extent of resection?

Adj RT has been shown to be beneficial with **myxopapillary ependymoma.**
MDACC data: +/– 50.4 Gy RT 10-yr LC GTR/STR (55%/0%) vs. GTR + RT/STR + RT (90%/67%), all SS (*Akyurek S et al., J Neurooncol 2006*)

What RT schedule is often used for high-grade ependymomas with CSF spread?

CSI to 36 Gy + boost to 50.4–54 Gy gross Dz

What anatomic region needs to be covered with RT in caudal ependymomas?

The **thecal sac down to S2–3** needs to be covered.

What are the typical sup-inf RT margins for SC tumors?

The typical sup-inf margin required for SC tumors is **3–5 cm.**

What is the Lhermitte sign? When does it occur, and what causes it?	The Lhermitte sign is **shocklike sensations in the extremities on neck flexion.** It occurs within **2–6 mos of RT** from **demyelination of the nerve tracts.**
When does RT myelopathy occur, and what is the temporal sequence of onset for neurologic deficits?	RT myelopathy occurs **13–29 mos** after RT, with paresthesia → weakness → pain/temperature loss → loss of bowel/bladder function.
Per QUANTEC, what is the risk of myelopathy with 1.8–2.0 Gy/fx to the full thickness of the cord at 54 Gy? At 61 Gy?	<1% at 54 Gy, <10% at 61 Gy (*Kirkpatrick JP et al., IJROBP 2010*)
Per QUANTEC, what is the risk of myelopathy with SRS to the cord to 13 Gy in 1 fx? To 20 Gy in 3 fx?	<1% with 13 Gy/1 fx, <1% with 20 Gy/3 fx (*Kirkpatrick et al., IJROBP 2010*)
Within what timeframe do SC astrocytoma pts usually relapse?	Relapse in SC astrocytoma pts usually occurs within **2 yrs** (most in-field).
How long of a follow-up is required after SC ependymoma resection?	**>10 yrs** follow-up is required, as **late recurrences (>12 yrs) have been reported** in 5%–10% of pts.
What region of the SC has traditionally been thought to be most sensitive to RT? Least sensitive?	The **lumbar SC is thought to be most sensitive** to RT, while the **cervical cord is thought to be least sensitive.**

21 Choroid Plexus Carcinoma and Papilloma

Updated by Jingya Wang

▶ **BACKGROUND**

What % of intracranial neoplasms do choroid plexus (CP) tumors represent in adults and children?	In adults, CP tumors account for <1% of primary intracranial neoplasms, whereas CP tumors represent up to 5% of pediatric brain tumors.

What are the most common locations of CP tumors in children vs. adults?	<u>Children</u>: Lat ventricles <u>Adults</u>: 4th ventricle

What is the name for the benign CP variant, and how frequent is it? How about the malignant variant?	<u>Benign variant</u>: choroid plexus papilloma (CPP)/
	    WHO grade I (60%–80% of cases)
	<u>Malignant variant</u>: choroid plexus carcinoma
	    (CPC)/WHO grade III (20%–40% of cases)

What are the pathologic features of WHO grade I papillomas vs. WHO grade II atypical papillomas vs. WHO grade III carcinomas?	WHO grade I CPP are characterized by papillary formation and lack of mitosis. WHO grade II atypical papillomas resemble WHO grade I papillomas but have increased mitoses. WHO grade III CPC are characterized by nuclear atypia, pleomorphism, frequent mitoses, and invasion of brain parenchyma. (*Louis D et al., Acta Neuropathol 2007*)
With what syndrome is CPC associated?	**Li-Fraumeni,** due to p53 mutation (*Tabori U et al., JCO 2010*)
What proportion of children present with metastatic Dz at Dx?	**One-third** of children present with metastatic Dz, all typically with CPC.
What is the most common age of presentation for these tumors?	70% of pts are **<2 yo.**
What % of CPCs can have CSF seeding? How about CPPs?	**Up to 40%** of CPCs have CSF seeding, but such seeding is **very rare for papillomas.**
What are the 2 most important prognostic/ predictive factors for CP tumors?	Histologic grade and extent of resection
How does age affect prognosis?	Patients >40 yrs have poorer prognosis, followed by children <10 yrs. Those in the 10–40 yo group fare the best. Sex is not a prognostic factor.

▶ WORKUP/STAGING

What are the 2 most common Sx at presentation in pts with CP tumors?	Hydrocephalus and HA (due to CSF overproduction and flow obstruction)
What studies need to be performed during the workup for CP tumors?	MRI of brain and spine and CSF cytology

What is the differential for an intraventricular mass?	Ependymoma, subependymoma, central neurocytoma, subependymal giant cell astrocytoma, CPP, CPC, meningioma, metastasis (*Koeller KK et al., Radiographics 2002*)
What are the radiologic features of CPPs vs. CPCs?	CPP: lobulated, solid, well-demarcated intraventricular mass that is isodense to mildly hyperdense on CT. On MRI, homogenous with intense contrast enhancement. CPC: usually larger than papillomas with heterogeneous signal patterns on CT and MRI; may contain calcifications, necrosis, and hemorrhage and frequently invade brain parenchyma.

▶ TREATMENT/PROGNOSIS

What is the general Tx paradigm for CP tumors?	CP tumor Tx paradigm: max safe resection (after embolization/chemo, if necessary) +/− chemo (younger pts) and/or RT (if age >3 yrs)
What are the indications for RT in pts with CP tumors?	Age >3 yrs and 1 of the following: carcinoma histology, +CSF/spine Dz (CSI), or recurrent tumors
What is the role of RT in CPPs after STR?	**No RT is necessary upfront,** as only 50% of STR pts require reoperation, surgical salvage is good, and reoperation may not be needed until yrs later. Consider RT if there is a STR after recurrence. (Mayo data: *Krishnan S et al., J Neurooncol 2004*)
What is the recommended EB dose for CPPs?	<u>Conventional RT</u>: **>50 Gy** to localized field <u>Stereotactic RT</u>: **12 Gy to 50% IDL** (Pittsburgh data: *Kim IY et al., J Neurosurg 2008*)
What is the strongest indication for CSI?	Positive neuroaxis staging. If pt >3 yo, CSI can be given to 36 Gy followed by boost to primary site and/ or mets.
What makes the resection of CPCs especially challenging?	CPCs are **very friable and extremely vascular.**
What can be attempted preoperatively to make resection easier?	Embolization (reduces intraoperative bleeding risk) or neoadj chemo
What agents may be used neoadjuvantly (after Bx and before 2nd-look surgery) for CPCs?	Ifosfamide, carboplatin, and etoposide (Toronto data: *Wrede B et al., Anticancer Res 2005*)
What data support the use of adj chemo and/or RT in CPCs?	Johns Hopkins Hospital data: 75 pts. GTR was better than STR (84% survival if GTR vs. 18% if STR). Adj RT offered a survival advantage after STR ($p = 0.004$) but not after GTR. (*Fitzpatrick LK et al., J Neurooncol 2002*)

What study supports delaying RT in very young children with CPCs?

"Baby" Pediatric Oncology Group study: 8 CPC pts treated with surgery, chemo, and delayed RT without any adverse sequelae (*Duffner PK et al., Pediatr Neurosurg 1995*)

What data support CSI over smaller RT fields in CPC?

Mazloom A et al. reviewed the literature and found 56 pts with CPC; 5-yr PFS with CSI was 44.2% vs. 15.3% with smaller fields (*IJROBP 2010*)

What do the data show with regard to RT after GTR for CPC?

Canadian data (*Wolff JE et al., Lancet 1999*): 5-yr OS was 70% with RT and 20% without RT.

What is the 5-yr survival rate for CPPs?

The 5-yr survival rate is 80%–100% following gross total resection and 68% following subtotal resection.

What is the 5-year survival rate for CPCs?

CPCs are significantly more aggressive, with greater tendency for leptomeningeal dissemination and/or recurrence. The 5-yr OS is only 20%–30%.

▶ TOXICITY

What are some prominent side effects from RT in the pediatric population with CP tumors?

Skull hypoplasia and neurocognitive/endocrine deficits

In patients with Li-Fraumeni syndrome, what long-term risk is of special concern after RT?

Radiation-induced 2nd malignancies

22 Arteriovenous Malformation
Updated by Sarah McAvoy

▶ BACKGROUND

What is the avg age at presentation for arteriovenous malformations (AVMs)?

30 yrs (10–40 yrs).

What is the nidus of an AVM?

The nidus is a **tangle of abnl arteries/veins connected by at least 1 fistula.**

What is the main histologic abnormality in the vasculature of an AVM?	**Absence of smooth muscle layer;** ↑ venous pressure (fibromuscular thickening with incomplete elastic lamina)
What is the morbidity and mortality per bleed for AVMs?	Morbidity: 30%–50%/bleed Mortality: 5%–10%/bleed (1%/yr)
What is the rate of hemorrhage per yr for AVMs?	AVMs have a **2%–4%** chance of hemorrhage/yr.
Are most AVM cases familial or sporadic?	Most AVMs are **sporadic.**
What familial/genetic syndromes are associated with AVMs?	**Osler-Weber-Rendu** (hereditary hemorrhagic telangiectasia; HHT) **and Sturge-Weber syndromes** are associated with AVMs.
What characteristics portend an increased risk of hemorrhage from AVMs?	Previous hemorrhage, increased age, aneurysm, deep venous sinus drainage, deep location, single draining vein, and venous stenosis
Aneurysms are found in what % of pts with AVMs?	**6%–8%** of AVM pts harbor aneurysms.

▶ **WORKUP/STAGING**

What are the common presenting signs of AVMs?	Intracerebral hemorrhage (42%–72%) > seizures (11%–33%) > HA > focal neurologic deficit. Children are more likely to present with hemorrhage than adults.
What imaging modality is ideal to r/o a bleed?	**CT** is ideal to r/o cerebral bleeds.
What is the gold standard imaging modality for AVMs?	**Angiography** is the gold standard modality for imaging AVMs.
What other imaging modalities can be used for AVMs? What are their advantages?	CT angiography (good vascular detail), MR angiography (good anatomy detail), functional MRI (eloquent areas), and diffusion tensor imaging (for white matter tracts)
What scale is used to evaluate AVM pts for surgery?	**Spetzler-Martin scale/grading system** (totals possible: I–V).

What 3 AVM characteristics in the Spetzler-Martin scale are predictive of surgical outcomes?

AVM characteristics that predict surgical outcome:

1. **Diameter** (<3 cm = 1, 3–6 cm = 2, >6 cm = 3)
2. **Location** (noneloquent area = 0, eloquent area = 1)
3. **Pattern of venous drainage** (superficial = 0, deep = 1)

How does AVM diameter/size scoring correlate with surgical outcomes?

The smaller the AVM diameter/size (<3 cm), the better the outcomes.

What brain areas are considered eloquent?

Eloquent areas include sensorimotor, language, visual, thalamus, hypothalamus, internal capsule, brainstem, cerebellar peduncles, and deep cerebellar nuclei.

▶ **TREATMENT/PROGNOSIS**

What are the 3 Tx options for AVMs?

Surgery, radiosurgery, and endovascular embolization

What is the goal of Tx with AVMs? Why?

Complete obliteration is the goal, since there is **no benefit or** ↑ **risk of bleed** if the obliteration is partial.

Is Tx of unruptured AVMs beneficial?

Controversial but likely not. Recent studies suggest tx if unruptured led to increased risk of hemorrhage, clinical impairment, and death (*Wedderburn CJ et al., Lancet Oncol 2008; van Beijnum J et al., JAMA 2011*)

Which lesions are most amenable to surgery?

Those with **low (I–III) Spetzler-Martin scores** are most amenable to surgery.

What is frequently done for grade III lesions before surgery?

Embolization can be performed for grade III lesions before surgery.

What is the main advantage of surgery?

Immediate cure and reduction in the risk of hemorrhage.

For what AVM lesions is SRS preferred?

Radiosurgery is preferred for **lesions <3 cm that are located in deep or eloquent regions of the brain.**

What is the main disadvantage of SRS for AVMs?

The main disadvantage of SRS is the **lag time of 1–3 yrs to complete obliteration** (i.e., continued bleeding risk).

How does RT lead to AVM obliteration?

Vascular wall thickening (fibrointimal hyperplasia) **and luminal thrombosis** from RT effect result in obliteration of the AVM.

Is the bleeding risk completely eliminated after SRS?

No. It is reduced by ~54% during latency period and 88% after obliteration but not eliminated. (*Maruyama K et al., NEJM 2005; Yen CP et al., Stroke 2011*)

On what do SRS cure rates for AVMs primarily depend?

Size of AVM: 81%–91% if <3 cm, lower if >3 cm (*Maruyama K et al., NEJM 2005*)

What can be done for high-grade AVMs (IV–V) not amenable for surgery?	**Staged SRS** (different components targeted at separate sessions) (*Sirin S et al., Neurosurg 2006*)
For which AVMs can embolization be curative?	**AVMs <1 cm that are fed by a single artery** can be cured by embolization alone.
How are AVMs with feeding artery aneurysms managed?	**If the aneurysm is >7 mm in diameter, clip or coil the aneurysm 1st, then treat the AVM.** The aneurysm is at greater risk for rupture if the AVM is treated 1st.
What did the randomized ARUBA trial investigate?	The ARUBA trial randomized patients with brain AVMs to medical management with interventional therapy (surgery, embolization, SRS alone or in combination) vs. medical management alone. Trial stopped early due to superiority of medical management group. Risk of death or stroke was significantly lower in medical management group rather than interventional group (HR 0.27, 95% CI 0.14–0.54) (*Mohr JP et al., Lancet 2014*).
What SRS doses are commonly used for AVMs?	Lesions <u><3 cm</u>: **21–22 Gy** to 50% IDL. If the lesion is in the brainstem, lower the dose to ≤16 Gy. Lesions <u>>3 cm</u>: **16–18 Gy** to 50% IDL

▶ TOXICITY

What are the reported rates of permanent weakness or paralysis, aphasia, and hemianopsia for grades I–III AVM pts treated with surgery?	The rate of serious postsurgical complications is **0%–15%.**
What are common early and delayed complications after SRS for AVMs?	<u>Early</u>: seizures (up to 10%), n/v, HA <u>Delayed</u>: seizures, hemorrhage, radionecrosis (1%–3% risk), edema, venous congestion, cyst formation
What is the incidence of transient vs. permanent neurologic complications after SRS for AVMs?	Complications after SRS for AVMs are as follows: **transient (5%) vs. permanent (1.4%).**
On what 2 factors do complication rates after SRS for AVMs primarily depend?	**Size of AVM and RT dose.**
What does the follow-up entail after Tx for AVMs?	Adequate follow-up includes routine H&P + MRI q6mos for 1–3 yrs, then annually.
What study needs to be performed once the MRI shows evidence of AVM obliteration?	An **angiogram** needs to be performed (in addition to MRI) to confirm complete AVM obliteration.

23

Vestibular Schwannoma/ Acoustic Neuroma

Updated by Sarah McAvoy

▶ BACKGROUND

What is the cell of origin for vestibular schwannomas and acoustic neuromas (ANs)?

The **Schwann cell** of the myelin sheath is the cell of origin for ANs.

Which CN do ANs affect?

ANs affect **CN VIII.** Most affect the vestibular portion of the nerve.

In which anatomic region do ANs arise?

Most ANs are found in the **cerebellopontine angle** (CPA).

What are the most common presenting symptoms, incidence, and what cranial nerves (CNs) are they associated with?

Hearing loss (95% of pts) and **tinnitus** (63%) → CN VIII; cochlear nerve unsteadiness/veering/tilting (61%) → CN VIII; vestibular nerve, facial paresthesia, or pain (17%) → CN V; facial paresis (6%) → CN VII (*Matthies C and Samii M, Neurosurg 1997*).

What is the median age at diagnosis?

50 yrs

Most people with symptomatic ANs will present between what ages?

Most symptomatic pts are **30–50 yo.**

What proportion of ANs are sporadic?

The **majority (90%)** are sporadic as well as unilateral.

What % of ANs are bilat, and with what genetic abnormality are they associated?

10% are bilateral and associated with **NF-2,** the tumor suppressor gene on chromosome 22.

What protein is abnl in NF-2 pts?

Merlin or schwannomin (involved in actin cytoskeleton organization)

What is the name of the anatomic layer of CN VIII that gives rise to most ANs?

The **Obersteiner-Redlich zone** (the junction between the central and peripheral myelin) gives rise to most ANs.

Subclinical ANs are present in what % of the general population?	**Up to 1%** (autopsy series) of the general population harbor subclinical ANs.
ANs account for what % of intracranial tumors?	**5%–8%** of intracranial tumors are ANs. Overall incidence is ~1/100,000 person-years.
Apart from NF-2, what are 2 other risk factors that predispose to the development of ANs?	Loud noise exposure (ORR 13) and parathyroid adenoma (ORR 3.4), childhood exposure to low-dose radiation (RR per Gy 1.14).
What are the Antoni A and Antoni B areas on histopathology?	Antoni A and B are **zones of dense and sparse cellularity,** respectively.
For what do ANs stain on immunohistochemistry?	Most ANs stain for **S100.**
How do bilat ANs fare after Tx when compared to unilat ANs?	Bilat ANs have **similar failure rates** to unilat lesions if treated adequately.

▶ WORKUP/STAGING

What tests are performed on physical exam for pts with CPA lesions?	Rinne test (mastoid bone, air conduction > bone conduction) and Weber test (occiput, vibratory sound louder on good side) to confirm sensorineural hearing loss; also need to check for other CN deficits (CN VII, hypesthesia, corneal twitching)
What CN is being tested when a pt is asked to tighten the ant neck muscles?	**CN VII** (innervates platysma muscle) can often be affected with large AN lesions.
Why are pts with CPA lesions often asked to march in place with their eyes closed on physical exam?	When the vestibular nerve is affected, **pts will often veer to the side of the lesion.**
What is the best initial screening test for ANs, and what does it usually show?	**Audiometry (asymmetric sensorineural loss,** more prominent at ↑ frequencies) is the best screening tool for ANs.
What is the avg growth rate per yr for ANs?	**~1 mm/yr.** Growth rates range from 0.5–2.5 mm/yr (slow-growing lesions) to ≥2.5 mm/yr (fast-growing lesions).
What % of ANs are stable (shrink/do not grow)?	**~20%–40%** of ANs are considered stable.

Is the size of the tumor at presentation predictive of the tumor's growth rate?	**No.** Tumor size is generally not predictive of the tumor's growth rate.
Does AN tumor size correlate with hearing loss?	**Usually not.** The location of the tumor (i.e., intracanalicular vs. not intracanalicular) is more predictive. Pts with tumor growth rate ≤2.5 mm/yr have higher hearing preservation than those with higher tumor growth (*Sughrue ME et al., J Neurosurg 2010*)
What do brainstem auditory evoked potentials typically show in pts with ANs?	A **delay of conduction time on the affected side** is seen with auditory evoked potentials.
What imaging study is typically performed for ANs?	**Thin-slice (1–1.5 mm) MRI with gadolinium.** MRI can detect tumors as small as 1–2 mm in diameter. If NF is suspected, neuraxis MRI is performed. If pt cannot undergo MRI, high-resolution CT scan +/– contrast is the alternative.
To what is the "ice cream cone" appearance of ANs on MRI due?	This AN appearance is due to **enhancing lesions in the canal (cone) and CPA (ice cream).**

▶ TREATMENT/PROGNOSIS

What options are available for AN pts?	Observation, surgery, or RT
When is observation appropriate for ANs?	Observation is appropriate with small tumors (<2 cm) or no/slow growth without Sx progression. 43% with growth, **51% stable,** and 6% regressed without treatment. (*Smouha EE et al., Laryngoscope 2005*)
What follow-up is required for AN pts opting for observation?	**Audiometry and MRI scans q6–12mo**
What are the 4 surgical approaches available for ANs, and what are the prominent disadvantages/advantages of each?	Retromastoid: may not be able to achieve GTR/ good facial nerve preservation, good **hearing preservation**, can be used for any size tumor
	Middle cranial fossa: GTR, facial nerve preservation moderate-**hearing preservation** better, good for small <1.5-cm tumors
	Translabyrinthine: sacrifices hearing/good facial nerve preservation, recommended if tumor >3 cm
	Retrolabyrinthine: sacrifices hearing
When is surgery the preferred Tx option for ANs?	Surgery is preferred for **large (>4 cm) symptomatic tumors or recurrence/progression after RT.**

What are the recurrence rates after GTR for ANs?

<1% (*Samii M et al., J Neurosurg 2001; Guerin C et al., Ann Acad Med Singapore 1999; Gormley WB et al., Neurosurgery 1997*)

What are the overall facial nerve and hearing preservation rates after surgery for ANs?

After surgery for ANs, there is an **80%–90% facial nerve preservation rate** and a **50% hearing preservation rate.**

What are the overall facial nerve and hearing preservation rates after RT for ANs?

With SRS: **facial nerve preservation rate >95%, hearing preservation 70%–90%**

With fractionated RT (FSR): **~95% facial nerve preservation rate** and **~55%–65% hearing preservation rate**

What are the long-term LC rates after RT for ANs?

Long-term LC after RT for ANs is **90%–97%.** (*Lunsford LD et al., J Neurosurg 2005; Combs SE et al., IJROBP 2006; Litre F et al., Radiother Oncol 2013; Hasegawa T et al., J Neurosurg 2013; Maniakas A et al., Otol Neurotol 2012*)

What are some commonly employed doses when SRS/Gamma Knife (GK) SRS is used for ANs?

12–13 Gy to 50% IDL is a commonly employed SRS regimen for ANs.

What has the dose trend been for the Tx of ANs with SRS?

The dose was **lowered from 16 Gy to 12–13 Gy.** Pittsburgh and Japanese data showed similar LC rates but less facial weakness and hearing loss with lower doses.

What doses are used with FSR?

50–55 Gy (in 25–30 fx at 1.8 Gy/fx) if larger (>2–3 cm) lesions Alternative approach: **25 Gy (5 Gy × 5 fx)** with smaller lesions

What are the hearing preservation rates with FSR?

This is **controversial,** but hearing preservation rates are thought to be slightly better with FSR than with SRS or surgery (**94%** in *Combs SE et al., IJROBP 2005;* **81%** in *Andrews DW et al., IJROBP 2001*). Other studies suggest outcomes are equivalent if SRS dose <13 Gy (*Combs SW et al., IJROBP 2011*)

What recent data suggest better hearing preservation and similar LC rates with lower-dose FSR therapy?

Thomas Jefferson data: a lower dose of 46.8 Gy (vs. 50.4 Gy) had 100% LC at 5 yrs with a better hearing preservation rate. (*Andrews DW et al., IJROBP 2009*)

What other RT modalities have been successfully employed in AN?

CyberKnife (*Chang SD et al., J Neurosurg 2005*) and protons (*Weber DC et al., Neurosurg 2003; Vernimmen FJ, Radiother Oncol 2009*): worse hearing preservation (not used with tumors >2 cm and if pt can hear well)

What important AN studies prospectively compared surgery to SRS? What did they show?

Mayo Clinic data: <3-cm tumors, same tumor control rates but worse pt QOL after surgery. (*Pollock BE et al., J Neurosurg 2006*)

French data: largest prospective study. GK pts had better function overall. (*Regis J et al., Neurochirurgie 2002*)

Meta-analysis: included 16 studies showed SRS better long-term hearing preservation (70% vs. 50%) but no difference in tumor outcome. (*Maniakas A and Saliba I, Otol Neurotol 2012*)

What AN study prospectively evaluated SRS vs. FSR?

Dutch data: dentate pts rcvd FSR (20–25 Gy in 5 fx) and edentate SRS (10–12.5 Gy), with similar LC and functional outcomes. (*Meijer OW et al., IJROBP 2003*)

What agent has recently been shown to be effective in NF-2 pts with refractory ANs?

Bevacizumab (Avastin) was recently shown to be effective in NF-2 pts with refractory ANs. (*Plotkin SR et al., NEJM 2009*)

▶ TOXICITY

The dose falloff to which structures needs to be carefully evaluated with GK SRS for ANs?

Cochlea and brainstem doses need to be carefully evaluated with GK SRS.

What IDL is prescribed in GK? Why? How about for LINAC-based SRS?

GK: **50%** (sharpest drop off in dose is at 50% IDL)
LINAC: **80%**

What is the difference in the onset of side effects after surgery vs. RT for ANs?

Side effects present **upfront/immediately after surgery vs. in a delayed/gradual (mos to yrs) fashion after RT.**

What is the dose threshold above which hearing preservation rates decrease with RT?

Preservation rates decrease at doses **>13 Gy.** (Japanese data: *Hasegawa T et al., J Neurosurg 2005*)

What mean cochlea dose is the threshold for hearing preservation with SRS?

Mean cochlea 3 Gy. 2-yr hearing preservation 91% if mean cochlea <3 Gy vs. 59% if >3 Gy (*Baschnagel J et al., Neurosurg 2013*)

What are some toxicities and rates of toxicities after SRS for ANs?

Trigeminal neuropathy/hyperesthesia: 0%–5%
Facial nerve neuropathy/palsy: 0%–5%
Hearing deficit: useful hearing preserved in 40%–60%

What are the main toxicity differences between RT and surgery?

RT carries a lower risk of facial nerve/trigeminal nerve injury.

Part III Eye

24 Ocular Melanoma

Updated by Vinita Takiar

▶ BACKGROUND

How does intraocular melanoma rank in terms of incidence among the various eye malignancies?

Intraocular melanoma is **#1** among primary cancers (#1 overall is ocular mets).

What is the incidence of ocular melanoma in the U.S.? Is there a race predilection?

4 in 1 million (~1,500–2,000 cases/yr of ocular melanoma)
Yes. 98% of pts are white.

What are some of the risk factors for developing ocular melanoma?

UV exposure, fair skin, family Hx of ocular melanoma, and personal Hx of cutaneous melanoma

What is the most common site in the eye where ocular melanomas arise?

Uvea, mostly choroidal (85%) > adnexa (10%) > conjunctiva (5%)

What is the cell of origin for ocular melanoma?

Ocular melanoma arises from **melanocytes of the uveal stroma** (neural crest origin).

What are the components of the uveal tract?

The **choroid, ciliary body, and iris** comprise the uveal tract.

Name the layers of the choroid from outer to inner.

Layers of the choroid (outer to inner):
1. Haller layer
2. Sattler layer
3. Choriocapillaris
4. Bruch membrane

What are the basic layers of the globe?

Outer fibrous layer (sclera), middle vascular layer (choroid), and inner nerve layer (retina)

What region in the retina is particularly important for color vision?

The **macula** is important for color vision.

Where is the optic disc relative to the macula?	The optic disc is **2 mm medial** to the macula (~1.5 mm in diameter).
What are the histologic subtypes of ocular melanoma, and which carry the best and worst prognosis?	**Spindle cell (best), epithelioid (worst),** and mixed (if <50% epithelioid histology)
What % of pts with ocular melanoma present with DM at Dx? What is the most common location?	**1%–2%** present with DM. The **liver** is the most common site (5%–20% DM rate over 5 yrs).
What are the different ways melanoma can spread within the globe?	Melanoma can spread <u>intraocularly</u> (through the vitreous, aqueous, or along ciliary vessels/nerves); <u>extraocularly</u> (through the optic nerve, transsclerally, vascular tracking), and through <u>extrascleral extension</u> (10%–15%)
What tumor characteristics predict for DM in ocular melanoma? What is the 5-yr mortality rate in these pts?	Epithelioid histology, large tumors, ant location (ciliary body invasion), monosomy 3, scleral penetration, ↑ mitotic rate, ↑ Ki-67, pleomorphic nucleoli, optic nerve invasion, ↑ MIB-1 index, vascular networks of closed vascular loops, extraocular extension The 5-yr mortality rate is **55%.**
What is the long-term (>10-yr) DM rate from ocular melanoma?	**50%** of ocular melanoma pts develop DMs at 15 yrs.

▶ **WORKUP/STAGING**

How do pts with ocular melanoma normally present?	Most (one-third) pts are **asymptomatic.** Ocular melanoma is usually found on routine exam; otherwise, pts detect it themselves due to vision loss, scotoma, flashing lights, or pain (rare).
What is the workup for a pt with suspected ocular melanoma?	H&P, CBC (LFTs), ophthalmic/funduscopic/slit lamp exam, visual acuity/visual field testing, US (Kretz A-scan, immersion B-scan), fluorescein angiography, MRI, PET/CT to r/o mets
Is Bx commonly done for ocular melanoma?	**No.** It is a clinical Dx made by exam and imaging. Historically, there is concern that Bx may cause tumor seeding. More recently, Bx is more common for risk stratification/mutational analysis.
What is the genetic alteration most associated with poor prognosis?	**BAP1** inactivation. Mutation of 1 allele results in loss of an entire copy of chromosome 3. This correlates with metastatic spread.

What are simulation lesions?	Simulation lesions are **lesions that may look like melanoma,** such as nevi, hemangiomas, retinal detachment, age-related disciform lesions, and mets.
What feature does ocular melanoma manifest on standard A-scan US?	An **acoustic "quiet" zone** (central hypoechoic area) vs. mets or hemangiomas (have higher internal reflectivity)
What features do ocular melanomas exhibit on fluorescein angiography?	On fluorescein angiography, ocular melanomas exhibit a **double circulation pattern and fluorescein leakage** (appearing as hot spots).

What is the T staging of choroidal/ciliary body melanoma based on the latest AJCC (7th edition, 2011) staging guidelines?

AJCC staging is based on 4 tumor size categories that depend on tumor diameter and height as follows (Fig. 24.1):

T1: tumor size category 1
T2: tumor size category 2
T3: tumor size category 3
T4: tumor size category 4

For the T staging of choroidal/ciliary body melanomas, what do the designations a–e represent?

a: no ciliary body involvement/extraocular extension
b: +ciliary body involvement
c: no ciliary body/+extraocular extension ≤5 mm
d: +ciliary body/+extraocular extension ≤5 mm
e: +extraocular extension >5 mm

Describe the AJCC staging for choroidal/ciliary body melanomas.

Stage I: T1aN0M0
Stage IIA: T1b-dN0M0 or T2aN0M0
Stage IIB: T2bN0M0 or T3aN0M0
Stage IIIA: T2c-d, T3b-c, T4aN0M0
Stage IIIB: T3d, T4b-cN0M0
Stage IIIC: T4d-eN0M0
Stage IV: any TN1M0, any T, any NM1

For the M staging of choroidal/ciliary body melanomas, what do the designations a–c represent?

Ma: largest diameter of met ≤3 cm
Mb: largest diameter of met 3.1–8 cm
Mc: largest diameter of met >8 cm

In the Collaborative Ocular Melanoma Study (COMS) staging system, what are COMS small, medium, and large lesions?

COMS staging is based on apical height (AH) and basal diameter (BD):
<u>Small</u>: AH <34 mm, BD up to16 mm
<u>Medium</u>: AH 35–38 mm, BD up to16 mm
<u>Large</u>: AH >8 mm, BD ≥16 mm when AH >2 mm

What are the 10-yr OS rates of COMS small, medium, and large tumors? Pts with DM?

10-yr OS for COMS tumors:
<u>Small</u>: 80%
<u>Medium</u>: 60%
<u>Large</u>: 30%–40%
<u>DM pts</u>: <7 mos

Thickness (mm)

> 15					4	4	4
12.1-15.0				3	3	4	4
9.1-12.0		3	3	3	3	3	4
6.1-9.0	2	2	2	2	3	3	4
3.1-6.0	1	1	1	2	2	3	4
≤ 3.0	1	1	1	1	2	2	4
	≤ 3.0	3.1-6.0	6.1-9.0	9.1-12.0	12.1-15.0	15.1-18.0	> 18

Largest basal diameter (mm)

FIGURE 24.1 Primary ciliary body and choroidal melanomas are classified according to the 4 tumor size categories shown. (Edge SD, Byrd DR, Compton CC, et al., eds. *AJCC cancer staging manual*. 7th ed. New York: Springer; 2010.)

What is the melanoma-related mortality for COMS small lesions after 8 yrs?	Mortality is **4%** for COMS small lesions after 8 yrs.

 TREATMENT/PROGNOSIS

In order of importance, what are the 3 main goals of Tx in the management of ocular melanoma?	Main goals of ocular melanoma Tx (in order of importance): 1. Preserve life 2. Preserve eye 3. Preserve vision
What is the preferred management approach for COMS category small uveal melanomas?	**Observation or local therapy** (transpupillary thermotherapy, photocoagulation, photodynamic therapy, local resection, or enucleation [pt choice])
When is RT employed in the management of COMS category small uveal melanomas?	RT is employed when there is **progression after conservative management** (i.e., observation or other local Tx).
What are the eligibility criteria for observing uveal melanomas?	COMS small, inactive lesions, and good baseline visual function
When should Tx for uveal melanomas be initiated after observation?	Tx for uveal melanomas should be initiated **when growth is detected or there are pigmentation changes.**
If resection is employed for small melanomas, for what ocular location is it generally reserved?	Resection is reserved for **lesions of the iris or ciliary body.** It is *not* used for uveal lesions due to impact on vision.

In the COMS trials, pts with small uveal melanomas were observed with close follow-up. What % of pts progressed after 5 yrs?

~**33%** of pts with small melanomas progressed. (**Report No. 4**, *JAMA Ophthalmol, 1997*):

What features of small uveal melanomas were found to be associated with growth after observation?

Orange pigmentation (6.4 times), no drusen and no adjacent retinal pigmentary changes (4.2 times), >2 mm thickness (4.4 times), >12-mm BD (5.2 times)

What are the Tx options for COMS medium melanomas?

Enucleation, plaque brachytherapy, and proton RT

When is enucleation a preferred approach for the management of uveal melanoma?

Pt choice, as salvage therapy, tumor involving >40% of intraocular volume, tumor in a nonfunctional eye, symptomatic pt (pain), eye with marked neovascularization, and extrascleral extension

What are the indications for the use of plaque brachytherapy?

Plaque brachytherapy is used for **organ preservation** for COMS medium lesions and **small progressive tumors** after observation.

What are the max AH and BD sizes allowed for plaque brachytherapy?

For plaque brachytherapy, max allowed sizes are ≤**10-mm (3–8 mm optimal) AH and 16-mm BD.**

Under what circumstances should notched plaques be used?

Notched plaques are typically used for **peripapillary tumors.**

What is the most common isotope used in plaque brachytherapy? What is the dose rate?

I-125, at a dose rate of **0.7–1 Gy/hr** (Tx times vary from 4–7 days)

What other isotope can be used for small-to medium-sized tumors? Why might it be preferred over I-125?

Ruthenium-106 (β-emitter). Ru-106 has limited dose penetration relative to I-125, so it results in less toxicity and is also easier to insert.

How is the dose prescribed with plaque brachytherapy?

85 Gy to the tumor apex (or 5 mm from the internal surface of the sclera if the height is <5 mm), with a 2-mm margin around the tumor (or a plaque size equal to 4 mm + greatest BD)

When is proton beam the preferred RT modality in the Tx of uveal melanoma?

Proton beam is used not only as a **substitute for plaque brachytherapy or enucleation** but also for large tumors, tumors near the optic nerve, tumors near the macula, or tumors under the orbital muscles.

How is proton beam RT prescribed in the Tx of uveal melanoma?	**70 cobalt gray equivalents (CGE) in 5 fx over 7–10 days**
What is the long-term LC rate of proton beam compared to plaque brachytherapy?	Proton beam: 95% Plaque brachytherapy: 92%–94%
What is the 5-yr DM rate of ocular melanoma after Tx with either protons or brachytherapy?	The 5-yr DM rate after local RT is **16%–20%.**
What is the randomized phase III study that compared the efficacy of enucleation vs. plaque brachytherapy for medium-sized uveal melanomas?	**COMS study** (*Report No. 28, Arch Ophthalmol, 2006*): 1,317 pts. There was no difference in all-cause mortality and melanoma-specific mortality. 12-yr OS was 17%–21%.
In the COMS medium trial, what is the 5-yr secondary enucleation rate after plaque brachytherapy? To what is it due?	The 5-yr secondary enucleation rate is **13%** due to **tx failure or ocular pain from brachytherapy complications.**
What is the standard management for large uveal melanomas?	**Enucleation.** Charged particles (protons) can also be used.
What % of pts present with large uveal melanomas?	**30%** of pts present with large uveal melanomas.
Per the COMS trial, does preop EBRT improve outcomes over enucleation alone for COMS large tumors?	**No.** In the COMS trial, there was no OS or DFS difference between the 2 groups.

▶ TOXICITY

What are some early and late complications associated with plaque brachytherapy?	Early: pain, bleeding, diplopia, infection, edema Late: **retinopathy (42% at 5 yrs, increasing to 80%–90% thereafter)**, decreased visual acuity, cataracts, keratitis, optic neuropathy
The use of what agent has recently been associated with a lower incidence of macular edema after plaque brachytherapy?	**Triamcinolone** (periocular injections). In a RCT, macular edema rates were 58% in the control group vs. 36% in the triamcinolone arm (SS). (*Horgan N, Ophthalmology 2009*)

What % of pts have loss of ≥6 lines of vision 3 yrs after plaque brachytherapy?	**~50%** of pts have significant vision loss after plaque brachytherapy.
What % of pts have cataracts 5 yrs after plaque brachytherapy?	**83%** of pts develop cataracts after plaque brachytherapy.
How should pts treated with plaque brachytherapy be followed?	Plaque brachytherapy follow-up: H&P, ocular US q3mos × 1 yr, q4mos in 2nd yr, q6mos in 3rd and 4th yrs, then annually; CT C/A/P or liver US q6mos with LFTs (can detect >95% of mets)
Are periodic LFTs alone adequate to r/o liver mets?	**No.** There is very poor sensitivity (15%), PPV (46%), and NPV (71%), with a specificity of 92%. Adding liver US to LFTs increases the detection rate to 95%. (*Eskelin S et al., Cancer 1999*)
What is the best way to detect liver mets? What is the main disadvantage of this modality?	**PET/CT** is the best imaging modality for the detection of liver mets. The **cost and availability of such testing** are the main disadvantages.

25 Orbital and Intraocular Primary Eye Lymphomas

Updated by Randa Tao

▶ BACKGROUND

Under what type of lymphomas are intraocular/orbital lymphomas classified?	Intraocular/orbital lymphomas are classified as **non-Hodgkin lymphomas** (B-cell histology > T-cell histology).
What is the median age of onset? What are the 2 main types of eye lymphoma?	The median age of onset is **50–60 yrs** (females > males). The 2 main types are **intraocular and orbital/ocular adnexa lymphoma**.

What are the most common histologies?	Intraocular: usually diffuse large B-cell lymphoma Orbital: extranodal marginal zone B-cell lymphoma or mucosal-associated lymphoid tissue (MALT) lymphoma
Which structures are involved in intraocular vs. orbital lymphomas?	Intraocular lymphomas involve the neural structures. Orbital lymphomas can involve the conjunctiva, ocular adnexa, lacrimal apparatus, uvea, and retrobulbar areas.
What % of pts with primary intraocular lymphomas develop CNS Dz within 3 yrs?	**60%–80%** of pts with intraocular lymphomas develop CNS Dz.
What % of pts with primary CNS lymphomas develop intraocular involvement?	**25%** of pts with primary CNS lymphoma develop intraocular involvement.
What is the recurrence rate after Tx of intraocular lymphomas?	The recurrence rate after Tx is ~**50%**.
Intraocular lymphoma is bilat in what % of pts? How about orbital/adnexa lymphoma?	Intraocular: 80% Orbital: 20%
What is a common chromosomal translocation in intraocular lymphoma? What % of pts have this translocation?	**t(14;18)** is a common translocation in intraocular lymphoma. **56%** of pts have this translocation.
Ocular lymphoma cells are usually positive for which 2 important immunohistochemical markers?	Ocular lymphomas usually stain positive for **CD20** and **bcl-2.**
What type of lymphoma accounts for most lymphomas of the ocular adnexa?	**MALT lymphoma** accounts for most lymphomas of the ocular adnexa.
Which ocular lymphoma has a male predominance and is associated with mycosis fungoides?	**Ocular lymphoma of T-cell histology** occurs predominantly in males and is associated with mycosis fungoides.

With what infectious agent has orbital MALT been associated? What site is often involved?

Chlamydia psittaci has been associated with orbital MALT lymphomas. The **lacrimal gland** is often involved. Treatment with doxycycline alone in a phase II trial of 47 pts (89% with biopsy + *Chlamydia* DNA) resulted in a 5-year PFS of 55% and lymphoma regression in 65% of pts (*Ferreri AJ et al., JCO 2012*).

Lymphoma of what orbital structure has a high propensity for LN spread?

Lacrimal gland lymphoma has a high propensity for LN spread (>40% are LN+).

Which lymphomas have a better prognosis: orbital or intraocular?

Orbital lymphomas tend to be indolent, whereas intraocular lymphomas are aggressive with a high propensity for CNS involvement.

▶ WORKUP/STAGING

What are the common presenting Sx of ocular/ orbital lymphomas?

Blurred vision, floaters, pain (uveitis/vitreitis), proptosis (if retro-orbital), and orbital lesion (e.g., salmon-colored conjunctival mass).

What must the physical exam portion of the workup include?

The physical exam portion must include an **ophthalmologic exam** (fundoscopy, slit lamp exam) as part of the workup.

What lab/pathology tests are required during the workup?

CSF/vitrectomy, BM Bx, CBC, LFTs, ESR

What imaging is recommended for ocular/ orbital lesions?

MRI brain/orbits, ocular US, CT C/A/P (PET/CT if MALT: *Perry C et al., Eur J Haematol 2007*)

What staging system is used for eye lymphomas?

Ann Arbor staging system:

Stage IE: localized eye lymphomas
Stage II: cancer located in 2 separate regions
Stage III: cancer on both sides of diaphragm, including 1 organ or area near LNs or spleen
Stage IV: diffuse or disseminated involvement of ≥1 extralymphatic organs (e.g., liver, BM, or nodular involvement of lungs)

What is the most widely used classification system for lymphomas of the eye?

REAL (Revised European-American Classification of Lymphoid Neoplasms): 3 classes—indolent, aggressive, and highly aggressive

▶ TREATMENT/PROGNOSIS

What is the Tx paradigm for orbital lymphoma?

Orbital lymphoma Tx paradigm: **RT alone** (low grade) **or CRT** (if intermediate/high grade)

What RT doses are used for orbital lymphoma?	**19.5–24 Gy at 1.5 or 2 Gy** (MALT, low grade) or even **4 Gy in 2 fx ("boom-boom") can be used as a palliative dose,** and **30–36 Gy** (high grade, based on chemo response)
Does radiation alone offer high rates of local control for low-grade orbital lymphoma? What rates have been reported?	Yes. A retrospective series of 31 orbital MALT lymphoma patients at Stanford treated with 30–40 Gy achieved a 10-year LC of 100% and freedom from relapse of 71%; no dose response was observed as there was no difference in pts treated with >34 Gy vs. ≤34 Gy (*Le Q et al., IJROBP 2002*).
What is the Tx paradigm for intraocular lymphoma?	Intraocular lymphoma Tx paradigm: **chemo +/– RT.** These are treated more like primary CNS lymphomas.
What area is irradiated in intraocular lymphoma?	The **orbits (+/– whole brain)** are irradiated in intraocular lymphoma.
Which chemo agent is typically used for intraocular lymphomas?	High-dose **methotrexate** (Mtx). Intraocular/intravitreal Mtx and rituximab (Rituxan) are usually employed.
What chemo regimens are typically used for high-grade orbital/ocular adnexa lymphomas?	Cyclophosphamide HCl/doxorubicin/Oncovin/prednisone + Rituxan **(R-CHOP) or** cyclophosphamide/vincristine/Adriamycin/dexamethasone) **(CVAD)** are typically used for high-grade orbital lymphomas.
What is 1 additional option for refractory/relapsed Dz?	Radioimmunotherapy (RIT) with Bexxar (I-131) or Zevalin (Yttrium-90) is another option for refractory/relapsed Dz.
What RT technique can be utilized for ant (eyelid, conjunctival) lesions?	**Ant orthovoltage or electron fields** can be employed for ant eye lesions.
How is lens shielding accomplished with an ant orthovoltage field?	A lead shield is **suspended in the beam** to shield the lens (limits lens dose to 5%–10%).
What are some poor prognostic factors for ocular/orbital lymphomas?	High-grade Dz, advanced Dz (stage IVE), and symptomatic Dz

▶ **TOXICITY**

Above what cumulative dose (standard fractionation) is lens opacification seen?	Lens opacification is seen with doses >**13–16 Gy.**
What toxicities are associated with RIT?	Myelosuppression, myelodysplastic syndrome, and acute myeloid leukemia

What is the min dose to induce cataracts with a single fx vs. multiple fx of RT?	Doses of **2 Gy** (single fx) and **4–5 Gy** (multiple fx) can induce cataracts.
Is cataract induction a stochastic or deterministic late effect? Explain.	**Deterministic.** There is a threshold and the severity/latency are dose related.
Which region of the lens is affected most by RT?	The **postsubcapsular region of the lens** is affected most by RT.
What is the dose tolerance of the retina/optic nerves?	The maximum dose tolerance of retina/optic nerves is **45 Gy (retina) and 54 (optic nerve) Gy, respectively.**
What is the dose tolerance of the lacrimal glands?	The mean dose tolerance of the lacrimal apparatus is **26–30 Gy.**
Above what dose can painful keratitis be seen?	Doses >**60 Gy** can cause painful keratitis.

26 Thyroid Ophthalmopathy

Updated by Randa Tao

▶ BACKGROUND

What causes thyroid ophthalmopathy (TO)?	T-cell lymphocytic infiltration of orbital and periorbital tissues (secondary to autoimmune antibody–mediated reaction against the TSH receptor)
Name 2 conditions associated with TO.	**Graves Dz** and **Hashimoto thyroiditis** are both associated with TO.
What is the end result of untreated TO?	Untreated TO will lead to **fibrosis,** which develops over the course of 2–5 yrs.
What are the signs/Sx of TO?	Exophthalmos, impaired extraocular movements/diplopia, periorbital edema, and lid retraction. In severe cases, compression of the optic nerves and decreased visual acuity can occur.

> ## WORKUP/STAGING

What does the general workup of TO include?

TO workup: H&P (Hertel exophthalmometer to measure proptosis), CBC, CMP, TFTs, and CT/MRI orbit

What is the staging/risk stratification?

There is **no formal staging/risk stratification.** Studies have grouped pts into mild, moderately severe, and severe TO, though the exact definition of these terms varies between studies.

> ## TREATMENT/PROGNOSIS

What is the general Tx paradigm for TO?

TO Tx paradigm: Treat underlying disorder. For <u>mild Dz</u>, consider observation vs. RT; for <u>moderately severe Dz</u>, consider high-dose steroids (generally 1st-line treatment with response in up to 60% of pts) vs. RT; and for <u>severe Dz unresponsive to steroids</u>, perform orbital decompression surgery (e.g., for acute visual acuity or color perception changes as these are symptoms of optic nerve compression).

RT should be initiated within how many mos from onset of TO?

RT should be initiated **within 7 mos** of TO onset for pts who fail or have contraindications to high-dose steroids. Delayed RT is not as effective based on retrospective data.

What are 2 common contraindications to high-dose steroids in pts with TO?

Optic neuropathy and corneal ulceration are 2 contraindications to steroids in pts with TO.

What are the typical RT dose/fractionations for TO? What evidence supports these doses?

Typical RT dose/fractionations for TO:

1. **20 Gy in 2 Gy/fx** (most common)
2. **10 Gy in 1 Gy/fx**
3. **20 Gy in 1 Gy/fx/wk × 20 wks**

Kahaly et al. prospectively compared the 3 regimens above and found that all were equally effective (the latter 2 were better tolerated). (*J Clin Endocrinol Metab 2000*)

What beam arrangement is used for TO?

Opposed lats, half-beam block anteriorly to minimize divergence into contralateral lens.

What RT technique is used to minimize the dose to the contralat lens?

Place the isocenter posterior to lenses and the half-beam block anteriorly (limits divergence to contralat lens).

What structures define the post, sup, and ant borders of the RT fields?

<u>Posterior</u>: ant clinoids
<u>Sup/Ant</u>: bony orbit

In pts with moderately severe TO, what drug should be used concurrently with RT?	Continue or start **steroids** with RT, as pts can develop edema and worsening Sx.
What evidence is there to support RT for mild TO?	***Prummel MF et al.:*** A double-blind RCT of 88 pts with Graves: 44 rcvd RT vs. 44 sham RT. RT improved clinical Sx (response rate 52% for RT vs. 27% for sham RT). There was no improvement in the QOL survey and no reduction in overall Tx costs. (*J Clin Endocrinol Metab 2004*)
What evidence is there against RT for mild TO?	***Gorman CA et al.:*** In an RCT with crossover, RT was administered to 1 orbit and then the opposite orbit after 6 mos. At 6 mos, there was no difference in results for either eye. At 12 mos, there was minor improvement in the 1st treated eye. The authors concluded that RT was not justified. (*Ophthalmology 2001*)
What evidence is there to support RT for moderately severe TO?	***Premmel MF et al.:*** In an RCT, all pts with Graves rcvd RT vs. 3 mos of prednisone. RT and prednisone were equally effective, but RT was better tolerated. (*Lancet 1993*) ***Mourits MP et al.:*** In an RCT, all pts with Graves rcvd RT vs. sham RT. RT improved diplopia and elevation but not proptosis or eyelid swelling. It was concluded that RT should be used to treat motility impairment only. (*Lancet 2000*)
Would a pt with diplopia or proptosis be more likely to see an improvement in Sx after RT?	**Diplopia** (*Mourits MP et al., Lancet 2000*); also supported by recent meta-analysis (*Stiebel-Kalish H et al., J Clin Endocrinol Metab 2009*)
Estimate the response rate of TO pts to RT.	Response rates to RT are **50%–70%** in pts with TO. (*Prummel MF et al., J Clin Endocrinol Metab 2004; Kahaly GJ et al., J Clin Endocrinol Metab 2000*)
What % of TO pts will require further therapy after RT?	**50%–75%** of TO pts will require further therapy. (*Mourits MP et al., Lancet 2000; Gorman CA et al., Ophthalmology 2001*)

▶ TOXICITY

What are the late side effects of orbital RT?	Cataracts, permanent dry eye, retinopathy, and optic neuropathy
What is the RT dose limit of the lenses?	Try to limit the dose to <8–10 Gy to prevent cataracts.
What other disciplines/ specialists should be actively involved in the follow-up of pts with TO?	The ophthalmologist and the endocrinologist should be actively involved in the follow-up of pts with TO.

27 Orbital Pseudotumor

Updated by Randa Tao

▶ BACKGROUND

What is an orbital pseudotumor (OP)? What are 2 other terms for OP?

A benign inflammatory process causing a mass lesion in the orbit with mature polyclonal lymphocytes. 2nd most common cause of exophthalmos after thyroid ophthalmopathy. Other terms for OP:

1. Lymphoid hyperplasia
2. Pseudolymphoma

What is the eponym given to OP with cavernous sinus involvement?

Tolosa-Hunt syndrome is OP with cavernous sinus involvement.

What % of pts with OP will subsequently develop a malignant lymphoma?

5%–25% will subsequently develop a malignant lymphoma. (*Orcutt JC et al., Br J Ophthalmol 1983; Mittal BB et al., Radiology 1986*)

Does OP affect children, adults, or both?

OP affects **both children and adults.** 5%–15% are pediatric cases. (*Smitt MC et al., Semin Radiat Oncol 1999*)

Name 5 signs/Sx associated with OP.

Signs/Sx associated with OP:

1. Orbital mass
2. Orbital pain
3. Proptosis
4. Abnl extraocular movements (e.g., diplopia)
5. Decreased visual acuity

▶ WORKUP/STAGING

What is the DDx for an orbital mass?

Rhabdomyosarcoma, malignant orbital lymphoma, thyroid ophthalmopathy, and nodular fasciitis. OP is a Dx of exclusion.

What is the workup for an orbital mass?

The workup is the same as for a suspected orbital lymphoma, including CT/MRI brain/orbit and tissue diagnosis to r/o malignancy.

Is there a formal staging system for OP?

No. There is **no formal staging system** for OP.

▶ **TREATMENT/PROGNOSIS**

What is the initial Tx for OP?

Steroids are the mainstay initial Tx for OP. (*Smitt MC et al., Semin Radiat Oncol 1999*)

What are the response rate and long-term control rate with a single steroid course?

Response rate: 80%
Long-term control rate: 33%
(*Mombaerts I et al., Ophthalmology 1996*)

What is the 2nd-line therapy for OP?

RT is the 2nd-line therapy for OP for pts with contraindications or unacceptable toxicity to steroid therapy.

What is the most common RT dose/fx schedule for OP?

20 Gy in 10 fx is the most commonly employed schedule for OP.

What are the estimated control rates for OP with RT?

Control rates with RT range from **66%–100%**. (*Smitt MC et al., Semin Radiat Oncol 1999*)

What is the standard RT setup for OP?

There is no standard RT setup, as the process may involve any aspect of the orbit. Tx must be individualized.

Can RT be repeated for OP?

Yes. RT can be repeated, if necessary.

What are the late side effects of orbital RT?

Cataracts, permanent eye dryness, retinopathy, and optic neuropathy

What is the RT dose limit of the lens?

Try to limit the lens to **<8–10 Gy** depending on the clinical situation.

Diabetic pts are at an increased risk for what complication after orbital RT?

After orbital RT, diabetic pts are at an increased risk for **RT retinopathy.** (*Wakelkamp IM et al., Ophthalmology 2004*)

28 Nasopharyngeal Cancer

Updated by Eva N. Christensen

 BACKGROUND

What is the prevalence of nasopharyngeal cancer (NPC) in the U.S. vs. in Asian countries?	NPC is rare in the U.S. (0.2–0.5 in 100,000 cases) but endemic in Asia (25–50 in 100,000 cases).
What are the environmental risk factors associated with NPC?	Consumption of salted fish and preserved meats, EBV infection, and smoking for keratinizing squamous cell type (no alcohol association)
What is the median age at Dx for NPC?	~50 yrs.
What are the anatomic boundaries that make up the nasopharynx (NPX)?	Superior: sphenoid bone Inferior: soft palate Posterior: clivus/C1–2 Anterior: post edge of choanae
From what anatomic location do most NPCs arise?	**Fossa of Rosenmuller** (fossa post to the torus tubarius, which is the cartilaginous prominence in the lat wall of the NPX that forms the opening of the eustachian tube)
What is the local pattern of spread for NPC superiorly, inferiorly, posteriorly, laterally, and anteriorly?	Superiorly: invades (via the **foramen lacerum**) the cavernous sinus with predominantly CN VI involvement Inferiorly/posteriorly: oropharynx (OPX) Laterally: parapharyngeal space Anteriorly: nasal cavity
What 2 CN syndromes are commonly associated with NPC, and what CNs are involved in each?	Petrosphenoidal syndrome: CNs III–IV and VI involvement (oculomotor signs/Sx) Retroparotidian syndrome: CN IX–XII involvement

What CNs or structures traverse through the base of skull sinuses/foramina (e.g., cavernous sinus, foramen rotundum, ovale, lacerum, jugular, hypoglossal)?	Cavernous sinus: CNs III–IV, V1 and V2, and VI Foramen rotundum: V2 Foramen ovale: V3 Foramen lacerum: cartilage of the eustachian tube Jugular foramen: CNs IX–XI Hypoglossal canal: CN XII
What are the 3 WHO histologic subtypes of NPC, and what is the prevalence of each?	**WHO I:** keratinizing squamous cell carcinoma (SCC) (20%) **WHO II:** nonkeratinizing SCC (nondifferentiated) (30%–40%) **WHO III:** undifferentiated or lymphoepithelial (40%–50%)
Which WHO type of NPC is endemic and prone to distant recurrence?	**WHO III** (undifferentiated or lymphoepithelial) is endemic (better LC but more distant spread).
Which WHO type of NPC is associated with smoking and has poor LC but a lower propensity for DM?	**WHO I** (keratinizing SCC) is associated with smoking, poor LC, and less distant spread.
Which WHO type of NPC is most strongly associated with EBV exposure?	**WHO III**
With what autoimmune condition can NPC be associated?	**Dermatomyositis**
What histologic feature of NPC is an *adverse* prognostic factor in terms of LC and OS?	**Presence of keratin**
What role does p53 play in the pathogenesis of NPC?	p53 alteration is seen in the minority of cases (unlike other H&N cancers).
What is a commonality between NPX and OPX cancers?	Viral-associated tumors (EBV-NPX: HPV-OPX) have better local control but more distant spread compared to nonviral associated tumors in these regions.

▶ WORKUP/STAGING

What are some common presenting Sx in pts with NPC?	Neck mass (>60%); epistaxis, otalgia, and nasal congestion. Trismus and/or CN deficits are seen with more advanced Dz.

What is the workup for a pt who presents with a neck node and a suspicious mass in the NPX according to the NCCN guidelines?

H&P, nasopharyngolaryngoscopy and Bx of the lesion, MRI with gadolinium of base of skull, NPX, and neck to clavicles, CT of skull base/neck with contrast as indicated; dental, speech and swallow, and audiology evaluations as indicated, and PET scan or other imaging to evaluate for DM

What is the DDx for a pt with a nasopharyngeal mass?

Carcinoma, lymphoma, melanoma, plasmacytoma, angiofibroma, rhabdomyosarcoma (children), and mets

What % of NPC pts present with palpable LAD?

60%–90%

What % of NPC pts present with bilat LAD?

Up to **50%**

Adenopathy near the mastoid tip is indicative of involvement of which nodal group?

Retropharyngeal nodes (node of Rouviere)

Pts with upper-level V LAD are most likely to have what kind of H&N primary?

NPC

What factors predict for DM in pts with NPC?

Lower neck nodal involvement, advanced nodal stage, and WHO type III histology

What are the common DM sites for NPC?

Bones, lungs, liver, and brain

What correlates better with DM spread in NPC: N stage or T stage?

N stage

T Stage	Description
T1	NPX ± OPX ± nasal cavity
T2	Parapharyngeal extension (i.e., posterolateral extension beyond the pharyngobasilar fascia)
T3	Base of skull bones ± paranasal sinuses
T4	intracranial extension, CN involvement, hypopharynx, orbit, or infratemporal fossa/masticator space

N Stage	Description
N1	Unilat ≤6 cm ± retropharyngeal LN ≤6 cm (unilat or bilat)
N2	Bilat ≤ 6 cm
N3a	>6 cm
N3b	Extension to supraclavicular (SCV) fossa

What defines the SCV fossa?

The triangle of Ho, defined by 3 points:

1. The point where the neck meets the shoulder
2. (The superior margins of) the sternal end of the clavicle
3. (The superior margins of) the lateral end of the clavicle

How does the latest AJCC 7th edition (2011) staging of NPC differ from previous staging schemes?

According to the latest AJCC staging, T2a lesions are now T1; T2b lesions are now T2; old stage IIA is now stage I; and old stage IIB is now stage II. Retropharyngeal LN involvement is now considered N1 Dz.

Stage grouping:

	N0	N1	N2	N3
Tis	0	—	—	—
T1	I	II	III	IVB
T2	II	II	III	IVB
T3	III	III	III	IVB
T4	IVA	IVA	IVA	IVB

M1: stage group IVC

► TREATMENT/PROGNOSIS

What is the typical Tx paradigm for pts with NPC?

RT alone for stage I, CRT for stages II–IVB, chemotherapy (with RT reserved for focal palliation) for stage IVC

What must be done before planning the NPC pt for RT?

Nutrition consult, PEG tube placement, and dental evaluation are all recommended before RT.

When is surgery indicated in the management of NPC?

To Bx the lesion and in cases of elective neck dissection for persistent Dz after CRT.

For early-stage NPC, what are the typical survival and control rates with RT alone?

With RT alone, the 3-yr OS is **70%–100% for stage I–II NPC** and LC rates are **70%–80% for T1–T2 lesions.**

What stages of NPC should be treated with concurrent chemoradiotherapy?

Per the **Intergroup 0099 study** (*Al Sarraf M et al., JCO 1998*), all T3–T4 or N+ pts should be considered for CRT. Per **RTOG 0225** (*Lee N et al., JCO 2009*), all pts with ≥T2b (old staging) or T2 (new staging) and N+ Dz should be considered.

What was the CRT regimen used for locally advanced NPC in the Intergroup 0099 (Al-Sarraf et al.) study?

Concurrent chemo with **cisplatin IV 100 mg/m²
days 1, 22, and 43** and **RT to 70 Gy** → adj chemo with cisplatin/5-FU × 3 cycles

What were the PFS and OS outcomes in the Intergroup 0099 (Al-Sarraf et al.) trial?

In **Intergroup 0099,** 3-yr PFS was 24% vs. 69%, and **3-yr OS was 46% vs. 76%** in favor of CRT over RT alone. B/c of these remarkable results, the study was closed early. This was 1 of the 1st studies to demonstrate a survival benefit with CRT.

What are the main criticisms of the Intergroup 0099 (Al-Sarraf et al.) study?

Major criticisms of **Intergroup 0099** include the large number (25%) of pts with WHO type I NPC (not typically seen in endemic areas) and the poor results of the RT alone arm. Single-institution studies with RT alone (Princess Margaret Hospital: *Chow E et al., Radiother Oncol 2002*) for locally advanced NPC had better 5-yr DFS (48%) and OS (62%). Other groups (New York University: *Cooper JS et al., IJROBP 2000*) also demonstrated better outcomes with RT alone (3-yr DFS was 43%, and 3-yr OS was 61%).

What are the 3 key confirmatory randomized trials from Asia that demonstrated a benefit with CRT vs. RT alone for locoregionally (LRC) advanced NPC?

Hong Kong (**NPC-9901:** *Lee AW et al., JCO 2005*): 348 pts, RCT, median follow-up 2.3 yrs; concurrent cisplatin + RT, <u>no adj chemo</u>; better DFS (72% vs. 62%), LRC (92% vs. 82%), but not DM or OS; greater toxicity in the CRT arm (84% vs. 53%); greater otologic toxicity (28% vs. 13%)

Singapore (**SQNP01:** *Wee J et al., JCO 2005*): 221 pts, RCT, median follow-up 3.2 yrs; <u>used</u> **Al-Sarraf** <u>regimen</u>: better DFS (72% vs. 53%), OS (80% vs. 65%), and DM rate (13% vs. 30%); greater toxicity with CRT; confirmed results of **Intergroup 0099** for endemic NPC

Taiwan (*Lin JC et al., JCO 2003*): 284 pts, median follow-up 5.4 yrs; cisplatin/5-FU + RT vs. RT alone: better PFS (72% vs. 53%) and OS (72% vs. 54%). The subgroup reanalysis (*Lin JC et al., IJROBP 2004*) showed that CRT benefited low-risk "advanced" NPC (LN <6 cm, no SCV) but not high-risk "advanced" pts.

Is there a benefit with the use of induction chemo followed by RT or CRT in NPC?

No. Multiple RCTs in Asia demonstrated no benefit in terms of DFS, OS, or DM with induction chemo.

Is there a benefit with the use of adj chemo after definitive RT or CRT in NPC?

No. Multiple RCTs in Asia and 1 Italian study did not demonstrate a benefit with adj chemo.

Estimate the LC of NPC treated with IMRT to 70 Gy in standard fx.

UCSF data (*Lee N, IJROBP 2004*) suggests LC rates as high as 97% for NPC pts treated with IMRT.

What is the typical IMRT dose painting technique, and what are the corresponding IMRT doses used in the Tx of NPC?

Many institutions (MSKCC/RTOG) employ the simultaneous integrated boost technique: **2.12 Gy × 33 = 69.96 Gy** to GTV, **1.8 Gy × 33 = 59.4 Gy** to intermediate-risk areas, and **1.64 Gy × 33 = 54 Gy** to low-risk areas.

How would you support the use of IMRT in NPC?

Better salivary outcomes with IMRT were demonstrated in data from Queen Mary Hospital (*Pow EH et al., IJROBP 2006*): 51 pts, stage II NPC, 2D vs. IMRT. At 2 mos, there was no difference in xerostomia; however, over time, QOL and objective salivary function improved for the IMRT group.

▶ **TOXICITY**

What are the RTOG 0225 dose constraints for the chiasm/optic nerves when using IMRT for NPC?

Per **RTOG 0225,** the dose constraints for the chiasm/optic nerves are **54 Gy** or 1% of the PTV not >60 Gy.

What are the accepted RTOG 0225 dose constraints for the parotids?

Per **RTOG 0225,** the dose constraints for the parotids are as follows: mean dose **<26 Gy** (should be achieved in at least 1 gland) or at least 20 cc of the combined volume of both parotid glands <20 Gy or at least 50% of 1 gland <30 Gy.

Why might sparing of the parotid glands not be sufficient to prevent xerostomia?	Sparing of the parotids alone may not be sufficient b/c **mucus production by minor salivary glands may be necessary for subjective improvement,** according to data from Prince of Wales Hospital (*Kam MK et al., JCO 2007*): 60 pts randomized to IMRT or 2D-RT. Objective improvement in both stimulated and unstimulated salivary flow was found, but not in the subjective improvement of xerostomia.
What is the RTOG 0615 dose constraint for the brainstem?	**54 Gy max dose** to the true structure, ≤1% of the planning risk volume (the volume that is at least 1 mm larger than the true brainstem) to exceed **60 Gy**
What is the follow-up paradigm for NPC pts?	NPC follow-up paradigm: H&P with nasopharyngolaryngoscopy (q1–3mos for yr 1, q2–4mos for yr 2, q4–6mos for yrs 3–5, and q6–12mos if >5 yrs), imaging (for signs/Sx), TSH (if neck irradiated), speech/hearing/dental evaluation, and smoking cessation

29 Sinonasal Tract Tumors

Updated by Vinita Takiar and Gopal K. Bajaj

▶ BACKGROUND

What is the incidence of sinonasal tract (SNT) tumors in the U.S.?	~**2,000 cases/yr** of SNT tumors (<1% of all tumors)
Is there a sex predilection for SNT tumors?	**Yes. Males** are more commonly affected than females (2:1).
SNT tumors are more common in what continents?	SNT tumors are more prevalent in **Asia and Africa.**
What histologies are typically seen with SNT tumors?	**Squamous (70%),** adenocarcinoma, adenoid cystic, melanoma, esthesioneuroblastoma (ENB), sinonasal undifferentiated (SNUC), small cell, sarcoma (rhabdomyosarcoma), lymphoma, plasmacytoma, and mets

What nonmalignant entities present as a mass in the paranasal sinuses (PNS) or the nasal cavity?	Sinonasal polyposis, choanal polyps, and juvenile angiofibromas
What sinuses make up the PNS?	The **frontal, ethmoid, sphenoid, and maxillary** sinuses make up the PNS.
What structures border the maxillary sinus?	Anterior: facial bone Anterolateral: zygomatic arch Posterolateral: infratemporal fossa Posterior: pterygopalatine fossa Superior: orbital floor Inferior: hard palate Medial: nasal cavity
What is the name for the thin bone in the medial wall of the orbit that is prone to erosion/breakthrough by ethmoid tumors?	The thin bone of the medial orbital wall is called the **lamina papyracea.**
What is the local invasion pattern of ethmoid tumors?	**Superiorly** through the cribriform plate to the ant cranial fossa or **medially** through the lamina papyracea into the orbit
Which is the most common sinus/site of origin for SNT tumors?	The **maxillary sinus** is the most commonly involved sinus/site for SNT tumors (70%–80%).
What is the most common site for ENB?	The **nasal cavity** is the most common site for ENB.
What environmental exposures are associated with the development of SNT tumors?	**Industrial fumes, wood dust,** nickel, chromium, hydrocarbons, nitrogen mustard

▶ WORKUP/STAGING

What are some presenting Sx of SNT tumors?	Facial pain, nasal obstruction, nasal discharge, epistaxis, sinus obstruction, trismus (pterygoid involvement), ocular deficits (diplopia, blurry vision), facial pain due to trigeminal neuralgia, midfacial hypesthesia from impingement of the infraorbital branch of CN V2, palatal mass/erosion, and otalgia
What is the basic workup for SNT tumors?	SNT tumor workup: H&P, labs, CT/MRI head/neck, Bx, and CT chest, dental consult if required (per NCCN, 2013)

Describe the T staging of maxillary tumors per the latest AJCC (7ᵗʰ edition, 2011) classification.

T1: confined to sinus, no bone erosion
T2: bone erosion *without* involvement of posterior wall of maxillary sinus or pterygoid plate
T3: invasion of posterior wall of max sinus, pterygoid fossa, floor/wall of orbit, ethmoid sinus
T4a: invasion of ant orbital structures, skin of cheek, pterygoid plate, infratemporal fossa, cribriform plate, sphenoid or frontal sinus
T4b: invasion of orbital apex, nasopharynx, clivus, intracranial extension, CN involvement (except V2), dura, brain

How are the nodes staged for SNT tumors?

N1: single, ipsi, ≤3 cm
N2a: single, ipsi, >3 and ≤6 cm
N2b: multiple, ipsi, ≤6 cm
N2c: bilat or contralat ≤6 cm
N3: >6 cm

How are the overall SNT stage groups broken down (based on TNM)?

Stage I: T1N0
Stage II: T2N0
Stage III: T3N0 or T1–3N1
Stage IVA: T4aN0–2 or T1–3N2
Stage IVB: T4b or N3
Stage IVC: M1

What is the T stage for a maxillary tumor with involvement of the pterygoid plate vs. the pterygoid fossa?

Pterygoid **plate** involvement: **T4a**
Pterygoid **fossa** involvement: **T3**

What is the Ohngren line, and why is it important?

The Ohngren line is a theoretic plane that extends **from the medial canthus of the eye to the angle of the mandible.** Tumors superoposterior to this line have deeper invasion, with many being unresectable (due to invasion of the orbit, ethmoids, and pterygopalatine fossa). The relationship of a tumor to Ohngren's line was an important prognostic factor, but with CT, MRI, and PET for imaging tumors, the significance of this line is principally historic.

For SNT tumors, what factors predict for nodal mets?

Neck nodal involvement is uncommon at Dx except **when tumors have progressed to involve the mucosal surfaces** (i.e., oral cavity, maxillary gingiva, or gingivobuccal sulcus). Histology is also predictive; squamous and undifferentiated tumors most commonly present with nodes, while nodal disease is very uncommon with adenoid cystic and adenocarcinomas.

What neck node groups are generally involved with SNT tumors?

Level Ib, II, retropharyngeal (1st echelon), and periparotid nodes are most commonly involved.

What subsite of SNT tumors has the highest rate of nodal mets?	**Maxillary sinus tumors** have the highest rate of nodal mets (10%–15%) of all SNT tumors.
What is the 5-yr OS rate for maxillary/ethmoid sinus tumors (all stages)?	The 5-yr OS rate for all stages of SNT tumors is **~45%**
What is the 5-yr OS rate for N+ maxillary sinus tumors?	The 5-yr OS rate for N+ maxillary sinus tumors is **<10%.**
What is the 5-yr OS rate for nasal cavity tumors (all stages)?	The 5-yr OS rate for all stages of nasal cavity tumors is **~60%.**
What is the overall LC rate for SNT tumors?	The overall LC rate is **50%–60%.**

▶ TREATMENT/PROGNOSIS

How are SNT tumors typically managed?	**Surgical resection and adj RT +/– chemo.** Consider induction chemo in SNUCs or in very advanced primary squamous carcinomas.
What type of surgery is necessary to manage a maxillary sinus tumor?	**Partial** (2 walls of maxilla removed) **or total maxillectomy to – margins.** For smaller tumors, endoscopic sinus surgery (ESS), with or without robotic assistance, is replacing open procedures. For larger medial tumors, a medial maxillectomy with a midfacial degloving technique is performed with an incision made under the lip (Caldwell-Luc). For tumors that are mainly inferior, an infrastructure maxillectomy is often performed. For larger tumors, access through the nasal crease/upper lip may be necessary. Tumors involving the orbital floor or orbit often require orbital exenteration. Reconstruction is done with skin grafting and obturator placement. Larger defects are filled with free flaps.
How are ethmoid sinus tumors managed surgically?	Ethmoid sinus tumors are surgically managed by either ESS for small tumors or **craniofacial resection,** requiring access both anteriorly through the sphenoethmoid area (through the nose) and superiorly with a craniotomy (neurosurgery) to address the skull base/dura.
When is orbital exenteration necessary in SNT tumors, and when is it not absolutely necessary?	It is **necessary if periorbital fat or extraocular muscles are involved.** It is **not necessary if there is only bone erosion.**

What are some indications for definitive radiotherapy in the management of SNT tumors?

Inoperable tumors (medically and technically)

What are the indications for adj radiotherapy after resection of SNT tumors?

Maxillary sinus T3–T4 lesions, ethmoid sinus T1–T4 lesions (per NCCN 2013), N+, + or close margins, +PNI, high-grade histology

How is radiotherapy delivered and to what dose?

IMRT, FSR, or SRS approaches, to **70 Gy (definitively) or 60–66 Gy (adj), to the tumor bed and margins; 50–56 Gy to low-risk areas.** Use image fusion (MRI/CT) for planning purposes.

Per the NCCN, what altered RT fractionation regimens can be employed for maxillary sinus tumors when definitive radiation is delivered without chemotherapy?

Per **NCCN (2013):**
  Accelerated (6 fx/wk during wks 2–6): 70 Gy for
    gross Dz and >50 Gy for subclinical Dz
  Concomitant boost (bid last 2 wks): 72 Gy over
    6 wks (1.8 Gy/fx large field and 1.5 Gy/fx
    same-day boost over last 2 wks)
  Hyperfractionated: 1.2 Gy/fx bid to 81.6 Gy
    over 7 wks

Is concurrent chemo a standard approach in the definitive management of SNT tumors with RT?

No. Prospective trials are evaluating CRT, and it can certainly be considered based on principles for other head and neck cancers for which concurrent chemotherapy is recommended (stages 3–4 treated definitively, or + margins or nodes with ECE in the adj setting)

For which tumors should elective neck management be considered (with surgery or RT)?

Elective neck management should be strongly considered for **tumors with squamous or undifferentiated histology and for T3 or T4 tumors of other histologies.** It is controversial for ENB, though recommended by many centers. It may be left out for other subsites with N0 Dz.

What studies/data support the use of ENI for maxillary sinus tumors?

Stanford data *(Le QT et al., IJROBP 2000)*: 97 pts (36 RT alone, 61 surgery + RT), 12% nodal failure overall in levels I–II; 5-yr nodal failure risk 20% – ENI, 0% +ENI; 5-yr distant relapse rate 29% with neck control, 81% if neck failure
MDACC data *(Bristol I et al., IJROBP 2007)* SCC/undifferentiated: nodal failure 36% in 36 patients without ENI vs 7% in 45 patients with ENI

What have recent studies demonstrated regarding the use of adj IMRT for SNT tumors?

There was **no significant improvement in terms of LC or OS;** however, there was a lower incidence of complications with IMRT. *(Madani I et al., IJROBP 2009; Dirix P et al., IJROBP 2010)*

What is the RT dose tolerance of the retina?	The maximum RT dose tolerance of the retina is **45–50 Gy.**
What is the RT dose tolerance of the optic chiasm?	The maximum RT dose tolerance of the chiasm is **50–54 Gy.**
What is the RT dose tolerance of the parotids?	The RT dose constraints for the parotids are as follows: **mean dose <26 Gy or V30 Gy <50%.**
What is the RT dose tolerance of the lacrimal gland?	The RT dose tolerance of the lacrimal gland is mean dose **<26–30 Gy,** similar to that of other glands (e.g., the parotids).
Describe the recommended follow-up schedule for pts treated for SNT tumors.	SNT tumor follow-up (per **NCCN** 2013): H&P (q1–3mos for yr 1, q2–4mos for yr 2, q4–6mos for yrs 4–6, and q6–12mos thereafter), baseline CT/MRI after Tx and regular chest imaging if indicated clinically, TSH every 6–12 mos if neck RT

30 Oral Cavity Cancer

Updated by Anna O. Likhacheva and Gopal K. Bajaj

► BACKGROUND

What is the incidence of oral cavity cancer (OCC) in the U.S.?	**~24,000 cases/yr** of OCC in the U.S.
What % of H&N cancers are OCCs?	OCCs comprise **25%–30%** of all H&N cancers.
Of what structures does the oral cavity (OC) consist?	Lips, gingiva, alveolus, buccal mucosa, retromolar trigone (RMT), hard palate, floor of mouth (FOM), and oral tongue
What is the most and least commonly involved site in OCC?	The lower **lip is the most common site** (38%), and the **buccal mucosa is the least common site** (2%). The tongue is involved 22% of the time. (*Krolls S. O. et al., J Am Dent Assn, 1976*)

What CNs provide motor and sensory innervation to the oral tongue?	<u>Motor</u>: CN XII <u>Sensory</u>: CN V (lingual branch)
What CNs provide the tongue with taste sensation?	<u>Ant two-thirds of tongue</u>: CN VII (chorda tympani) <u>Posterior one-third of tongue</u>: CN IX
Which nerve provides motor innervation to the lips?	The **facial nerve** (CN VII) provides motor innervation to the lips.
Where is the ant-most border of the OC?	The **vermilion border of the lips** is the ant-most border of the OC.
Where is the posterior-most border of the OC?	The **hard/soft palate border superiorly and the circumvallate papillae inferiorly** are the posterior-most borders of the OC.
What are some premalignant lesions of the OC, and which type has the greatest propensity to progress to invasive cancer?	**Erythroplakia** (~30% progression rate) **and leukoplakia** (4%–18% progression rate) are premalignant lesions of the OC.
What are some risk factors that predispose to OCC?	Tobacco (smoked or chewed), betel nut consumption, alcohol, poor oral hygiene, HPV infection, and vitamin A deficiency
What are the sup and inf spans of levels II–IV LN chains/levels?	<u>Level II</u>: skull base to bottom of hyoid <u>Level III</u>: bottom of hyoid to bottom of cricoid <u>Level IV</u>: bottom of cricoid to clavicles
Where are the levels IA–IB nodes located?	Level IA nodes are **submental,** and level IB nodes are **submandibular.**
Where are the levels V–VI nodes located?	Level V nodes are in the **posterior triangle,** and level VI nodes are in the **paratracheal/prelaryngeal region.**
What is the Delphian node?	The Delphian node is a **midline prelaryngeal level VI node.**
What is the estimated risk of LN involvement with a T1–T2 primary of the lip, FOM, oral tongue, and buccal mucosa?	The risk of LN involvement is **~5% for the lip, 20% for the oral tongue, and 10%–20% for the other OC T1–T2 primaries.**
What is the estimated risk of LN involvement with a T3–T4 primary of the lip, FOM, oral tongue, and buccal mucosa?	The risk of LN involvement is **~33% for the lip and 33%–67% for the other OC T3–T4 primaries.**

What is the nodal met rate for a T1 vs. T2 lesion of the oral tongue?

The nodal met rate is **14% for T1 tongue lesions and 30% for T2 tongue lesions.** (*Lindberg R et al., Cancer 1972*)

What is the overall and stage-by-stage nodal met rate for FOM lesions?

Overall: 20%–30%
T1: 10%
T2: 30%
T3: 45%
T4: >50%

(*Lindberg R et al., Cancer 1972*)

Lesions located where in the OC predispose to bilat LN mets?

Midline and anterolat OC lesions (tongue, FOM) predispose to bilat LN mets.

Which OC cancer has the greatest propensity for LN spread?

Oral tongue cancer has the greatest propensity for LN spread.

What OC subsite is 2nd only to the oral tongue in propensity for nodal spread?

The **alveolar ridge/RMT** has the 2nd highest propensity for LN spread (3rd highest is FOM).

Can ant oral tongue lesions involve other LN levels without involving level I LNs?

Yes. ~13% of ant tongue lesions skip the level I LNs. (*Byers RM et al., Head Neck 1997*)

Which anatomic structure divides the oral tongue from the base of tongue (BOT)?

The **circumvallate papillae** divide the oral tongue from the BOT (per the AJCC 7th edition, 2011). Some use the sulcus terminalis as the border.

What is the most common site of minor salivary cancers?

Hard palate

What are common sites of DM for cancers of the OC?

Lungs, bones, and liver

What anatomic structure divides the FOM anteriorly into 2 halves?

The **lingual frenulum** divides the FOM anteriorly.

Where is the Wharton duct located, and what gland does it drain?

The Wharton duct **opens at the ant FOM** (midline) and **drains the submandibular gland.**

From where in the OC do most gingival cancers arise?

Most (80%) gingival cancers arise from the **lower gingiva.**

Do most lip cancers arise from the upper or lower lip?

Most (~90%) lip cancers arise from the **lower lip.**

What are some benign lesions that arise from the lip?

Benign lip lesions include **keratoacanthoma, actinic keratosis, hemangiomas, fibromas, HSV, and chancre.**

What nodal groups drain the tip of the tongue, the ant tongue, and the post tongue?

Tip of tongue: level IA
Anterior tongue: level IB and level III (midjugular)
Posterior tongue: level IB and level II

Which OC site lesions are notorious for skipped nodal mets?

Anterior oral tongue lesions can skip levels II–III and involve only level IV (so a full neck dissection is typically needed).

What features of lip cancer predict for nodal spread?

DOI, high grade, large size, invasion of buccal mucosa/dermis, or recurrent Dz after resection

What nodal stations are involved with upper vs. lower lip lesions?

Upper lip lesions spread to preauricular, facial, parotid, and IA–IB LNs; lower lip lesions spread to levels IA–IB and level II LNs.

▶ WORKUP/STAGING

A pt presents with tongue deviation to the left. What CN is involved?

The **left CN XII** (hypoglossal) is involved with left tongue deviation (deviation is toward the involved nerve).

A pt presents with an OC lesion and ipsi ear pain. What nerve is responsible?

The **auricotemporal nerve** (branch of **CN V3**) causes ear pain in OCC.

Which lesions in the OC are most and least likely to present with +LNs?

Most likely: tongue, FOM
Least likely: lips, buccal mucosa, gingiva

What are some common presenting signs with OC lesions?

Asymptomatic red/raised lesion, ill-fitting dentures, bleeding mass, pain, dysphagia (due to tongue fixation), trismus (pterygoid/masticator space involvement), and otalgia

What does the typical workup of OC lesions entail?

OC lesion workup: H&P with palpation, direct endoscopy + Bx, CBC, CMP, CT/MRI H&N, and CT or PET/CT

What is the DDx for lesions of the OC?

Squamous cell carcinoma (SCC), minor salivary gland tumors, lymphoma, melanoma, sarcoma, plasmacytoma, and ameloblastoma

What defines T1–T3 lesions of the OC?

T1: <2 cm
T2: 2–4 cm
T3: >4 cm

What defines T4a vs. T4b lesions of the OC?	**T4a:** invasion of adjacent structures (bone, deep tongue muscles, maxillary sinus), resectable **T4b:** very advanced (invasion of masticator space, pterygoid plates, skull base, carotid artery) and typically unresectable
What is the nodal staging breakdown for OCC?	The nodal staging breakdown is the same system used for other H&N cancers (except for that of the nasopharynx): **N1:** single, ipsi, ≤3 cm **N2a:** single, ipsi, >3 cm, ≤6 cm **N2b:** multiple, ipsi, ≤6 cm **N2c:** bilat or contralat, ≤6 cm **N3:** >6 cm
What defines stages I–II OCC?	**N0 OCC** is either stage I or II (T1N0 or T2N0).
What defines stage III Dz in the OC?	**T3N0** or **T1–3N1** OC lesions are considered stage III.
What defines stages IVA–IVC OCC?	<u>Stage IVA</u>: T4a or N2 Dz <u>Stage IVB</u>: T4b or N3 Dz <u>Stage IVC</u>: M1 Dz
If RT is anticipated for OCC, what should be done and when should it be done before starting Tx?	Dental evaluation (teeth extractions, fluoride trays) should be done 10–14 days before RT.
What is the most common location involved in oral tongue cancers?	The **lat undersurface of the tongue in the middle to posterior 3rd** is most commonly involved.
What is the overall bilat nodal involvement rate for oral tongue cancers?	**5%** of oral tongue cancers present with bilat neck Dz (most nodal Dz is ipsi). If N1–N2 ipsi Dz, there is an ~30% risk for bilat Dz.
What 2 factors are most predictive of nodal involvement in oral tongue cancers?	**DOI and tumor thickness** (not T stage) are most predictive of LN mets in oral tongue cancers.
What are the 2 most important prognostic factors after surgery alone for buccal mucosa cancers?	**DOI ≥3 mm or tumor thickness ≥6 mm** are the most important prognostic factors for buccal mucosa cancers. (*Urist MM et al., Am J Surg 1987*)

▶ **TREATMENT/PROGNOSIS**

In general, what is the Tx paradigm for OCC?

OCC Tx paradigm: **surgery +/− PORT (+/− chemo)**

What pathologic features of the OCC primary lesion call for prophylactic/elective neck management?

Tumor thickness >2 mm, grade III Dz, +LVI, lower alveolar ridge and RMT, and a recurrent lesion are features that increase the need for prophylactic neck management.

What are the indications for PORT?

>N2a (>3-cm LN), low neck nodes or >2 LN levels, T3/T4, close margins, no neck dissection in high-risk pts, DOI >2mm, and LVI, PNI are indications for PORT.

In what circumstances should chemo be added to PORT?

Chemo should be administered with RT if there is a **+margin, +ECE** (per Bernier and Cooper adjuvant RCT of PORT vs. PORT + chemotherapy) (*Bernier J et al., NEJM 2004, Bernier J et al., J Head Neck 2005 and Cooper JS et al., IJROBP 2012*).

When is bilat neck dissection recommended for lesions of the OC?

Bilat neck dissection is recommended with **≥N2c Dz** (bilat or bulky LNs).

For what OC sites is definitive RT preferred and why?

Definitive RT is preferred (over surgery) for **lip commissure and RMT lesions with tonsillar pillar involvement.**

What is considered a close margin?

<5 mm

What are the indications for PORT to the primary site for OC lesions?

+ or close margin, PNI/perivascular invasion, and T3–T4 Dz are indications for PORT.

What RT doses are typically used in OCC?

<u>PORT</u>: **60 Gy** (−margins) to **66 Gy** (+margins) in 2 Gy/fx
<u>Definitive RT</u>: **70 Gy** to gross Dz +/− chemo

When is brachytherapy indicated for OCC?

<u>Definitive</u>: early (T1–T2) lip/early oral tongue/FOM lesions—LDR to **66–70 Gy** in 1 Gy/hr
<u>As a supplement</u>: T4 tongue/FOM lesions, 40% of total dose or **~30 Gy**

For oral tongue lesions, which modality is associated with better LC: LDR or HDR?

Both modalities yield similar results. 5-yr LC was 76%–77% for both HDR and LDR techniques in a phase III comparison. (*Inoue T et al., IJROBP 2001*)

What are the common LDR and HDR doses used with an interstitial implant for OCC?

<u>LDR</u>: 60–70 Gy (0.4–0.6 Gy/hr)
<u>HDR</u>: 60 Gy (5 Gy bid × 12 fx)

What alternate teletherapy modalities can be employed for superficial OC lesions?

An **intraoral cone** can be employed for superficial OC lesions: orthovoltage (100–250 keV) or electrons (6–12 MeV).

Why is a tongue depressor/bite block used when irradiating the OC?

A tongue depressor is used to **spare the sup OC/hard palate and to surround the lat oral tongue lesion with other mucosa** to minimize air tissue interfaces and maximize dose buildup.

What kind of surgical resection is typically performed for leukoplakia or CIS of the lip?

Vermilionectomy with advancement of the mucosal flap ("lip shave"), which involves simple excision from the vermilion to the orbicularis muscle

When is surgery an option for cancers of the lip?

Surgery is an option **if the lesion involves <30% of the lip, if it is a T1 lesion, or the lesion does *not* involve the oral commissure;** otherwise, use RT. Surgery is typically WLE with primary closure (W-shaped excision) and with a 0.5-cm gross margin.

When is definitive RT used for cancers of the lip?

Definitive RT is used for lip tumors **>2 cm, large lesions (>50% of the lip), upper lip lesions, or if the lesion involves the oral commissure.**

Is elective nodal RT of the neck required for T1–T2 cancers of the lip?

No. Elective nodal RT is not needed b/c the occult nodal positivity rate is only ~5%.

What are the doses used for the Tx of T1–T2 cancers of the lip?

T1: 50 Gy (2.5 Gy × 20)
T2: 60 Gy (2.5 Gy × 24) with 100–250 keV
photons or 6–9 MeV electrons + 1-cm bolus

When is PORT indicated for lip cancers?

PORT is indicated for lip cancers in case of **T4 Dz (bone invasion), +margin, extensive PNI, +ECE, ≥2 nodes+, or T3–T4 Dz without dissection of the neck.**

What randomized evidence supports PORT over surgery alone for stages III–IV SCC of the buccal mucosa?

Indian data. *Mishra RC et al.* showed improved 3-yr DFS with PORT (68% vs. 38%). (*Eur J Surg Oncol 1996*)

Is bilat neck RT required for stage III–IV buccal mucosa lesions?

No. Ipsi RT may be sufficient for stages III–IV buccal mucosa lesions. (*Lin CY et al., IJROBP 2008*)

What must the PORT field include for gingival lesions with PNI?

PORT fields for gingival lesions with PNI must include the **entire hemimandible** (from the mental foramen to the temporomandibular joint).

What randomized data support the need for PORT for OC lesions based on specific risk factors?

MDACC series (*Ang KK et al., IJROBP 2001*): pts with a +margin, PNI, and ECE had higher failure rates.

For RMT/alveolar ridge tumors, in what circumstances is RT preferred over surgery and vice versa?

Definitive RT preferred if there is no bone erosion or if the lesion extends to the ant tonsillar pillar, soft palate, or buccal mucosa. If there is bone erosion, then surgery is preferred → PORT.

What is the preferred management approach for hard palate lesions?

Generally, initial surgery is preferred for all cases, except if there is extension to the soft palate or RMT, in which case definitive RT can be considered.

Per NCCN guidelines, what is the recommended time interval between surgery and PORT for OCC?

Per **NCCN** guidelines, the recommended time interval between surgery and PORT for OCC is **6 wks.**

▶ TOXICITY

Why is brachytherapy generally avoided for gingival lesions?

There is a **high risk of osteoradionecrosis** with brachytherapy for gingival lesions.

To avoid malnutrition during a course of RT or CRT, pts need at least how many calories/day?

To avoid malnutrition during a course of RT or CRT, pts need at least **2,000 calories/day**

The mandible should be kept at or below what RT dose?

The maximum mandibular RT dose should be **≤70 Gy.**

What does the follow-up for OCC pts entail?

OCC follow-up: H&P + laryngoscopy (q1–3mos for yr 1, q2–4mos for yr 2, q4–6mos for yrs 3–5, and q6–12mos if >5 yrs), imaging (for signs/Sx), annual TSH (if the neck is irradiated), speech/hearing/dental evaluation, and smoking cessation

31 Oropharyngeal Cancer

Updated by Gary V. Walker

▶ BACKGROUND

What is the incidence of oropharyngeal cancer (OPC) in the U.S.?
~**36,000 cases/yr** of OPC in the U.S. with 6,850 deaths (2013 data)

How does the incidence of OPC compare to that of other H&N sites?
The incidence of **OPC is increasing,** whereas **cancer of other H&N sites is decreasing.**

Is there a sex predilection for OPC?
Yes. Males are more commonly affected than females (3:1).

What are the 4 subsites of the oropharynx (OPX)?
Soft palate, tonsils, base of tongue (BOT), and pharyngeal wall

From which subsite do most OPCs arise?
The **tonsil** (ant tonsil pillar and fossa) is the most common primary site.

What are the borders of the OPX?
Anterior: oral tongue/circumvallate papillae
Superior: hard palate/soft palate junction
Inferior: valleculae
Posterior: pharyngeal wall
Lateral: tonsil

What 3 structures make up the walls of the tonsillar fossa?
Walls of the tonsillar fossa:
1. Ant tonsillar pillar (palatoglossus muscle)
2. Post tonsillar pillar (palatopharyngeus muscle)
3. Inf glossotonsillar sulcus

What are the 4 most important risk factors for the development of OPC?
Risk factors for developing OPC:
1. Smoking
2. Alcohol
3. HPV infection (up to 80% of cases now)
4. Betel nut consumption

What is the 1st-echelon drainage region for most OPCs?
The 1st-echelon drainage site for most OPCs is the **level II (upper jugulodigastric) nodes.**

Are skipped mets common for OPC?
No. Skipped mets are **extremely rare** in OPC (<1%).

What are the 2 most common histologies encountered in the OPX? Rare histologies?
Most common histologies: squamous cell carcinoma (SCC) (90%), non-Hodgkin lymphoma (10% tonsil, 2% BOT)
Rare histologies: lymphoepithelioma, adenoid cystic carcinoma, plasmacytoma, melanoma, small cell carcinoma, mets

What proportion of pts with OPC fail locoregionally vs. distantly?

1:1 proportion of locoregional:distant failures

How prevalent is HPV infection in OPC?

Depending on the series, **40%–80%** of OPCs are associated with HPV infection.

Which HPV serotype is most commonly associated with OPC?

HPV 16 is the most common serotype in OPC (80%–90%).

What is a surrogate marker of HPV infection in OPC that can be used as an indirect indication of HPV seropositivity?

The surrogate marker for HPV infection is **p16 staining;** E7 protein inactivates Rb, which upregulates p16.

Which pt population is most likely to present with HPV-related OPC?

Nonsmokers and nondrinkers are most likely to have HPV+ SCC of the OPX.

Do HPV+ or HPV– OPC pts have a better prognosis?

HPV+ OPC pts have a better prognosis. Data from **RTOG 0129** (*Ang KK et al., NEJM 2010*) showed better 3-yr OS (82.4% vs. 57.1%) and risk of death (HR 0.42) for HPV+ pts. Smoking was an independent poor prognostic factor.

What is the hypothesis behind why HPV+ OPC pts have a better prognosis?

HPV+ H&N cancers are **usually in nonsmokers and nondrinkers, so p53 status is usually nonmutated;** p53 mutation (which is common in non–HPV-related H&N cancers) predicts for a poor response to Tx.

▶ WORKUP/STAGING

What nerves are responsible for otalgia in cancers of the oral tongue, BOT, and larynx/hypopharynx (HPX)?

Oral tongue: CN V (auriculotemporal) → preauricular area
BOT: CN IX (Jacobson nerve) → tympanic cavity
Larynx/HPX: CN X (Arnold nerve) → postauricular area

What is the most common presentation of OPC?

The most common presentation is a **neck mass,** especially with HPV+ OPC.

What are additional common presenting Sx by OPX subsite?

Base of tongue: sore throat, dysphagia, otalgia, neck mass
Tonsils: sore throat, trismus (T4b), otalgia, neck mass
Soft palate: leukoplakia, sore throat with swallowing, trismus/perforation, phonation defect with advanced lesions
Pharyngeal wall: pain/odynophagia, bleeding

Describe the workup for a pt with an OPX mass (per NCCN).

OPX mass workup: H&P (bimanual exam of the floor of mouth), labs, direct laryngoscopy, CT/MRI with contrast H&N, tissue Bx (EUA if necessary), and CXR (or CT chest), consider PET/CT for stages III–IV disease, nutrition, speech/swallow, audiogram, Bx with HPV testing

If the neck mass Bx is positive, is an additional Bx of the primary lesion necessary?

Yes. A Bx of the primary (or suspected primary) should also be done.

What % of OPC pts have clinically occult nodal mets?

30%–50% of OPC pts have clinically occult nodal mets.

What % of OPC pts present with clinically+ nodes, and what % present with bilat nodal Dz?

~75% of OPC pts have clinically+ nodes at presentation, with **~30%** having bilat Dz (especially if lesions are BOT/midline).

What is the T staging of OPC?

T staging of OPC is similar to other **SOOTH** (mnemonic: **S**alivary, **O**ral cavity, **O**ropharynx, **T**hyroid, **H**ypopharynx) H&N cancers:
  T1: ≤2 cm
  T2: >2 cm, ≤4 cm
  T3: >4 cm or extension to lingual surface of epiglottis
  T4a (moderately advanced): invades larynx, deep/extrinsic tongue muscles, medial pterygoid, hard palate, mandible
  T4b (very advanced): invades lat pterygoid muscle, pterygoid plate, lat nasopharynx, skull base, carotid encasement

What are the 4 extrinsic tongue muscles, and what are their anatomic spans?

Extrinsic tongue muscles (-glossus) and anatomic spans:
  1. Genioglossus (ant mandible to tongue)
  2. Styloglossus (styloid process to tongue)
  3. Palatoglossus (palate to tongue; also forms ant tonsillar pillar)
  4. Hyoglossus (hyoid bone to tongue)

What is the nodal (N) staging of OPC?

The N staging of OPC is the same as other H&N sites (except for nasopharyngeal):
  N1: single, ipsi, ≤3 cm
  N2a: single, ipsi, >3 cm and ≤6 cm
  N2b: multiple, ipsi, ≤6 cm
  N2c: bilat or contralat, ≤6 cm
  N3: any >6 cm

Describe the overall stage groupings for OPC.	**Stage I:** T1N0 **Stage II:** T2N0 **Stage III:** T3N0 or T1–3N1 **Stage IVA:** T4a or N2 **Stage IVB:** T4b or N3 **Stage IVC:** M1
Broadly speaking, what OPC pts/stage groups are deemed early, intermediate, and advanced?	<u>Early</u>: stages I–II (cT1–2N0) and select III (T2N1) <u>Intermediate/favorable</u>: HPV+ stages III–IV (without T2N1) in nonsmokers/drinkers, T3N0 (exophytic) regardless of HPV/smoking status <u>Advanced/unfavorable</u>: HPV– smokers with stages III–IV Dz, T4 Dz regardless of HPV/smoking status

▶ **TREATMENT/PROGNOSIS**

What are the Tx paradigms for early (e.g., cT1-T2, cN0) oropharyngeal tumors?	Early oropharyngeal tumor Tx paradigm: **surgical resection with selective neck dissection +/– PORT or definitive RT alone**
What are the Tx paradigms for intermediate-group oropharyngeal tumors?	Intermediate-group oropharyngeal tumor Tx paradigms: **surgery +/– postop CRT, altered fractionation RT, and CRT** (conventional fractionation)
What are the Tx paradigms for advanced/ unfavorable oropharyngeal tumors?	Advanced/unfavorable oropharyngeal tumor Tx paradigm: **CRT (conventional)**
When is WLE alone appropriate for OPC?	**Rarely.** WLE may suffice in the rare instance of a small (<1 cm), ant tonsillar pillar lesion.
Is tonsillectomy ever adequate as a definitive Tx for tonsillar cancers?	Generally, **no.** Simple tonsillectomy is considered an excisional Bx and thus needs further definitive Tx. Radical tonsillectomy may be adequate in select cases but results in worse functional outcomes than RT.
What type of surgery is required for the surgical management of OPC?	The **"commando" procedure** is typically required for OPC, which consists of composite resection of the mandible with en bloc removal of the tumor and deep structures.
When is PORT indicated for OPC?	PORT is generally indicated in OPC with a **+margin,** T3 or T4 disease, **N2 disease, +ECE, PNI, and LVSI.**
When can unilat neck Tx be considered for OPC pts?	Unilat neck Tx can be considered **if the lesion is well lateralized** (at least 1.5 cm from midline) **and the N stage is <N2a based on multiple retrospective reviews showing a very low contralateral failure rate (<3%).**

Which LN regions/levels should be irradiated in pts with an early T stage but N+ OPC?

Levels II–IV should always be included/irradiated; however, recent data (*Sanguineti G et al., IJROBP 2009*) suggest that levels I and V may be omitted due to a significantly lower incidence of nodal spread.

What is the main indication for a neck dissection after definitive CRT for OPC?

The main indication for a neck dissection after CRT is **persistent nodal Dz** that can be documented by fine-needle sampling, CT (at 4–6 wks), or PET/CT (at 10–12 wks).

What is the recommended timing for a neck dissection after CRT?

Neck dissection should typically occur at **6–8 wks** (**12–15 wks** if evaluated by PET/CT).

How should OPC pts be set up for simulation?

OPC pts should be simulated **supine, with arms pulled inferiorly and the head extended with a bite block or stent.** Contrast is recommended with CT.

What type of custom stent can be used?

Mouth opening, tongue depressing stent

What should the pre-RT evaluation/preparation include?

Dental evaluation/fluoride prophylaxis, speech and swallow evaluation/exercises, and nutrition evaluation with a PEG tube if the pre-Tx weight loss is >10% over 3 mos

What are the typical CTVs for IMRT planning?

CTV high dose (CTVHD): primary tumor and nodal GTV with 0.5–1-cm margin

CTV intermediate dose (CTVID): soft palate, adjacent parapharyngeal space, superior tonsillar pillars for lateral tumors, and nodal levels adjoining involved nodes

CTV elective dose (CTVED): levels II–IV, RP nodes. If node+, include ipsi IB and V.

What are the typical RT doses and volumes used for OPC?

T1 and superficial T2N0: **66–70 Gy to CTVHD, 60 Gy to CTVID, and 54 Gy to CTVED, given in 30–35 fx over 6–7 wks**

>T2+ without chemo: (1) 70 Gy to CTVHD, 63 Gy to CTVID, and 56 Gy to CTVED given in 35 fxs over 6 wks (per Danish Head and Neck Cancer Group [DAHANCA]); (2) 70 Gy to CTVHD, 60 Gy to CTVID, and 57 Gy to CTVED given in 33 fx

>T3 or >N2 with chemo: 70 Gy to CTVHD, 63 Gy to CTVID, and 59.5 Gy to CTVED in 35 fx

What is the 2-yr LF rate after IMRT alone for early (T1–2N0–1) OPC?

RTOG 00–22 (*Eisbruch A et al., IJROBP 2010*) demonstrated excellent results with accelerated hypofractionated IMRT for early OPC: **2-yr LF rate was 9%** (if major deviations, 50%; otherwise, 6%, SS).

What were the RT techniques and doses employed in RTOG 00–22?

In **RTOG 00–22** (*Eisbruch A et al., IJROBP 2010*), RT was delivered with accelerated hypofractionated IMRT as follows: 66 Gy in 30 fx (2.2 Gy/fx) to the primary PTV and 54–60 Gy in 30 fx (1.8–2 Gy/fx) to the secondary PTV.

How was the N stage established in RTOG 00–22 for eligibility purposes?

For **RTOG 00–22** (*Eisbruch A et al., IJROBP 2010*), **neck staging was clinical** (not from CT); however, pts "upstaged" by CT (e.g., cN1 but N2 after CT) were also eligible.

What did the RTOG 90–03 study demonstrate about the use of altered fractionation in H&N cancers?

RTOG 90–03 (*Fu KK et al., IJROBP 2000*): 1,073 pts with H&N cancers (10% oral cavity [OC], 60% OPX, 13% HPX) with stage III (28%) or stage IV (68%) Dz randomized to (a) conventional 70 Gy qd, (b) 81.6 Gy in 1.2 Gy/fx bid, (c) accelerated with split, and (d) concomitant boost (1.8 Gy/fx qd × 17, with last 12 fx bid with 1.8 Gy am, 1.5 Gy pm to 72 Gy). There was better LC with altered fx (54% vs. 46%) but no OS/DFS benefit. There was worse acute toxicity but no difference in late toxicity.

What randomized studies demonstrated better outcomes with hyperfractionated RT over conventional RT for OPC?

RTOG 90–03 (*Fu KK et al., IJROBP 2000*): see above.

EORTC 22791 (*Horiot JC et al., Radiother Oncol 1992*): 325 pts (all OPX, but no BOT): 70 Gy vs. 80.5 Gy at 1.15 Gy bid. There was better LC (60% vs. 40%) but no OS benefit. LC was best for T3 Dz.

What data showed good LC rates with RT alone for select advanced (stages III–IV) OPCs?

MDACC data (*Garden AS et al., Cancer 2004*): pts with small primaries but stages III–IV Dz by virtue of +LNs; treated with RT alone. There were acceptable 5-yr LF (15%), DM (19%), and OS (64%) rates.

What are 2 important randomized trials that demonstrated the importance of adding chemo to conventionally fractionated RT in OPC?

GORTEC 94–01 (*Calais G et al., JNCI 1999*): 222 pts with stages III–IV OPC randomized to conventional RT alone vs. conventional RT + carboplatin/5-FU, no planned neck dissection for N2–3 Dz. The CRT arm had better 3-yr OS (51% vs. 31%), DFS (30% vs. 15%), and LC (66% vs. 42%); however, there was significantly worse grades 3–4 mucositis and weight loss/feeding tube use in the CRT arm.

Cleveland Clinic data (*Adelstein DJ et al., JCO 2003*): 295 pts with unresectable stages III–IV H&N cancers (15% OC, 55% OPX, 20% HPX), RT alone vs. CRT with cisplatin 100 mg q3wks × 3. 3-yr OS was better in the CRT arm (37% vs. 23%). There also was improved DFS (51% vs. 33%) in the CRT arm.

What are the indications for adding chemo to PORT in H&N cancers, and what are 2 important RCTs that support this?

Pooled analysis suggests **+margin and ECE** as the most important indications.

EORTC 22931 (*Bernier J et al., NEJM 2004*): 334 pts randomized to PORT 66 Gy vs. PORT + cisplatin 100 mg/m^2 on days 1, 22, and 43. Eligibility: ECE, +margin, PNI, LVI, and levels 4–5 +N from OCC/OPC. There was better OS, DFS, and 5-yr LC with CRT but ↑ grades 3–4 toxicity.

RTOG 95–01 (*Cooper JS et al., NEJM 2004*): 459 pts randomized to 60–66 Gy PORT vs. PORT + cisplatin 100 mg/m^2 on days 1, 22, and 43. Eligibility: >2 LN, ECE, +margin. There was better DFS (43% vs. 54%) and 2-yr LRC (72% vs. 82%) but only a trend to improvement in OS (57% vs. 63%).

What study demonstrated improvement in OS with the addition of cetuximab (C225) to RT in H&N cancers?

Bonner JA et al. (*NEJM 2006*): 424 pts with stages III–IV SCC of the OPX, laryngeal cancer (LCX), or hypopharynx randomized to RT vs. RT + C225. RT options were conventional to 70 Gy, 1.2 bid to 72–76.8 Gy, or concomitant boost to 72 Gy. There was better 3-yr LRC (47% vs. 34%) and OS (55% vs. 45%) with C225 + RT. Subset analysis showed improvement mostly in OPC and in the altered fractionation RT arms (~50% treated with altered fractionation).

What studies are looking at HPV+ OPX?

E1308: stages III/IV resectable, HPV+ receive induction (paclitaxel, cisplatin, cetuximab). If CR: IMRT to 54 Gy/27 fx with concurrent cetuximab. If PR: 69.3gy/33 fx with concurrent cetuximab
RTOG 1016: stages III–IVB, HPV+ treated with accelerated IMRT to 70 Gy/6 wks randomized to concurrent cisplatin vs. cetuximab

What 2 randomized studies demonstrated a benefit with induction taxane/platinum/5-FU (TPF) chemo over PF in pts with unresectable H&N cancers?

TAX 324 study (induction chemo → CRT) (*Posner MR et al., NEJM 2007*): 501 pts, unresectable stages III–IV H&N cancers (52% OPX, 13%–18% OC, larynx, HPX) randomized to induction platinum + 5-FU or TPF → CRT with carboplatin. There was better 3-yr OS (62% vs. 48%), MS (71 mos vs. 30 mos), and LRC (70% vs. 62%) in the TPF arm.
Pts in the TPF arm had fewer Tx delays than in the platinum/5-FU arm despite higher myelotoxicity in the TPF arm (98% rcvd planned Tx in the TPF arm vs. 90% in the PF arm).

TAX 323 study (induction chemo → RT)
(*Vermorken JB et al., NEJM 2007*): 358 pts,
unresectable stages III–IV H&N cancers (46% OPX,
18% OC, 29% HPX, 7% larynx) randomized to
induction platinum + 5-FU or TPF → RT alone. TPF
resulted in better median PFS (11 mos vs. 8.2 mos),
MS (18.8 mos vs. 14.5 mos), and HR 0.73. The rate
of toxic deaths was greater in the platinum/5-FU
group (5.5% vs. 2.3%). Also, there was more grades
3–4 thrombocytopenia, anemia, stomatitis, n/v,
diarrhea, and hearing loss in the platinum/5-FU arm.
Neutropenia, leukopenia, and alopecia were more
common in the TPF arm.

What study compared induction chemotherapy vs. upfront chemoradiation?

PARADIGM study (induction TPF → CRT vs CRT) (*Haddad H et al., Lancet Oncol 2013*): 145
patients, stages III–IV (55% OPX), randomized to
induction TPF → CRT vs. CRT. At a median
follow-up of 49 mos, there was no difference in 3-yr
OS (73% for induction vs. 78% for CRT), with a
higher rate of febrile neutropenia observed in the
induction arm.

What are some advantages and disadvantages of split-field IMRT (vs. whole-field IMRT) in the Tx of H&N cancers?

There is potentially **better laryngeal sparing with split-field IMRT techniques;** however, the drawback
is that the **practitioner may have to junction the RT dose through involved nodes.**

What are the advantages and disadvantages of IMRT "dose painting" (vs. sequential plans) in the Tx of H&N cancers?

The main advantage of IMRT dose painting is that
better conformality can be achieved in a single plan.
The drawback, however, is that **nonstandard doses/fx are required.**

How do unplanned RT interruptions in H&N cancer affect LC rates and why?

Each wk of Tx time prolongation **reduces the LC rate by ~10%–12%** in H&N cancer pts b/c of **accelerated repopulation.**

What is the best way to compensate for several/ few missed RT sessions and avoid Tx time prolongation in H&N cancer pts?

According to *Bese NS et al.,* the best way to compensate
is by preserving total time, dose, and dose/fx (i.e.,
can treat bid on Fridays or extra fx on Saturdays).
Alternatively, dose/fx can be increased (e.g., by
0.5–0.7 Gy/day). (*IJROBP 2007*)

▶ **TOXICITY**

What is the approximate long-term PEG tube dependency rate after CRT for OPC?

The long-term PEG tube dependency rate after CRT can be as high as **15%–20%,** which is reduced with efforts on sparing swallowing structures (pharyngeal constrictors, larynx) with swallowing exercises and the use of PEG on demand.

What are some typical RT dose constraints for the parotid glands?

Typical RT dose constraints for the parotid glands are (a) mean dose to either parotid **<26 Gy** or (b) at least 50% of either parotid gland **<30 Gy.**

What is the typical RT dose constraint for the inner ears?

The mean dose to the inner ears should be ≤**35 Gy.**

Approximately what % of pts receiving cisplatin-based chemo will experience hearing loss as a result of ototoxicity?

~**30%** of pts will experience hearing loss.

What is the typical RT dose constraint for the larynx?

Approximately one-third of the larynx should not exceed a dose of 50 Gy (**V50 <30%**).

What were the xerostomia rates for OPC pts treated with IMRT in RTOG 00–22?

Xerostomia rates in **RTOG 00–22** (*Eisbruch A et al., IJROBP 2010*) were **55% at 6 mos, 25% at 1 yr, and 16% at 2 yrs.** Salivary output did not recover over time.

What was the observed rate of osteoradionecrosis with accelerated hypofractionated IMRT in RTOG 00–22?

The observed rate of osteoradionecrosis was **6%** in **RTOG 00–22** (*Eisbruch A et al., IJROBP 2010*), which is higher than expected for IMRT (potentially b/c of the accelerated hypofractionated approach). Other toxicities were acceptable (grade 2+ for mucosa [24%], salivary [67%], esophagus [19%]).

What oral care do all patients need to be instructed on?

Fluoride trays. Consult a dental oncologist before any dental procedures.

What is the follow-up paradigm for OPC pts?

OPC follow-up paradigm: H&P + pharyngolaryngoscopy (q1–3mos for yr 1, q2–4mos for yr 2, q4–6mos for yrs 3–5, q6–12mos if >5 yrs), imaging (for signs/Sx), TSH (if neck irradiated), speech/hearing/dental evaluation, and smoking cessation.

32 Salivary Gland Cancer

Updated by Vinita Takiar

▶ BACKGROUND

What is the incidence of salivary cancers in the U.S.?

~**2,500 cases/yr** of salivary cancers (~3% of all H&N cancers)

What is the sex predilection and median age at presentation for benign vs. malignant tumors?

<u>Benign</u>: female > male, 40 yo
<u>Malignant</u>: female = male, 55 yo

What is the most common type of benign tumor of the salivary gland, and where is it most commonly found?

Pleomorphic adenoma (65%). It is most commonly found in the **parotid glands.**

In addition to pleomorphic adenoma, what are some other benign salivary gland tumors?

Warthin tumor (papillary cystadenoma lymphomatosum), Godwin tumor (benign lymphoepithelial lesion, associated with Sjögren), and monomorphic adenoma (oncocytoma, basal cell)

What is the most common malignant salivary gland tumor, and where is it most commonly found?

Mucoepidermoid carcinoma. It most commonly arises in the **parotid** (most are low grade, but if the tumor is high grade, it needs to be managed with surgery + LND + adj RT).

How are tumors of the salivary gland separated into low vs. intermediate vs. high grade by histology?

Tumors should be assigned a grade by the pathologist. Some tumors are assumed a grade unless specified, though it should always be verified. Acinic cell carcinoma is typically a low-grade tumor. Carcinoma ex-pleomorphic adenoma (CexPA), and salivary ductal carcinomas are almost always high grade. Mucoepidermoid carcinoma must be graded. Adenoid cystic carcinoma (ACC) is often low grade, but rather than grading, pathologists will describe ACC as either tubular, cribriform (low), or solid (high). ACC is often grouped with high-grade tumors as its propensity for poorly defined borders and neurotropism almost always requires multimodal therapy. The nomenclature for salivary gland tumors is also evolving. Thus, mixed malignant tumors are rarely seen as the majority are CexPA, and most adenocarcinomas seen are aggressive salivary duct carcinoma or low-grade polymorphous adenocarcinoma (most commonly seen in the hard palate).

What is the relationship between the gland size and malignant nature of the salivary tumor?	Typically, **the smaller the gland, the more malignant the tumor.**
What is the approximate incidence ratio of benign to malignant tumors in the various salivary glands?	Approximate incidence ratios of benign to malignant tumors: 1. Parotid, ~75:25 2. Submandibular gland, ~50:50 3. Sublingual gland, ~10:90 4. Minor salivary, ~20:80
What is the most common malignant histology arising in the submandibular gland?	**Adenoid cystic carcinoma** is the most common malignant histology of the submandibular gland.
What is the most common malignant histology arising in the minor salivary glands?	**Adenoid cystic carcinoma** is the most common malignant histology of the minor salivary glands.
Where are the minor salivary glands found in the H&N?	Minor salivary glands are found in the **mucosal lining of the aerodigestive tract.** Most are in the oral cavity (OC) (85%–90%), with the palate (especially the hard palate) being the #1 site. They can be found in all sites of the OC, nasal cavity, paranasal sinus, oropharynx, and larynx.
What are the risk factors for developing salivary gland tumors?	Ionizing RT, personal Hx of tumor, and family Hx
What is the lymphatic drainage predilection of the parotid, submandibular/ sublingual, and minor salivary glands?	Lymphatic drainage predilection: Parotid: preauricular, periparotid, and intraparotid, with deep intraparotid nodes draining sequentially along the jugular nodes (levels II–IV) Submandibular/sublingual: levels I–II nodes, less often levels III and IV Minor salivary: depends on site of involvement and histology
How does the propensity for cervical LN mets relate to the site of origin of the salivary tumor?	The propensity for LN spread is **greatest for the minor salivary gland > submandibular/sublingual > parotid gland malignancies.**
What is the natural Hx of ACC?	ACC is often low grade (cribriform or tubular), but **is very locally infiltrative. Perineural invasion with skipped lesions and involvement of large nerves is common, as is DM. Recurrence can be very late,** though high-grade tumors (solid type) tend to have a more aggressive course. **Nodal mets are uncommon** (5%–8%).

What % of pts with adenoid cystic carcinoma ultimately go on to develop lung mets?	**~40%** of pts with adenoid cystic carcinoma ultimately develop lung mets.

▶ WORKUP/STAGING

What is the most common presentation of parotid gland tumors?	A **painless, solitary mass** is the most common presentation of parotid gland tumors.
For what does a painful growth/mass in the salivary gland predict?	It predicts for **malignancy or an inflammatory etiology/condition.**
What are some other presenting Sx in pts with salivary gland tumors?	Pain, facial weakness from CN VII involvement, rapid growth of mass, skin involvement, neck nodes. Sensory changes of the face can occur from involvement of the trigeminal nerve branches (CN V), and dysarthria/dysphagia can occur from CN XII being affected.
What is the DDx for a parotid mass?	Primary tumor, mets, lymphoma, parotitis, sarcoid, cyst, Sjögren syndrome, stone, lipoma, hemangioma
What are the 2 most important factors that predict for nodal mets in salivary gland malignancies?	**Grade and size** are the 2 most important factors that predict for nodal mets: high grade (50%) vs. intermediate/low grade (<10%) and size (>4 cm: 20% vs. <4 cm: 4%).
What is the typical workup performed for salivary gland tumors?	Salivary gland tumor workup: H&P (CNs/nodes), CBC, CMP, CXR, CT/MRI H&N, and FNA Bx
How should Bx be obtained for pts who present with a salivary gland mass?	Some argue that a salivary gland mass should be removed regardless, so do not biopsy. However, FNA should be done (despite a false negative rate of 20%), as knowledge of the histology may impact the type of surgery.
What does the mnemonic *SOOTH* stand for in terms of tumor (T) staging of the H&N?	**S**alivary **O**ral cavity **O**ropharynx **T**hyroid **H**ypopharynx (Mnemonic: **SOOTH**) SOOTH tumors are the H&N tumors with similar size-dependent T staging.
What is the T-staging breakdown for major salivary gland tumors?	**T1:** ≤2 cm **T2:** >2 cm, ≤4 cm **T3:** >4 cm (and/or extraglandular extension) **T4(a-b):** local invasion of adjacent structures (see below)

What salivary gland tumors are considered T3?

T3 salivary gland tumors are **tumors with extraglandular extension or tumors >4 cm.**

What is the distinction between T4a vs. T4b major salivary gland tumors?

T4a: usually still resectable; skin, mandible, ear, facial nerve invasion

T4b: usually unresectable; skull base, pterygoid plate, carotid artery invasion

What is the nodal staging system used for major salivary gland tumors?

Nodal staging is the same as for other H&N sites (except for the nasopharynx):

Per the latest AJCC 7th (2011) edition classification, what are the stage groupings for major salivary gland tumors?

N1: single, ipsi, ≤3 cm
N2a: single, ipsi, >3 cm, ≤6 cm
N2b: multiple, ipsi, ≤6 cm
N2c: bilat or contralat ≤6 cm
N3: >6 cm
Stage I: T1N0
Stage II: T2N0
Stage III: T3N0 or T1–3N1
Stage IVA: T4aN0–1 or T1–4aN2
Stage IVB: T4b any N or any TN3
Stage IVC: any T any NM1

On what is the staging system for the minor salivary gland tumors based?

Staging of the minor salivary gland tumors is based on the **site of origin.**

What are some important prognostic factors in salivary gland tumors?

Size, grade, histology, nodal status, and "named" nerve involvement are important prognostic factors.

What is the 5-yr OS for stages I–IV cancers of the salivary gland?

Stage I: 80%
Stage II: 60%
Stage III: 50%
Stage IV: 30%

What is the 5-yr OS of pts who present with facial nerve involvement?

The 5-yr OS is **65% with simple invasion and 10% if pts have nerve dysfunction** (i.e., if symptomatic).

▶ TREATMENT/PROGNOSIS

What is the general management paradigm for benign mixed/ pleomorphic adenoma of the parotid?

Benign mixed/pleomorphic adenoma management paradigm: **WLE, or superficial parotid lobectomy →** **observation** (even if +margin or with extraglandular extension)

What is the management paradigm for low- to intermediate-grade tumors of the salivary gland?

Low- to intermediate-grade salivary gland tumor management paradigm: **surgical resection with PORT** for close (<2 mm) or +margin, unresectable Dz, pT3–4, PNI, capsule rupture, +nodes, or recurrent Dz

What is the management paradigm for high-grade tumors of the salivary gland?

High-grade salivary gland tumor management paradigm: **surgical resection** (facial nerve sparing if possible for parotid tumors), **including LND if node+ → PORT**

What is the role of concurrent chemoradiation (CRT)?

The level of evidence for CRT is weak. NCCN guidelines recommend **consideration** of definitive CRT for T4b disease or PORT + chemo for pathologic adverse features including intermediate or high grade, inadequate margins, PNI, +LN, and LVI.

What is the management paradigm for ACC with pulmonary mets?

ACC (cribriform or tubular) with pulmonary mets (typically asymptomatic with low tumor burden) management paradigm: **same local therapy as in patients without mets** because pulmonary mets have a long natural Hx

What is the difference between superficial, total, and radical parotidectomy?

Superficial: en bloc resection of gland superficial to CN VII

Total: en bloc resection of entire gland with nerve sparing

Radical: en bloc resection of entire gland + CN VII + skin + fascia +/– muscle

What are the indications for LND with salivary gland tumors?

A clinically+ neck. LND is often done for high-grade and large tumors, but in the clinically negative neck, if the patient is to get PORT, the role of LND is questionable.

What are the indications for PORT in the management of salivary gland cancers?

Adj RT is indicated for the following: **high grade (regardless of margin), close/+ margin, pT3-T4 Dz, PNI, capsule rupture, tumor spillage, ECE, N2-N3 Dz, unresectable tumor/gross residual Dz, and recurrent tumor**

For which cN0 salivary gland tumors, by histology, does elective nodal RT significantly reduce the incidence of nodal relapse?

Elective nodal RT is more likely to reduce the incidence of nodal relapse in **pts with squamous, undifferentiated, or adenocarcinoma histologies.** (*Chen AM et al., IJROBP 2007*)

When should bilat neck coverage with RT be considered for salivary gland neoplasms?

Treatment of the ipsi neck should be adequate for major salivary gland cancers. Bilat nodal treatment is indicated for high-grade minor salivary gland cancers affecting midline structures.

What are some ways to deliver RT/set up the RT fields in the Tx of parotid gland tumors?

RT delivery and set up of RT fields:

1. **AP/PA wedge pairs** (120-degree hinge angle) but difficult setup, exit through OC
2. **Sup/Inf wedge pair** (with 90-degree couch kick), avoids exit through OC but exits through brain
3. **Single direct field with mixed energy beam** (80% 15 MeV electron: 20% 6 MV photon) with bolus, electron portal 1 cm larger than the photon field b/c of IDL constriction with depth, higher dose to bone, keep contralat parotid at <30 Gy
4. **IMRT**

What are the PORT doses used in the management of salivary gland tumors?

60 Gy for –margin, **66 Gy** for close/+margin, **70 Gy** for gross residual, and **50–56 Gy** to a low-risk neck

What RT techniques are used in the management of the ipsi neck?

RT techniques for the ipsi neck:

1. Single lat appositional electron field
2. Mixed electron-photon beam technique
3. Half beam block technique
4. IMRT

What key retrospective data demonstrated the importance of adding PORT for stages III–IV and high-grade salivary gland tumors?

MSKCC data (*Armstrong JG et al., Arch Otolaryngol Head Neck Surg 1990; Harrison L et al., J Surg Oncol 1990*) showed improved LC and survival.

What is the largest retrospective study demonstrating a benefit of adj RT for malignant salivary gland neoplasms?

Dutch NWHHT study (*Terhaard CHJ et al., IJROBP 2005*): 498 pts. Adj RT significantly improved LC in pts with T3-T4 Dz, a close margin, incomplete resection, bony invasion, and PNI.

What is the best RT modality for managing unresectable salivary gland tumors?

Neutrons (superior LC, with photons showing LC of 25% for inoperable cases). If no access to neutrons, many advocate concurrent CRT

When is surgical resection alone adequate in the management of recurrent salivary gland tumors?

If tumors are of low/intermediate grade, <3 cm, and there are no other risk features, then surgery alone may suffice.

 TOXICITY

What is Frey syndrome, and from what does it result?

Auriculotemporal nerve syndrome (gustatory sweating or redness and sweating on the cheek area when the pt eats, sees, or thinks about or talks about certain kinds of food). It is a **postop complication of parotidectomy.**

What are some possible Tx sequelae from RT for parotid cancers?	The main concerning sequelae are related to the ear. Acute effects include otitis externa or media with mild hearing loss. Late effects include dry cerumen, otitis media, and hearing loss. ORN of the temporal bone (parotid cancer) is uncommon as is mandibular ORN. Since treatment is mostly unilateral, xerostomia is mild.
Above which RT doses can salivary gland function be compromised, resulting in xerostomia?	The parotid is the most sensitive gland due to a large component of serous glands which are highly radiosensitive. There is no dose threshold. Minimum doses to effect parotid function start at ~14 Gy. Based on older data, mean doses of 26–30 Gy are still used as planning goals with IMRT, although doses as high as 40 Gy can still allow some recovery. The doses that result in damage to other salivary glands have not been well studied.
What is the general follow-up for pts with salivary gland neoplasms?	Per 2013 NCCN guidelines, H&P (q1–3mos for yr 1, q2–4mos for yr 2, q4–6mos for yrs 3–5, and q6–12mos thereafter), chest imaging if clinically indicated, and TSH q6–12mos if neck RT

33 Laryngeal and Hypopharyngeal Cancers

Updated by Anna O. Likhacheva and Gopal K. Bajaj

▶ BACKGROUND

What is the incidence of laryngeal cancer (LCX) in the U.S.?	~12,000 cases/yr of LCX (20% of all H&N cancers; 2013 data)
What are the risk factors for developing LCX?	Smoking, alcohol use, and voice abuse
What are the subsites of the larynx?	Supraglottic, glottic, and subglottic
What is the incidence/ distribution of LCX according to subsite?	Glottic: 69% Supraglottic: 30% Subglottic: 1%

What % of premalignant lesions (leukoplakia/ erythroplakia) progress to invasive laryngeal lesions?	**20%** of premalignant laryngeal lesions ultimately progress to invasive cancer (higher for erythroplakia than leukoplakia).
What is the most common LCX histology?	**Squamous cell carcinoma** (SCC) makes up >95% of LCX. Other histologies include verrucous carcinoma (1%–2%), adenocarcinoma, lymphoma, chondrosarcoma, melanoma, carcinoid tumor, and adenoid cystic carcinoma
What are the subdivisions of the supraglottic larynx?	Subdivisions of the supraglottic larynx include the **epiglottis (suprahyoid and infrahyoid), aryepiglottic folds, arytenoids, ventricles, and false vocal cords** (FVCs)
What are the subdivisions of the glottic larynx?	Subdivisions of the glottic larynx include the **ant/post commissures and the true vocal cords** (TVCs)
What are the anatomic borders of the subglottic larynx?	The subglottic larynx lies **0.5 cm below the TVCs down to the 1ˢᵗ tracheal ring.**
What are the nodal drainage pathways of the various laryngeal subsites?	<u>Supraglottic</u>: levels II–IV <u>Glottic</u>: virtually no drainage <u>Subglottic</u>: pretrachea and Delphian (level VI)
What is the incidence of hypopharyngeal cancer (HPC) in the U.S.?	There are **~2,500 cases/yr** of HPC in the U.S.
What is the median age at Dx for HPC?	The median age at Dx is **60–65 yrs** for HPC.
What are the subsites of the hypopharynx (HPX)?	**P**yriform sinus **P**ostcricoid area **P**osterior pharyngeal wall (Mnemonic: "**3 Ps**")
What are the anatomic boundaries of the HPX?	The HPX spans from **C4–6 or from the hyoid bone to the inf edge of the cricoid cartilage.**
What is the sex predilection for HPC based on the different subsites?	The sex predilection is **predominantly male for pyriform sinus and post pharynx primaries,** but **predominantly female for postcricoid area tumors.**
What are the classic risk factors for the development of HPC?	Smoking, alcohol, betel nut consumption, nutritional deficiency (vitamin C, Fe [Fe deficiency is associated with 70% of postcricoid cancers in northern European women]), and prior Hx of an H&N cancer
Is nodal involvement common with HPC?	**Yes.** Nodal involvement is common due to abundant submucosal lymphatic plexus drainage to the retropharyngeal nodes, cervical LNs, paratracheal LNs, paraesophageal nodes, and supraclavicular nodes.

What are the most commonly involved nodal stations in HPC?	**Levels II, III, and the retropharyngeal nodes** are most commonly involved in HPC. **Level VI** can also be involved and therefore should be covered when planning these cases for RT.
What is the name for the most sup of the lat retropharyngeal nodes?	The most sup of the lat retropharyngeal nodes is the **node of Rouviere.**
What % of HPC pts have nodal involvement at Dx?	**~75%** overall have nodal involvement at Dx (~60% for T1).
What is the typical histology seen in HPC?	The predominant histology is **SCC** (>95%) → adenoid cystic, lymphoma, and sarcoma.
What are the most common subsites of origin for HPC?	The **pyriform sinus (70%–80%), post pharyngeal wall (15%–20%), and postcricoid (5%)** are the most common subsites of origin.
At what cervical spine levels are the hyoid bone and the TVCs located?	The **hyoid bone is at C3,** whereas the **TVCs are located near C5–6.**

▶ **WORKUP/STAGING**

How do pts with LCX typically present?	Hoarseness, odynophagia/sore throat, otalgia (via the Arnold nerve/CN X), aspiration/choking, and neck mass
What is the typical workup for pts presenting with a possible laryngeal mass?	Possible laryngeal mass workup: H&P (voice change, habits, indirect/direct laryngoscopy), CXR, CT/MRI, PET, basic labs, EUA + triple endoscopy, and Bx of the primary +/– FNA of the neck mass
What does the loss of the laryngeal click on palpation of the thyroid cartilage indicate?	Loss of the laryngeal click on exam indicates **postcricoid extension/involvement.**
What does pain in the thyroid cartilage indicate on exam?	Pain on palpation of the thyroid cartilage indicates **tumor invasion into the thyroid cartilage.**
What imaging device is best to assess for bony or cartilage erosion in pts with LCX?	**CT scan** is best for assessing bony/cartilage erosion.
What is the incidence of nodal involvement for T1, T2, and T3–T4 glottic cancer?	**T1:** 0%–2% **T2:** 2%–7% **T3–T4:** 15%–30%

What is the incidence of nodal involvement for supraglottic lesions according to T stage?

T1–T2: 27%–40%
T3–T4: 55%–65%

(*Wang CC, Radiation therapy for head and neck neoplasms,* 1996)

What proportion of pts with supraglottic cancer present with unilat vs. bilat nodal Dz?

~**55%** of supraglottic cancer pts present with unilat nodal Dz, and **16%** present with bilat nodal involvement. (*Lindberg R et al., Cancer 1972*)

What % of pts with subglottic cancer present with nodal involvement?

20%–50% of subglottic pts present with nodal Dz (generally the prelaryngeal/Delphian, lower jugular, pretracheal, or upper mediastinal nodes).

Describe the T staging for cancers of the supraglottic larynx AJCC (7th edition, 2011).

T1: 1 subsite
T2: 1 adjacent subsite or outside supraglottis (base of tongue [BOT], vallecula, pyriform sinus) without fixation of larynx
T3: cord fixation and/or invasion of postcricoid area or pre-epiglottic tissue
T4a (resectable): through thyroid cartilage, trachea, soft tissue of neck, deep/intrinsic muscles of tongue, thyroid, esophagus
T4b: invasion of prevertebral space, mediastinum, carotid

Describe the T staging for cancers of the glottic larynx AJCC (7th edition, 2011).

T1: limited to TVCs +/− ant/post commissure involvement with normal mobility (1a, 1 TVC; 1b, both cords)
T2: extends to supra- or subglottis or impaired vocal cord mobility
T3: fixed vocal cords
T4a-b: same as above/for supraglottic lesions

What is the T-staging breakdown for cancers of the subglottic larynx AJCC (7th edition, 2011)?

T1: tumor limited to subglottis
T2: extension to vocal cords, with normal or impaired mobility
T3: limited to larynx with vocal cord fixation
T4a-b: same as above

Describe the overall stage groupings for LCX.

Stages I–II: T1–2N0
Stage III: T3N0 or N1
Stage IVA: T4a or N2
Stage IVB: T4b or N3
Stage IVC: M1

With what stage of Dz do most pts with HPC present?

Most pts (>80%) present with **stage III or IV Dz** (lesions remain asymptomatic until the advanced stages).

What % of pts with HPC present with DMs?

~**2%–4%** of HPC pts present with DMs. ~20%–30% develop DMs within 2 yrs despite Tx.

With what Sx do most HPC pts present?	Neck mass, sore throat, dysphagia, hoarseness (**direct vocalis or cricoarytenoid joint invasion**), and otalgia (Arnold nerve/CN X involvement)
What is the typical workup for pts who present with hoarseness?	Hoarseness workup: H&P (check for thyroid click), labs, CT/MRI, PET, neck FNA, EUA + triple endoscopy, and Bx of the primary mass
Describe the T staging of HPC AJCC (7th edition, 2011).	**T1:** <2 cm or 1 subsite **T2:** 2–4 cm or >1 subsite **T3:** >4 cm or fixation of hemilarynx **T4a:** invades thyroid/cricoid cartilage, hyoid bone, thyroid gland, esophagus, or central soft tissue **T4b:** invades prevertebral fascia, carotid artery, or mediastinal structures
What is the nodal staging breakdown for HPC?	Same system as used for other H&N cancers (except for nasopharynx): **N1:** single, ipsi, ≤3 cm **N2a:** single, ipsi, >3, ≤6 cm **N2b:** multiple, ipsi, ≤6 cm **N2c:** bilat or contralat ≤6 cm **N3:** >6 cm
Describe the overall stage groupings for HPC.	**Stages I–II:** T1–2N0 **Stage III:** T3N0 or N1 **Stage IVA:** T4a or N2 **Stage IVB:** T4b or N3 **Stage IVC:** M1

▶ TREATMENT/PROGNOSIS

What does total laryngectomy entail?	It entails the **removal of the hyoid, thyroid and cricoid cartilage, epiglottis, and strap muscle with reconstruction of the pharynx as well as a permanent tracheostomy.**
What structures are removed with a supraglottic laryngectomy?	A supraglottic laryngectomy sacrifices the **FVCs, epiglottis, and aryepiglottic folds.**
What is the preferred surgical option for dysplastic lesions on the glottic larynx?	**Mucosal stripping** is typically curative for dysplastic lesions. Close follow-up is needed.
What are the Tx options for Tis lesions of the glottic larynx?	**Cord stripping/laser excision** (need close follow-up; cannot r/o microinvasive Dz) **or definitive RT**
What are the ~5-yr LC rates for glottic CIS with the use of stripping vs. laser vs. RT?	Stripping: 72% Laser: 83% RT: 88%–92% (all >95% after salvage)

What are the Tx options for T1–T2 glottic cancer?

Cordectomy (CO_2 laser)/partial laryngectomy, or definitive RT

What are the 5-yr control and survival rates after hemilaryngectomy for T1–T2 glottic cancer?

After hemilaryngectomy, the ~**5-yr LC is 83%** and the **DFS is 88%** for T1–T2 glottic cancer. (*Scola B et al., Laryngology 1999*)

What is the salvage Tx of choice for glottic lesions after RT failure?

The salvage Tx of choice is **total laryngectomy +/– neck dissection.**

What is the ~5-yr CSS rate for T1 glottic cancers treated with definitive RT?

The 5-yr CSS rate with RT is **>90%** (95% with salvage; organ preservation rate is >90%).

What are the advantages and disadvantages of using RT for early glottic cancer?

<u>Advantages</u>: better voice quality, noninvasive, organ preservation

<u>Disadvantages</u>: long Tx duration, RT changes could obscure post-Tx surveillance

What is the voice quality preservation rate for early glottic tumors/pts treated with laser vs. RT?

The Johns Hopkins Hospital data (*Epstein BE et al., Radiology 1990*) suggest **better voice quality after RT** (laser: 31%, RT: 74%, $p = 0.012$).

What are the initial and ultimate (after salvage) LC rates for T2 glottic lesions?

Initial LC is 70%–90% and **50%–70% after salvage** for T2 glottic lesions.

What are the currently accepted dose fractionation and total dose Rx for CIS and T1 glottic lesions?

The currently accepted RT doses are **56.25 Gy for CIS** and **63 Gy for T1**, at **2.25 Gy/fx.**

What is the typical RT dose used for T2 glottic lesions?

The typical RT dose for T2 lesions is **70 Gy at 2 Gy/fx** or **65.25 Gy at 2.25 Gy/fx.**

What randomized data/trial highlighted the importance of hypofractionation for early glottic cancers?

Japanese data (*Yamazaki H et al., IJROBP 2006*): 180 pts, 2 fractionations: 2 Gy/fx (60–66 Gy) vs. 2.25 Gy/fx (56.25–63 Gy). 5-yr LC rate was better with 2.25 Gy/fx (92% vs. 72%). The greater toxicity for the hypofractionation regimen was acute skin erythema (83% vs. 63%).

What RT field sizes/spans are employed for Tis/T1 glottic cancers?

5 × 5 cm opposed lat fields are typically employed (from the upper thyroid notch to the lower border of the cricoid, post border at the ant edge of the vertebral body, and flash skin at the ant border).

What RT planning technique can be used when treating T1 glottic lesions with ant commissure involvement?

Generally, for T1 glottic lesions, **wedges** are used (heel anteriorly, usually 15 degrees) to reduce ant hotspots due to curvature of the neck. However, if there is ant commissure Dz, the wedges can be removed, or wedge angle reduced, to add hotspots to this region. Alternatively, a bolus/beam spoiler can be added for additional coverage.

What structures must be encompassed by the 95% IDL when irradiating T1 glottic cancer?

The 95% IDL must encompass the **TVCs, FVCs, and the sup subglottis.**

What RT fields are used for T2 glottic lesions?

This is **controversial** and may depend on the degree of supraglottic/subglottic extension. Most advocate using 6 × 6 cm opposed lat fields; others advocate covering levels II–III nodes (2 cm above the angle of the mandible, splitting vertebral body, down to the bottom of the cricoid) to **50–54 Gy**, with CD to the 5 × 5 cm box covering the larynx to **70 Gy.**

What are the Tx options for early-stage supraglottic LCX?

Supraglottic laryngectomy, transoral laser resection, or definitive RT

What are the 5-yr LC and OS rates for early supraglottic cancers treated with surgery and LND?

The **5-yr LC rate is ~85%**, whereas the **5-yr OS is ~100% for T1 and ~80% for T2** supraglottic lesions.

What are the LC rates for early-stage supraglottic cancers after definitive RT alone?

Retrospective series demonstrate LC rates of **73%–100% for T1 and 60%–89% for T2 lesions** (e.g., University of Florida and Italian data).

Describe the standard RT fields used in treating supraglottic cancers.

Because 20%–50% of T1–T2 supraglottic cancers have +LNs (occult), necks need to be covered for all pts (levels II–IV). This requires an off-cord CD after 45 Gy and a boost to the post neck to 50 Gy with electron fields.

What definitive RT doses are typically recommended for early-stage supraglottic cancers?

T1 dose: **70 Gy** in 2 Gy/fx
T2 dose: hyperfractionated dosing to **76.8 Gy** in 1.2 Gy/fx or with concomitant boost techniques to **72 Gy** (1.8 Gy in a.m. × 30 fx to 54 Gy to areas of subclinical Dz, and 1.5 Gy in p.m. for the last 12 days of Tx to boost GTV + 1.5–2 cm to 72 Gy)

What data support the use of reirradiation for previously treated early-stage LCX pts?

Massachusetts General Hospital data (*Wang CC et al., IJROBP 1993*): 20 pts treated with 1.6 Gy bid to 65 Gy. 5-yr OS was 93%, and LC was 61% after reirradiation.

What are the Tx options for pts with advanced LCX?

Total laryngectomy (with adj RT or CRT for +margin, +ECE) or organ preservation with definitive CRT **(RTOG 91–11)** or RT alone (altered fractionation)

What are the Tx options for pts with advanced HPC?

Induction chemo → RT or surgery depending on response for T1–3N+ Dz; total laryngectomy/laryngoesophagectomy (with CRT for +margin, +ECE) for T4 Dz

What are the typical RT doses used to treat advanced LCX/HPC?

Subclinical Dz (2nd echelon nodal regions) to **50–54 Gy; high-risk regions (1st-echelon or involved nodal regions) to 60–63 Gy,** primary tumor to **70 Gy** (in 2 Gy/fx)

What are the 3 indications for boosting the stoma with PORT?

Indications for boosting the stoma with PORT:

1. Emergency tracheostomy
2. Subglottic extension
3. Ant soft tissue extension

What are some indications for performing an elective neck dissection after definitive RT?

This is controversial, but elective neck dissection should be done for persistent Dz and can be considered with >N2 Dz, although it is now common to observe if clinical and radiographic CR is obtained after RT.

What randomized data/ study compared preop RT to PORT for (predominantly) HPC?

RTOG 73–03 (*Tupchong L et al., IJROBP 1991*): 354 pts, 50 Gy preop vs. 60 Gy postop; 69% of pts had advanced supraglottic or HPC. LC was better with PORT but not OS.

What are the 2 randomized phase III trials that demonstrated a benefit with postop CRT vs. PORT alone for high-risk H&N pts?

EORTC 22931 (*Bernier J et al., NEJM 2004*): 334 pts randomized to PORT 66 Gy vs. PORT + cisplatin 100 mg/m^2 on days 1, 22, and 43. Eligibility: ECE, +margin, PNI, LVI, and levels 4–5 +N from oral cavity cancer (OCC)/oropharyngeal cancer (OPC). There was better OS, DFS, and 5-yr LC with CRT but ↑ grades 3–4 toxicity.

RTOG 95–01 (*Cooper JS et al., NEJM 2004*): 459 pts randomized to 60–66 PORT vs. PORT + cisplatin 100 mg/m^2 on days 1, 22, and 43. Eligibility: >2 LNs, ECE, +margin. There was better DFS (43% vs. 54%) and 2-yr LRC (72% vs. 82%) with CRT but only a trend to improvement in OS (57% vs. 63%).

What are the presumed reasons why EORTC 22931 showed an OS benefit while RTOG 9501 did not?

The EORTC trial included more margin+ pts (28% vs. 18%), pts with worse tumor differentiation (19% vs. 7%), more HPX cases (20% vs. 10%), and more pts who started RT 6 wks or later after surgery (32%).

Which randomized trials demonstrated a benefit with altered fractionation RT in advanced H&N cancer?

EORTC 22851 (*Horiot JC et al., Radiother Oncol 1997*): 512 pts (all H&N except the HPX) randomized to conventional RT to 70 Gy (7 wks) or 1.6 Gy tid to 72 Gy (5 wks). There was better 5-yr LRC with tid RT (59% vs. 46%) but not OS.

RTOG 9003 (*Fu KK et al., IJROBP 2000*): 1,073 pts (all H&N sites) randomized to (1) standard fx 70 Gy/2 qd; (2) 81.6 Gy/1.2 bid; (3) accelerated with split 67.2 Gy/1.6 bid; and (4) accelerated with concomitant boost 72 Gy/1.8 qd × 17 → 1.8 Gy am + 1.5 Gy pm × 33 fx. All altered fx schemes were better than conventional RT in terms of LRC (54% vs. 46%) but not OS.

Which studies investigated induction CRT for organ preservation in pts with LCX?

Department of Veterans Affairs (VA) larynx study (*Wolf GT et al., NEJM 1991*): stages III–IV resectable LCX; 332 pts randomized to total laryngectomy + PORT vs. induction CRT. If after induction chemo × 2 cycles the tumor had <PR, salvage surgery + PORT was the next step. If there was a CR or >PR, 1 more cycle was added, then RT was initiated if there was no progression. 2-yr larynx preservation rate was 64%. There was no OS difference (there were less DMs but more local relapses in the chemo arm).

GETTEC (*Richard JM et al., Oral Oncol 1998*): early closure due to poor accrual; only 68 pts, mostly T3N0, design similar to the VA study. There was poorer 2-yr survival for the chemo group (69% vs. 84%). 3-yr laryngectomy-free survival was 20%.

What is the only randomized study that investigated organ preservation for advanced HPC with induction CRT?

EORTC 24891 (*Lefebvre JL et al., JNCI 1996 and Ann Oncol 2012*): 194 pts randomized to surgery + PORT vs. induction chemo (5-FU/cisplatin) + RT; if NR to induction chemo, then salvage laryngectomy + PORT. 5-yr larynx preservation rate was 35%. At 3 yrs, OS was better with induction therapy, but there was no difference at 5 and 10 yrs (DMs were less in the chemo arm; no difference in LRF).

What are the key studies demonstrating a benefit with concurrent CRT over RT alone for resectable LCX?

Cleveland Clinic (*Adelstein DJ et al., Cancer 2000*): randomized phase III, 100 pts with stages III–IV H&N cancer (50% larynx/HPX); RT alone vs. chemo (platinum/5-FU) + RT. 5-yr larynx preservation rate was 77% vs. 45%, 5-yr laryngectomy-free survival was 42% vs. 34% (no OS difference).

RTOG 91–11 (*Forastiere AA et al., NEJM 2003*): 547 pts, T2–T4 (excluded T4 with thyroid cartilage invasion or >1-cm BOT invasion) randomized to (1) CRT (platinum 100 mg/m² on days 1, 22, and 43), (2) induction chemo → RT (like the VA study), and (3) RT alone (all to 70 Gy). There was a better rate of laryngeal preservation at 3.8 yrs with concurrent CRT (84% vs. 72% vs. 67%); better 2-yr LRC (78% vs. 61% vs. 56%); and better DM rate with any chemo arm than with RT alone. There was no OS benefit. There was ↑ acute grades 3–4 toxicity but no ↑ late toxicity with concurrent CRT.

What are the survival/LC numbers based on the latest update of RTOG 91–11? Exclusion criteria for 91–11?

The latest update of **RTOG 91–11** (*Forastiere AA et al., JCO 2013*) had a median follow-up of 10.8 yrs. CRT improved larynx preservation over chemo → RT (HR, 0.58; $p = 0.005$) and over RT alone ($p < 0.001$), while chemo → RT and RT were equivalent (HR = 1.26; $p = 0.35$). Late effects were not different. The 10-yr OS was the same (27.5% CRT, 38.8% chemo → RT, and 31.5% RT). Deaths not attributed to larynx cancer or treatment were higher with CRT. The exclusion criteria were T1 primaries and high-volume T4 primaries (invasion >1 cm into the base of tongue or penetration through cartilage).

What is the only randomized study that compared total laryngectomy + RT to CRT in advanced LCX?

Singapore study (*Soo KC et al., Br J Cancer 2005*): 119 pts, the majority with bulky T4 (56%) or stage IVA (78%) Dz; closed early due to poor accrual; nonstandard chemo (platinum 20 mg/m²; 5-FU 1,000 mg/m²), nonstandard RT (66 Gy). There was no difference in 3-yr DFS, with a larynx preservation rate of 45%. Pts with LCX or HPC had higher organ preservation rates (68% vs. 30%).

What study demonstrated an OS and DFS benefit with CRT over RT alone for unresectable H&N cancers?

Cleveland Clinic (*Adelstein DJ et al., JCO 2003*): 295 pts with unresectable stages III–IV H&N cancers (15% oral cavity [OC], 55% oropharynx [OPX], 20% HPX), RT alone vs. CRT with cisplatin 100 mg q3wks × 3. 3-yr OS (37% vs. 23%) and DFS (51% vs. 33%) were better with CRT.

What study demonstrated improvement in OS with the addition of cetuximab (C225) to RT in H&N cancers?

Bonner et al. (*NEJM 2006*): 424 pts with stages III–IV SCC of the OPX, larynx, or HPX randomized to RT vs. RT + C225; RT options were conventional to 70 Gy, 1.2 bid to 72–76.8 Gy, or concomitant boost to 72 Gy. There was better 3-yr LRC (47% vs. 34%) and OS (55% vs. 45%) with RT + C225. Subset analysis showed improvement mostly in OPC and in the altered fractionation RT arms (~50% with altered fractionation).

What 2 randomized studies demonstrated a benefit with induction taxane/platinum/5-FU (TPF) chemo over PF → in pts with unresectable H&N cancers?

TAX 324 study (induction chemo → CRT)
(*Posner MR et al., NEJM 2007*): 501 pts, unresectable stages III–IV H&N cancers (52% OPX; 13%–18% OC, larynx, HPX) randomized to induction platinum + 5-FU or TPF → CRT with carboplatin. There was better 3-yr OS (62% vs. 48%), MS (71 mos vs. 30 mos), and LRC (70% vs. 62%) in the TPF arm. Pts in the TPF arm had fewer Tx delays than those who rcvd platinum/5-FU despite higher myelotoxicity in the TPF arm (98% rcvd planned Tx in TPF vs. 90% in the platinum/5-FU arm).

TAX 323 study (induction chemo → RT)
(*Vermorken JB et al., NEJM 2007*): 358 pts, unresectable stages III–IV H&N cancers (46% OPX, 18% OC, 29% HPX, 7% larynx) randomized to induction platinum + 5-FU or TPF → RT alone. TPF resulted in better median PFS (11 mos vs. 8.2 mos), MS (18.8 mos vs. 14.5 mos), with an HR of 0.73. The rate of toxic deaths was greater in the platinum/5-FU group (5.5% vs. 2.3%). There was also more grades 3–4 thrombocytopenia, anemia, stomatitis, n/v, diarrhea, and hearing loss in the platinum/5-FU arm. Neutropenia, leukopenia, and alopecia were more common in the TPF arm.

Which study compared induction chemotherapy vs. upfront chemoradiation?

PARADIGM study (induction TPF → CRT vs. CRT) (*Haddad H et al., Lancet Oncology 2013*): 145 patients, stages III–IV (25% larynx and hypopharynx), randomized to induction TPF → CRT vs. CRT. At a median follow-up of 49 mos, there was no difference in 3-yr OS (73% for induction vs. 78% for CRT), with a higher rate of febrile neutropenia observed in the induction arm.

▶ **TOXICITY**

What are some acute and late toxicities with RT in the Tx of LCX?

Acute: hoarseness, sore throat, odynophagia, skin irritation

Late: laryngeal edema, glottic stenosis, hypothyroidism, xerostomia, L'hermitte syndrome, myelitis, laryngeal necrosis

What are the main late toxicities after organ preservation with concurrent CRT for LCX?

Moderate speech impairment, dysphagia (25% of pts; <5% cannot swallow), and xerostomia (advanced cases)

What are some approximate RT dose constraints for laryngeal edema?	Recent data suggest that the incidence of laryngeal edema ↑ significantly with mean doses ≥**44 Gy.** (*Sanguineti G et al., IJROBP 2007*)
What is the QOL impact of larynx preservation when compared to laryngectomy in the Tx of LCX?	VA data demonstrated better social, emotional, and mental health function with larynx preservation (swallowing and speech function were similar), which suggests that better QOL is not due to preservation of speech but due to freedom from pain, emotional well-being, and less depression. *Hanna et al.* demonstrated that pts had worse social functioning, greater sensory disturbance, more use of pain meds, and coughing after total laryngectomy than those treated with CRT. (*Arch Otolaryngol H&N Surg 2004*)
What is the follow-up paradigm for LCX pts?	LCX follow-up paradigm: H&P + laryngoscopy (q1–3mos for yr 1, q2–4mos for yr 2, q4–6mos for yrs 3–5, q6–12 mos if >5 yrs), imaging (for signs/Sx), TSH (if neck is irradiated), speech/hearing evaluation, and smoking cessation

34 Thyroid Cancer

*John P. Christodouleas
and Updated by Mark Edson*

▶ BACKGROUND

Name the anatomic subdivisions/lobes of the thyroid.	Subdivisions/lobes of the thyroid: 1. Right lobe 2. Left lobe 3. Isthmus 4. Pyramidal lobe (in 50% of individuals is remnant of thyroglossal duct)
In the thyroid follicle, what are the normal functions of the epithelial follicular cells and the parafollicular cells?	<u>Epithelial follicular cells</u>: remove iodide from the blood and use it to **form T_3 and T_4** thyroid hormones <u>Parafollicular cells (C cells)</u>: lie just outside of the follicle cells and **produce calcitonin**

What is the most common endocrine malignancy?

Thyroid cancer (TCa) is the most common endocrine malignancy, but is only 1% of all diagnosed malignancies.

What is the incidence of new TCa Dx and deaths in the U.S.?

There are an estimated 60,000 new Dx and 1,850 deaths in 2013.

What are the 3 main TCa histologies in decreasing order of frequency?

Differentiated (follicular-derived) thyroid carcinoma (DTCa) (~94%) > **medullary** (2%–4%) > **anaplastic** (2%)

What are the 3 subtypes of DTCa in decreasing order of frequency?

Papillary (80%–90% of all TCa) > **follicular** > **Hürthle cell carcinoma**

What is happening to the incidence of diagnosed papillary TCa?

The incidence of papillary TCa is **increasing** (by ~15% over the past 40 yrs, largely driven by better surveillance/detection).

What is the typical age at Dx for follicular vs. papillary TCa?

Follicular incidence peaks at 40–60 yrs of age, whereas **papillary peaks at 30–50 yrs of age.**

Is there a sex predilection for papillary or follicular TCa?

Yes. Both papillary and follicular TCa more commonly affect **females** than males (3:1).

What is the strongest risk factor for papillary TCa?

RT exposure to the H&N as a child is the strongest risk factor for papillary TCa. There is no increased risk if exposure is after age 20 yrs. Most papillary cases are sporadic.

Name 4 genetic disorders associated with papillary TCa.

Genetic disorders associated with papillary TCa:
1. Familial polyposis
2. Gardner syndrome
3. Turcot syndrome
4. Familial papillary carcinoma

Name a genetic disorder associated with follicular TCa.

Cowden syndrome (*PTEN* gene mutation) is associated with follicular TCa.

Medullary TCa arises from what precursor cell?

Medullary TCa arises from the calcitonin-producing **parafollicular C cells.**

Name 2 genetic syndromes associated with medullary TCa.

MEN 2a and **MEN 2b** (*RET* gene mutation) are associated with medullary TCa.

What % of medullary TCa is related to a genetic syndrome?

~25% of medullary TCa is related to a genetic syndrome.

Name the nerve that lies in the tracheoesophageal (TE) groove, post to the right/left thyroid lobes.

The **recurrent laryngeal nerve** lies in the TE groove.

What are the primary, secondary, and tertiary lymphatic drainage regions of the thyroid?	<u>Primary</u>: central compartment (**level VI**), **TE groove, Delphian** (prelaryngeal) LNs <u>Secondary</u>: cervical, supraclavicular, and upper mediastinal LNs (levels III–IV, VII) <u>Tertiary</u>: upper cervical (level II)/retropharyngeal LNs

▶ WORKUP/STAGING

What % of palpable thyroid nodules are malignant?	Only **5%** of palpable thyroid nodules are malignant.
In a pt with low TSH and a nodule that shows uptake by I-123 or Tc-99 scan, what is the likely Dx?	**Adenomas** commonly present with low TSH and increased uptake on I-123 or Tc-99 scans.
Which DTCa subtypes are difficult to distinguish from adenomas on FNA?	**Follicular and Hürthle subtypes** are difficult to distinguish from adenomas. Histologically, they show only follicular structures. Papillary TCa shows both papillary and follicular structures, which helps to distinguish it from adenomas.
What pathologic criteria must be met to make the Dx of Hürthle cell TCa?	The Dx requires **hypercellularity with >75% Hürthle cells** (also referred to as oncocytic cells), which are characterized by abundant eosinophilic granular content.
Which TCa subtype is more likely to present with N+ Dz: papillary or follicular?	**Papillary** TCa (**~30%** node+) is more likely to spread to LNs than follicular (~10% node+).
Name the 2 major and 3 minor prognostic factors for DTCa.	<u>Major</u>: age and tumor size (15–44 yo, ≤4 cm, respectively, have better prognosis) <u>Minor</u>: histology, local tumor extension, LN status
What variables constitute the mnemonic AMES risk group system?	**A**ge, **M**etastasis, **E**xtent, **S**ize
Which pts are low risk?	1. Young (males <41 yo, females <51 yo), no DMs 2. Older with minor tumor capsule involvement *and* tumor <5 cm *and* no DMs
For DTCa, what sizes distinguish AJCC 7ᵗʰ edition T1, T2, and T3 tumors?	**T1:** <2 cm (T1a if <1 cm; T1b if >1 cm) **T2:** 2–4 cm (limited to thyroid) **T3:** >4 cm with only min extrathyroidal extension
What is the difference between T4a and T4b TCa lesions?	**T4a:** local extension but still technically resectable **T4b:** unresectable Dz

What is the difference between N1a and N1b in TCa?	**N1a:** mets to **level VI** LNs (pre-/paratracheal, prelaryngeal)
	N1b: mets to **levels I–V, VII** (cervical neck, upper mediastinal) or retropharyngeal LNs
List the latest AJCC 7th-edition (2011) stage groupings for papillary and follicular TCa.	**Stage I:** M0 and age <45 yrs or T1N0 and age ≥45 yrs
	Stage II: M1 and age < 45 yrs or T2N0 and age ≥45 yrs
	Stage III: T3N0 or T1–3N1a and age ≥45 yrs
	Stage IVA: T4a or N1b and age ≥45 yrs
	Stage IVB: T4b and age ≥45 yrs
	Stage IVC: M1 and age ≥45 yrs
What is unique about the staging of DTCa?	It is **age dependent;** it differs for pts > or <45 yo.
Can a pt <45 yo with follicular or papillary TCa have stage III or IV Dz?	**No.** A pt <45 yo with follicular or papillary TCa cannot have stage III or IV Dz.
What is the stage of a 37-yo pt with DTCa and a solitary bone met?	**Stage II.** If the pt were 65 yo, he or she would be stage IVc.
What is the stage of a 45-yo pt with an unresectable primary DTCa and no mets?	**Stage IVb.** If the pt were 44 yo, he or she would be stage I.
What must be done prior to an I-123 or I-131 scan?	**TSH stimulation** must be done prior to an iodine scan.
What are 2 ways to do TSH stimulation?	TSH stimulation can be accomplished through **thyroid hormone withdrawal or by using recombinant TSH.**
What are some advantages of recombinant TSH stimulation?	**Fewer side effects and a shorter period of elevated TSH** (theoretically, a lower risk of tumor progression)
What are the approved indications for recombinant TSH stimulation?	Recombinant TSH is approved for **follow-up iodide scans and** for the **I-131 Tx of low-risk pts.**
What sites of the body show a physiologic uptake of iodide?	The **salivary glands and the GI tract** show physiologic uptake due to the presence of iodide transporters.
Which DTCa subtype has a better long-term prognosis: papillary or follicular?	**Papillary** has a better 10-yr OS at ~93% (vs. 85% for follicular).

Is the presentation and Tx of Hürthle cell carcinoma more similar to that of papillary or follicular TCa?	It is more similar to **follicular TCa;** however, Hürthle cell carcinoma has a slightly higher DM rate and worse prognosis (10-yr OS ~76%).
Estimate the 10-yr OS for pts with localized vs. N+ medullary TCa.	For localized medullary TCa, the 10-yr OS is ~**90%.** If N+, the 10-yr OS is ~**70%.**
What are the stage groupings for anaplastic TCa?	All anaplastic TCa is **stage IV.** Stage IVA is resectable, stage IVB is unresectable, and stage IVC is metastatic.
Estimate the MS and the 1-yr OS for pts with anaplastic TCa.	**MS is ~6 mos** and the 1-yr **OS is ~20%** for pts with anaplastic TCa.
Does the tall cell variant have a more favorable or unfavorable prognosis when compared to classic papillary TCa?	The tall cell variant has an **unfavorable prognosis** (10-yr OS ~75%) when compared to classic papillary carcinomas.
What is the most frequent site of DM in papillary and follicular TCa?	**Lung** (~50%), followed by bone, CNS.

▶ TREATMENT/PROGNOSIS

Generally, what is the Tx paradigm for DTCa?	DTCa Tx paradigm: **primary surgery** (even in M1 Dz) → **observation vs. adj Tx**
What are the 3 surgical options in TCa?	Surgical options in TCa are: 1. Lobectomy + isthmusectomy 2. Near-total thyroidectomy 3. Total thyroidectomy
What is the difference between near-total and total thyroidectomy?	**Near-total is less aggressive** around the recurrent laryngeal nerve.
For which pts with papillary TCa is a lobectomy + isthmusectomy adequate?	This is **controversial.** It is a good option for pts with none of the following risk factors: age >45 yrs, tumor >4 cm, aggressive histology variant, prior Hx of RT, DM, N+, local extension, and +margins.
In addition to improved LC, what is another reason to advocate for a total thyroidectomy even in low-risk pts?	It allows for **easier follow-up** with whole-body iodide scans and serum thyroglobulin.

Per NCCN guidelines (Version 2.2013), what are 4 indications for recommending adj Tx after GTR in DTCa?

Indications for adj Tx after GTR in DTCa are (if any present):

1. >4-cm tumor
2. DM
3. Extensive vascular invasion
4. pT4 (gross extrathyroidal extension)

What are the 5 aggressive histologic subtypes of DTCa that merit consideration of adj Tx?

Aggressive histologic subtypes that merit consideration of adj Tx are:

1. Tall cell
2. Columnar cell
3. Insular cell
4. Oxyphilic
5. Poorly differentiated

Generally, what is the adj Tx paradigm for DTCa?

DTCa adj Tx paradigm: **long-term TSH suppression alone or with I-131 +/− EBRT**

What are the indications for adj I-131 in addition to TSH suppression for DTCa?

Suspected or proven residual normal thyroid tissue or residual tumor are indications for adj I-131.

What is the mCi dose range to ablate residual normal thyroid tissue?

30 mCi is as effective as 100 mCi to ablate residual normal thyroid tissue in low-risk DTCa (*Mallick U et al., NEJM 2012*).

What is the mCi dose range to ablate a residual DTCa lesion?

The dose to ablate a residual DTCa lesion is **100–200 mCi.**

What are the 4 indications for adj EBRT in addition to TSH suppression and I-131 in TCa?

Indications for adj EBRT in addition to TSH suppression and I-131 are:

1. pT4 papillary and ≥ 45 yo
2. Gross residual Dz in the neck after I-131
3. Bulky mets after I-131
4. Lesions with inadequate iodide uptake

What 3 regions should be irradiated with EBRT in a pt ≥45 yo with pT4 papillary TCa?

Thyroid bed, bilat neck, and the upper mediastinal nodes

What is the prognosis for pts with locoregional vs. distant recurrence of DTCa?

The prognosis is **excellent if recurrence is locoregional** (long-term OS is 80%–90%). It is much **worse with distant recurrences.**

What are the typical EBRT doses for DTCa?	<u>Gross Dz</u>: **66–70 Gy,** positive margins: 63–66 Gy <u>Microscopic Dz</u>: **60 Gy** –<u>Nodal basins</u>: **50–54 Gy**
Generally, what is the Tx paradigm for medullary TCa?	Medullary TCa Tx paradigm: **definitive surgery and EBRT for palliation**
Generally, what is the Tx paradigm for anaplastic TCa?	Anaplastic TCa Tx paradigm: **max safe resection → adj CRT;** taxane, and/or doxorubicin, and/or platin chemo with conventional or hyperfractionated EBRT (*Smallridge RC et al., Thyroid 2012*)
For which group of anaplastic TCa pts does PORT improve survival?	Per a recent SEER analysis (*Chen J et al., Am J Clin Oncol 2008*), PORT improved survival in pts with **T4b/extrathyroid extension of Dz** but not for those with T4b/thyroid-confined or stage IVC/metastatic Dz.

▶ TOXICITY

What are the acute side effects of >100 mCi of I-131?	GI irritation, sialadenitis, and cystitis
What are the 3 most important long-term side effects of >100 mCi of I-131?	Pulmonary fibrosis, oligospermia, and leukemia
What does the follow-up of TCa pts entail?	TCa follow-up: H&P + TSH/thyroglobulin levels at 6 and 12 mos, then annually if no Dz; neck US; TSH-stimulated iodine scans if clinically indicated
What kind of additional imaging can be considered if the I-131 scan is negative but the stimulated thyroglobulin level is elevated?	If the I-131 scan is negative but the stimulated thyroglobulin level is elevated, **PET/CT** can be considered.
What is the max recommended lifetime dose for I-131?	The max recommended lifetime dose is **800–1,000 mCi.**

35 Head and Neck Cancer of Unknown Primary

*Boris Hristov, Giuseppe Sanguineti,
and Updated by Gary V. Walker*

▶ BACKGROUND

H&N cancers of an unknown primary represent what % of H&N cancers?

~3%–5% of all H&N cancers are of an unknown primary.

What is the most commonly presumed general site of origin for H&N cancers of an unknown primary?

The **oropharynx** (OPX) is the presumed site of origin for most cases (less common are the nasopharynx [NPX], hypopharynx [HPX], and larynx).

What are the 2 most common originating sites/primary locations if the cancer is presumed to be of oropharyngeal origin?

Tonsils and base of tongue (BOT). Up to 80% of presumed oropharyngeal tumors are thought to originate from these 2 sites.

Approximately what % of pts with tonsillar primaries harbor Dz in both tonsils?

~5%–10% of pts with tonsillar primaries harbor Dz in both tonsils.

A primary can be identified in what % of H&N cancers of unknown primary?

A primary site of origin can ultimately be identified in ~20%–40% of pts.

▶ WORKUP/STAGING

What is the most common presentation for H&N cancers of an unknown primary?

Painless upper neck LAD (IB–III) is the most common presentation.

What is the T staging if no primary H&N site is found after workup?

T0 (not TX) is the assigned T stage if no primary is found.

On what are the overall stage groupings based if the primary is not known?

LN involvement determines the stage groupings:
  Stage III: N1
  Stage IVA: N2
  Stage IVB: N3
  Stage IVC: M1

What % of pts with an unknown primary present with bilat LAD (N2c)?

~10% of pts present with bilat neck Dz.

What does the workup include for pts with an unknown H&N primary?

Unknown H&N primary workup: H&P, CT/MRI, FNA of involved node, panendoscopy + directed Bx with HPV testing, and bilat tonsillectomy (+/– PET, bronchoscopy, esophagoscopy)

If FNA is negative in H&N pts with an unknown primary, what other kind of nodal Bx can be attempted?

If FNA is negative, a **core Bx** can be attempted next. Avoid incisional/excisional Bx, b/c this would result in "neck violation."

What does cystic appearance of the involved LNs suggest in pts with H&N cancers?

Cystic appearance on imaging suggests **HPV positivity/etiology.**

What is the significance of nodal location in terms of likely primary sites?

If <u>upper neck nodes</u> are involved, they are more likely to be due to a H&N primary (e.g., if level I LNs, oral cavity [OC]; if upper level V, NPX primary). If <u>lower neck or supraclavicular nodes</u> are involved, they are more likely to be due to a chest or abdominal primary.

What is the significance of histology in terms of likely primary sites?

<u>Squamous cell</u>: more likely to be a H&N primary
<u>Adenocarcinoma</u>: more likely to be a chest or abdominal primary

What sites are traditionally biopsied for level II nodal involvement?

The **BOT, NPX, pyriform sinus, and tonsils** are typically biopsied with level II LN involvement.

Why is it problematic to obtain the PET scan after endoscopy and Bx in pts with an unknown H&N primary?

Post-Bx inflammation may lead to false+ results. This is why some advocate that if used, PET scans should be done initially.

When is triple endoscopy indicated in pts with neck Dz and an unknown primary?

Triple endoscopy is generally **done in pts with levels IV–V LAD** (more likely to be lung/abdominal primary). Also, PET/CT C/A/P should be considered in such cases.

Site-directed Bx will reveal the primary in roughly what % of unknown primary cases?

Site-directed Bx will reveal the H&N primary in ~50% of cases.

Unilat tonsillectomy will reveal the primary in approximately what % of cases?

Unilat tonsillectomy will reveal the primary in ~25% of cases.

PET/CT will reveal the primary in approximately what % of unknown H&N primary cases?

PET/CT will reveal the primary in ~20%–25% of cases.

What do the data show in regard to bilat tonsillectomy for pts with an unknown H&N primary?

Data from the **Johns Hopkins Hospital** (*McQuone S et al., Laryngoscope 1998*) showed **improved diagnostic yields with bilat tonsillectomy.** Additionally, it **may render follow-up with PET/CT easier.**

When should tonsillectomy be performed in pts being worked up for an unknown primary?

Tonsillectomy is generally performed **at the time of direct laryngoscopy.**

What are the approximate predictive values of PET for pts with an unknown primary?

The **PPV is ~90%** and the **NPV is ~75%** for pts with an unknown primary.

What % of pts with an unknown H&N primary have metastatic Dz on PET/CT?

~10% have metastatic Dz on PET/CT—yet another reason to consider upfront PET.

▶ **TREATMENT/PROGNOSIS**

What is the general Tx paradigm for H&N cancers if a primary is found vs. if there is an unknown primary?

H&N cancer Tx paradigm:
  If primary found: treat according to the primary location
  If no primary found: surgery +/– RT, RT alone, or RT +/– neck dissection

Which unknown primary pts can be treated with neck dissection alone?

Generally, **N1 (<3 cm) pts.** B/c of this and b/c it allows for better staging, some advocate upfront neck dissection at the time of direct laryngoscopy. (*Coster JR et al., IJROBP 1992*)

For which H&N pts is upfront neck dissection a reasonable approach?

Upfront neck dissection is reasonable **if better staging is desired** (e.g., if the path is unclear), **if the neck has been "violated"** (i.e., after incisional Bx), and **with a small, unilat, single +node** (N1).

What % of pts with N1 Dz fail at the primary site after neck dissection alone?

~25% of N1 pts ultimately fail at the primary site after neck dissection alone. However, this can vary from 10%–50%.

What is the approximate overall neck failure rate after neck dissection alone?

The overall neck failure rate is ~15% after neck dissection alone. (*Coster JR et al., IJROBP 1992*)

What is the approximate neck failure rate after neck dissection if there is evidence of ECE?

The approximate neck failure rate after neck dissection alone is ~60% with ECE. (*Coster JR et al., IJROBP 1992*)

What are the indications for PORT in pts with an unknown H&N primary?

≥N2 Dz, ECE/+margin, or neck violation (e.g., after open/excisional Bx)

What do the standard RT fields include in pts with an unknown H&N primary?

The fields generally include **both neck and the mucosal sites at risk** (NPX, OPX, HPX, larynx). Some advocate omission of the HPX/larynx from the RT fields, especially if HPV+.

What are the historical 5-yr LC and OS rates after definitive RT for pts with an unknown H&N primary?

University of Florida data (*Erkal HS et al., IJROBP 2001*): LC 78% and OS 47%
Danish data (*Grau C et al., Radiother Oncol 2000*): OS 37%

What factors have been traditionally associated with inferior OS after definitive RT for H&N tumors of an unknown primary?

More advanced N stage, ECE, and lower RT doses have been associated with inferior outcomes. (*Erkal HS et al., IJROBP 2001*)

What standard RT fields have been traditionally used for H&N tumors of an unknown primary?

Opposed lats matched with an ant low neck/supraclavicular field (with post neck electron fields after 40–44 Gy). However, conformal techniques such as IMRT should be used as standard of care.

What were the anatomical borders of the traditional setup for the 2D lat fields used for H&N tumors of an unknown primary?

Anterior: behind OC/hard palate
Superior: to base of skull to include NPX
Posterior: below tragus to post edge of spinous processes
Inferior: sup edge of thyroid cartilage; if level III or IV, inf edge of cricoid to cover larynx

What RT doses are generally employed?

66–70 Gy to gross Dz with margin, **60 Gy** to intermediate-risk areas 1 nodal station above and below in ipsi side, and **50–54 Gy** to low-risk areas (including mucosal sites) (all in 2 Gy/fx)

What evidence supports the omission of the larynx/HPX from the standard RT fields?

University of Florida data (*Baker CA et al., Am J Clin Oncol 2005*): larynx-sparing RT is just as effective with less toxicity.

What is the evidence in favor of bilat neck irradiation for H&N tumors of an unknown primary?

Loyola data (*Reddy SP et al., IJROBP 1997*): contralat nodal failure is higher (44%) in pts receiving unilat nodal RT (vs. 14% for bilat nodal RT). Also, there is a higher primary emergence rate with unilat RT (44% vs. 8%).

What are a few of the advantages of IMRT for H&N tumors of an unknown primary?

Greater parotid sparing, can consider concurrent chemo (*Klem ML et al., IJROBP 2008*), dose painting to avoid sequential cone downs, **can use simultaneous integrated boost dosing** (e.g., 212 × 33 = 69.96 Gy, 180 × 33 = 59.4 Gy, and 170 × 33 = 56.1 Gy)

When is neck dissection entertained after definitive RT for H&N tumors of an unknown primary?

Post-RT neck dissection is considered with **persistence of Dz** (e.g., on PET or clinically). Some still consider it standard for all pts with ≥N2 Dz, although more commonly, elective neck dissection after RT is not performed if there is no clinical evidence of disease on clinical exam and radiographic restaging.

Within what timeframe after RT should neck dissection be performed if decided upon upfront (i.e., regardless of response to RT)?

Neck dissection should occur ~3–4 mos (and no later than 6 mos) after RT.

▶ TOXICITY

What are common acute side effects from RT to the H&N region?

Mucositis, hoarseness, and malnutrition (weight loss)

What are common long-term complications from RT to the H&N region?

Xerostomia, dysphagia, neck scarring and edema (especially if combined with neck dissection), hypothyroidism, and laryngeal dysfunction (aspiration, hoarseness, etc.)

After what dose must the practitioner come "off-cord" when irradiating the post neck with standard fields?

The practitioner must come off-cord **after a dose of 40–44 Gy** (in 2 Gy/fx). Use matching electron fields or IMRT if greater post neck doses are desired.

After RT, when should PET be performed to assess for nodal response?

PET should be performed no sooner than ~2–3 mos after RT. (TROG analysis: *Corry J et al., Curr Oncol Rep 2008*)

36

Neck Management and Postoperative Radiation Therapy for Head and Neck Cancers

Updated by Gary V. Walker

What is a radical neck dissection?

Radical neck dissection is a **procedure that removes all LN levels ("comprehensive") from levels I–V and other structures** (the sternocleidomastoid, jugular vein, and spinal accessory nerve).

What is a modified radical neck dissection?

Modified radical neck dissection is a **comprehensive nodal dissection** that spares at least 1 of the following structures: sternocleidomastoid, jugular vein, or spinal accessory nerve.

What is considered a selective neck dissection?

Selective neck dissection is **dissection of selective neck areas** based on the understanding of the common pathways of spread according to the H&N site.

What is a supraomohyoid neck dissection?

Supraomohyoid neck dissection is **removal of nodes above the omohyoid muscle** (levels I–III and sup V), common for cancers of the oral cavity (OC).

What is a lat neck dissection?

Lateral neck dissection is **elective dissection of levels II–IV,** traditionally for cancers of the larynx and pharynx.

What is an anterolat neck dissection, and when should it be done?

Anterolat neck dissection is **elective neck dissection of levels I–IV,** typically **done for cN0 oropharyngeal cancer** (OPC).

What is an ant neck dissection, and when should it be done?

Ant neck dissection is **selective neck dissection of levels II–IV,** typically **done for cN0 laryngeal/ hypopharyngeal cancers.**

What is a posterolat neck dissection, and when is it done?

Posterolat neck dissection is **elective neck dissection of the retroauricular, suboccipital, upper jugular, and post cervical nodes.** It is **used for skin cancers** (squamous cell carcinoma, melanoma) **located post to the ear canal.**

What is an ant compartment dissection, and when is it done?	Ant compartment dissection is **selective level VI dissection,** traditionally **performed for thyroid cancers.**

▶ WORKUP/STAGING

Which 3 H&N sites have the highest rates of clinical nodal positivity?	The **nasopharynx** (NPX) (87%), **base of tongue** (78%), **and tonsil** (76%) have the highest rates of clinical nodal positivity. (*Lindberg R et al., Cancer 1972*)
Which 2 H&N sites have the highest rates of retropharyngeal nodal positivity on CT/MRI?	On CT/MRI, **nasopharyngeal and pharyngeal wall primaries** have the highest rates of retropharyngeal involvement (74% and 20%, respectively). (*McLaughlin MP et al., Head Neck 1995*)

▶ TREATMENT/PROGNOSIS

When is a selective neck dissection appropriate?	When there is a **clinically negative neck but ≥10% risk of subclinical Dz;** otherwise, do at least a modified radical neck dissection (rarely is a radical neck dissection done anymore).
When is an elective neck dissection necessary after definitive RT?	Elective neck dissection is necessary whenever there is a **partial response/residual Dz after RT (any nodal stage).**
When can an elective neck dissection be omitted for a pt with ≥N2 Dz?	This is **controversial.** The decision may be guided by PET response 10–12 wks after RT. If a CR, elective neck dissection may be left out. However, at some institutions, any pt with ≥N2 Dz would get neck dissection regardless of the response to RT. The use of elective neck dissection in the absence of disease after RT is increasingly less common.
What are the indications for adj RT after a neck dissection?	After a neck dissection, adj RT should be used with **≥3 cm +nodes, ≥2 +nodes, if ≥2 nodal levels are involved, with +ECE, or if there is an undissected high-risk nodal area.**
When should chemo be added to PORT in the management of H&N cancers?	Absolute indications: +margin, +ECE (category 1 per the NCCN) Relative (weaker) indications: multiple nodes, PNI/LVI, T4a, or OC primary with level IV nodes
How should cisplatin be dosed when given with RT for H&N cancers?	The cisplatin dosing with RT is **100 mg/m^2 intravenously on days 1, 22, and 43.**

How did the 2 seminal H&N trials supporting the addition of chemo to RT in the adj setting differ, and what did they show?

EORTC 22931 (*Bernier J et al., NEJM 2004*): 334 pts randomized to PORT 66 Gy vs. PORT + cisplatin 100 mg/m^2 on days 1, 22, and 43. Eligibility: ECE, + margin, PNI, LVI, and levels 4–5 + N from OC cancer/OPC. There was better OS, DFS, and 5-yr LC with CRT but ↑ grades 3–4 toxicity.

RTOG 95–01 (*Cooper JS et al., NEJM 2004*): 459 pts randomized to 60–66 PORT vs. PORT + cisplatin 100 mg/m^2 on days 1, 22, and 43. Eligibility: >2 LNs, ECE, + margin. There was better DFS (43% vs. 54%) and 2-yr LRC (72% vs. 82%) but only a trend to improvement in OS (57% vs. 63%).

What are the presumed reasons why EORTC 22931 showed an OS benefit while RTOG 9501 did not?

The EORTC trial included more margin+ pts (28% vs. 18%), more pts with worse tumor differentiation (19% vs. 7%), more hypopharynx cases (20% vs. 10%), and more pts that started RT ≥6 wks after surgery (32%).

What important study compared preop RT to PORT for advanced H&N (mostly hypopharyngeal) cancers?

RTOG 73–03 (*Tupchong L et al., IJROBP 1991*): 354 pts, 50 Gy preop vs. 50–60 Gy postop. LC improved with PORT but not OS. Both LC and OS improved with PORT in OPC pts.

What are the indications for boosting the tracheostomy stoma with PORT?

Indications for boosting the stoma with PORT are:

1. Emergency tracheostomy/tracheostomy prior to definitive surgery if close to tumor
2. Subglottic extension
3. Ant soft tissue extension
4. T4 laryngeal tumors

What are the dose recommendations for PORT to the neck and primary?

In 2 Gy/fx: **50–54 Gy:** undissected clinically negative area, **60 Gy:** postop (–margin) and dissected neck, **66 Gy:** postop (+margin, +ECE), **70 Gy:** gross residual,

When should the retropharyngeal nodes be covered/irradiated?

Nasopharyngeal, hypopharyngeal, and pharyngeal wall primaries or N2 or greater disease all merit prophylactic irradiation of the lateral retropharyngeal nodes.

What are the indications for treating the sup mediastinal nodes in H&N cancer?

T3-T4, hypopharyngeal/thyroid primaries, and involvement of the supraclavicular nodes are indications for treating the sup mediastinal nodes.

What is the inf extent of the RT fields if sup mediastinal nodes are to be treated?

The inf extent encompasses **nodes to the level of the carina or 5 cm below the clavicular heads.**

What are some contraindications to neck dissection as the primary management of the neck in pts with H&N cancers?

Base of skull invasion, satellite skin nodules/dermal invasion, and medically unstable/inoperable pts. Relative contraindications include internal carotid invasion, bone invasion, and skin ulceration.

What did the TROG 98.02 study suggest regarding the utility of planned neck dissections after definitive CRT for H&N cancer?

TROG 98.02 determined that neck dissection may not be needed for N2–N3 pts who have a CR on PET 12 wks post-CRT. These pts have low rates (4%–6%) of LRF despite the omission of neck dissection. (*Corry J et al., Head Neck 2008*)

 TOXICITY

What are some common late sequelae of RT (+/– neck dissection) in H&N cancer?

Neck fibrosis/scarring, submental edema, hypothyroidism, and xerostomia

According to the RTOG combinatorial analysis, what factors were associated with severe late toxicity after CRT in advanced H&N cancer pts?

Per the RTOG combinatorial analysis, advanced age, advanced T stage, laryngeal/hypopharyngeal primaries, and neck dissection were all associated with severe late sequelae after CRT. (*Machtay M et al., JCO 2008*)

37 Early-Stage (I–II) Non–Small Cell Lung Cancer

Updated by Nikhil G. Thaker and Steven H. Lin

▶ BACKGROUND

What are the estimated annual # of new lung cancer cases diagnosed in the U.S. and the # of deaths from lung cancers?

In 2013, there were **228,190 newly diagnosed cases** of lung cancers in the U.S., **accounting for 159,480 deaths.** This accounts for more deaths than all colon, breast, and prostate cancers combined.

What is the median age at diagnosis of lung cancer? What is the lifetime risk of developing lung cancer—in men and women?

The median age at diagnosis is ~70 yrs. The lifetime risk of developing lung cancer is 1 in 13 for men and 1 in 16 for women. (*American Cancer Society [ACS] Lung Cancer Key Statistics; NCI SEER Stat Fact Sheets*)

Overall, what is the 5-yr survival rate for lung cancer pts?

The overall 5-yr survival rate for non–small cell lung cancer (NSCLC) is **15.9%.** (*Goldstraw P et al., J Thorac Oncol 2007*)

What is the median and 5-yr OS for stages I–II patients who do not undergo treatment?

The median and 5-yr OS for stages I–II patients who do not undergo treatment is ~12 months and ~10%, respectively.

What is the most common nonskin-related cancer in the world and the leading cause of cancer-related mortality in the U.S. and worldwide?

Lung cancer is the most common nonskin cancer in the world and the leading cause of cancer-related mortality in the U.S. and worldwide.

How many lobes are there in the lung? How many segments are there per lobe?

There are **5 lobes in the lung**—3 on the right and 2 on the left: RUL, RML, RLL, LUL, and LLL. Lingula is the anatomic equivalent of LML and is part of the LUL. There are **5 segments per lobe, except for the RUL and RML, which are divided in 3 and 2 segments,** respectively, supplied by tertiary bronchi.

Name the 9 N2 nodal stations.	N2 nodal stations: <u>Station 1</u>: highest mediastinal <u>Station 2</u>: upper paratracheal <u>Station 3</u>: prevascular (3A) and retrotracheal/ prevertebral (3P) <u>Station 4</u>: lower paratracheal <u>Station 5</u>: subaortic (AP window) <u>Station 6</u>: para-aortic <u>Station 7</u>: subcarinal <u>Station 8</u>: paraesophageal <u>Station 9</u>: pulmonary ligament
Where are the intrapulmonary and hilar nodes located?	Intrapulmonary nodes are nodes **along the secondary bronchi,** whereas hilar nodes are those **along the main stem bronchi.** These are all considered N1 nodes.
Name the 5 N1 nodal stations.	N1 nodal stations (*Note:* N1 nodes are all **double digits**): <u>Station 10</u>: hilar <u>Station 11</u>: interlobar <u>Station 12</u>: lobar <u>Station 13</u>: segmental <u>Station 14</u>: subsegmental
What are the 3 histologic subtypes of NSCLC in decreasing order of frequency?	Histologic subtypes of NSCLC are: **adenocarcinoma** (50%) > **squamous cell carcinoma** (35%) > **large cell** (15%)

In addition to tobacco smoke, what are 3 other environmental exposure risk factors for developing lung cancers?	Environmental exposure risk factors for lung cancer:
	  1. Radon
	  2. Asbestos (*Note:* Smoking and asbestos exposures are synergistic in early reports, but more recent studies suggest less than a multiplicative effect.)
	  3. Occupational exposure (arsenic, bis-chloromethyl ether, hexavalent chromium, mustard gas, nickel, polycyclic aromatic hydrocarbon)

What is the estimated RR for lung cancer in heavy smokers vs. nonsmokers?	**Heavy smokers have a 20-fold excess of lung cancer** (*ACS cohort study*). There is also a 2%–3% per yr risk of tobacco-induced 2nd primary cancer.
What is the risk of lung cancer in former smokers compared to current smokers?	The risk of developing lung cancer in former smokers is **around half** (9 times vs. 20 times) that of current smokers. (*ACS cohort study*)
What is the risk of lung cancer from passive smoke exposure?	There is an RR of 1.2–1.3 for developing lung cancer from passive smoke exposure.
Approximately what % of smokers develop lung cancer?	**<20%** of smokers actually develop lung cancer (in the Carotene and Retinol Efficacy Trial, 10-yr cancer risk was 1%–15%).

What histology subtype of NSCLC is least associated with smoking?

Adenocarcinoma is the histologic subtype that is least associated with smoking.

Name 3 histologic variants of adenocarcinoma of the lung.

Adenocarcinoma in situ (previously bronchoalveolar), acinar, and papillary

Discuss the natural history and Tx response of adenocarcinoma in situ (formerly bronchoalveolar) carcinoma.

Adenocarcinoma in situ is typically not associated with smoking. It can present as a solitary nodule or multifocally. The pneumonitic form may spread along alveoli without basement membrane invasion. These tumors may have a good response to tyrosine kinase inhibitors (TKIs).

Name 2 variants of large cell cancer of the lung.

Giant cell and clear cell

What is the race and sex predilection for NSCLC?

Blacks have the highest incidence of lung cancer. **Males** also are historically at greater risk, but as females continue to start smoking, the incidence in females is rising.

What is the most common stage at initial presentation?

The most common stage of presentation for lung cancer is **metastatic Dz** (around one-third of pts).

What are the most common sites of DMs for lung cancer?

Bone, adrenals, and brain

What are the paraneoplastic syndromes associated with lung cancers?

Hypercalcemia of malignancy due to PTHrP, syndrome of inappropriate secretion of antidiuretic hormone (SIADH) → ↓ Na, Cushing (due to ↑ ACTH), Lambert-Eaton syndrome, other neurologic disorders, hypercoagulability (adenocarcinoma), gynecomastia (large cell), carcinoid (including vasoactive intestinal peptide → diarrhea), and hypertrophic osteoarthropathy (adenocarcinoma).

What is the cause of Lambert-Eaton syndrome? Clinically, how can Lambert-Eaton be distinguished from myasthenia gravis?

Lambert-Eaton syndrome is caused by **circulating autoantibodies against presynaptic P/Q calcium channel. Lambert-Eaton strength improves with serial effort** but not myasthenia gravis.

Which histologic subtypes of lung cancer are associated with peripheral and central locations?

Peripheral: adenocarcinoma, large cell
Central: SCC

With which histologic subtypes of lung cancer is thyroid transcription factor-1 (TTF-1) staining associated?	**Adenocarcinoma, nonmucinous bronchioalveolar carcinoma (adenocarcinoma in situ), and neuroendocrine tumors** (i.e., small cell lung cancer, carcinoid). TTF-1 is rare in SCC. A thyroid cancer primary must be excluded.
In NSCLC, what is the role of CXR or CT screening for high-risk pts?	This topic remains complex and controversial as of 2013. The U.S. Preventive Services Task Force (USPSTF) has issued a draft statement (July 30, 2013) recommending high-risk individuals to get a low-dose CT scan every year. CXR is not recommended for screening for lung cancer.
Who are the high-risk individuals that the USPSTF recommends undergo lung cancer screening?	Current smokers or those who have quit within the past 15 years, who are aged 55–79 yrs, and who have a smoking history of 30 pack-years or greater.
What RCT have reported on low-dose CT screening for lung cancer among high-risk groups?	The National Lung Cancer Screening Trial (NLST, *N Engl J Med 2011*) was a prospective, RCT of lung ca screening comparing low-dose CT vs. annual CXR for 3 years in patients at high risk for lung cancer. Results suggested that low-dose CT decreased the relative risk of lung cancer death by 20%. To prevent 1 death from lung cancer, 320 high-risk individuals needed to be screened with low-dose CT. The Dutch Belgian NELSON trial is currently ongoing.
What factors define the high-risk group for lung cancer according to the NCCN guidelines?	Per **NCCN 2014:** Age 55–74 yrs and ≥30-pack-year smoking history and smoking cessation <15 years (category 1) OR age ≥50 and ≥20 pack year history of smoking and 1 additional risk factor (other than 2nd-hand smoking) (category 2B). Additional risk factors include cancer Hx, lung disease Hx, family Hx of lung cancer, radon exposure, and occupational exposure. Exposure to 2nd-hand smoking is not an independent risk factor.
What is lead-time bias and how could it affect the results of a screening trial?	The lead time in diagnosis is the length of time between detecting the cancer from screening and when the diagnosis would have otherwise have occurred (i.e., through symptoms or imaging studies). This could lead to an apparent increase in survival.
What is length-time bias and how could it affect the results of a screening trial?	Length-time bias occurs when a screening test detects cancers that take **longer** to become symptomatic (i.e., due to the detection of slower-growing or indolent cancers). This too could lead to an apparent increase in survival.

What is the single most clinically significant acquired genetic abnormality in NSCLC?

EGFR mutation in exon 19 (in-frame deletion of 4 amino acid, LREA) **and exon 21** (L858R point mutation); results in a constitutively active receptor.

Among pts with NSCLC, in what particular groups are the EGFR mutations common, and for what do these mutations predict?

In the overall lung cancer population, EGFR mutations are **seen in only ~10%,** but this occurs at high rates (30%–70%) in nonsmokers, adenocarcinomas, and Asians. These mutations **predict for a high response rate of ~80% to TKIs;** gefitinib, erlotinib).

Is EGFR overexpression more common in SCC or adenocarcinoma?

EGFR may be overexpressed in 80%–90% of SCCs vs. 30% of adenocarcinomas.

What point mutation in the *EGFR* gene is associated with TKI resistance?

T790M is the point mutation in the *EGFR* gene associated with TKI resistance.

What other testing results predict well for response to TKI?

EGFR amplification (by FISH) and the VeriStrat test (serum protein test from Biodesix based on a phase III trial (PROSE, *Gregorc V et al., ASCO 2013*) is a good predictor for TKI response.

For what does the *KRAS* mutation or *ERCC1* expression predict?

The *KRAS* mutation or high *ERCC1* expression predicts for **resistance to platinum-based chemo.** However, **low *ERCC1* expression** is an indicator of better prognosis (better overall survival).

▶ WORKUP/STAGING

What is the initial workup for a pt suspected of having lung cancer?

Lung cancer initial workup: H&P + focus on weight loss >5% over prior 3 mos, Karnofsky performance status (KPS), tobacco Hx, neck exam for N3 Dz, CBC, CMP, CT chest to include adrenals, PET/CT scan), MRI brain for presumed stages II–III, MRI for paraspinal/sup sulcus tumors, Dx of lung cancer rendered by Bx via transbronchial endoscopic or transthoracic FNA (intraop preferred, mediastinoscopy or endobronchial US (EBUS) for suspected hilar or N2 nodes, PFTs prior to Tx, and smoking cessation counseling

What are the 3 most common presenting Sx of NSCLC?

Dyspnea, cough, and weight loss (others include chest pain and hemoptysis)

What is the sensitivity and specificity of sputum cytology for Dx of lung cancer?

Sensitivity <70%, specificity >90%. Accuracy increases with increasing # of specimens analyzed. At least 3 sputum specimens are recommended for the best accuracy.

What is the sensitivity and specificity of FDG-PET compared to CT for the staging of lung cancers?

<u>PET</u>: sensitivity 83%, specificity 91%
<u>CT</u>: sensitivity 64%, specificity 74%

What is the estimated % of pts who will have false+ N2 nodes based on PET/CT?

~10%–20%. PPV ~80%. +N2 nodes by PET/CT need pathologic confirmation before deferring to potentially curative surgery.

What is the estimated % of pts who will have false–N2 nodes based on PET/CT?

~5%–16%. NPV ~95%. –N2 nodes by PET/CT for clinical T1 lesions may not need mediastinoscopic evaluation (this is controversial).

What is the rate of occult mets from lung cancer detected by FDG-PET?

In many series, the range is **~6%–18%.**

If a PET scan is being ordered, should a bone scan be obtained to evaluate for bone mets as well?

No. In NSCLC, PET is just as sensitive as bone scan but more specific. However, consider pathologic confirmation for solitary PET+ lesions given the risk of a false+.

What clinical characteristics are important to focus on to determine the nature of a solitary pulmonary nodule?

Nodule size (and whether there are changes in size in the past 2 yrs), **Hx of smoking, age,** and **nodule margin on CT** (i.e., spiculation)

Stage for stage, does adenocarcinoma or SCC have a worse prognosis? Why?

Adenocarcinoma. It has a **greater propensity to metastasize,** particularly to the brain.

Does large cell carcinoma have a natural Hx and prognosis more similar to SCC or adenocarcinoma?

Large cell carcinoma has a natural Hx and prognosis more similar to **adenocarcinoma.**

Describe the T staging of NSCLC using the AJCC 7th edition (2011) of the TNM stage.

T1: ≤3 cm, surrounded by lung parenchyma (T1a ≤2 cm; T1b 2.1–3 cm)
T2: >3–7 cm, +visceral pleura, >2 cm from carina, +atelectasis of lobe (T2a 3.1–5 cm; T2b 5.1–7 cm)
T3: >7 cm, tumor invading main stem bronchus <2 cm from carina; invasion to diaphragm, chest wall (CW), pericardium, mediastinal pleura; or associated atelectasis or obstructive pneumonitis of entire lung or satellite nodule in same lobe

T4: any size, invading mediastinum, heart, great vessels, trachea, recurrent laryngeal nerve, esophagus, vertebral body, carina, or with separate tumor nodules in a different ipsi lung lobe

Describe the N staging of NSCLC.

N1: ipsi hilar or peribronchial nodes
N2: ipsi mediastinal or subcarinal nodes
N3: any supraclavicular/scalene nodes or contralat mediastinal/hilar nodes

What is the AJCC 7th edition (2011) of the TNM stage for malignant pleural/pericardial nodules/effusion or opposite lung tumor nodules in NSCLC?

Malignant pleural/pericardial nodules/effusion or opposite lung tumor nodules in NSCLC is characterized as **M1a,** whereas DM is M1b.

What is considered early-stage NSCLC? Categorize the appropriate TNM stratification.

Stages I and II are considered early-stage NSCLC.
Stage IA: T1aN0, T1bN0
Stage IB: T2aN0
Stage IIA: T2bN0 or T1–2aN1
Stage IIB: T2bN1 or T3N0

What procedures prior to thoracotomy can be used to evaluate the following nodal stations: (1) left and right stations 2, 4, and 7; (2) stations 5–6?

1. **Mediastinoscopy** to evaluate left and right stations 2, 4, and 7 **or EBUS** to evaluate left and right stations 2, 3, 4, 7, and 10
2. **Video-assisted thoracic surgery (VATS) or ant mediastinotomy** (Chamberlain procedure) for stations 5–6

When should pre-Tx mediastinal nodal assessment be done?

1. To confirm PET or CT + nodes
2. All superior sulcus tumors
3. If T3 or central T1–T2 lesions

As per NCCN 2014, invasive mediastinal staging should be performed for most patients with stages I or II lung cancer, preferably during and just before the planned resection.

What routine PFT results (FEV$_1$ and DLCO) indicate that the pt needs further testing prior to undergoing resection?

If the **FEV1 is <80%** predicted for the age and size of the pt **or the DLCO is <80%** predicted, then the pt may need quantitative lung scans/exercise testing to carefully predict postop pulmonary function.

What is the min absolute FEV1 necessary for pneumonectomy and lobectomy?

Pneumonectomy: >2 L
Lobectomy: Postop >1.0 L
Any <1.5-L pt may be a candidate for wedge resection. The marginal % FEV1 for surgery is 40% of the predicted value.

Which subsets of lung cancer pts are at high risk for surgical morbidity?	Subsets at high risk for surgical morbidity: 1. pCO_2 >45 mm Hg (hypercapnia controversial) 2. pO_2 <50 mm Hg 3. Preop FEV_1 <40% of predicted value 4. Poor exercise tolerance 5. DLCO <40% of predicted value (desired >60%) 6. Postop FEV_1 <0.71 or <30% of predicted value 7. Cardiac problems (left ventricle ejection fraction <40%, myocardial infarction within 6 mos, arrhythmias) 8. Obesity
What are some factors that predict for postop complications (i.e., mortality, infection)?	**Active smoking (6 times higher), poor nutrition, advanced age, and poor lung function.** It is advised that pts should quit smoking for at least 4 wks prior to resection and have a nutrition evaluation.
What % of lung cancer pts clinically at stage I are upstaged at surgery?	~5%–25% of stage I lung cancer pts are upstaged at surgery.
In addition to stage, name 3 other poor prognostic factors in lung cancer pts.	Poor prognostic factors in lung cancer: 1. KPS <80% 2. Weight loss >5% in 3 mos (10% in 6 mos) 3. Age >60 yrs

▶ TREATMENT/PROGNOSIS

Generally, what is a Tx paradigm for a stage I–II medically operable NSCLC pt?	Stages I–II medically *operable* NSCLC Tx paradigm: surgical resection (lobectomy) + mediastinal LND → adj chemo for stage II (and chemo perhaps for stage IB, depending on risk factors including grade, LVSI, >4 cm size, visceral pleural involvement, incomplete LN staging). (per NCCN 2014)
Generally, what is the Tx paradigm for a stage I–II medically inoperable NSCLC pt?	Stages I–II medically *inoperable* NSCLC Tx paradigm: if T1–2N0, consider definitive hypofractionated stereotactic body radiation therapy (SBRT) or stereotactic ablative radiotherapy (SABR). Otherwise, use definitive conventional RT alone.
Name 3 surgical options to resect a T1-T2 tumor.	Surgical options to resect a T1-T2 tumor: 1. Wedge or segmental resection 2. Lobectomy 3. Pneumonectomy
For a T1N0 NSCLC, what is the estimated LC for wedge/segmental resection vs. lobectomy?	Wedge/segmental LC is **82% vs.** lobectomy LC is **94%** (LF 18% vs. 6%) based on RCT **LCSG 821.** (*Ginsberg RJ et al., NEJM 1995*) Lobectomy is preferred when feasible. However, CALGB 140503 is a currently ongoing phase III trial of lobectomy vs. sublobar resection for ≤2 cm peripheral NSCLC (smaller tumors than those treated in LCSG 821).

For a T1N0 NSCLC, what is the estimated LC for wedge/segmental resection +/− intraop brachytherapy?

LC is **97% with brachytherapy** compared to **83% without brachytherapy.** The outcomes may be equivalent to lobectomy. (*Fernando HC et al., J Thorac Cardiovasc Surg 2005*)

What % of stage I NSCLC pts will develop a 2nd primary after definitive surgical resection?

Up to 30% of pts develop a 2nd primary.

What is the estimated 5-yr OS of completely resected T1–2N0 NSCLC with no adj chemo?

T1N0 ~80%; T2N0 ~68% (*Martini N et al., J Thorac Cardiovasc Surg 1999*)

What is the 5-yr OS, CSS, and MS for pts who refuse any Tx for T1–2N0 NSCLC?

5-yr OS is 6%, CSS is 22%, and MS is 13 mos. (*Raz DJ et al., Chest 2007*) Tumor size is a prognostic factor, independent of T stage.

What are the indications for adj chemo after definitive resection for stages I–II NSCLC?

Indications for adj chemo after definitive resection for stages I–II NSCLC:
1. Stages II–IIIA Dz after resection (category 1)
2. N1 Dz (category 1)
3. T2N0 (stage IB), if the tumor is >4 cm as per unplanned analysis of **CALGB 9633** (surgery +/− carboplatin/paclitaxel). (*Strauss GM et al., JCO 2008*) Other risk factors include poorly differentiated tumor, LVSI, wedge resection, visceral pleural involvement, and incomplete nodal sampling.

What is the estimated 5-yr OS benefit with adj chemo for pts with completely resected stage I or II NSCLC?

~5% at 5 yrs for adj cisplatin-based chemo based on **LACE meta-analysis** of recent trials. (*Pignon JP et al., JCO 2008*) However, HR for stages IA and IB were not significant.

Is there a role for preop chemo in early-stage lung cancer pts?

No. Based on a meta-analysis, the survival gain is the same as for adj chemo (5%). The largest randomized trial (**MRC LU22/EORTC 08012**) for 519 pts randomized to preop chemo vs. surgery alone found good RR (49%) and downstaging (31%) but no survival benefit to preop chemo. (*Gilligan D et al., Lancet 2007*) **The CHEST Trial** tested preop gemcitabine + cisplatin and found no significant benefit for stages IB/IIA but improved OS for stages IIB and IIIA. (*Scagliotti DV et al., JCO 2012*) The **NATCH Spanish Trial** tested surgery vs. preop chemo + surgery vs. surgery + adj chemo and found no significant differences. However, more patients were able to receive chemo in the neoadj setting. (*Felip E et al., JCO 2010*)

Is there a benefit of full mediastinal dissection vs. nodal sampling in early-stage pts undergoing surgical resection?

Possibly. A recent pooled analysis of 3 trials demonstrated a 4-yr OS benefit in stages I–IIIA NSCLC pts (HR 0.78). Mediastinal dissection involves removal of the right 2R, 4R, 7, 8R, and 9R and the left 5, 6, 7, 8L, and 9L. (*Manser R et al., Cochrane Database Syst Rev 2005*)

What are the indications for postop mediastinal RT (PORT) after definitive resection for stages I–II NSCLC?

+Margins, +ECE, and unexpected N2 Dz. Per NCCN 2014, give concurrent CRT for an R2+ margin and sequential for R1 Dz (chemo → RT). Although not specified in NCCN, chemo → RT may also be considered for ECE.

What RT dose is used for a +margin after surgery?

Microscopic +margin: **54–60 Gy**
Gross +margin: **60–70 Gy**

Which randomized study demonstrated improved LC and survival with PORT after surgical resection for early-stage (stages Ia and Ib) NSCLC?

Italian study: 104 pts, stage I, resected with LND (pN0), randomized to PORT vs. observation; PORT encompassed the bronchial stump + ipsi hilum (mean area, 50 cm^2) to 50.4 Gy. There were better LF rates (2% vs. 23%) with a trend to improved 5-yr survival (67% vs. 58%, $p = 0.048$). There was minimal toxicity and no worsened pulmonary function. (*Trodella L et al., Radiother Oncol 2002*)

What is the max RT dose that has been used for definitive RT alone in stages I–II NSCLC?

Up to 84 Gy in standard fractionation if lung dose volume constraints are respected. RTOG 9311 dose-escalation study found that 90.3 Gy dose level was too toxic. (*Bradley J et al., IJROBP 2005*)

What is the 2-yr local recurrence rate for RT alone using standard fractionation?

A **50%–78%** 2-yr local recurrence is based on **RTOG 9311,** but this study included stage III pts as well.

In stages I–II NSCLC pts being treated with definitive RT alone, should elective nodal regions be treated? What is the estimated elective nodal failure rate if untreated?

No. Elective nodal failure rate was <10% in **RTOG 9311.** In most series with stage I lung cancer treated with hypofractionated SBRT, the regional nodal failure rate ranged from 5%–10%. From the Indiana University dose escalation study using SBRT for stage I lung cancer, regional nodal failure as the site of 1st failure was 10%. (*Hoopes DJ et al., Lung Cancer 2007*) Multiple retrospective reviews have shown low elective nodal failure rates and the resultant possibility of dose escalation.

What is the estimated 3- to 5-yr LC and OS for medically inoperable stage I pts treated with definitive hypofractionated SBRT?

In most series using hypofractionated SBRT for stage I lung cancer pts, the **3-yr LC ranged from 85%–95%** and the **3-yr OS was 55%–91%.**

What biologic effective dose (BED) should be achieved to attain max LC and survival in pts with stage I lung cancer treated with SBRT?

According to Japanese data, if the **BED is ≥100 Gy,** then the 5-yr LC rate is 92% and the 5-yr OS is 71%. However, if the BED is <100 Gy, then the 5-yr LC rate is 57% and the 5-yr OS is 30%. (*Onishi H et al., JTO 2007*)

What is the estimated 5-yr rate of DM in early-stage NSCLC after definitive SBRT?

~15%–25%, which is very similar to the rate seen after surgical resection.

What is the SBRT technique that was evaluated in RTOG 0236? What is the 2-yr LC and OS rate for this group of inoperable pts?

SBRT using **20 Gy × 3** (without homogeneity correction) given in 1.5–2 wks. Dose was 18 Gy × 3 with homogeneity correction. 3-yr primary tumor control is 97.6%, but the 3-yr primary tumor and involved lobe control is 90.6%, DFS was 48.3%, and OS was 55.8%. (*Timmerman R et al., JAMA 2010*)

Are centrally located or peripherally located lesions a relative contraindication for hypofractionated SBRT?

Lesions located **centrally** (i.e., **within 2 cm** of the central bronchial tree) are not good hypofractionated RT candidates using 20 Gy × 3 fx due to the risk of grades 3–5 toxicity. (*Timmerman R et al., JCO 2006*) **MDACC** (*Chang JY et al., IJROBP 2008*) proposed 12.5 Gy × 4, with LC at 17 mos of 100%. There was grades 2–3 dermatitis and CW pain in 11%. There was no pneumonitis for newly diagnosed stage I pts.

What CTV and PTV margins are used for SBRT?

At **MDACC,** there is no GTV to CTV expansion. ITV (around GTV) + 5 mm → PTV when 4D-CT simulation and daily CBCT are used. According to RTOG 0915, GTV + 5 mm in axial plane and GTV + 1 cm in longitudinal plane if no 4D-CT used.

What studies have attempted to address the role of SBRT in both operable and inoperable early-stage lung cancer pts?

Operable:

RTOG 0618: phase II, operable stages I–II NSCLC, accrued 33 pts using 18 Gy × 3 (with heterogeneity correction) (*Timmerman R et al., ASCO 2013*): Median f/u 25 mos, 2-yr LF (primary tumor + involved lobe) 19.2%, PFS 65.4%, and OS 84.4%.

ROSEL (Dutch): phase III SBRT vs. surgery for operable stage I pts. RT 20 Gy × 3 for T1, 12 Gy × 5 for T2, and 7.5 Gy × 8 for central tumors. Primary endpoint is 2- and 5-yr LC, QOL, and cost. Trial closed to lack of accrual.

STARS (Accuray/MDACC): phase III SBRT (CyberKnife) vs. surgery in operable stage I pts. RT 12.5 Gy × 4 for central lesions and 16.7 Gy × 3 fx for peripheral tumors. Primary endpoint is OS, DFS, and toxicity at 3 yrs closed to poor accrual. Now a single arm phase II trial in operable patients.

JCOG 0403: phase II study for stage IA medically inoperable or operable pts. 48 Gy in 4 fx over 4–8 days with heterogeneity corrections. Primary endpoint: 3-yr OS and target size of 165 pts.

Inoperable:

TROG 09.02: phase III. T1/T2aN0 for pts who are medically inoperable/refuse surgery. 54 Gy in 3 fx over 2 weeks vs. conventional RT 60–66 Gy in 30–33 fx +/– concomitant carboplatin/paclitaxel. Primary endpoint: time to local failure.

RTOG 0915: phase II study in inoperable stage T1/T2 (<5 cm) NSCLC and peripherally located lesions. 34 Gy single fraction vs. the Japanese regimen of 12 Gy × 4 fx. The winning arm will be compared to the current RTOG reference 20 Gy × 3 fx in a future phase III trial. Early results in ASTRO 2013 showed trial met pre-specified 1-yr toxicity endpoint. Longer follow-up needed.

SPACE (Scandinavian): phase II randomized trial of 3D-CRT 70 Gy in 35 fx vs. SBRT 45 Gy in 3 fx.

RTOG 0813: trial has completed accrual to the phase I/II study of dose-escalated SBRT (9, 10, 11, and 12 Gy × 5 fx over 2 wks) for centrally located tumors. 1 pt developed grade 3 RP in the 12 Gy group. No Tx-related grade 3 or greater toxicity from 9–11 Gy. Phase II completed at 11 Gy × 5 fx. No local failures presented at ASTRO 2011. Final results pending.

▶ TOXICITY

What is the typical follow-up schedule of pts treated for lung cancer?	Typical lung cancer follow-up: H&P + CT chest with contrast q6–12 mos for 2 yrs, then noncontrast CT chest annually; continued smoking cessation counseling. PET or brain MRI is not indicated. (per NCCN 2014)
What are the toxicities seen with SBRT for early-stage lung cancer?	Pneumonitis, lung fibrosis/consolidation, cough, dermatitis, CW pain, esophagitis, and hemoptysis
What is the total lung V20 dose-volume constraint for RT alone?	The total lung V20 dose-volume constraint is <**35%.** (per NCCN 2014)
What is the mean lung dose (MLD) constraint for definitive RT to lung cancer?	The MLD constraint is ≤**20 Gy.** (per NCCN 2014)

What is the distinction between grade 2 and 3 RTOG pneumonitis?

Grade 2 pneumonitis: symptomatic with the need for steroids
Grade 3 pneumonitis: dyspnea at rest and oxygen supplementation needed
Other grades of pneumonitis include grade 1: asymptomatic, seen only on CT; grade 4: hospitalized and intubated; grade 5: death

What are the heart dose-volume constraints for conventionally fractionated RT?

Heart V40 ≤**80%**, V45 ≤**60%** and **V60 ≤30%, mean ≤35 Gy.** (per NCCN 2014)

What is the dose constraint for the brachial plexus with conventional fractionation?

The max dose to the brachial plexus should be kept at ≤**66 Gy.** (per NCCN 2014)

What is the rate of brachial plexopathy seen for pts treated with SBRT for early-stage lung cancer?

The recommended max dose to the brachial plexus is <**26 Gy in 3–4 fx.** (*Forquer JA et al., Radiother Oncol 2009*) Of the 37 apical tumors for the 253 pts treated, 19% of pts developed grades 2–4 plexopathy. A dose >26 Gy resulted in 46% risk vs. 8% risk if the dose was <26 Gy.
At MDACC, for 70 Gy in 10 fx, max dose to the brachial plexus should be <60 Gy, ≤1 cc reaching 50 Gy and ≤10 cc 40 Gy. For 50 Gy in 4 fx, max dose to the brachial plexus should be <40 Gy, ≤1 cc, reaching 35 Gy and ≤5 cc 30 Gy.

At a minimum, what other normal tissue constraints should be closely examined during SBRT?

Location and size are important factors when considering normal tissue toxicity and constraints. Other tissues to monitor closely include esophagus, brachial plexus, trachea, main bronchus and bronchial tree, heart, total lung, major vessels, skin, CW, and spinal cord.

What is the esophageal dose constraint for conventionally fractionated RT?

Ideally, the mean dose of RT to the esophagus should be ≤34 Gy and max ≤105% of Rx dose. (per NCCN 2014) Try to minimize the V60 as much as possible (V60 <33%, V55 <66%, ≤45 Gy to the entire esophagus).

What is the max BED for SBRT resulting in significant complications when centrally located tumors were treated?

180–210 Gy with grade 3 pulmonary complications. (*Timmerman R et al., JCO 2006*) Keeping the BED ≥100 Gy may be sufficient for LC and may avert toxicities for central lesions. (*Onishi H et al., J Thorac Oncol 2007*)

Is a normal SUVmax of FDG-PET required to be considered a good clinical response in the follow-up of stage I NSCLC pts treated with SBRT?

No. Prospective and retrospective reviews suggest that the SUVmax remains elevated for an extended period after SBRT due to an inflammatory response, but there is no evidence of correlation with recurrence. (*Timmerman R et al., IJROBP 2009; Henderson MA et al., IJROBP 2009*)

What % of pts treated with SBRT for early-stage lung cancer have grades 3–5 toxicities?

15% of pts have grades 3–5 toxicities in a review of 15 studies (683 pts). (*Sampson JH et al., Semin Radiat Oncol 2006*)

In **RTOG 0236,** 16.3% of pts experienced grades 3–4 toxicity but no grade 5 toxicity. (*Timmerman R et al., JAMA 2010*)

What factors predict for grades 3–5 toxicities after SBRT for early lung cancer seen on the Indiana University phase II study?

Location (46% hilar/pericentral vs. 17% peripheral) and **tumor size** (GTV >10 cc had 8 times the risk of grades 3–5 toxicity). (*Timmerman R et al., JCO 2006*)

What are the PFT changes before and after SBRT for early-stage lung cancer?

Very minimal based on an institutional review of 92 pts (*Stephans KL et al., JTO 2009*): mean FEV_1 −0.05 (−1.88%), DLCO −2.59% of predicted value; no association with central vs. peripheral location or the dose administered.

38 Advanced-Stage (III–IV) Non–Small Cell Lung Cancer
Updated by Steven H. Lin

▶ BACKGROUND

What is the most common hallmark of locally advanced Dz?

Mediastinal or supraclavicular nodal involvement

What % of pts present with stage IIIA non–small cell lung cancer (NSCLC)?

~30% of all NSCLC pts have stage IIIA Dz at presentation.

What % of pts will have occult N2 Dz found at the time of surgery?	**25%** of pts will have occult N2 Dz found at surgery.
After definitive Tx of a primary lung tumor, what is the time period after which it is considered a 2nd primary tumor?	A tumor that develops **≥2 yrs** after definitive Tx of primary lung cancer is likely a 2nd primary. Whenever a recurrence with identical histology occurs at <2 yrs, it is considered a met. 5-year survival after Dx of a 2nd primary can be as high as 40% if early stage.
What % of pts with locally advanced NSCLC develop brain mets as a 1st site of relapse?	**~15%–30%** of NSCLC pts develop brain mets as a site of 1st relapse.
What is Pancoast syndrome?	Pancoast syndrome is a **result of apical tumors (aka, superior sulcus tumors) invading the thoracic inlet,** with compression on structures such as the sympathetic ganglion, brachial plexus, recurrent laryngeal nerve and vasculature causing shoulder/arm pain, Horner syndrome, paresthesias of the hand in ulnar nerve distribution, hoarseness, and SVC syndrome. Tumors that cause these Sx are referred to as Pancoast tumors.
What is Horner syndrome?	Horner syndrome is a result of tumor compression on the sympathetic ganglion, resulting in a triad of symptoms: **ipsi miosis, ptosis, and anhidrosis.**
How prevalent are superior sulcus tumors?	Superior sulcus tumors account for **~3% of NSCLC.**

▶ WORKUP/STAGING

What is the TNM staging (AJCC 7th ed. (2011)) that defines advanced NSCLC?	**Stage IIIA:** T3N1, T1-T3N2, T4N0-1 **Stage IIIB:** TXN3, T4N2 **Stage IV:** TXNXM1
What is the MS of pts who present with malignant pleural effusion with NSCLC?	MS is **3–9 mos.** These pts are staged as M1a Dz in the new staging system.
What are the survival outcomes of stage IIIA Dz with T3N1 vs. TXN2 Dz?	Stage IIIA is a heterogeneous group, with 5-yr survival ranging from **20%–25%** for T3N1 and **3%–8%** for T1–3N2 Dz. There is a lot of heterogeneity in the prognosis of the T1–3N2 group due to the # and bulk of LNs involved.

What is the utility of PET/CT to determine the resectability of the lung cancer pts?

PET/CT **may improve the staging** to spare pts from futile thoracotomies b/c of unresectable Dz that is not detectable by conventional imaging. A Danish RCT (*Fischer B et al., NEJM 2009*) randomized 189 pts using either conventional staging with CT + mediastinoscopy or conventional staging and PET/CT staging. PET reduced the # of futile thoracotomies and the total # of thoracotomies (both statistically significant). But the overall mortality did not differ between groups.

▶ **TREATMENT/PROGNOSIS**

What are the Tx options for pts with cN2, stage IIIA Dz?

Tx options with cN2, stage IIIA Dz:
1. Induction chemo → surgery ± PORT (*Roth J et al., JNCI 1994; Rosell R et al., NEJM 1994*)
2. Neoadj CRT → lobectomy (**INT-0139**) (*Albain KS et al., Lancet 2009*)
3. Definitive CRT (**RTOG 9410,** Curran W et al., JNCI 2011)

What are the Tx options for pts with cN3, stage IIIB Dz?

Definitive CRT is the only Tx option for cN3, stage IIIB Dz.

Which clinical trials have demonstrated a survival benefit with adding induction chemo to surgery for stages IIIA–B NSCLC pts?

MDACC data (*Roth JA et al., JNCI 1994; Roth JA et al., Lung Cancer 1998*): 60 pts randomized to surgery alone vs. cisplatin/etoposide/ cyclophosphamide × 1 cycle → surgery. MS was 21 mos (induction chemo) vs. 14 mos for surgery alone.

Madrid data (*Rosell R et al., NEJM 1994; Rosell R et al., Lung Cancer 1999*): 60 pts randomized to surgery alone vs. cisplatin/ifosfamide/ mitomycin-C × 3 cycles → surgery. MS was 22 mos (chemo) vs. 10 mos for surgery alone.

Spanish Lung Cancer Group Trial 9901 (*Garrido P et al., J Clin Oncol 2007*): phase II study, 136 pts, all with stage IIIA (N2) or stage IIIB (T4N0–1) Dz. Pts underwent cisplatin/ gemcitabine/docetaxel × 3 cycles → surgery. There was pCR in 13%. MS was 48.5 mos for R0 resection vs. 12.9 mos for R1-R2 resection. The overall complete resection rate was 69%. MS was 16 mos, 3-yr OS was 37%, and 5-yr OS was 21%.

Did any trial fail to demonstrate a benefit for induction chemo followed by surgery?

JCOG 9209 (Japan: *Nagai K et al., J Thorac Cardiovasc Surg 2003*): trial closed early due to poor accrual. 62 pts with stage IIIA N2 NSCLC randomized to surgery alone vs. cisplatin/vindesine × 3 cycles → surgery. There was no difference in MS (16–17 mos) or 5-yr OS (10% with chemo vs. 22% with surgery).

Are there data to demonstrate the need for adding PORT to adj chemo in pts with completely resected stage IIIA N2 NSCLC?

This cannot be adequately answered at this point. CALGB 9734 attempted to address this question (adj chemo alone vs. chemo → RT), but the trial was closed due to poor accrual. (*Perry C et al., Lung Cancer 2007*) There was no difference in DFS or OS. However, some evidence suggests that pts with N2 Dz should be evaluated for chemo → PORT

What is the evidence for PORT? What subset of pts may benefit from PORT?

In subset analysis from randomized trials and meta-analysis, pts with N2 Dz **may benefit from PORT.** There are ongoing prospective phase III trials testing the role of PORT in pN2 pts.

LCSG 773 (*Weisenburger TH et al., NEJM 1986*): RCT, 210 pts, stages II–IIIA (T3 or N2), margin– resection, randomized to PORT or observation. RT: ≥Co-60 to the mediastinum to 50 Gy on postop day 28 (turned out to be nearly all squamous cell carcinoma). Overall LR was better in PORT (3% vs. 41%), and DFS was better in N2 pts. There was no difference in OS between the arms.

PORT Meta-Analysis Trialist Group, Cochrane database, 2005 (*Burdett S et al., Lung Cancer 2005*): meta-analysis of 10 trials of pts treated after 1965. Suggested OS was a detriment to PORT overall. Subset analysis showed a detriment in resected stages I–II Dz but no adverse effect in N2 Dz.

Criticisms: (1) 25% of pts were T1N0; (2) the staging technique is no longer used; (3) the RT technique is no longer used (large fields and fx, high total doses, Co-60 machines); (4) >30% of the meta-analysis relied on a poorly done study using poor techniques/technology (*Dautzenberg B et al., Cancer 1999*) that showed PORT to be detrimental due to a high 5-yr mortality from PORT (31% vs. 8%), mostly due to Tx-related cardiac or respiratory deaths.

SEER analysis (*Lally BE et al., JCO 2006*): 7,465 pts, stages II–III NSCLC from 1988–2002, PORT vs. observation, median follow-up 3.5 yrs. Overall, PORT did not affect OS. However, for the N2 subset, PORT was associated with better OS (HR 0.85) but detrimental for N0-N1.

Reanalysis of the ANITA trial (*Douillard JY et al., IJROBP 2008*): RCT of adj cisplatin/vinorelbine vs. observation for stages IB–IIIA pts after resection. 232 pts rcvd PORT. Overall, as a group, PORT was detrimental on survival (HR 1.34). In subset analysis based on pN stage, PORT was detrimental for pN0 pts. However, there was improved survival in pN1 Dz in the observation arm but detrimental in the chemo arm. PORT improved survival for both observation and chemo arms in pN2 pts.

Is there an advantage of postop CRT vs. PORT alone for stage III N2 NSCLC?

No. INT-0115/RTOG 9105/ECOG (*Keller MB et al., NEJM 2000*) tested PORT vs. CRT in resected stage II or III NSCLC. There was no difference in OS (3.2 yrs) or LC.

What are the anatomic areas targeted with PORT when given for unexpected N2 NSCLC? What is the recommended dose?

Bronchial stump, ipsi hilum, and ipsi mediastinum. Standard doses after complete resection are 50–54 Gy but a boost can be administered to areas of positive margins or extracapsular extension (per NCCN 2014). Doses between 60–70 Gy are appropriate for gross residual disease.

What should be the rate of Tx-related deaths (death from intercurrent disease [DID]) following PORT for NSCLC?

Based on old data with old techniques, DID was 20%–30%, mainly due to pulmonary or cardiovascular excess deaths from PORT. New data suggest much lower rates (2%–3%).

Penn retrospective (*Machtay M et al., JCO 2001*): 202 pts, Tx with surgery + PORT; 4-yr DID PORT (13.4%), vs. matched controls (10%). If <54 Gy, DID was 2%; but ≥54 Gy, DID was 17%.

ECOG 3590 reanalysis (*Wakelee H et al., Lung Cancer 2005*): 488 pts randomized to PORT vs. PORT + chemo; 50.4 Gy RT. Overall, 4-yr DID was 12.9% vs. matched controls at 10.1%.

Is preop chemo alone adequate as an induction regimen in stages IIIA–B lung cancer pts or is preop CRT better?

Two trials have attempted to address this question:
1. **RTOG 0412/SWOG 0332:** pts randomized to induction chemo +/– RT → surgery. Unfortunately, this trial was closed due to poor accrual.

2. **German Lung Cancer Cooperative Group Trial**
(*Thomas M et al., Lancet Oncol 2008*): 558 pts,
stages IIIA–B NSCLC, randomized to induction
chemo etoposide/cisplatin (EP) × 3 cycles →
surgery → RT (arm 1) vs. chemo → CRT (bid RT
with carboplatin/vindesine) → surgery (arm 2).
If +margin/unresectable Dz, the pt rcvd more
bid RT. There was greater pCR (60% vs. 20%)
and mediastinal downstaging (46% vs. 29%) in
the CRT group but no difference in PFS or
survival. If pts required a pneumonectomy,
postop mortality ↑ in the CRT group. This study
has been criticized for its nonstandard RT
regimen.

If CRT is given for stage IIIA Dz upfront, is there a clear benefit to consolidation with surgery?

For all-comers, there may be an improvement in LC, but there is no survival benefit. Subset analysis
demonstrates that those receiving lobectomy may have
an improved survival outcome.

INT-0139 (*Albain KS et al., Lancet 2009*): 396
technically resectable stage IIIA pts randomized to
induction CRT to 45 Gy (50.4 Gy with heterogeneity
correction) + surgery vs. definitive CRT (61 Gy)
alone. Both therapies were proceeded with 2
additional cycles of chemo, which was cisplatin
(50 mg/m^2 days 1, 8) with etoposide (50 mg/m^2 days
1–5), q28day cycle. In the group overall, local relapse
was much better for the surgery arm (10% vs. 22%,
$p = 0.002$), but there was no difference in DM and no
OS benefit. There was OS benefit in subset analysis in
matched pts with lobectomy (5-yr OS 36% vs. 18%;
MS 34 mos vs. 22 mos, $p = 0.002$) but not in pts
who had pneumonectomy. 26% of pts with
pneumonectomy died, but only 1% died from
lobectomy.

What is the RT dose for neoadj CRT if consolidative surgery is planned?

45 Gy. >50 Gy has been shown to have complications
of bronchopleural fistula, prolonged air leak with
empyema, and prolonged postop ventilation.

After an objective response to induction chemo for a pt with stage IIIA Dz, is adding postinduction surgical resection more beneficial than adding sequential radiotherapy?

No. In this circumstance, resection is not more beneficial than radiotherapy.

EORTC 08941 (*Van Meerbeeck J et al., JNCI 2007*): randomized trial for stage IIIA-N2 Dz. Patients responding to platinum-based induction chemotherapy were randomized to RT 60 Gy in 2 Gy/fx (arm 1) vs. surgery (arm 2). Only 50% had radical resection, with only 5% pCR (42% pathology downstage). Operative 30-day mortality was 4%. There was only 55% compliance in the RT arm. There was no difference in OS or PFS.

In light of all the evidence above, does including surgical resection in therapy for stages IIIA–B lung cancers improve outcomes?

The studies above do not show a clear benefit to adding surgery to CRT for locally advanced NSCLC. Both INT-0139 and EORTC 08941 failed to find superior outcomes with surgery over definitive radiation in stage III disease (albeit in different contexts). Definitive CRT is probably preferred over trimodality therapy in most pts with stages IIIA–B lung cancers.

Is there a subset of patients that is likely to benefit from trimodality therapy?

Patients with minimal, nonbulky N2 disease who can get lobectomy are the best candidates based on the INT-0139 subgroup analysis.

What randomized study established a min dose of 60 Gy for definitive RT for stage III NSCLC?

RTOG 7301 (*Perez C et al., Cancer 1980*): stages IIIA–B pts, dose escalation trial with RT alone of 40 Gy, 50 Gy, and 60 Gy vs. 40 Gy (split course), all in 2 Gy/fx. LC improved with 60 Gy. 60 Gy was established as the standard.

Is there a benefit of altered fractionation of definitive RT (without chemo) for stage III NSCLC?

Yes. Several phase II–III trials have demonstrated this benefit.

RTOG 8311 (*Cox JD et al., J Clin Oncol 1990*): randomized phase I–II, 848 pts with unresectable N2, 1.2 Gy bid to 60, 64.8, 69.6, 74.4, and 79.2 Gy. Patients with good performance status who received ≥69.6 Gy had significantly better 3-yr OS.

CHART (*Saunders MI et al., Lancet 1997*): phase III, 563 pts randomized to 54 Gy at 150 tid (450/day) × 12 consecutive days vs. 60 Gy for 6 wks. There was 10% improvement in 3-year absolute survival for CHART compared to standard RT. Severe esophagitis was common (19% vs. 3%).

What were the 2 seminal studies that demonstrated the importance of adding chemo to radiotherapy compared to radiotherapy alone?

CALGB 8433 "Dillman regimen" (*Dillman RO et al., NEJM 1990*): 155 pts with stage IIIA Dz (T3 or N2) treated with (1) RT alone (60 Gy) or (2) sequential chemo (cisplatin [CDDP]/vinblastine) → RT (60 Gy). Sequential chemo → RT improved MS from 10 mos to 14 mos, 2-yr OS from 13% to 26%, and 5-yr OS from 7% to 19%.

RTOG 88–08 (*Sause W et al., Chest 2000*): 458 pts with unresectable NSCLC (stages II–IIIB) randomized to 3 arms: 2 Gy qd/60 Gy alone (arm 1); 1.2 bid/69.6 Gy alone (arm 2); or sequential chemo (CDDP/vinblastine) + 60 Gy RT (arm 3). There was improved MS in arm 3 with sequential chemo → RT (13.2 mos) compared with conventional RT (11.4 mos) or bid RT (12 mos).

Which 2 randomized studies demonstrated the superiority of concurrent CRT over sequential CRT for unresectable or medically inoperable stages II–III NSCLC?

West Japan Lung Cancer Study Group (*Furuse K et al., JCO 1999*): 320 stages II–III pts randomized to sequential vs. concurrent CRT. Concurrent arm: CDDP/vindesine/MMC split-course RT (28 Gy × 2). Sequential arm: same chemo → RT (56 Gy conventional, nonsplit course). There was better OS and PFS in pts with concurrent CRT. MS was 16.5 mos vs. 13.3 mos (SS); 5-yr OS was 15.8% vs. 8.9% (SS).

RTOG 9410 (*Curran W et al., JNCI 2011*): 610 pts randomized to 3 arms: sequential (Dillman regimen with RT to 63 Gy) (arm 1); concurrent CRT (to 63 Gy) (arm 2); and concurrent hyperfractionated RT (1.2 bid/69.6 Gy) + chemo (arm 3). Chemo was CDDP/vinblastine (except EP for arm 3). Definitive concurrent CRT (arm 2) had a better outcome in MS (17 mos) vs. 14.6 mos (arm 1) or 15.6 mos (arm 3) and 5-yr OS (16% vs. 10% vs. 13%). However, there was ↑ toxicity in the concurrent CRT arm.

Which chemo regimen allows a full dose and which would need to be dose reduced during the course of concurrent CRT?

Cisplatin/etoposide and cisplatin/vinblastine allow a full dose to be administered with RT. Carboplatin/paclitaxel, gemcitabine, or vinorelbine require a significant dose reduction during RT administration.

Is there a benefit of adding induction chemo → CRT for pts with unresectable stages IIIA–B NSCLC?

No. Two prospective studies (**LAMP** and **CALGB 39801** trials) demonstrated no benefit to neoadj chemo. Definitive CRT alone is the standard of care.

LAMP trial (*Belani CP et al., JCO 2005*): randomized phase II, 276 pts with stages IIIA–B NSCLC randomized to arm 1: chemo × 2 cycles → 63 Gy RT (Dillman regimen); arm 2: induction chemo × 2 cycles → concurrent CRT (63 Gy); and arm 3: concurrent CRT → consolidation chemo × 2 cycles. Chemo was carboplatin/paclitaxel. Arm 3 (concurrent CRT) had a better outcome, where MS was 16.3 mos vs. 13 mos (arm 1) or 12.7 mos (arm 2).

CALGB 39801 (*Vokes E et al., JCO 2007*): randomized phase III trial, enrolled 366 pts with unresectable stages IIIA–B randomized to arm 1: CRT vs. arm 2: induction chemo × 2 cycles → CRT. Chemo was carboplatin/paclitaxel. There was no difference in MS or OS. MS 12 mos (CRT) vs. 14 mos (induction) (p = NS), 2-yr OS 29% vs. 31% (p = NS). Upfront chemo ↑ grades 3–4 heme toxicity.

What about consolidation chemo after definitive CRT?

This is **uncertain, at least for docetaxel.** Despite initial enthusiasm with the **SWOG 9504** phase II study showing ↑ MS with consolidation docetaxel in stage IIIB pts after definitive CRT (26 mos), the randomized phase III trial (*Hanna N et al., JCO 2008*) demonstrated no benefit of consolidation chemo with docetaxel but only ↑ toxicities and Tx-related deaths. Thus, there may not be a role of consolidation with docetaxel, but there may be a role for other agents, such as pemetrexed, as maintenance therapy. However, when low dose carboplatin/paclitaxel is used as concurrent regimen with RT, consolidation full dose carboplatin/paclitaxel × 2 cycles is often recommended after completing CRT.

Is there a role for elective nodal irradiation for the Tx of inoperable, locally advanced NSCLC?

No. The current recommendation is to treat with CRT only the involved areas (assessed either by imaging or pathology) to improve dose escalation and improve toxicity.

MSKCC data (*Rosenzweig K et al., JCO 2007*): retrospective analysis of pts treated with IFRT alone. 524 pts treated with definitive 3D-CRT to areas of gross Dz; mean dose 66 Gy. Total elective nodal failures (ENF) (initial uninvolved nodal areas that fail) were 6.1%. The 2-yr primary tumor control rate was 51%. Overall, 2-yr ENF was 7.6%. Pts with local Dz control had a 2-yr ENF of 9%. Ipsi mediastinum had ↑ nodal failures (3%).

Prospective phase III trial (*Yuan et al., ASCO 2007*): inoperable stage III NSCLC randomized to involved-field irradiation vs. elective nodal irradiation. Involved-field irradiation achieved better overall response and improved 5-yr LC of 51% vs. 36% ($p = 0.032$).

What are the volumes and Tx techniques used for RT of locally advanced NSCLC?

GTV is defined by +FDG uptake areas, Bx-proven LN areas, or any LN >15 mm on CT. PTV = GTV + 1–1.5 cm. 3D-CRT or IMRT technique to 60 Gy or higher in 1.8–2 Gy/fx should be given.

Is there a benefit of dose escalation in locally advanced NSCLC?

No, there is currently no evidence that a dose >60 Gy is beneficial based on results from RTOG 0617 (see below). Prior studies suggested that dose escalation improves LC and possibly survival.

RTOG 73–01: RCT testing 40 Gy split vs. 40 Gy continuous vs. 50 Gy continuous vs. 60 Gy continuous. The 60 Gy continuous had the best survival. 60 Gy became standard b/c of this trial, and since then 55–66 Gy is standard.

RTOG 93–11: dose escalation without chemo to 70.9 Gy, 77.4 Gy, 83.8 Gy, and 90.3 Gy. The 90.3 Gy is too toxic, but 77.4 Gy and 83.8 Gy are safe if V20 is 25%–36% and <25%, respectively. LC 50% to 78%, with LF in elective nodal areas <8%.

Michigan study (*Kong FM et al., IJROBP 2005*): 106 pts, stages I–III NSCLC, treated with 63–103 Gy in 2.1 Gy/fx with 3D-CRT; primary tumor + LN + ≥1 cm; no chemo in 81%. MS was 19 mos. MVA showed that the RT dose was the only predictor of better survival.

What was the design of RTOG 0617?

RCT phase III comparison for stages IIIA-B NSCLC treated with CRT with 2 randomizations:
1. 60 Gy vs. 74 Gy
2. Carboplatin/paclitaxel +/− cetuximab

What was the outcome of the dose escalation portion of the study?

Closed early at interim analysis. Patients receiving 74 Gy had worse grade 5 toxicity and grade 3 esophagitis, higher rate of LFs, and worse OS.

What are some possible explanations for the counterintuitive findings in the higher-dose arm?

1. Too tight margins in the high-dose arm → higher local failures → worse survival
2. Unmeasured or underreported toxicities → more treatment deaths → worse survival
3. Extended therapy duration → worse local control → worse survival
4. Combination of the above

Was there a benefit of adding cetuximab to CRT in RTOG 0617?

No. There was no survival benefit except for worse toxicities in the cetuximab arm. In a subset analysis, there was suggestion that higher tumor H-score for EGFR predicted for better outcome with cetuximab.

What should be done in NSCLC pts with incidental N2 Dz found at the time of surgery?

If technically resectable, with only an occult, single-station mediastinal nodal met at surgery, **surgical resection should proceed with lung resection + mediastinal LND → adj chemo, with consideration of PORT.**

For patients who receive surgery upfront, what is the role of adj platinum-based chemo?

It should be given for patients with N+ disease or primary tumors >4 cm in pts with T2N0 (stage IB) tumors.

 LACE meta-analysis for 5 adj trials demonstrated 5-yr OS advantage of 5.4%. (*Pignon JP et al., JCO 2008*)

 CALGB 9633 unplanned subset analysis demonstrated a survival benefit for stage IB pts with tumors >4 cm. (*Strauss GM et al., JCO 2008*)

What is considered bulky, unresectable Dz in NSCLC pts?

Pts with a **histologically involved LN >2 cm on CT, +extranodal involvement, or multistation nodal Dz** (regardless of size)

What is the preferred Tx strategy for pts with stage IIIB T4N0 Dz?

Neoadj chemo or CRT, or definitive CRT. 5-yr OS may approach 25%–30%. R0 resection should be attempted if this is technically feasible.

What is the 5-yr OS of pts with satellite nodules in the same lobe?

5-yr OS is **33%** if pts undergo lobectomy. Careful nodal assessment to exclude N2 Dz must be done.

What is the Tx paradigm for resectable T3-4N0-1 superior sulcus tumors?

Resectable T3–4N0–1 superior sulcus tumor Tx paradigm: preop CRT → surgery → chemo × 2 (**SWOG 9416/INT-0160**) or surgery → PORT to at least 55 Gy (**MDACC:** *Komaki R et al., IJROBP 2000*). If surgical margin is positive, postop CRT should be done using hyperfractionation b/c of potential toxicity to the brachial plexus (60 Gy at 1.2 Gy bid).

What trial established the role of induction CRT for superior sulcus NSCLC? What was the induction regimen and the primary outcome of this study?

A single-arm phase II trial by SWOG 9416/INT-0160 (*Rusch VW et al., JCO 2007*) evaluated induction CRT + surgery for resectable T3-4N0-1 superior sulcus tumors. The induction regimen was with concurrent cisplatin, etoposide, and RT to 45 Gy → restage; if no progression, then surgery → chemo × 2 cycles. Chemo was cisplatin (50 mg/m^2 days 1 and 8) with etoposide (50 mg/m^2 days 1–5), repeated q28days for a total of 4 cycles. 95% completed induction therapy. Of the pts who had thoracotomy (88 of 110 pts [80%]) based on preop judgment of resectability, 94% had complete resection (83 pts). The study showed a 56% pCR or near CR rate and a 5-yr OS of 44% (compared to 30% for historical controls). Survival was better with complete resection (54%). There was no difference between T3-T4 tumors.

What are the appropriate Tx volumes, dose, and field arrangement for a superior sulcus tumor?	GTV defined by PET + 2 cm and ipsi supraclavicular region. AP/PA to 41.4 Gy, then off-cord to 45 Gy. Cord should not exceed 110% of the Rx dose.
Are all pts with stage IIIB NSCLC unresectable?	**No.** Pts with T4 Dz with invasion of vertebral bodies and multiple nodules in different ipsi lung lobes are still resectable.
What are the Tx options for pts with malignant pleural effusion?	Treat as a stage 4 pt: thoracentesis, chest tube + drainage, sclerotherapy with talc or bleomycin, or placement of a chronic indwelling catheter. Depending on performance status, chemo can be considered.
What should be done for pts with 2 synchronous nodules of NSCLC (i.e., occurring in different lobes)?	If there is identical histology, consider M1. If a different histology or genetic signature, it can be considered synchronous stage I NSCLC and definitive surgery can be considered after full workup for nodal/distant involvement is excluded.
How should pts with newly diagnosed NSCLC with a solitary brain lesion be managed?	Surgical resection should be considered, especially if the pt is symptomatic or to exclude a possible primary brain tumor, then either SRS or WBRT. Otherwise, SRS +/– WBRT should be used (per NCCN). The primary lung tumor should be managed according to the appropriate TN stage.
Overall, what is the 5-yr OS in this group of pts?	5-yr OS is 20%–40% as a group.
Is there a role for PCI after Tx for locally advanced NSCLC?	**No.** 4 older randomized trials showed only improvement in brain relapse rates (9% vs. 19%) but no survival benefit in adding PCI. (*Cox JD et al., JAMA 1981; Umsawasdi T et al., J Neurooncol 1984; Miller TP et al., Cancer Ther 1998; Russell AH et al., IJROBP 1991*) A meta-analysis summarizes these data. (*Lester JF et al., IJROBP 2005*) **RTOG 0214** is a modern phase III randomized trial testing the utility of PCI for locally advanced NSCLC. The trial was closed due to futility after enrolling 356 pts (planned 1,058). There was a significant improvement for brain relapse with PCI (1-yr relapse 7.7% vs. 18.0%, $p = 0.004$) but no difference in 1-yr OS or PFS. (*Gore EM et al., JCO 2011*)
What is the role of endobronchial/ intraluminal brachytherapy for palliation for lung cancer?	Various fractionation schemes (15 Gy × 2 or 8–10 Gy × 1, prescribed to 0.5 cm) have been used in prior irradiated pts with endobronchial Dz causing Sx. Sx relief can be seen in 80% of pts. Complications included fatal hemoptysis (5%–10%), bronchoesophageal fistula (2%), and bronchial edema (1%).

MDACC published a series of 81 previously irradiated lung cancer pts who were treated with palliative HDR endobronchial brachytherapy, 15 Gy × 2, 6 mm depth, over 2 wks. Response was seen in 84%. Pts with excellent response had better survival (MS 13.3 mos) vs. those with poor response (MS 5.4 mos) ($p = 0.01$). 2 fatal complications were due to fistula and tracheomalacia. (*Delclos ME et al., Radiology 1996*)

What fractionation scheme is optimal for pts with lung cancers treated with palliative RT for Sx such as hemoptysis, cough, pain, and shortness of breath?

Conventional fractionation is probably no better than hypofractionation. In a Norwegian RCT, *Sundstrom S et al.* tested 30 Gy in 10 fx vs. 17 Gy in 2 fx (1 wk apart) vs. 10 Gy in 1 fx. All achieved equivalent palliation. (*JCO 2007*)

▶ TOXICITY

What is the typical follow-up schedule of pts treated for lung cancer?

Typical lung cancer follow-up: H&P, CT chest with contrast q4–6mos for yrs 1–2, then noncontrast CT chest annually yrs 3–5, and continued smoking cessation counseling (per NCCN 2014)

What are the expected acute and late toxicities of RT for lung cancer?

Acute: Skin reaction, fatigue, dysphagia, odynophagia, cough

Subacute and late: RT pneumonitis, lung fibrosis, brachial plexopathy, Lhermitte syndrome, RT myelitis, esophageal fibrosis/stricture, pericarditis, 2nd cancers

What are the signs and Sx of RT pneumonitis, and how is it managed?

RT pneumonitis is a subacute reaction that begins as early as 3–6 mos after RT. Typically, Sx include **chest pain, shortness of breath, fever, and hypoxia.** CT scan shows ground glass changes within the RT port. Check oxygenation and supplement if necessary. **If symptomatic, treat with prednisone 1 mg/kg/day for at least 3 wks with a very slow taper. Bactrim can be used for PCP prophylaxis.**

What is the total lung V20 dose-volume constraint for RT alone and concurrent CRT in definitive lung cancer Tx?

NCCN: V20 <37%
MDACC: RT alone → V20: <40%; CRT → V20: <35% (based on *Lee HK et al., IJROBP 2003*)

What is the mean lung dose (MLD) constraint for definitive RT to lung cancer?

MLD ≤**20 Gy.**

What is the heart RT dose-volume constraint for RT alone and concurrent CRT?	**NCCN:** V40 <100%, V45 <67%, V60 <33% **MDACC:** RT alone → V40: <50%; CRT → V40: <40%
What is the dose constraint for the brachial plexus?	The dose constraint is **1 cc below 60 Gy;** the max dose point should be <66 Gy. Two retrospective studies showed that the dose could be higher (MDACC, *Amini A et al., IJROBP 2012*; median dose >69 Gy, max dose >75 Gy to 2 cc; and *UPenn, Eblan MJ et al., IJROBP 2013*: V76<1 cc).
What is the max esophageal dose?	Ideally, **MLD <34 Gy.** Try to minimize the V60 as much as possible (V60 <33%, V50 <50%, ≤45 Gy to the entire esophagus, max dose point <70 Gy).
What is the expected grade 3–4 esophagitis rate in pts treated with sequential CRT vs. concurrent CRT in locally advanced NSCLC?	Sequential: ~4% Concurrent: ~22% (*Choy H, ASTRO 2003* [summary of multiple studies])
What are the strategies for delivering external radiation to lung tumors if dose constraints cannot be met?	1. Induction chemotherapy for debulking 2. Adaptive radiation during treatment 3. Alternative modalities (i.e., protons)

39 Small Cell Lung Cancer and Bronchial Neuroendocrine Tumor

Updated by Shervin M. Shirvani and Ritsuko Komaki

▶ BACKGROUND

Small cell lung cancer (SCLC) accounts for what % of new lung cancer Dx in the U.S.? What % of lung cancer deaths?	**~15%** (~33,000 cases/yr) of new lung cancer is SCLC, accounting for **25% of lung cancer deaths** annually.

What % of SCLC is linked to smoking?

>90% of SCLC cases are linked to smoking.

What is the median age of Dx of SCLC? What % of pts are >70 yo at Dx?

The median age of SCLC Dx is **64 yrs,** with **25%** of pts presenting at age >70 yrs.

What % of pts with SCLC presents with metastatic Dz?

67% of SCLC pts present with mets, most commonly to the contralat lung, contralat or bilat malignant pleural effusion, liver, renal, adrenals, bone, BM, and brain.

What are the pathologic characteristics of SCLC?

Small round blue cells of epithelial origin with neuroendocrine differentiation, ↑ **mitotic count,** and ↑ **N/C ratio**

What are the markers that characterize SCLC?

Markers that characterize SCLC include **S100, synaptophysin+, chromogranin+, and neurotensin + EGFR–.**

What pathology finding is often associated with SCLC?

Crush artifact

What are some common neurologic and endocrine paraneoplastic syndromes associated with SCLC?

Neurologic: Lambert-Eaton syndrome (antibody to presynaptic voltage-gated calcium channels), encephalomyelitis, sensory neuropathy (anti-Hu antibody)

Endocrine: Cushing Dz (↑↑ ACTH), syndrome of inappropriate secretion of antidiuretic hormone (SIADH) (↑↑ ADH)

What is the most common chromosomal abnormality associated with SCLC but not seen with extrapulmonary small cell carcinomas?

Deletion of 3p (95% of cases, particularly 3p14–25 region, with inactivation of at least 3 tumor suppressor genes, including *FHIT* and *RASSF1A*)

What is the most common genetic alteration seen in SCLC?

Amplification of the bcl-2/C-myc family of oncogenes is most common but likely is not the initiating event. Other common abnormalities include loss of p16, loss of Rb, and mutation in p53.

▶ **WORKUP/STAGING**

How do pts with SCLC usually present?

Large hilar mass with bulky mediastinal LAD that causes cough, shortness of breath, weight loss, postobstructive pneumonia, and debility. Other common presentations include paraneoplastic syndromes such as Lambert-Eaton, SIADH, or ectopic ACTH production.

Classically, does SCLC present centrally or peripherally in the lung?

Classically, SCLC presents **centrally** in the lung.

What histology is most commonly associated with superior vena cava obstruction (SVCO) syndrome?

SCLC is most commonly associated with SVCO syndrome.

Do SCLC pts present with solitary peripheral nodules without mediastinal LAD?

This is very **uncommon** (<3%).

How should pts be managed whose FNA results cannot clearly differentiate between small cell and atypical carcinoid histology?

Surgical staging, with mediastinoscopy → surgical resection if the mediastinum nodes (MN) are negative (per NCCN 2014)

Once SCLC has been diagnosed in a pt who presents with a large hilar mass, what further workup is necessary besides the basic H&P and labs?

LDH levels, CT C/A/P +/– PET, **MRI brain,** bone scan if PET is not done, **BM Bx** (for pts with elevated LDH), thoracentesis with cytopathologic exam for pts with pleural effusion, and smoking cessation counseling

What % of pts with SCLC at the time of Dx present with brain mets, BM involvement, and bone mets?

Brain mets: 10%–15% (30% are asymptomatic)
BM involvement: 5%–10%
Bone mets: 30%

What is the latest AJCC system for staging SCLC?

The same as for non-SCLC, but this system is not commonly used.

How is SCLC most commonly staged?

SCLC is commonly staged using the **International Association of Lung Cancer system,** which is a modification of the Veterans Administration Lung Cancer Study Group (VALCSG) system. There are 2 stages: limited and extensive. Tumors are staged according to whether the Dz can be encompassed within an RT port. Limited stage Dz is typically confined to the ipsi hemithorax, without malignant pleural effusion, contralat Dz, or mets; other presentations are usually extensive stage.

What % of pts present with limited-stage SCLC?

~33% of pts present with limited-stage SCLC.

What are some adverse prognostic factors in SCLC?

Poor performance status (PS); weight loss (>5% in prior 6 mos); ↑ LDH; male gender; endocrine paraneoplastic syndromes (controversial), variant, or of mixed cell type; metastatic Dz

What is the MS of untreated limited-stage and extensive-stage SCLC?	**~12 wks** for limited stage and **~6 wks** for extensive stage, based on a VALCSG trial comparing cyclophosphamide to placebo.
What is the MS for pts with limited- vs. extensive-stage SCLC?	Limited stage: 19–23 mos (*Turrisi AT et al., NEJM 1999*) Extensive stage: 5–7 mos (*Slotman B et al., NEJM 2007*)
What is the long-term survival rate in limited-stage SCLC treated with a combined modality?	**~20%–30%** long-term survival (5-yr OS)
What additional workup should be considered for pts with carcinoid tumors of the lung?	Consider **octreotide scan.**

▶ TREATMENT/PROGNOSIS

What are some important poor prognostic factors for limited stage SCLC?	Karnofsky PS <70, weight loss, ↑ **LDH**
What is the Tx paradigm for pts with limited-stage SCLC?	Limited-stage SCLC Tx paradigm: 4 cycles of EP chemo (etoposide [120 mg/m^2, days 1–3] + cisplatin [60 mg/m^2, day 1, q3wks]) + concurrent RT (only 1 cycle is concurrent). Current standard RT regimen is based on INT-0096: 45 Gy in 1.5 Gy bid × 30 fx.
What is the OS and LC benefit of adding RT to chemo in limited-stage SCLC?	There is an **OS benefit of 5%** based on *Pignon J-P et al.* meta-analysis (*NEJM 1992*), with **LC benefit of 25%–30%** (*Warde P et al., NEJM 1992* [meta-analysis]).
What is the benefit of smoking cessation prior to Tx in pts with limited-stage SCLC?	↓ **Toxicity and** ↑ **survival,** based on a retrospective review (*Videtic GMM et al., IJROBP 2003*)
What are the typical response rates seen after concurrent CRT for limited-stage SCLC?	Typical response rates are **80%–95% with** CR rates of 40%–60%.
What is the median duration of response for pts with LS-SCLC after definitive Tx?	**6–8 mos** is the median duration of response.
What is the preferred Tx approach for elderly pts (age >70 yrs) with LS-SCLC?	**Depends on PS.** In pts with good PS, combined CRT is preferred. Otherwise, standard combination chemo is better than single-agent cytotoxic agents.

What is the MS of SCLC pts after recurrence if treated with salvage chemo?

4–5 mos is the MS for these pts.

Why is EP the preferred regimen in concurrent CRT for limited-stage SCLC?

EP causes little mucosal toxicity, offers low risk of interstitial pneumonitis, and has lower cardiac toxicity compared to doxorubicin. Full systemic doses can be administered with RT, and there is modest hematologic toxicity. EP has a better therapeutic ratio over the older regimen of CAV (cyclophosphamide, doxorubicin, and vincristine), but it confers no survival benefit.

What are the benefits and disadvantages of substituting carboplatin for cisplatin in EP for Tx of SCLC?

Carboplatin is less emetic, neuropathic, nephropathic, ototoxic, but there is **more heme toxicity.**

Is there a benefit to maintenance chemo after the initial 4–6 cycles in the Tx of SCLC?

No. Maintenance chemo only produces minor prolongation of response without improving survival and increasing cumulative toxicity.

Is there a benefit of irinotecan compared to etoposide when added to cisplatin in the Tx of SCLC?

No. A Japanese RCT demonstrated a survival benefit with irinotecan, but this was not reproduced in a U.S. trial that used a modified (lower) dose from that used in the Japanese regimen. A phase III randomized trial of IP using the same Japanese full dose regimen was compared to EP, and with 651 pts randomized, there was no survival benefit of IP, with less hematologic and greater GI toxicity with IP (*Lara PN et al., JCO 2009*).

What is the optimal sequence of combining chemo with RT?

Concurrent is better than sequential (JCOG: *Takada M et al., JCO 2002*): MS 27 mos vs. 20 mos; 5-yr OS 30% vs. 20% (10% OS benefit)

What evidence supports early concurrent CRT → chemo over late RT with induction CT → CRT?

NCIC data (*Murray N et al., JCO 1993*): phase III, 308 pts. 5-yr OS was 20% (early RT) vs. 11% (late RT).

Yugoslavia data (*Jeremic B et al., JCO 1997*): an early vs. late RT trial showed better MS (34 mos vs. 26 mos) and 5-yr OS (30% vs. 15%) for early.

Meta-analysis of 7 trials (*Fried DB et al., JCO 2004*): early (<9 wks) vs. late (>9 wks) after chemo. There was **5.2%** better 2-yr OS with early RT.

What is the recommended RT dose in CRT for limited-stage SCLC?

45 Gy in 1.5 Gy bid or 60–70 Gy in 2 Gy qd (per NCCN 2014). 61.2 Gy in 5 wks is an alternative regimen (1.8 Gy qd × 16 fx → bid as in **RTOG 97–12**) (*Komaki R et al., IJROBP 2005*)

What randomized trial demonstrated a clear superiority of altered fractionation with chemo compared to qd RT in the Tx of SCLC?

INT-0096 (*Turrisi AT et al., NEJM 1999*): phase III, 381 pts, EP × 4 cycles + RT at 1st cycle; randomization with 1.5 Gy bid × 3 wks vs. 1.8 Gy qd × 5 wks (both to 45 Gy); all rcvd prophylactic cranial irradiation (PCI) to 25 Gy. There was better 5-yr OS (26% vs. 16%) and LC (64% vs. 48%) in the bid arm. There was increased grade 3 esophagitis (27% vs. 11%) in the bid regimen, but not in the grade 4 toxicity. *Criticism:* 45 Gy qd is not biologically equivalent to the accelerated hyperfractionation of 45 Gy in 30 fx.

Do any studies support dose escalation with conventional fractionation rather than traditional bid approach?

CALGB 8837 (*Choi H et al., JCO 1998*): phase I maximum tolerated dose (MTD) in 50 pts of 2 RT regimens: 1.5 Gy/fx bid or 2.0 Gy/fx qd; MTD of bid was 45 Gy, whereas MTD of qd regimen was >70 Gy. Updated survival results were that 6-yr OS was better in the qd regimen compared with bid (36% vs. 20%). A phase III trial is ongoing (**CALGB 30610/RTOG 0538**) to compare 45 Gy in 3 wks (arm A: **INT-0096**) vs. 70 Gy in 35 fx (arm B: CALGB regimen) vs. 61.2 Gy in 5 wks (arm C: MTD in dose escalation study **RTOG 97–12** also used in **RTOG 0239**).

Describe classic RT targets for limited-stage SCLC?

Gross tumor, ipsi hilum, bilat MN from thoracic inlet (1st rib) down to 5 cm below the carina. CTV = GTV + 1.5 cm (and elective hilum and MN regions + 8 mm), PTV = CTV + 1 cm.

CALGB 30610/RTOG 0538: **3D-CRT or IMRT allowed. CTV** needs to include **GTV** plus potential occult Dz defined as (1) ipsi hilum (level 10 LN) and (2) N2-N3 levels from the top of the aortic arch down to 3 cm below the carina encompassing levels 3, 4R, 4L, and 7 (and levels 5–6 for left-sided tumors). These areas are treated electively except for the supraclavicular fossa. **PTV** is CTV + 0.5 cm if daily setup imaging is used and if **ITV** assessment is done during simulation and the planning process (either breath-hold or 4D-CT imaging). If a free-breathing non-ITV approach is used (non–4D-CT simulation), the PTV is CTV + 1.5 cm (sup-inf direction) and 1.0 cm in the axial direction. If a breath-holding non-ITV, PTV is CTV + 1.0 cm (sup-inf direction) and 0.5 cm in the axial direction.

What thoracic RT field arrangements are classically used for treating limited-stage SCLC?

Minimize contralat lung exposure with AP/PA to 15 Gy (1.5 Gy bid × 5 days) with oblique field to 45 Gy (AP/PA in a.m. and obliques for p.m. sessions).

Are there circumstances where IMRT may be beneficial?

Consider IMRT if V20 >30% or FEV_1 <1 L.

Is IMRT associated with worse outcomes compared to 3D-CRT?

Retrospective review of MDACC experience demonstrated no difference in local control or overall survival when IMRT was compared to 3D-CRT. PEG tube placement was significantly lower in IMRT cohort. (*Shirvani SM et al., Int J Radiat Oncol Biol Phys 2013*)

Is there a group of patients who can potentially be treated with involved field RT only?

Patients staged with PET-CT. The occurrence of isolated elective nodal failure in this group is ~5% among those treated with involved field radiation. (*van Loon J et al., Int J Radiat Oncol Biol Phys 2010; Shirvani SM et al., Int J Radiat Oncol Biol Phys 2012*) Patients staged with only CT have higher rates of elective nodal failure.

What is the role of PCI in limited-stage SCLC? Is there an OS benefit with it?

Auperin meta-analysis of 7 RCTs (*NEJM 1999*) compared PCI vs. no PCI after CR following induction chemo +/– RT and no evidence of brain mets before randomization. There was ↓ 3-yr incidence of brain mets (33% vs. 59%) and **5.4%** better 3-yr OS (20.7% vs. 15.3%) and improved DFS. There was a trend to a better outcome with ↑ doses and RT <4 mos from the start of chemo.

What PCI dose is now standard for limited-stage SCLC?

25 Gy in 10 fx is now the standard dose for PCI for limited-stage SCLC. (**RTOG 0212-Intergroup:** *Le Pechoux C et al., Lancet Oncol 2009*)

For pts with limited-stage SCLC, what PCI doses were compared in RTOG 0212?

Standard doses (25 Gy in 10 fx) **vs. higher doses** (36 Gy in either 18 fx qd or 24 fx bid). There was **no difference in the 2-yr incidence of brain mets,** but there was an **OS and chest relapse advantage for the standard arm** (42% vs. 37%, $p = 0.05$) due to greater cancer-related mortality in the high-dose group. (*Le Pechoux C et al., Lancet Oncol 2009*)

What is the effect of PCI timing after the initiation of chemo for SCLC?

Based on **Auperin meta-analysis,** there was a ↓ in risk of brain mets with earlier PCI (<4–6 mos vs. >6 mos) without an effect on risk of death.

Are there data demonstrating greater neuropsychologic complications after PCI for SCLC?

No. The data actually demonstrate no difference with or without PCI in a randomized trial addressing the question of neuropsychologic changes after PCI. (*Arrigada et al., JNCI 1995*) Most pts (97%) actually have abnl neuropsychologic testing after chemo and before PCI, without a difference after PCI. (*Komaki R et al., IJROBP 1995*)

Is there evidence to use surgery for limited-stage disease?

The NCCN guidelines (2014) allow surgery as an option for peripheral nodules. Retrospective studies suggest that with modern staging, T1–2N0 SCLC pts have reasonable outcomes with surgery and adj platinum-based chemo. The situation is uncommon (~5% of cases). (*Brock MV et al., J Thorac Cardiovasc Surg 2005*) For more advanced lesions, two randomized studies (LCSG 832 [*Lad T, Chest 1994*] and the Medical Research Council [*Fox W et al., Lancet 1973*]) showed no benefit to surgery over definitive radiation.

What is the recommended adj Tx for SCLC if the mediastinal nodes are found to be involved after attempted surgical resection?

Concurrent CRT directed at the MN (per NCCN 2014); if node–, adj chemo alone

What is the Tx paradigm for pts with extensive-stage SCLC?

Extensive-stage SCLC Tx paradigm: **multiagent chemo regimen including etoposide/cisplatin (EP) or Cytoxan/doxorubicin/vincristine (CAV).** Consider consolidation RT to the thorax for pts who achieve a CR to distant Dz after initial chemo. (*Jeremic B et al., JCO 1999*) Also, PCI found to offer survival benefit even if extensive stage disease.

What additional chemo agents, when added to EP, have been shown to modestly improve the survival of pts with extensive-stage SCLC?

Ifosfamide or cyclophosphamide + an anthracycline have been shown to modestly improve survival.

Is there evidence to support consolidative RT to thoracic Dz in extensive-stage SCLC?

Yes. *Jeremic et al.* enrolled 210 extensive-stage pts. All rcvd EP × 3. The subset of 109 pts who achieved a CR at all distant sites was randomized to rcv consolidative RT (accelerated hyperfractionation to 54 Gy) with concurrent carboplatin/etoposide or not. In both arms, pts rcvd PCI and consolidative EP. Consolidative CRT improved 5-yr OS (9.1% vs. 3.7%) and MS (17 mos vs. 11 mos). There was a trend in favor of LC but not DM-free survival. (*JCO 1999*)

What are some salvage chemo agents used at the time of recurrence for SCLC?

Oral topoisomerase I inhibitors are standard for postchemo failure. (Topotecan was tested in RCTs showing doubling of survival [26 wks vs. 14 wks] compared with supportive care; irinotecan as a single agent was not tested.) The old combo chemo of CAV can be used (if EP is used as 1st line). Paclitaxel, docetaxel, vinorelbine, and gemcitabine as single agents are not standard since activity is low against SCLC.

What seminal study demonstrated a survival benefit with PCI in pts with extensive-stage SCLC with any response to chemo? What are some main criticisms of this study?

EORTC 08993 RCT (*Slotman BJ et al., NEJM 2007*): 286 pts with extensive-stage SCLC treated with chemo; primary endpoint was time to symptomatic brain mets; pts randomized to +/– PCI after *any* response to chemo; most PCI pts given 20 Gy in 5 fx. PCI lowered the risk of symptomatic mets and improved DFS and OS (5.4 mos –PCI vs. 6.7 mos +PCI). 1-yr OS nearly doubled (13% –PCI vs. 27% +PCI).

Criticisms: There was no pre-Tx MRI. The RT group was more likely to rcv chemo at the time of extracranial progression (68% vs. 45%). Only about half (59%) of pts in the control group rcvd WBRT for intracranial progression of Dz.

What was the greatest QOL alteration after PCI in the EORTC trial for extensive-stage SCLC?

3-mo QOL assessment showed that the largest negative impact of PCI was **fatigue and hair loss.** Worsening role, emotional, and cognitive function were also seen after PCI. (*Slotman BJ et al., JCO 2009*)

What is the current recommendation for PCI in pts with SCLC?

Limited or extensive stage, CR/PR after chemo +/– RT, +/– MRI brain, PS of ECOG 0–2, within 3–6 wks of last cycle of chemo, 25 Gy in 10 fx. In pts with less than a CR, PCI is at the discretion of the treating physician.

In SCLC pts with SVCO, cord compression, or brain mets, what regimen is preferred as upfront palliative Tx: RT or chemo?

In a chemo-naive pt presenting with SVCO, RCTs have shown a similar symptomatic response rate with chemo compared with RT. But in a chemo-refractory pt, RT is the preferred regimen. In pts with cord compression/brain mets, RT is standard (in both chemo-naive and chemo-refractory pts).

How is palliative RT delivered for SVCO syndrome in pts with SCLC?

Generally, **a few large fx upfront** (3–4 Gy × 2–3) → **more definitive dosing in conventional fractionation** (qd or bid regimen)

What fractionation scheme is optimal for pts with lung cancers treated with palliative RT for Sx such as hemoptysis, cough, pain, and shortness of breath?	**Conventional is probably no better than hypofractionation.** In a Norwegian RCT, *Sundstrom et al.* tested 30 Gy in 10 fx vs. 17 Gy in 2 fx (1 wk apart) vs. 10 Gy for 1 fx. All achieved similar levels of palliation. (*JCO 2007*)
How should a tumor characterized as a high-grade neuroendocrine carcinoma, or as large cell neuroendocrine carcinoma, be managed?	Treat per non-SCLC guidelines. (per NCCN 2014)
How should a pt with a carcinoid tumor of the lung be managed?	**Surgery is 1st line if it is resectable.** Some centers will treat atypical carcinoid per the SCLC paradigm (nonsurgical). Per NCCN 2014: 1. Stages I–III typical carcinoid tumor can be observed after R0 resection. 2. For unresectable or medically inoperable stage III typical carcinoid tumors, RT alone is recommended. 3. For atypical carcinoid tumors, resected stage I can be observed. However, for resected stages II–IIIa tumors, chemo (EP) and RT adjuvantly is recommended.
How should stages IIIB–IV or unresectable carcinoid of the lung be managed?	**Systemic therapy (EP),** or octreotide if octreotide scan positive or symptomatic from paraneoplastic syndrome (per NCCN 2014)

▶ **TOXICITY**

What is the recommended follow-up schedule for SCLC pts?	SCLC follow-up schedule: H&P, CT chest, and labs at each visit (visits q2–3mos for yr 1, q3–4mos for yrs 2–3, q4–6mos for yrs 4–5, then annually). PET scan should be considered whenever CT findings suggest recurrence or mets.
What is the total lung V20 dose-volume constraint for RT alone and concurrent CRT in definitive lung cancer Tx?	RT alone: V20 <40% CRT: V20 <35% (per NCCN 2014)
What is the recommended mean lung dose (MLD) constraint with definitive RT for lung cancer?	MLD is <**15 Gy** ideally but not >20 Gy.

What is the max cord dose allowed on INT 0096 ("Turrisi regimen")?

On INT 0096, the max cord dose was **36 Gy** (but according to **RTOG 0538,** the max allowable cord dose is **41 Gy**).

What is the main toxicity associated with using bid RT as done in the Turrisi regimen?

Grade 3 acute **esophagitis:** 27% (bid) vs. 11% (qd). Other toxicities (myelosuppression, nausea) were the same as the qd regimen.

What is the distinction between grade 2 and 3 pneumonitis (per the RTOG)?

Grade 3 pneumonitis: dyspnea at rest or oxygen
    supplementation needed
Grade 2 pneumonitis: symptomatic and not
    requiring oxygenation

What is the heart dose-volume constraint for RT alone vs. concurrent CRT?

RT alone: V40 <50%
CRT: V40
According to **RTOG 0538,** the following limits are also acceptable: 60 Gy less than one-third, 45 Gy less than two-thirds, and 45 Gy <100%.

What is the esophageal dose-volume constraint for RT alone vs. concurrent CRT?

RT alone: V60 <50%
CRT: V55 <50% (ideally, keep the mean dose to
    <34 Gy per **RTOG 0538**)

40 Thymoma and Thymic Carcinoma

Updated by Shervin M. Shirvani and Melenda D. Jeter

▶ BACKGROUND

What is the embryonic derivation of the thymus?

The embryonic derivation of the thymus is the **3rd pharyngeal pouch.**

Where is the thymus located, and what is its function?

The thymus is in the **ant mediastinum** (MN), involved in the **processing and maturation of T lymphocytes to recognize foreign antigens from "self" antigens.**

What structures are located in the ant, middle, and post MN?

Anterior: LNs, thymus, mesenchymal tissues
Middle: heart and great vessels, trachea, esophagus, most mediastinal LNs, vagus and phrenic nerves
Posterior: paraspinal tissues, sympathetic and peripheral nerves

What proportion of tumors of the MN are malignant?

One-third of mediastinal tumors are malignant.

How prevalent is thymoma relative to other mediastinal tumors?

Thymoma comprises **20% of all mediastinal tumors** but **50% of all ant mediastinal tumors.**

What is the median age and sex predilection for thymomas?

The median age for thymomas is **40–60 yrs.** There is **no sex predilection** (male = female).

Are thymomas common in children?

No. Thymomas are extremely rare in children, but if present they are extremely aggressive with poor survival.

Pathologically, what is the most important defining feature of thymomas?

Coexistence of nonneoplastic lymphoid cells with **neoplastic epithelial cells** (spindle to polygonal types)

How do thymic carcinomas differ from thymomas?

Much less prevalent (<1% of thymic tumors), **very aggressive,** with **poorer survival** (5-yr OS 30%–50%)

What are the WHO designations of thymomas vs. thymic carcinomas?

WHO type is based on shape and the lymphocyte/epithelial ratio.
WHO types A–AB: benign thymoma, medullary, spindle cell
WHO types B1–B3: malignant thymoma, lymphocytic, cortical, epithelial
WHO type C: highly malignant, thymic carcinoma, clear cell/sarcomatoid types

What is the LN metastatic rate of thymomas vs. thymic carcinomas?

Thymoma: ~1%–2%
Thymic carcinoma: ~30%
(*Kondo K et al., Ann Thorac Surg 2003* [review of 1,320 pts with thymic tumors])

What is the hematogenous dissemination of thymomas vs. thymic carcinomas?

Thymoma: ~1% (mostly to lung)
Thymic carcinoma: 12% (lung > bone, liver)

▶ **WORKUP/STAGING**

What is the DDx of a mediastinal mass by location in the ant, middle, and post MN?

Anterior: thymoma, thymic carcinoma, carcinoid, germ cell tumors, lymphomas (Mnemonic: **TTT**: **T**hymoma, **T**eratoma, **T**errible lymphoma)
Middle: cysts > lymphoma, teratomas > sarcomas (osteosarcoma, fibrosarcoma, angiosarcoma, rhabdomyosarcoma of the heart), granuloma
Posterior: neurogenic tumors (PNET, schwannoma, neurofibroma, neuroblastoma, ganglioneuroma), pheochromocytoma

What clinical presentations are common for pts with mediastinal tumors?

About one-half are diagnosed incidentally on imaging studies. The remainder present with local symptoms (**cough, shortness of breath, pain, stridor, Horner,** SVC **syndrome) or as an association with myasthenia gravis** (MG) if thymoma.

How do pts with thymomas or thymic carcinomas usually present?

50% are incidental findings; but if there are Sx, they reflect either **locally advanced Dz, metastatic sequelae, or paraneoplastic disorders** (in 50%–60% of thymomas but hardly seen in thymic carcinomas).

What paraneoplastic disorders are commonly seen in thymomas?

MG (35%–50% of cases), **red cell aplasia** (5%), **immune deficiency syndromes** such as hypogammaglobulinemia (5%), autoimmune disorders (collagen vascular, dermatologic, endocrine, renal Dz), and **other malignancies** (lymphomas, GI/breast carcinomas, Kaposi sarcoma)

What workup should be employed for a mediastinal mass?

Mediastinal mass workup: H&P (ask about B Sx [fever >38°C, drenching night sweats, weight loss >10% in preceding 6 mos] to r/o lymphoma, physical to assess nodal status, MG Sx), basic labs (LDH, ESR, AFP/HCG to r/o germ cell tumor, as needed), imaging (PA/lat CXR, CT chest, MRI, PET if lymphoma suspected), Bx (FNA, but preferably Tru-Cut core Bx) or surgical (video-assisted thoracoscopic surgery, Chamberlain), PFTs to assess lung function

The Dx of thymoma is essentially established clinically if the pt presents in what way?

Ant mediastinal mass with Sx of MG, red cell aplasia, or hypogammaglobulinemia

Approximately what % of pts with thymoma present with MG?

35%–50%. Conversely, 10%–15% of pts with MG have thymoma.

What are the pathogenesis, presentation, Dx, and Tx of MG?

Autoantibody to the acetylcholine receptor at the postsynaptic endplate. Pts present with **easy fatigability, ptosis, and diplopia** (worse with movement, whereas the opposite is true for Lambert-Eaton). Dx is by the **Tensilon test** (edrophonium). Tx is by **anticholinesterase** (pyridostigmine) **or thymectomy** (reverses in 40% of pts with thymoma).

What is the Modified Masaoka system used to stage thymomas?

Stage I: fully encapsulated, no microscopic capsular invasion

Stage IIA: microscopic invasion into capsule

Stage IIB: macroscopic invasion into surrounding fat or mediastinal pleura

Stage III: macroscopic extension to surrounding organs (lung, pericardium) without great vessel invasion (A) or with great vessel invasion (B).

Stage IVA: pleural or pericardial dissemination

Stage IVB: +LN or DM

Is there controversy regarding the Masaoka staging system for thymoma?

Yes. UCLA retrospective meta-analysis of ~2,500 patients showed no difference in DFS or OS between stages I and II patients (*Gupta R, Arch Pathol Lab Med 2008*)

What are the 5-yr survival rates for thymomas based on the Masaoka staging?

5-yr survival for thymomas (Masaoka staging):
Stage I: 95%
Stage II: 90%
Stage III: 60%
Stage IV: 11%–50%

What is the 5-yr survival rate of invasive vs. noninvasive thymomas?

Invasive: 50%
Noninvasive: 70%

What are the most important prognostic factors for thymomas?

The **Masaoka stage and completeness of resection** are the most important prognostic factors for thymomas.

Based on modern surgical series, what are the rates of complete resection, the recurrence rate, and 5-yr OS based on Masaoka staging?

Kondo et al. reported outcomes for 1,320 pts. The % of complete resection, % of recurrence, and 5-yr OS, respectively, were as follows:
Stage I: 100%, 1%, 100%
Stage II: 100%, 4%, 98%
Stage III: 85%, 28%, 89%
Stage IVA: 42%, 34%, 71%

(*Ann Thorac Surg 2003*)

Is the Masaoka staging useful for thymic carcinoma?

Controversial. Although the Masaoka staging is also applied for thymic carcinomas, a MSKCC series of 43 patients failed to find association of Masaoka staging with survival. (*Blumberg D, J Thorac Cardiovasc Surg 1998*)

What are the most important prognostic factors for thymic carcinomas?

The **completeness of resection, invasion of innominate vessels, and presence of LN mets** are the most important prognostic factors for thymic carcinomas.

What is the 5-yr survival rate for thymic carcinoma?

The 5-yr OS for thymic carcinoma is **20%–30%.**

▶ **TREATMENT/PROGNOSIS**

What is the most important modality in the management of thymomas?

Surgery is the mainstay of Tx, with complete resection being the primary goal. The outcome is fully dependent on the extent and completeness of the resection, regardless of stage or histology. Surgical clips can help identify areas difficult to resect or possible residual Dz. It may even be reasonable to resect pleural mets since prolonged survival is possible.

What is the usual approach for the surgical management of thymomas?

Median sternotomy, but more extensive resections may be required depending on the stage at presentation, including partial or total pneumonectomy or pericardiectomy.

In a thymoma pt with MG, what should be done preoperatively?

Signs + Sx should be controlled medically prior to undergoing surgical resection.

How is thymic carcinoma generally managed?

If possible, **max surgery → CRT postoperatively.** If inoperable, consider induction therapy with chemo, RT, or combination CRT.

When is adj radiotherapy a reasonable indication for the management of thymic malignancies?

Adj radiotherapy should be considered with **stages III–IVA, +/close margins, or any thymic carcinoma.**

Is adj radiotherapy necessary for a stage II thymoma after complete resection?

This is **controversial.** It initially was recommended based on a classic review (*Curran W et al., JCO 1988*) in 103 pts with thymomas, finding that pts without PORT had ↑LR (6 of 19 pts for stage II) vs. no LR in PORT (0 of 1 pt for stage II, 0 of 4 pts for stage III). More recent data out of the Massachusetts General Hospital (*Mangi A et al., Ann Thorac Surg 2002*) and Japan (*Haniuda M et al., Ann Surg 1996*) showed that PORT may not be necessary after complete resection for stage II pts. *Haniuda et al.* demonstrated that stage II thymoma with macroscopic adherence to the pleura did benefit from PORT (LR 36% vs. 0%), but PORT was not useful for microscopic invasion of the pleura or pericardium.

Meta-analysis (*Korst RJ et al., Ann Thorac Surg 2009*): 1981–2008 systematic review of 13 studies, 592 pts, ~42% had surgery + PORT. The LR rate did not benefit from PORT for stages II–III thymoma (OR 0.87 for both stages II–III, $p = 0.69$).

Forquer JA et al.: 901 pts, SEER data 1973–2005; 92% thymoma, 8% thymic carcinoma (TC); localized Dz in 274 pts, regional Dz in 626 pts. 5-yr OS benefited from surgery + PORT for regional Dz (76% vs. 66%, $p = 0.01$); for localized Dz, surgery alone was more favorable (98% vs. 91% [PORT], $p = 0.03$). (*IJROBP 2009*)

Current recommendation for adj RT for stages II–III thymoma: +/close margin (<1 mm), gross fibrous adhesion to pleura, or ↑ WHO grade (B3) tumors (*Wright CD et al., Hem Oncol 2008*)

What should the postop target volume include?

The postop target volume should include the **entire bed of resection and any involved organs.** It is imperative to have a preop CT scan available to help delineate tumor bed volumes. Also, information from operative and pathology reports may help determine areas that might have had adherent, invasive Dz. For high-risk disease, consider elective LN coverage.

What are the RT doses used for the postop management of thymic malignancies?

Depends on the extent of resection:
If R0: **45–54 Gy**
If R1: **55–60 Gy**
If R2: **60–70 Gy**

When should postop concurrent chemotherapy be considered with RT for the management of thymic malignancies?

Per NCCN 2014, thymoma with gross residual Dz (R2 resection) or thymic carcinoma with R1-R2 resection

What are some management approaches for unresectable thymic tumors?

Management approaches for unresectable thymic tumor:
1. Induction chemo → RT only
2. Induction chemo → surgery → PORT
3. Induction RT/CRT → surgery → ± more RT

What are the results of definitive RT for unresectable thymic tumors?

RT can be used as the sole modality, with **5-yr OS 50%–87%.** Surgery should be done whenever possible, however, since resectability is still the most important prognostic factor.

Given the good response rates seen with platinum-based chemo, what is the current preferred Tx paradigm for unresectable thymic malignancy?

Unresectable thymic malignancy Tx paradigm:
1. **Chemo → RT (no surgery)** (*Loehrer PJ et al., JCO 1997*). Cisplatin/doxorubicin/cyclophosphamide (PAC) 2–4 cycles → RT to ≥54 Gy to primary + regional LN. 5-yr OS was 53%.

2. **Chemo → surgery (if possible) → PORT**
(MDACC: *Shin DM et al., Ann Int Med 1998*).
3 cycles induction chemo (Cytoxan/Adriamycin/
cisplatin [CAP] + prednisone) → max surgery →
RT. 7-yr follow-up showed 100% OS and 73%
DFS.

What RT dose can be used for the neoadjuvant management of unresectable thymomas?

24–30 Gy with chemo → surgery → then consideration for more RT depending on resection status

What are the 1st-line combination chemo regimens used for the management of thymic malignancies?

CAP +/– prednisone; VP-16/ifosfamide/cisplatin (VIP); cisplatin/VP-16 (EP); carboplatin/Taxol; cisplatin/Adriamycin/vincristine/Cytoxan (ADOC); Cytoxan/Adriamycin/vincristine/prednisone (CHOP)

What are the typical response rates with induction chemo for the management of thymic malignancies?

Typical response rates with induction chemo are **50%–60%.**

▶ **TOXICITY**

What is the follow-up for pts who have had a complete resection of a thymoma?

Completely resected thymoma follow-up: H&P + annual CT chest

Is 5 yrs of follow-up sufficient for a pt treated for thymomas?

No. Late recurrences can occur at >10 yrs. Pts need lifelong follow-up.

What are the expected early and late toxicities after adj RT for the management of thymic tumors?

Early: skin reaction, fatigue, dysphagia/
odynophagia, cough
Late: RT pneumonitis/fibrosis, pericarditis,
esophageal stricture, myelitis

What are the dose-limiting structures and dose limits when the MN is irradiated?

Lung: RT alone → V20 <40%; CRT → V20<35%,
V5<65%, mean lung dose <20 Gy (per NCCN
2014)
Heart: V40 <50% (V40 <40% if CRT)
Spinal cord: ≤45 Gy
Esophagus: Ideally, the mean dose of RT to the
esophagus should be <34 Gy. Try to minimize
the V60 as much as possible (V60 <33%, V50
<50%, ≤45 Gy to the entire esophagus, max
dose point <70 Gy).

41 Pleural Mesothelioma

Updated by Nikhil G. Thaker and Steven H. Lin

▶ BACKGROUND

Approximately how many cases of malignant mesothelioma are diagnosed in the U.S. annually?

~2,500 cases/yr of malignant mesothelioma in the U.S. (per NCCN 2014)

In which body sites can mesothelioma arise?

Mesothelioma commonly arises in the **pleura** but also occurs in the **peritoneum, pericardium, and tunica vaginalis testis.**

What is the most common cause of malignant pleural mesothelioma (MPM)?

The greatest risk factor for developing mesothelioma is **asbestos exposure** (amphiboles [rodlike] > chrysotile [serpentine form]). Asbestos is commonly found in insulation material, brake pads, and shipyards.

What is the MS of patients with MPM?

The MS of patients with MPM is approximately **12 months** (MS in most series is **4–20 mos**).

What is the major difference between the incidence of mesothelioma in the U.S. vs. the developing world?

B/c of early adoption of asbestos regulations, the incidence of **mesothelioma in the U.S. peaked in 2004 and has subsequently declined.** The incidence **has not yet peaked in the developing world** and is not expected to for the next 10–20 yrs. However, the U.S. still has more cases than anywhere else in the world.

What is the estimated latency between asbestos exposure and mesothelioma?

The estimated latency between asbestos exposure and mesothelioma is **20–40 yrs.** (*Lanphear BP et al., J Occup Med 1992*)

What % of mesothelioma cases are related to asbestos exposure?

~70%–80% of cases have documented asbestos exposure.

What is lifetime risk of mesothelioma for someone with an occupational asbestos exposure Hx?

The lifetime risk with asbestos exposure **~10%.**

Does smoking cause mesothelioma?

No. Smoking alone is not associated with mesothelioma, but smoking increases the risk associated with asbestos exposure.

Is there a sex predilection for mesothelioma?

Yes. Males are more commonly affected than females, likely related to occupational exposure differences.

At what age does the incidence of mesothelioma peak?

The **incidence does not peak.** It continuously increases with age.

What are the 3 most common histopathologic subtypes of mesothelioma in decreasing order of frequency?

Histopathologic subtypes of mesothelioma: **epithelioid (favorable,** 40%) > **mixed or biphasic** (35%) > **sarcomatous or mesenchymal** (25%)

What are some common genetic changes seen in mesothelioma?

Loss of tumor suppressor genes p16, p14, and NF-2 are common genetic changes in mesothelioma.

▶ **WORKUP/STAGING**

What are the common initial presenting Sx of mesothelioma?

Dyspnea and nonpleuritic chest pain. Other common symptoms include cough, pleural effusion, chest wall mass, weight loss, fever, and sweating. **Recurrent pleural effusion and/or pleural thickening** may be found incidentally on CXR.

What is the initial workup of a pleural-based mass seen on CXR?

Pleural-based mass initial workup: H&P, CBC, CMP, serum mesothelin-related peptide (SRMP) and osteopontin levels (optional), CT chest + contrast, thoracentesis for cytology, and pleural Bx (thoracoscopic Bx [preferred], open Bx, or CT-guided core Bx). Consider talc pleurodesis or a pleural catheter for management of effusion.

What additional workup should be done with a Dx of malignant mesothelioma?

Malignant mesothelioma workup: CT C/A/P + contrast, PET/CT, and MRI chest to determine if there is chest wall (CW) or diaphragmatic invasion. Consider mediastinoscopy or EBUS with FNA for suspicious nodes. Consider laparoscopy to r/o transdiaphragmatic extension if suggested by imaging. Use video-assisted thoracoscopic surgery to r/o contralat Dz, if necessary. Use PFTs to assess lung function.

How does malignant mesothelioma appear on a CT of the thoracic chest?

On CT of the thoracic chest, malignant mesothelioma appears as **pleural thickening with involvement of interlobar fissures/atelectasis, with possible pleural plaques and calcification.** Effusions and contracted ipsilateral hemithorax may also be seen.

What is the DDx of tumors of the pleura?

Primary tumors (benign or malignant), thymoma, sarcoma, or more commonly, **metastatic Dz** (i.e., adenocarcinoma).

What is the diagnostic yield of mesothelioma from the fluid cytology of the pleural effusion?

Fairly poor, only ~23%. Often, cytology finds atypical mesothelial cells only.

With a needle Bx, what entity is often confused with mesothelioma?

Adenocarcinoma (metastatic) is often confused with mesothelioma.

What pathologic features distinguish mesothelioma from adenocarcinoma?

Mesothelioma is negative for periodic acid-Schiff stain, carcinoembryonic antigen, and Leu-M1. It is positive for calretinin, vimentin, WT1, and cytokeratin 5/6. In mesothelioma, electron microscopy reveals that cells have long microvilli, in contrast to adenocarcinomas, which have short microvilli.

What biomarker is elevated in mesothelioma?

SRMP and osteopontin in serum. It may be elevated in >80% of pts.

What is the AJCC 7th edition (2011) T staging of mesothelioma?

Tis: CIS

T1a: limited to ipsi parietal pleura, *no* visceral pleural involvement

T1b: +ipsi parietal pleura and focal involvement of visceral pleura

T2: involves ipsi pleural surfaces with at least 1 of the following: (a) confluent visceral pleural tumor, (b) invasion of diaphragmatic muscle, or (c) invasion of lung parenchyma

T3: involves any ipsi pleural surfaces with at least 1 of the following: (a) invasion of endothoracic fascia, (b) invasion into mediastinal fat, (c) solitary focus of tumor invading soft tissues of CW, and (d) nontransmural involvement of pericardium

T4: involves any ipsi pleural surfaces with at least 1 of the following: (a) diffuse or multifocal invasion of soft tissues of CW, (b) any rib involvement, (c) invasion through diaphragm to peritoneum, (d) invasion of any mediastinal organs, (e) direct extension to contralat pleura, (f) invasion into spine, (g) extension to internal surface of pericardium, (h) pericardial effusion with +cytology, (i) invasion of myocardium, and (j) invasion of brachial plexus

Describe the N staging of mesothelioma.

N1: mets involving bronchopulmonary or hilar nodes

N2: mets to ipsi mediastinum (MN) or to subcarinal or **internal mammary nodes**

N3: mets to contralat MN, internal mammary nodes, or hilar LNs, or to ipsi or contralat supraclavicular nodes

Describe the overall stage groupings for mesothelioma.

Stage IA: T1aN0
Stage IB: T1bN0
Stage II: T2N0
Stage III: T1–2N1–2 or T3N0–2
Stage IV: T4 or N3 or M1

Which histologic subtype has a worse prognosis?

The **sarcomatous** type has the worse prognosis.

Name the 4 EORTC poor prognostic factors for mesothelioma.

EORTC poor prognostic factors for mesothelioma:
1. WBC >8.3 × 10^9/dL
2. Performance status (PS) 1–2
3. Sarcomatoid histology
4. Male gender

Other poor prognostic factors include N2 disease, DM, thrombocytosis, and hypercoagulability.

What are the estimated 1- and 2-yr OS rates for EORTC low- and high-risk mesothelioma?

<u>Low risk</u>: 1-yr OS 40%; 2-yr OS 14%
<u>High risk</u>: 1-yr OS 12%; 2-yr OS 0%

Is death from mesothelioma usually due to local progression or DM?

Death is usually due to **local progression** resulting in respiratory failure or infection.

> **TREATMENT/PROGNOSIS**

What is the Tx paradigm for resectable mesothelioma?

For stages I–III, resectable mesothelioma Tx paradigm:
1. Extrapleural pneumonectomy (EPP) → chemo → hemithorax RT *or*
2. Neoadj chemo → EPP → hemithorax RT

What is removed with an EPP for mesothelioma?

Parietal and visceral pleura, lung, mediastinal nodes, pericardium, and ipsi diaphragm, with a graft to prevent herniation of abdominal contents through the diaphragmatic defect. Mediastinal nodal dissection should be done.

What is the Tx paradigm for unresectable mesothelioma, clinical stage IV, or sarcomatoid histology?

Unresectable mesothelioma Tx paradigm: **combination chemo,** perhaps with cisplatin/pemetrexed, and then re-evaluation for surgery. If remains unresectable, continue chemo.

What % of mesothelioma pts are surgically resectable at Dx?

<5% of pts are surgically resectable at Dx.

What TNM stage of Dz determines surgical resectability using EPP for mesothelioma?

T1–3N0–1. Therefore, mediastinoscopy to r/o N2-N3 Dz will be important.

What are the chemos of choice for the Tx of mesothelioma?

Preferred Tx includes the combination chemo of choice incorporated into trimodality regimens utilizing antifolate agents such as pemetrexed (Alimta)/cisplatin or gemcitabine/cisplatin.

Pemetrexed/cisplatin is based on an RCT (*Vogelzang NJ et al., JCO 2003*) of unresectable mesothelioma pts to cisplatin vs. pemetrexed/cisplatin. There was improved response rate (17% vs. 41%) and survival (9 mos vs. 12 mos) with pemetrexed/cisplatin. This trial led to FDA approval for use in unresectable Dz. Cisplatin/gemcitabine use is based on several phase II studies.

When is a decortication/ pleurectomy a preferred procedure over EPP in a pt with mesothelioma?

Decortication/pleurectomy is preferred over EPP in pts with **more advanced Dz** ($\uparrow$ nodal Dz, areas of local invasion), **mixed histology,** and **medically high-risk pts.** Periop mortality is 2%–5%. It is considered palliative because it is not a negative margin surgery. LF 44%–73% vs. 13%–40% for EPP.

What is the mortality rate of EPP? What is the MS for mesothelioma after EPP?

The mortality rate of EPP ranges from **4%–31%** (~8% at MDACC) and depends largely on the experience of the center and preop selection. MS in most series is **4–20 mos.** *Rice et al.* reported 10.2 mos OS. If IMRT, 14.2 mos and if LN– and epithelioid, 28 mos. (*Ann Thorac Surg 2007*)

What study supports adj RT after EPP for mesothelioma?

MSKCC phase II trial with hemithorax RT to 54 Gy after EPP improved LC and OS compared to historical controls (*Rusch V et al., IJROBP 2003*). 2-yr OS was 33%. MS was 34 mos for stages I–II and 10 mos for later stages.

What study supports the role of trimodality therapy for mesothelioma?

Harvard retrospective review (*Sugerbaker D et al., J Thorac Cardiovasc Surg 1999*) of 183 pts treated with EPP + adj chemo (Cytoxan/Adr/cisplatin [CAP] or carboplatin/Taxol) + RT → adj chemo. Overall, MS was 19 mos; 5-yr OS was 15%. 3 factors predicted for best outcomes: epithelial histology, negative resection margin, and negative extrapleural nodes.

Name 2 RT techniques used for adj Tx of mesothelioma after EPP.

AP/PA or IMRT to 45–54 Gy, with a boost to 60 Gy for a close/+ margin. Traditional prescription for AP/PA technique: 54 Gy in 1.8 Gy/fx, off-cord at 41.4 Gy. Electrons given concurrently. Radiation initiated 3–6 wks after EPP.

Describe the conventional RT field borders for adj RT Tx of mesothelioma after EPP.

Based on *Yajnik S et al.* (*IJROBP 2003*):
  Superior: Top of T1
  Lateral: Flash the skin
  Medial: Contralateral edge of vertebral body if MN
      negative or 1.5–2.0 cm beyond contralateral edge
      of vertebral body if MN positive for Dz
  Inferior: bottom of L2

Need to block critical structures anteriorly and posteriorly from the incidental AP/PA photon beam such as the heart, stomach, and liver and supplement blocked areas with electrons.

An **abdominal block** to shield liver (right side) or stomach (left side) is present anteriorly and posteriorly throughout treatment with electron supplementation at 1.53 Gy/fx (15% scatter from photon fields under blocks). These blocks extend 1.5 cm from ipsi border of vertebral body to within 2 cm from edge of chest wall. Blocks are present only where diaphragm abutted the abdominal wall anteriorly/posteriorly, but not where the diaphragm was oblique to the abdominal wall.

For **left-sided** tumors, the kidney is blocked throughout, and the heart block is present after 19.8 Gy.

The **spinal cord** is blocked after 41.4 Gy by shifting the medial border to the ipsilateral edge of the vertebral body.

Include scars with bolus in the field and boost if necessary.

How is IMRT delivered for the adj Tx of mesothelioma?

MDACC experience (*Ahamad A et al., IJROBP 2003, 2004*), using 13–27 fields with 8–11 angles, with ~100 segments/field. Target volume was the entire hemithorax, all surgical clips, all sites of instrumentation, and the ipsi MN; initial dose to 45–50 Gy, with a boost to 60 Gy for a close/+ margin. 2-yr survival was 62%, and 3-yr DFS was 45% for LN–, epithelioid histology. 5 pts with stage I Dz had 3-yr DFS of 100%.

What is often recommended after a decortication/ pleurectomy procedure for mesothelioma?

B/c of the high LR rate, **adj RT is advocated.** (*Gupta V et al., IJROBP 2005*) At MSKCC, 125 pts were treated with pleurectomy → interstitial RT or EBRT. MS was 13.5 mos; 2-yr OS was 23%. Those with epithelioid or earlier-stage Dz did better. <40 Gy, left-sided Dz, use of an implant, or nonepithelioid histology did worse. LC rate was 40%. However, 12 pts developed pneumonitis, 8 pts pericarditis, and 2 pts died from grade 5 toxicity within 1 mo of Tx.

What is a palliative surgical procedure to consider for the management of poor-risk mesothelioma?

Pleurodesis with talc can be considered as palliative care with poor-risk mesothelioma.

What is the role of RT in unresectable mesothelioma Dz?

Palliative RT is used only for temporary pain relief. Use either 30 Gy in 10 fx or 20 Gy in 5 fx. In retrospective studies, the 2 regimens gave similar palliation.

What RT doses are used for palliation of chest pain associated with skin nodules in the CW?

Daily doses ≥4 Gy appear more efficacious than fx dose <4 Gy, for a total dose of 20–40 Gy.

What is the role of RT after invasive procedures for mesothelioma? What study evaluated the role of prophylactic RT, and what were the results?

Historically, RT was given to areas of invasive procedure (including thoracentesis and chest tube) to avoid needle tract seeding with tumor. RT was 7 Gy × 3, **for a total of 21 Gy** (*Boutin C et al., Chest 1995*). However, *O'Rourke N et al.* showed in a randomized trial that **prophylactic RT to drain sites did not statistically reduce the rate of seeding.** However, b/c recurrence is morbid, prophylaxis is still generally done. (*Radiother Oncol 2007*)

▶ TOXICITY

What is the estimated contralat lung V20 associated with the development of fatal pneumonitis in the Tx of mesothelioma?

RR was 42 for fatal pneumonitis if the V20 was >7% in the contralat intact lung based on MDACC data. (*Rice DC et al., Ann Thorac Surg 2007*)

What are the dose-volume constraints for the contralat lung in RT for mesothelioma?

In the remaining lung, with the V20 <7%, **mean lung dose ≤8.5 Gy, V5 <50%.**

What is the dose constraint for the liver? Heart? Spinal cord? Esophagus? Kidney?

Liver: V30 <30%
Heart: V40 <50%
Spinal cord: V45 <10%, no volume >50 Gy
Esophagus: V55 <30%
Kidney: V15 <20%

What are 5 acute and long-term complications from treatment?

Acute: fatigue, n/v, dysphagia/odynophagia, skin reactions, cough, dyspnea, pneumonitis, infection, Lhermitte syndrome
Late: cardiac (pericarditis, cardiomyopathy, MI, CHF) and lung (fibrosis, pneumonitis).

Part VI Breast

42 General Breast Cancer

Updated by Katherine Osusky Castle

▶ BACKGROUND

What are the 3 most commonly diagnosed cancers in women in decreasing order of incidence?

Most commonly diagnosed cancers in women: breast > lung > colorectal (*Siegal R et al., Cancer Stats 2013*)

What are the 3 most common causes of cancer death in women in decreasing order of incidence?

Most common causes of cancer death in women: lung > breast > colorectal (*Siegal R et al., Cancer Stats 2013*)

Approximately how many women are diagnosed with invasive and noninvasive breast cancer, and how many will die of breast cancer annually?

Incidence: ~232,000 invasive breast cancers and ~60,000 noninvasive breast cancers annually (*Siegal R, Cancer Stats 2013*)
Mortality: ~40,000

What is median age of Dx for invasive breast cancer?

The median age for invasive breast cancer is **61 yrs.** (*Siegal R et al., Cancer Treatment and Survivorship Stats 2013*)

What race has the highest rate of breast cancer Dx? What race has the highest rate of breast cancer mortality?

Highest Dx: whites
Highest mortality: blacks

(*Siegal R, Cancer Stats 2013*)

For women born in the U.S. in 2009, approximately what % will be diagnosed with breast cancer in their lifetimes?

~**12%** (1 in 8) of U.S. women born in 2009 will be diagnosed with breast cancer. (*Siegal R et al., Cancer Stats 2013*)

In the U.S. in 2009, was the incidence of breast cancer Dx increasing or decreasing?	The incidence of Dx was **increasing.** (*Siegal R et al., Cancer Stats 2013*)
In the U.S. in 2009, was the incidence of breast cancer mortality increasing or decreasing?	The incidence of mortality was **decreasing.** (*Siegal R et al., Cancer Stats 2013*)
What % of breast cancers are due to known hereditary mutations in single genes?	**≤10%** (*Foulkes WD et al., NEJM 2008*)
What are the 2 most common hereditary mutations that predispose to breast cancer?	*BRCA1* and *BRCA2* are the most common mutations. (These are most common in the Ashkenazi Jewish population, where they are found in as many as 1 in 40.) (*Metcalfe KA et al., JCO 2010*)
Mutations in which gene, *BRCA1* or *BRCA2*, confers a higher risk of ovarian cancer?	Both *BRCA1* and *BRCA2* are associated with increased risk of ovarian cancer, but risks are higher with *BRCA1* (45% lifetime risk) compared to *BRCA2* (15% lifetime risk). (*Chen S et al., JCO 2007*)
What are 2 other hereditary syndromes associated with an increased risk of breast cancer and their related germ line mutations?	Both are a result of mutations in tumor suppressor genes: 1. Li-Fraumeni syndrome: *TP53* 2. Cowden syndrome: *PTEN*
Is HRT with estrogen and progestin associated with an increased or decreased risk of breast cancer?	HRT with estrogen and progestin is associated with an **increased** RR of 1.7.
Separate the following factors into those that increase or decrease the risk of breast cancer: younger age at menarche, younger age at menopause, nulliparity, prolonged breastfeeding, use of HRT.	<u>Increase risk</u>: younger age at menarche, nulliparity, use of HRT <u>Decrease risk</u>: younger age at menopause, prolonged breastfeeding
Estimate the annual risk of a contralat breast cancer in the 10 yrs following a primary Dx.	<u>Premenopausal</u>: 1%/yr <u>Postmenopausal</u>: 0.5%/yr
What is the definition of natural menopause and what is the median age at which is occurs?	Definition: permanent cessation of menstrual periods (12 mos of amenorrhea) without other obvious pathologic or physiologic cause. Median age: 51 yrs

What are the U.S. Preventive Services Task Force (USPSTF) screening recommendations for normal-risk women age <50 yrs, age 50–74 yrs, and age >74 yrs?

For normal-risk women age ≤50 yrs: avoid routine mammographic screening (individualized use acceptable)

For normal-risk women age 50–74 yrs: biennial mammogram

For normal-risk women age >74 yrs: insufficient evidence to assess balance of benefits and harms

For all women: insufficient evidence for or against clinical breast exam (CBE) as a supplement to mammography.

For all women: recommend against breast self-exam (harms outweigh benefits) (*USPSTF, Ann Intern Med 2009*)

What are the ACS screening recommendations for normal-risk women age 20–39 yrs and women ≥40 yrs?

For normal-risk women age 20–39 yrs: CBE at least every 3 yrs and optional breast self-exam.

For normal risk women ≥40: annual CBE and mammogram as well as optional breast self-exam with decision to discontinue routine screening individualized (no strict age cutoff)

(The USPSTF recommends biennial screening mammography beginning at ≥50 yo and discontinuation at age 74.)

For a woman with prior thoracic RT during the 2ⁿᵈ and 3rd decades of life, when should screening begin for breast cancer and how?

According to NCCN guidelines:

Age ≤25: annual CBE beginning 8–10 yrs after RT

Age >25: annual mammogram + CBE every 6–12 mos and annual breast MRI beginning 8–10 yrs after RT or age 40 (whichever comes 1st).

When should a woman be screened for breast cancer using MRI?

ACS guidelines (2011) recommend screening MRI as a supplement to yearly mammography **beginning at age 30 for** women who have a high lifetime risk (>20%–25% risk). This includes those with *BRCA1/2* mutations or a 1ˢᵗ-degree relative with *BRCA1/2* but who have not had personal genetic testing, those with high lifetime risk according to risk assessment tools based primarily on family Hx, those who had radiation to the chest at 10–30 years of age, and those with Li-Fraumeni or Cowden syndrome or with a 1ˢᵗ-degree relative with 1 of these syndromes. This does *not* include women with a personal Hx of breast cancer without other risk factors or women with dense breast tissue.

According to NCCN 2013, what are the potential clinical indications and applications of dedicated breast MRI testing?

1. Define extent of cancer, multifocal or multicentric Dz in the ipsi breast.*
2. Screen for contralat breast cancer in a newly diagnosed breast cancer pt.

*Available data do not demonstrate that MRI improves local recurrence, survival, or detection in dense breasts.

3. Evaluate before and after neoadj therapy to define extent of Dz, response to Tx, and potential for breast conservation.
4. Detect additional Dz in women with mammographically dense breasts.*
5. Detect primary Dz in pts with +axillary LNs or Paget Dz of the nipple when primary is not identified on mammogram, US, or physical exam.

Breast MRIs should be performed only where there is a dedicated breast coil, an experienced radiologist, and capacity for MRI-guided biopsy. Since false+ findings on MRI are common, surgical decisions should not be based solely on MRI; additional tissue sampling should be performed in areas of concern identified by MRI.

Name the 5 rare histologic types of breast cancer that have a more favorable overall prognosis than invasive ductal/lobular carcinoma.

Rare types of breast cancer with a more favorable prognosis:
1. Tubular
2. Mucinous
3. Medullary (not including atypical medullary)
4. Cribriform
5. Invasive papillary

Name the 1 rare histologic type of breast cancer that has a less favorable overall prognosis than invasive ductal/lobular carcinoma.

Micropapillary carcinoma has a less favorable overall prognosis.

What is the Oncotype DX, and which breast cancer pts are eligible for its use?

Oncotype DX is a 21-gene assay that quantifies the likelihood of distant recurrence in tamoxifen-treated ER+, node– breast cancer patients. (*Paik S et al., NEJM 2004*) Evaluation of Oncotype DX in pts from NSABP B20 suggests that the recurrence score also predicts the magnitude of chemo benefit. (*Paik S et al., JCO 2006*) NCCN currently recommends the use of Oncotype DX in **early stage, ER+, node–** pts.

What are the 5 subtypes of the tissue microarray classification system for breast cancer? Which 2 subtypes carry poor prognoses?

Subtypes of the tissue microarray classification system:
1. Luminal A ($\uparrow$ ER expressing, $\downarrow$ proliferation)
2. Luminal B ($\uparrow$ ER expressing, $\downarrow$ proliferation)
3. *HER2* overexpressing
4. Normal-like
5. Basal type (ER/progesterone receptor (PR)/*HER2N*–)

Basal and luminal B carry relatively poor prognoses.

What are phyllodes tumors of the breast, and what is the most important factor that determines risk of recurrence?

Phyllodes tumors are rare tumors containing both stromal and epithelial elements. Although the subtypes range from benign to malignant, the most important prognostic factor for recurrence is a clear margin after resection.

▶ WORKUP/STAGING

What view(s) comprise a screening mammogram?

1. Mediolateral oblique: allows localization of tumor in superior-inferior dimensions
2. Craniocaudal: allows localization of tumor in medial-lateral dimensions

What is the workup for a breast lesion detected on screening mammogram?

Breast lesion workup: H&P (family Hx of breast and ovarian cancer, prior abnl mammograms, Hx of atypical ductal or lobular hyperplasia), diagnostic bilat mammogram (additional views including spot compression and magnification), and Bx of lesion (if mass nonpalpable, a stereotactic Bx should be performed).

What is the rate of axillary nodal positivity by T stage for breast cancer pts undergoing axillary dissection? What if the primary tumor is palpable vs. nonpalpable on exam?

ALL (nonpalpable/palpable)

Overall:	30%	(8%/40%)
Tis:	0.8 %	(0.7%/1.1%)
T1a:	5%	(3% /7%)
T1b:	16%	(8%/22%)
T1c:	28%	(18%/32%)
T2:	47%	(23%/50%)
T3:	68%	(46%/69%)
T4:	86%	(—/86%)

(*Silverstein M et al., World J Surg 2001*)

What are the 5 regional LN stations in breast cancer?

Regional LN stations in breast cancer:
Station I: nodes inf/lat to pectoralis minor muscle
Station II: nodes deep to pectoralis minor
Station III: nodes sup/med to pectoralis minor
Station IV: supraclavicular nodes
Station V: internal mammary (IM) nodes

Infraclavicular nodes typically refer to the level III axillary nodes by radiation oncology.

What is the T staging for invasive breast cancer according to the AJCC 7th edition (2011)?

Tis: in situ (ductal carcinoma in situ [CIS], lobular CIS, or isolated Paget)
T1mi: microinvasion ≤1 mm
T1a: >0.1–0.5 cm
T1b: >0.5–1 cm
T1c: >1–2 cm
T2: >2–5 cm
T3: >5 cm
T4a: extension to chest wall, not including pectoralis muscle
T4b: edema (including peau d'orange) or ulceration of skin of breast, or ipsilateral satellite nodules, not meeting T4d criteria
T4c: both T4a and T4b
T4d: inflammatory carcinoma (erythema and edema over at least one-third of the breast, present for less than 6 mos, in conjunction with biopsy proof of invasive carcinoma)

(*Note:* T classification is the same whether it is based on clinical judgment or pathologic assessment. In general, pathologic determination should take precedence for determination of T size.)

Does involvement of the dermis alone qualify as T4 disease?

No. Involvement of the skin by breast cancer qualifies as T4 only if there is edema, ulceration, or skin nodules.

What is the clinical N staging for invasive breast cancer according to the AJCC 7th edition (2011)?

N1: movable ipsi level I/II axillary LN
N2a: ipsi level I/II axillary LNs fixed/matted
N2b: clinically apparent IM node in absence of clinically evident axillary nodes
N3a: ipsi infraclavicular LNs
N3b: ipsi IM and axillary nodes
N3c: ipsi supraclavicular nodes

What is the pathologic N staging for invasive breast cancer according to the AJCC 7th edition (2011)?

pN0(i–): negative by immunohistochemistry (IHC)
pN0(i+): positive by IHC only, but no cluster >0.2 mm (also called isolated tumor cell clusters)
pN0(mol–): negative by reverse transcription-polymerase chain reaction (RT-PCR)
pN0(mol+): positive by RT-PCR only
pN1mi: all nodal mets >0.2 mm or > 200 cells but ≤2 mm
pN1a: 1–3 axillary LNs involved, at least 1 >2 mm
pN1b: IM node detected by sentinel LND, but not clinically apparent

pN1c: 1–3 axillary nodes and IM node detected by sentinel LND, but not clinically apparent

pN2a: 4–9 axillary LNs involved, at least 1 >2 mm

pN2b: clinically apparent IM nodes in the absence of axillary LN mets

pN3a: >10 axillary LN or mets to infraclavicular (axillary level III) LNs

pN3b: clinically apparent IM node in the presence of axillary nodes; or ≥3 axillary LNs and IM node detected by sentinel LND, but not clinically apparent

pN3c: ipsi supraclavicular node

Define the AJCC breast cancer stage groupings using TNM status.	**Stage 0:** Tis, N0
	Stage IA: T1, N0
	Stage IB: T1, N1mic
	Stage IIA: T2, N0 or T0-T1, N1
	Stage IIB: T3, N0 or T2, N1
	Stage IIIA: T3, N1 or T0-T3, N2
	Stage IIIB: T4, N0-N2
	Stage IIIC: any T, N3
	Stage IV: any T, any N, M1

What are the 5-yr relative survival rates for breast cancer?

The 5-yr relative survival rates (observed survival in women with breast cancer vs. expected survival in women without breast cancer) according to the SEER registry of pts diagnosed 2003–2009
Localized (confined to primary site): 98.6%
Regional (spread to LNs): 84.4%
Distant (cancer has metastasized): 24.3%

▶ TOXICITY

What are the acute and late toxicities of whole breast RT?

<u>Acute toxicities</u>: fatigue, dermatitis, hyperpigmentation, pneumonitis

<u>Late toxicities</u>: soft tissue fibrosis, telangiectasias, rib fractures, pulmonary fibrosis, cardiovascular Dz, 2nd RT-induced malignancy

What is the rate of acute skin breakdown, and where does it typically occur with whole breast RT?

25%–30% of pts experience skin breakdown, most often in the **inframammary fold or axillary sulcus.**

What % of women have a less than good or excellent cosmetic result after whole breast RT and lumpectomy?

20%–30% of pts have a more unfavorable cosmetic result.

In a pt with breast cancer, what is the rate of lymphedema after whole breast RT ± axillary LND? How does the RT technique affect risk?

15%–35% after RT + axillary LND; 5%–10% after RT and sentinel node Bx only. It is difficult to determine the RT effect b/c of other confounding tumor and Tx factors. However, retrospective studies suggest that tangent-only RT is associated with lower risk than directed nodal RT.

What is the RR of cardiovascular Dz death after RT to left-sided breast cancer compared to right-sided breast cancer?

Studies from the **pre-3D planning era** suggest that RT for left-sided breast cancer is associated with an **RR of 1.5–2 for cardiovascular Dz death** compared to RT for right-sided breast cancer. This has not been confirmed in women treated using modern RT techniques.

What is the risk of 2nd malignancy after whole breast RT?

The lifetime risk of 2nd malignancy after whole breast RT is **1%–2%**.

43 Ductal and Lobular Carcinoma In Situ

Updated by Emma B. Holliday

▶ BACKGROUND

Ductal carcinoma in situ (DCIS) represents what % of all breast malignancies?

DCIS represents ~20% of all breast malignancies.

Which is more common: DCIS or lobular carcinoma in situ (LCIS)?

DCIS is 5 times more common than LCIS.

Name the 5 most common histologic subtypes of DCIS.

Most common subtypes of DCIS:
1. **C**ribriform
2. **C**omedo
3. **P**apillary
4. **M**edullary
5. **S**olid

(Mnemonic: **C²PMS**)

Which histologic subtypes of DCIS have the worst and 2nd worst prognosis?	The DCIS subtype that has the worst prognosis is comedo, and the 2nd worst is solid. DCIS is often grouped into comedo and noncomedo subgroups.
How many pathologic grades are there for DCIS?	There are 3 pathologic grades for DCIS: low, intermediate, and high.
What % of DCIS are estrogen receptor (ER)+?	**75%–85%** of DCIS cases are ER+.
What is the most common clinical presentation of DCIS?	DCIS most commonly presents with **microcalcifications** on a mammogram.
What is the most common clinical presentation of LCIS?	LCIS most commonly presents as an **incidental finding.** LCIS typically does not result in mammographic or clinical abnormalities.
What is the incidence of progression of DCIS to invasive Dz if left untreated?	Very difficult to determine; **15%–50%** of DCIS cases will progress to invasive Dz if left untreated.
For a pt with LCIS, what is the risk of the pt to be diagnosed with invasive Dz by 10 yrs?	A pt with LCIS has an ~7% risk of developing invasive cancer at 10 yrs (~1%/yr), but the risk of subsequent invasive Dz is **equal in both breasts,** suggesting that LCIS is primarily a predictor of invasive Dz development, rather than a precursor lesion. (*Chuba PJ et al., JCO 2005*)
What % of pts with LCIS who subsequently develop invasive Dz develop invasive lobular cancers?	**25%–50%** of subsequent cancers are invasive lobular cancers (i.e., though LCIS is a proliferative lesion of the lobules, it is mostly a marker for subsequent ductal proliferative lesions).
Which subtype of LCIS has the worst prognosis?	Of LCIS subtypes, **pleomorphic** LCIS has the worst prognosis. It is more commonly associated with invasive Dz and hormone receptor negativity. Consider complete excision with negative margins.

▶ WORKUP/STAGING

What is the initial workup after a DCIS Dx?	DCIS workup: H&P (with emphasis on risk of hereditary breast cancer), diagnostic bilat mammogram, path review and assessment of ER status, genetic counseling if high risk (per NCCN 2014).
What is the T stage for DCIS as per AJCC 7th edition (2011)?	DCIS has its own designation: **Tis.**

What is the definition of DCIS with microinvasion, and what is the significance for workup?

DCIS with microinvasion refers to invasion ≤1 mm in size. If microinvasion is present, then a sentinel **LN Bx is indicated, as the LN+ rate is ~4%–8%.** (*Solin LJ et al., IJROBP 1992*)

For a pt with DCIS, if there is <1-mm margin at excision, what is the rate of residual Dz at the time of re-excision?

For a pt with DCIS and a <1-mm margin at excision, **~30% will have residual Dz at re-excision.** Notably, low- and intermediate-grade DCIS is more likely to grow in a discontinuous pattern. (*Faverly DR et al., Semin Diagn Pathol 1994*) B/c of this, margin status may be, paradoxically, more important in these lesions. In these discontinuous type lesions, gaps of uninvolved tissue between DCIS are typically small (<5 mm in 80% of cases).

For a pt with DCIS, in which situation would re-excision not be indicated with a margin <1 mm?

If a pt with DCIS has an **excisional margin <1 mm at the fibroglandular border** of the breast (skin or chest wall), then re-excision is not indicated.

▶ **TREATMENT/PROGNOSIS**

What is the Tx paradigm for unifocal DCIS?

There are 3 Tx paradigms for unifocal DCIS:
1. Lumpectomy + postop RT (PORT) +/– tamoxifen (if ER+)
2. Lumpectomy alone +/– tamoxifen (if ER+)
3. Mastectomy

Radiation can be delivered to the whole breast using standard fractionation or hypofractionation or could be delivered using accelerated partial breast irradiation.

Is an axillary sentinel node Bx needed for DCIS?

No. Surgical axillary evaluation is not needed for DCIS. However, per NCCN 2014, consider if (1) the pt is undergoing mastectomy for Tx or (2) if the location of lumpectomy will compromise future sentinel Bx should it be necessary.

For a pt with DCIS, what is rate of LR after mastectomy alone?

For a pt with DCIS, the rate of LR after mastectomy is **~1%–5% at 10 yrs.**

What are considered adequate surgical margins in pts receiving breast conservation surgery for DCIS?

For patients who will undergo postoperative RT: 2 mm. For patients who will not receive postoperative RT: 3 mm. A systematic review of published trials in DCIS with breast conservation therapy (BCT) involving 4,660 pts found that a **2-mm margin** was superior to a margin <2 mm (ORR 0.53), without any LC benefit in margins >2 mm. (*Dunne C et al., JCO 2009*) RTOG 9804 (RCT of omission of RT) and ECOG 5194 (observational study of omission of RT) both required a minimum 3-mm margin.

What are the contraindications for BCT for DCIS?

Contraindications for BCT for DCIS: multicentric Dz, persistently +margins, cosmetic limitations, and, potentially, the inability to get PORT (pregnancy or prior RT).

Is there a benefit of mastectomy over BCT for DCIS?

This is **undetermined.** No prospective study has directly compared mastectomy vs. BCT for DCIS. Indirect comparisons suggest that mastectomy results in lower LR than BCT. However, there is no expectation that mastectomy would improve OS compared to BCT, because the risk of breast cancer–related death after a diagnosis of DCIS is <2%.

For a pt with DCIS treated with lumpectomy, what is the impact of PORT on ipsi breast recurrence (invasive and noninvasive) and OS?

For DCIS treated with lumpectomy, PORT **reduces LR by 50%, but there is no evidence for OS benefit.**

Name 4 prospective studies that support the addition of RT after lumpectomy in pts with DCIS.

1. **NSABP B-17** (*Fisher B et al., Semin Oncol 2001*)
2. **EORTC 10853** (*Bijker N et al., JCO 2006*)
3. **United Kingdom Co-ordinating Committee on Cancer Research (UKCCCR)** (*Houghton J et al., Lancet 2003*)
4. **SweDCIS** (*Holmber L et al., JCO 2008*)

Describe the Tx arms and the invasive and noninvasive LR outcomes in NSABP B-17 and EORTC 10853.

In **NSABP B-17,** 818 DCIS pts treated with lumpectomy with no tumor at inked margins were randomized to 50 Gy whole breast RT or no RT. At 10 yrs, the overall ipsilateral breast tumor recurrence (IBTR) rate was 30.8% vs. 14.9% in favor of RT. Both the invasive and noninvasive recurrence rate was approximately halved by RT.

In **EORTC 10853,** 1,010 DCIS pts treated with lumpectomy with no tumor at inked margins were randomized to 50 Gy whole breast RT or no RT. At 10 yrs, RT reduced LF from 26% to 15%. Half of all recurrences were invasive.

What is the traditional target, dose, and fractionation for PORT for DCIS?

Target the whole breast to 50 Gy in 25 fx.

Could hypofractionated radiation to the whole breast be considered?

Yes. The RCTs that established the efficacy of hypofractionation excluded women with DCIS, and the ASTRO task force on hypofractionated whole breast RT (*Smith BD et al., IJROBP 2011*) chose not to offer recommendations for or against hypofractionation for DCIS as these patients were excluded from the randomized trials. **However, subsequent completed and ongoing trials using hypofractionation have included women with DCIS. Caution should be used in pts with very large volume DCIS or very large breasts.**

Could accelerated partial breast irradiation be considered?

Possibly. The **ASTRO APBI consensus statement** placed DCIS in the "cautionary" group for APBI outside of a clinical trial. (*Smith BD et al., IJROBP 2009*) The European Society of Therapeutic Radiology likewise placed DCIS in the "intermediate-risk" group for APBI. (*Polgar C et al., Radiother Oncol 2010*) The **NSABP B 39/RTOG 0413** trial to assess the role of APBI included patients with DCIS as well as stage 1 or 2 breast cancer with tumors ≤3 cm and ≤3 +LNs.

For a pt with ER+ DCIS, is there a benefit to tamoxifen? What studies support this?

Yes. 2 trials provide evidence to support the use of tamoxifen in DCIS: NSABP B-24 and UKCCCR. **NSABP B-24** compared lumpectomy + RT +/– tamoxifen. Patients were enrolled without respect to ER status. At 5 yrs, the overall incidence of breast events (ipsi and contralat, invasive and noninvasive) was decreased with tamoxifen (8.2% vs. 13.4%). (*Fisher B et al., Lancet 1999*) A subsequent analysis of tamoxifen effect by ER status analyzed 732 of the 1,801 pts on NSABP B24. (*Allred DC et al., JCO 2012*) At 10 yrs, the HR for any breast event was 0.49 for ER+ pts who received tamoxifen.

The UKCCCR was a 2×2 factorial trial of RT, tamoxifen, both, or neither after lumpectomy for DCIS or microinvasive disease, without respect to ER status. At a median follow-up of 52 mos, tamoxifen marginally reduced overall DCIS events only. (*UKCCCR Working Group, Lancet 2003*) However, on 12-yr follow-up analysis, tamoxifen significantly reduced overall breast events (HR 0.71). (*Cuzick J et al., Lancet 2011*)

To summarize, in current practice, ER+ DCIS pts are offered adj tamoxifen.

Is there evidence supporting the use of aromatase inhibitors (AIs) for DCIS?

No. There are no published randomized trials for AIs in DCIS. NSABP B-35 and IBIS-II both compared 5 yrs of either tamoxifen or anastrozole for patients with DCIS after lumpectomy and RT; NSABP B-35 was closed to accrual and IBIS-II is currently accruing.

What about trastuzumab?

There is currently no role for trastuzumab in the treatment of DCIS. NSABP B-43 is evaluating the use of 2 cycles of concurrent trastuzumab (Herceptin) with whole breast radiation after lumpectomy for DCIS.

For a pt with DCIS, what is the effect of adj tamoxifen on contralateral breast tumor recurrence (CBTR)?

NSABP B-24 showed that the addition of tamoxifen to BCT in DCIS pts significantly reduced CBTR as the 1st site of recurrence from 4.9% to 2.3% at 7 yrs.

For a pt with ER– DCIS, is there benefit to adj tamoxifen after lumpectomy + RT?

Probably not. Retrospective subset analysis of **NSABP B-24** showed that the benefit of adj tamoxifen was limited to ER+ pts. (*Allred DC et al., JCO 2012*)

For a pt with ER+ DCIS, does adj tamoxifen obviate the benefit of RT after lumpectomy? What study evaluated this?

RT is still beneficial for pts with DCIS treated with lumpectomy even with adj tamoxifen. UKCCCR was a 2 × 2 factorial study looking at the benefit of RT and tamoxifen in DCIS pts after lumpectomy. After a median follow-up >4 yrs, RT reduced IBTR in women given adj tamoxifen (6% vs. 18%). (*Houghton J et al., Lancet 2003*)

For a pt with DCIS, name some risk factors associated with LR and which is most important.

Risk factors for LR in a pt with DCIS:
1. Decreased margin width (most important)
2. Increased size of tumor
3. High grade
4. Young age (<50 yrs)
5. Postmenopausal status
6. Comedo necrosis
7. Multifocality

What is the purpose of the Van Nuys Prognostic Classification system, and what are its limitations?

The Van Nuys Prognostic Classification system is meant to identify DCIS pts who are at low risk for recurrence after RT alone using width of margins, size, grade, and age. The system was developed retrospectively and has not been validated in prospective studies or in different retrospective datasets. (*Silverstein MJ et al., Am J Surg 2003*)

Do all DCIS pts require PORT?

Some patients with low-risk DCIS can probably be safely observed. Pts can be considered for omission of RT if they have grades 1–2 DCIS no larger than 2.5 cm, with margins at least 3 mm. 2 studies provide the main evidence for omission of RT:

> **ECOG 5194** (*Hughes KK et al., JCO 2009*): prospective single-arm observational trial. 711 patients with nonpalpable DCIS measuring at least 3 mm and conservatively resected with ≥3 mm microscopic margins (606 with G1–2 disease measuring up to 2.5 cm, 105 with G3 DCIS measuring up to 1 cm). Patients were followed without RT; 31% declared an intent to take tamoxifen. At a median follow-up of 62 months, 5-yr ipsilateral breast event rate was 6.1% (G1–2) and 15.3% (G3).

> **RTOG 9804** (*McCormick B et al., JCO 2012* [abstract only]): prospective randomized trial of whole breast RT (50 Gy, no boost) vs. no RT for G1–2 DCIS conservatively resected with ≥3 mm margins. 585 eligible pts enrolled (accrual target 1,790 pts); 62% took tamoxifen. At a median follow-up of 6.46 yrs, the 5-yr local failure rate was 0.4% with RT vs. 3.2% without RT ($p = 0.0023$).

What whole breast dose and boost dose are used for a pt with DCIS after lumpectomy?

For DCIS, the whole breast dose is 42–50 Gy with a 10–16 Gy lumpectomy bed boost. The role of a boost in DCIS is controversial. The practice is extrapolated from results of the EORTC and Lyon boost trials for invasive cancers, but there have been no prospective trials of the role of boost in DCIS pts. ~44% of pts from **B-24** were given a boost, mainly for +margins. A recent population-based analysis showed that the addition of a boost was not associated with a lower risk of local or invasive recurrence. (*Rakovitch E et al., IJROBP 2013*)

What is the Tx paradigm for LCIS?

LCIS Tx paradigm: for pure LCIS after lumpectomy, pts can be observed +/– risk reduction procedures. Occurrence of invasive Dz after LCIS is low and is often in the contralat breast. In addition, invasive Dz after LCIS is generally relatively favorable, and deaths subsequently are rare. The exception may be pleomorphic LCIS, although data are limited.

For a pt with LCIS, what are 2 options to reduce the risk of development of an invasive cancer?

Options to reduce the risk of development of an invasive cancer:
1. Antiestrogen therapy with tamoxifen or raloxifene (raloxifene only if postmenopausal) (**NSABP P1 trial**)
2. Bilat mastectomy

What is the management for a woman with LCIS detected on percutaneous core needle Bx?

LCIS on core needle Bx should typically prompt a surgical excision to confirm pure LCIS.

Is LCIS associated with invasive cancer a contraindication for BCT?

No. Current literature supports the safety of BCT in the presence of coexisting LCIS in the specimen, and no special effort needs to be made to obtain –margins on LCIS.

For a pt with LCIS, what is the benefit of primary tamoxifen?

For a pt with LCIS, tamoxifen halves the risk of invasive recurrence in either breast. (*Fisher B et al., Lancet 1999*)

In a pt with DCIS or invasive Dz, what is the most common contraindication for adj tamoxifen therapy?

In a pt with DCIS or invasive Dz, the most common contraindication for adj tamoxifen therapy is **Hx of stroke or other coagulopathy.**

▶ **TOXICITY**

What is the recommended follow-up schedule after Tx for DCIS?

Recommended follow-up schedule after Tx for DCIS: interval H&P exam every 6–12 mos for 5 yrs, then annually. Bilateral mammogram annually.

For a pt with LCIS, what is the recommended observation strategy?

Recommended observation strategy for a pt with LCIS: H&P every 6–12 mos and bilat mammogram annually

What is the role of MRI screening in a patient with previous LCIS or DCIS?

Per NCCN 2014, MRI should only be used for screening if there is a >20% chance of a 2nd primary breast cancer. In the absence of other risk factors, Hx of DCIS or LCIS alone does not confer a 20% risk.

44 Early-Stage (I–II) Breast Cancer

Updated by Emma B. Holliday

▶ BACKGROUND

What histologic subtypes of invasive ductal carcinoma (IDC) are associated with favorable outcomes?

Tubular, medullary, mucinous (colloid), and papillary

What is a phyllodes tumor of the breast?

Previously known as cystosarcoma phyllodes, phyllodes tumor ranges from benign to malignant and is a **rare tumor with leaflike, lobulated appearance on microscopic section.** Surgery is the primary treatment: wide local excision (with at least 1-cm margins) or total mastectomy; surgical axillary evaluation is not indicated in clinically node-negative pts. Per NCCN 2014, there is no standard role for RT after either mastectomy or wide local excision with adequate margin. The role of RT after breast conservation surgery (BCS) for large and/or malignant phyllodes tumors is still undefined, however.

What is Paget Dz of the breast? What is the clinical presentation?

Paget Dz of the breast is caused by **malignant epithelial cells (Paget cells) infiltrating the epidermis of the nipple-areolar complex.** The clinical presentation is **crusting, scaling, itching, and redness on the skin of the nipple** that can progress to ulceration and bleeding. **80%–90%** of Paget Dz is associated with underlying ductal carcinoma in situ (DCIS) or invasive breast cancer.

What % of invasive cancers are lobular carcinomas?

10%–15% of invasive cancers are lobular carcinomas.

According to the NSABP B04 trial, what % of women with a clinically – axilla were found to have axillary mets at LND?

Per **NSABP B04, 40%** of these women had axillary mets at LND.

Of the women who had a clinically − axilla and did not have a nodal dissection, what % eventually developed a clinically + axilla?	**20%** of these women developed a clinically + axilla.

▶ WORKUP/STAGING

What is the workup for invasive breast cancer?	Per NCCN 2014, H&P (including family Hx of breast or ovarian cancer, personal Hx of atypical ductal or lobular hyperplasia), CBC, LFTs, diagnostic bilat mammogram, estrogen receptor (ER)/progesterone receptor (PR)/*HER2* status, and β-HCG (if premenopausal), and offer genetic counseling if at risk for hereditary breast cancer. Other imaging **only for suspicious Hx, physical, or lab findings.**
What is the role of MRI for pts with known invasive breast cancer?	Per NCCN 2014, MRI can be used to define the extent of Dx/multifocal Dz in the ipsi breast or for contralat Dz (cat. 2B). There is no evidence that MRI improves LR or OS.
How should the axilla be staged?	If palpable or radiologically visible LN, FNA/core Bx to confirm → full axillary lymph node dissection (ALND) (levels I and II) at the time of surgery. If no palpable or radiologically visible LN, sentinel lymph node dissection (SLND) is preferred over ALND in early-stage Dz.
Which major trials showed SLND Bx as an alternative to ALND for sentinel node–negative pts?	The **NSABP B-32** trial randomized 5,611 pts undergoing mastectomy or lumpectomy to SLN Bx + immediate completion axillary LND vs. SLN Bx alone. The OS, DFS, and regional control were statistically similar between groups. The 10-yr OS was 87.8% vs. 88.9%, DFS 76.9% for both, and LR rate 4.3% vs. 4.0%, for SLND alone vs. SLND + ALND, respectively. (*KragDN et al., Lancet Oncol 2010; 10-yr update ASCO 2013*) The **ALMANAC trial** (*Mansel RE et al., JNCI 2006*) and **Milan trial** (*Veronesi U et al., NEJM 2013; Lancet Oncol 2006; 10-yr update Ann Surg 2010*) also showed comparable outcomes. Both NSABP B32 and ALMANAC showed a decreased risk of lymphedema and arm numbness with SLN Bx.

What should be done if the SLND is positive?	If T1 or T2 tumor, 1 or 2 + SLN, whole breast irradiation (WBI) is planned after lumpectomy and no neoadj systemic therapy was given, no further surgery may be considered (NCCN 2014). American College of Surgeons Oncology Group (ACOSOG) Z0011 randomized ALND (n = 445) vs. no dissection (n = 445) for +SLND Tx with WBI (tangents) but no dedicated axillary RT. Study closed (891 of 1,900) early b/c of low accrual and no expected change in results with full accrual. SLND alone did not result in inferior 5-yr OS (91.8% vs. 92.5%), DFS (83.9% vs. 82.2%), or LRR-free survival (96.7% vs. 95.7%). (*Giuliano AE et al., JAMA 2011*)
List the subsets of T1 breast cancers per the 7th edition of AJCC.	**Per AJCC 7th edition (2011):** **T1mic:** ≤0.1 cm **T1a:** >0.1 but ≤0.5 cm **T1b:** >0.5 cm but ≤1 cm **T1c:** >1 cm but ≤2 cm
Define T2 and T3.	**T2:** >2 cm but ≤5 cm **T3:** >5 cm
What is the pathologic staging for N0?	**pN0(i–):** no LN met histologically, negative **immunohistochemistry** (IHC) **pN0(i+):** malignant cells/cell clusters ≤0.2 mm or ≤200 cells (detected by H&E or IHC, including **isolated tumor cells**)
What is the clinical staging for N1?	**cN1:** mets to any number of movable ipsi levels I–II axillary nodes
What is the pathologic staging for N1?	**pN1mic:** micrometastases (>0.2 mm or 200 cells but ≤2.0 mm) **pN1a:** 1–3 axillary nodes, at least 1 with >2.0 mm mets **pN1b:** micro- or macrometastases in internal mammary nodes, detected only by SLN Bx **pN1c:** micro- or macrometastases in internal mammary nodes, detected only by SLN Bx AND in 1–3 axillary nodes
What is the TNM staging for stage I breast cancers?	**IA:** T1 N0 **IB:** T1 N1mic
What is the TNM staging for stage II breast cancers?	**IIA:** T1 N1, T2 N0 **IIB:** T2 N1, T3 N0
What % of breast cancer pts are diagnosed with stages 0–II Dz?	~**80%** of breast cancer pts are diagnosed with stages 0–II Dz according to the most recent SEER statistics

How should Paget Dz associated with an underlying breast cancer be staged?

Per the AJCC 7th edition (2011), Paget Dz associated with underlying breast cancer should be staged **according to the T stage of the underlying cancer** (Tis, T1, etc.).

▶ **TREATMENT/PROGNOSIS**

What are the management options for early-stage breast cancers?

Early-stage breast cancer management options:
1. Total mastectomy +/– systemic therapy +/– RT
2. Breast conservation therapy (BCT = breast conservation surgery [BCS] + RT) +/– systemic therapy

Options for delivery of RT as a component of BCT include WBI +/– boost, hypofractionated WBI +/– boost, or accelerated partial breast irradiation via external beam, interstitial, or intracavitary brachytherapy.

When should adj chemo be utilized in the management of early-stage node-negative breast cancers?

1. TN or HER2/neu (H2N +): tumor >1 cm (consider for tumor 0.6–1 cm)
2. ER+ AND H2N- AND tumor >0.5 cm: consider using 21 gene assay (Oncotype DX to determine role of adj chemo).

What does the Oncotype DX score tell you?

Risk of distant recurrence within 10 yrs of Dx with 5 yrs endocrine therapy alone in ER+, N0 pts who undergo upfront surgery.
Low recurrence score (<18) → adj endocrine Tx
Intermediate recurrence score (18–30) → adj endocrine +/– chemo
High recurrence score (≥31) → adj endocrine + chemo

When should adj endocrine therapy be used in early-stage breast cancer?

ER+ AND tumor >0.5 cm (consider for tumors ≤0.5 cm)

What are some general principles of administering adj endocrine therapy?

General principles for administration of adj endocrine therapy:
1. If the pt is premenopausal, tamoxifen (20 mg/day) is given for 5 yrs. Consider an additional 5 yrs of tamoxifen (if pt remains premenopausal) or an aromatase inhibitor (AI).
2. If the pt is postmenopausal, AI × 5 yrs is the most common approach. For women who cannot or will not take an AI, tamoxifen × 5 yrs and consider an additional 5 yrs of tamoxifen

What is the major contraindication to the use of AIs?

Premenopausal status or unknown menopausal status. AIs are not effective in women with estrogen-producing ovaries.

What are the major side effects of tamoxifen and AIs?

Tamoxifen: blood clots, strokes, uterine cancer, and cataracts. Gyn exam every 12 mos should be performed in women with a uterus.

Aromatase inhibitors: bone loss and osteoporosis, as well as joint pain and stiffness. Bone mineral density should be assessed at baseline and monitored periodically.

What are the major chemo agents used in breast cancer?

A: doxorubicin
E: epirubicin
C: cyclophosphamide or carboplatin
T: paclitaxel or docetaxel
F: 5-FU
H: trastuzumab

What are the major chemo combinations used in breast cancer?

AC: doxorubicin + cyclophosphamide
EC: epirubicin + cyclophosphamide
FAC/FEC: 5-FU, doxorubicin/epirubicin, cyclophosphamide
AC/EC/FAC/FEC + T: the T is paclitaxel
TC: docetaxel + cyclophosphamide
TCH: docetaxel + carboplatin + trastuzumab

What chemo regimens are recommended for *HER2–* tumors?

The preferred chemo regimens are:
1. Dose-dense AC (q2wk × 4 instead of q3wk × 4–6) followed by paclitaxel q2wk × 4
2. Dose-dense AC followed by paclitaxel q1wk × 12
3. TC q3wk × 4–6

What chemo regimens are recommended for *HER2+* tumors?

The preferred chemo regimens are:
1. AC followed by T plus concurrent trastuzumab (various schedules), followed by single-agent trastuzumab q3wk for a total of 1 yr
2. TCH q3wk × 6, followed by single-agent trastuzumab q3wk for a total of 1 yr

What data support the equivalence of BCT (lumpectomy + radiotherapy) to mastectomy with regard to survival?

Several large randomized trials (**NSABP B06, Milan III, Ontario, Royal Marsden, EORTC 10801**) support this, but B06 has the longest (20-yr) follow-up data. Recent Oxford meta-analysis summarizes the data and survival outcomes:

NSABP B06 (*Fisher B et al., NEJM 2002*): 1,851 stages I–II pts randomized to (a) total mastectomy, (b) lumpectomy alone, or (c) lumpectomy + RT (50 Gy). 20-yr follow-up results showed that there was no difference in DFS, OS, or DM.

EBCTCG Oxford meta-analysis (*EBCTCG Collaborators, Lancet 2011*): 10,801 women enrolled in 17 trials for BCS +/– RT. The 10-yr 1st recurrence risk reduction was 15.7% (19.3% in RT vs. 35% in BCS alone). The 15-yr breast cancer mortality was reduced by 3.8% (21.4% vs. 25.4%) with RT. Pts with pN0 Dz had 15.4% and 3.3% absolute reduction in recurrence and breast cancer mortality. Pts with pN+ Dz had 21.2% and 8.5% absolute risk reduction in recurrence and breast cancer mortality, respectively. For all risk groups, RT halves the risk of recurrence and decreases breast cancer mortality by one-sixth. For every 4 women prevented to have LR, 1 woman is saved (4:1 ratio).

What % of pts are eligible for BCT for early-stage breast cancers?

In early-stage breast cancers, **75%–80%** of pts are eligible for BCT. (*Morrow M et al., Cancer 2006*)

What are the contraindications for BCT for pts with early-stage breast cancer?

Contraindications for BCT in early-stage breast cancer:

1. Prior RT to the chest
2. Extent of Dz that excision could not achieve – margins with an acceptable cosmetic result (note that multicentricity and multifocality are not necessarily contraindications to BCT).
3. Diffuse microcalcifications
4. 1st or 2nd trimester of pregnancy
5. Persistently +margin
6. Collagen vascular Dz (esp scleroderma)

(*NCCN 2014*)

Is there a contraindication for BCT in pts with a positive family Hx of breast cancer?

No. There is no evidence that demonstrates increased ipsi or contralat breast cancers in pts with a positive family Hx after BCT. (*Vlastos G et al., Ann Surg Oncol 2007*)

Are *BRCA* mutations a contraindication for BCT?

No. Multiple case-control studies have not established a higher ipsi breast tumor recurrence (IBTR) rate in *BRCA1/BRCA2* mutation carriers compared to wild-type individuals, particularly if oophorectomy is performed in *BRCA* carriers. However, contralat breast cancer development is a major risk for *BRCA* carriers. Contralat breast cancer risk can be reduced with tamoxifen, oophorectomy, or both, but is most effectively reduced with prophylactic total mastectomy. *BRCA*+ breast cancer pts who elect contralat prophylactic total mastectomy will frequently also choose an ipsi total mastectomy for Tx of their known breast cancer.

What are the dose fractionation schedules for WBI?

Standard fractionation schedules:
1. **50 Gy** in 2 Gy fx
2. **45–50.4 Gy** in 1.8 Gy fx

Hypofractionated schedules:
1. **42.56 Gy** in 2.67 Gy fx
2. **40.05 Gy** in 2.67 Gy fx

What data support the use of hypofractionated WBI?

4 randomized trials with ≥10-yr follow-up suggest the same outcomes using a hypofractionated approach, with potentially better side effect profile. (*Canadian, START pilot, START A/B trials*).

Canadian regimen (*Whelan TJ et al., JNCI 2002; Whelan TJ et al., NEJM 2010*): RCT using 42.5 Gy in 16 fx (2.65 Gy/fx) vs. 50 Gy in 25 fx (2 Gy/fx) with no boost; 1,234 T1-2N0 pts, all with −surgical margins (SMs). **Women with >25-cm breast width were excluded** (to reduce heterogeneity of dose to the breast). 10-yr follow-up: no difference in LR, DFS, or cosmesis. Good to excellent cosmesis was equivalent (71.3% standard vs. 69.8% hypofractionated).

British regimen (*START A/B trials, Lancet 2008*): 2,215 women with pT1-3N0-1 s/p surgery randomized to 50 Gy in 25 fx vs. 40 Gy in 15 fx (2.67 Gy/fx). Boost and adj systemic Tx were optional. After 6-yr follow-up, there was no difference in IBTR (3% vs. 2%). 10-yr results published in abstract form at the San Antonio Breast Cancer Symposium in 2012 (*Cancer Res, 72(24), 2012, suppl. 3):* no difference in locoregional relapse between the 50-Gy and 40-Gy arms. Physician assessed markers of cosmetic outcome better with hypofractionation. Outcomes did not vary by age, BCS vs. mastectomy, nodal status, tumor grade, or the receipt of boost or adj chemo.

According to ASTRO guidelines, who can be offered hypofractionated WBI?

ASTRO guidelines (*Smith BD et al., IJROBP 2011*) state task force consensus for pts meeting all these criteria:
1. ≥50 yo
2. pT1-2N0, treated with BCS
3. No systemic chemo
4. Good homogeneity: dose along central axis +/− 7% of Rx dose.

What data support the use of a tumor bed boost?

2 studies have demonstrated an improved LC rate with a 10–16 Gy boost after initial whole breast dose to 45–50 Gy:

EORTC boost trial (*Bartelink K et al., JCO 2007*): 5,318 women with BCT, 10-yr update: 50 Gy vs. 50 Gy + 16 Gy boost (SM–) or + 26 Gy boost (SM+). 10-yr LF: 6.2% + boost vs. 10.2% – boost. Absolute benefit was greatest in women <50 b/c they have a higher risk of LR (24% – boost vs. 13.5% + boost for women <40 yo), but **proportional benefits were seen across all age groups.**

Lyon boost trial (*Romestaing P et al., JCO 1997*): 1,024 pts, 50 Gy vs. 50 Gy + 10 Gy boost. At 3-yr follow-up, LF was reduced in the boost arm (3.6% vs. 4.5%).

In general, a boost of 10–16 Gy should be considered for all pts, and should always be administered for pts at higher risk for LR (age <50 yrs, +LVI, or close SMs). This can be administered with brachytherapy, electrons, or photons.

Is there a need for a higher tumor boost dose in pts with incomplete tumor excision after BCS?

No. In the EORTC boost trial, 251 pts with microscopically incomplete tumor excision were randomized to low (10 Gy) vs. high (26 Gy) boost. With median follow-up of 11.3 yrs, there was no difference in LC or survival. There was significantly more fibrosis in the high-dose arm. (*Poortmans PM et al., Radiother Oncol 2009*)

What is the next step in the management for a pt who undergoes a lumpectomy with a focal +margin?

This is **controversial.** Most would advocate taking the pt back to surgery for re-excision, which may diminish the 10-yr risk of LR to baseline levels (initial SM–: 7%, SM+: 12%; SM close: 14%; re-excision SM–: 7%, re-excision persistent SM+: 13%, re-excision persistent SM close: 21%). (*Freedman G et al., IJROBP 1999*)

Is there a subset of women whose LR risk may not be substantially influenced by margin positivity after BCS?

Possibly. There are data to suggest that the effect of margin positivity on LR **may be dependent on age <40 yrs.** In an analysis of 1,752 pts, 193 were SM+. Overall 10-yr LR rate was 6.9% (SM–) vs. 12.2% (SM+). 5-yr LR rate for pts ≤40 yo was 8.4% (SM–) and 37% (SM+) ($p = 0.005$); for pts >40 yo, the LR rate was 2.6% (SM–) and 2.2% (SM+). (*Jobsen JJ et al., IJROBP 2003*)

Should women with T1-2N0 invasive breast cancer treated with mastectomy to a +margin be treated with adj RT to the chest wall as well?

In a **British Columbia retrospective study** (*Truong PT et al., IJROBP 2004*), of 2,570 women with early-stage breast cancer treated with mastectomy, 94 pts had a +margin. About half (41 pts) were treated with postmastectomy RT (PMRT). B/c of the small numbers, there was a trend to improvement with PMRT in pts **≤50 yrs, T2 tumor, grade III, and LVI.** In pts without these features, there was no LR without PMRT.

What is EIC?

EIC (extensive intraductal component) is defined as **DCIS both admixed and adjacent to invasive Dz, and comprising >25% of the total tumor mass.** DCIS with focal microinvasive Dz also fits this category.

Does EIC have prognostic significance in the LR risk of pts treated with BCT?

Yes, but it is largely dependent on SM status. From studies mainly out of JCRT, EIC is only prognostic for LF if the margin status is considered. If there is a close or +margin, EIC is associated with a higher risk of recurrence. (*Gage I et al., Cancer 1996*)

What data suggest that results of BCT can be further improved with the use of tamoxifen?

NSABP B21 (*Fisher B et al., JCO 2002*): 1,009 pts with ≤1-cm tumors s/p lumpectomy randomized to 3 arms: (a) tamoxifen alone (10 mg bid × 5 yrs), (b) RT alone (50 Gy), and (c) RT + tamoxifen. After 8-yr follow-up, the IBTR was 16.5% with tamoxifen alone vs. 9.3% with RT alone vs. 2.8% with RT + tamoxifen. There was no difference in OS. No benefit was seen in ER– tumors. Contralat breast tumor recurrence was 0.9%, 4.2%, and 3.0% in the 3 arms, respectively.

Are there pt subgroups with a low risk of LR who can be treated with BCS and systemic therapy alone without RT?

Yes. Recent trials suggest that pts with advanced age (≥60–70 yrs) and ER+ T1N0 tumors have an acceptably low rate of LR with surgery and endocrine Tx, although LR risk is further reduced by RT. The data suggest that the risk is very low only for **pts >70 yo** and possibly in those with **very small tumors (<1 cm)**, so a discussion can be made about withholding RT if the pt is being treated with tamoxifen. The 2 most important trials are the Toronto and CALGB 9343/ Intergroup trials:

> **Princess Margaret Hospital/Canadian trial** (*Fyles AW et al., NEJM 2004*): 769 women ≥50 yo (median age 68 yrs) with T1 or T2 (≤5 cm) – nodes (in women age ≥65 yrs, either clinical or pathologic evaluation was sufficient and SLN Bx was not routinely done) underwent lumpectomy to –margins and were randomized to (a) tamoxifen alone (20 mg/day × 5 yrs) vs. (b) tamoxifen + RT (40 Gy in 16 fx with a boost of 12.5 Gy in 5 fx). After 8-yrs follow-up, RT reduced LR from 17.6% to 3.5%. But for tumors ≤1 cm, the risk of relapse was 2.6% vs. 0% for the RT group ($p = 0.02$). In those ≥60 yo with ≤1-cm tumor, the risk was no different between the 2 arms (1.2% vs. 0%), but this was unplanned analysis with a short follow-up.

CALGB 9343/Intergroup trial (*Hughes KS et al., NEJM 2004; updated JCO 2013*): 636 women ≥70 yo with T1, clinically N0, ER+ tumors were randomized to tamoxifen vs. tamoxifen + RT after lumpectomy with –margins. Axillary dissection was allowed but not encouraged. RT was 45 Gy to the whole breast with a boost of 14 Gy. At a median of 12.6 yrs follow-up, the 10-yr LF rate in the tamoxifen alone arm was 10% vs. 2% in tamoxifen + RT. There was no difference in time to mastectomy, DM, breast cancer survival, or OS.

Can RT be used in the Tx of axillary nodes in place of surgery if axillary nodal dissection is not performed?

Possibly. Previous era trials in clinically node– pts (esp *NSABP B04* and *Institut Curie*) have demonstrated equivalent LC, DM, and OS with nodal RT vs. axillary dissection. In the modern era, the AMAROS (After Mapping of the Axilla: Radiation or Surgery) trial randomized SLN+ pts to completion ALND or nodal RT; 5-yr results showed no significant difference in LRR, DM, or OS and overall better arm function in the RT arm (data not yet published).

Are there data supporting WBI + regional nodal irradiation (RNI) for early-stage breast cancer?

Yes, although the data are not yet published in manuscript form. NCIC-CTG MA.20 is a randomized trial that enrolled 1,832 N+, T3N0, or high risk T2N0 pts treated with BCS + axillary surgical evaluation, adj chemo in >90%, +/– endocrine Tx. Randomized to WBI (50 Gy/25 fx +/– boost) or WBI + RNI (45 Gy/25 fx) to axillary apex, internal mammary chain and supraclavicular. 85% had 1–3 +LN. WBI + RNI had improved 5-year locoregional DFS (96.8% vs. 94.5%), distant DFS (92.4% vs. 87%), and a trend toward OS (92.3% vs. 90.7%). (*Whelan T, JCO 29: 2011, suppl; abstr LBA1003*)

How should chemo be sequenced with radiotherapy after BCS?

JCRT sequencing trial ("Upfront-Outback" trial) (*Bellon J et al., JCO 2005*): per the initial report (*Recht A et al., NEJM 1996*), the 5-yr crude rate of distant recurrence was better in the chemo 1st arm (20% vs. 32%). However, in the 11-yr follow-up update, there was no difference in DFS, LR, DM, or OS. For those with a –margin, the crude LR rate was 6% in the chemo 1st arm vs. 13% in the RT 1st arm. However, the study was not powered to show any differences. Thus, either sequence is acceptable. However, convention is to give chemo 1st.

What U.S. trial investigated the role of accelerated partial breast irradiation (APBI)?

NSABP B39/RTOG 0413, which randomized women with stage 0, 1, or 2 breast cancer with tumors ≤3 cm and ≤3 +LN to whole breast RT vs. APBI by any of 3 methods (interstitial, intracavitary, or EBRT).

What is the dose and duration of Tx for APBI?

34 Gy in 3.4 Gy bid fx for interstitial and intracavitary treatments and 38.5 Gy in 3.85 Gy bid fx for EBRT. All APBI is given over 5 days. The volume treated is the surgical cavity plus a 1-cm margin for brachytherapy and a 2–2.5 cm for EBRT.

Who can be offered PBI off trial?

ASTRO has published guidelines on who may be considered for PBI off trial. (*Smith BD et al., IJROBP 2009*) "Suitable" pts are >60 yo, ER+, IDC ≤2 cm (no DCIS or invasive lobular carcinoma), N0, unicentric, ≥2-mm margin, no LVSI, no EIC, and *BRCA1/ BRCA2*–. The ABS updated guidelines (*Shah C et al., Brachytherapy 2013*) state "acceptable" pts are **≥50 yo, ≤3-cm tumor,** invasive subtypes **and DCIS, either ER+ or ER–,** no LVSI, N0.

Is there good evidence to support the use of IMRT for WBI for early-stage breast cancer?

Emerging data seem to indicate that homogeneous dose distribution of IMRT benefits pts in terms of acute effects and late-term cosmesis.
Canadian study (*Pignol JP et al., JCO 2008*) demonstrated in 358 pts that IMRT reduced the occurrence of moist desquamation compared with standard wedge technique (31.2% vs. 47.8%, $p = 0.002$). MVA shows breast IMRT and smaller breast size were associated with decreased risk of moist desquamation.
British study (*Mukesh MB et al., JCO 2013*) showed in 1,145 pts with 5-yr follow-up that overall cosmesis was improved with IMRT compared with standard techniques (OR 0.68, $p = 0.027$) as well as skin telangiectasia (OR 0.58, $p = 0.021$). This benefit was maintained on multivariable analysis.

Are there subsets of women who undergo mastectomy for early-stage breast cancers (T1-2N0) who may benefit from PMRT?

Only in limited circumstances. NCCN 2014 guidelines recommend consideration of RT for node– T1-T2 close or positive margins. Retrospective data suggest that some margin– high-risk pts (LVSI, high grade, T2 tumors, young age) have an excess risk of LRR after mastectomy. However, PMRT in node– pts does not improve survival per EBCTCG 2005 meta-analysis data, and at this time PMRT for high risk T1-2N0 in the absence of close or +margins is counter to standard of care.

How should a Dx of breast cancer be managed in a pregnant woman?	**Management depends on the stage of pregnancy.** Timing of surgery depends on need for chemo and relative risks to fetus and mother. Chemo can be used to delay surgery until after delivery. Nontaxane chemo (most commonly, FAC) can be used in the 2nd and 3rd trimesters of pregnancy; chemo should be discontinued 3 wks before expected delivery to reduce infection and bleeding risks. RT and endocrine therapy must be deferred until postpartum.

▶ **FOLLOW-UP/TOXICITY**

See Chapter 45 for follow-up and toxicity questions.

45 Locally Advanced Breast Cancer

Updated by Jingya Wang

▶ **BACKGROUND**

What is locally advanced breast cancer (LABC)?	**Typically, the term refers to stage III Dz** (T3N1, N2-3, or T4). However, stage IIB pts with T3N0 Dz may be included. Inflammatory breast cancer (IBC) is included, but met Dz is not. LABC can be separated into those cancers that are operable and those that are not.
What are the epidemiologic trends and incidence of LABC?	The incidence of **T3-4 Dz decreased by 27% from 1980–1987** (coincident with the institution of mammography). Analysis of the SEER database from 1992–1999 indicated that **LABC (stage III other than IBC) and IBC made up 4.6% and 1.3% of all female breast carcinomas, respectively.**
What are the diagnostic criteria for IBC?	The AJCC uses the following clinical diagnostic criteria to identify IBC: (a) diffuse erythema, (b) edema (peau d'orange), (c) erythema/edema of less than one-third skin overlying breast, (d) rapid clinical onset (≤3 mos). Tissue Dx is also required to demonstrate invasive carcinoma of breast parenchyma or dermal lymphatics.

What is the pathognomonic feature that is more characteristic of IBC than other forms of LABC?	Presence of tumor emboli (also known as dermal lymphatic invasion [DLI]) in the dermis of the skin overlying the breast; however, DLI is not necessary for the Dx of IBC.
What is the prevalence of IBC?	**1%–4%** of breast cancer cases are IBC. 70% present with regional Dz and 25% with distant Dz.
What are the histologic subtypes of LABC?	The histologic subtypes are the **same for LABC as for earlier-stage Dz.** Infiltrating ductal carcinoma is still the most common, but favorable histologies, such as tubular, medullary, and mucinous, are less frequently represented.
Are there genetic/ molecular factors associated with LABC?	**No.** There are no molecular markers that define LABC. However, tumors with *HER2*/Neu positivity, *BRCA1* mutation, and triple-negative status (estrogen receptor [ER]–, progesterone receptor [PR]–, *HER2*–) are associated with aggressive phenotypes. A genomic profile of basal and *HER2* subtypes is associated with a poor prognosis as well. The use of trastuzumab in *HER2*+ tumors has improved outcomes, though.

► **WORKUP/STAGING**

What is the workup for locally advanced invasive breast cancer?	Invasive breast cancer workup: H&P, CBC, liver profile, ER/PR/*HER2* status; bilat diagnostic mammogram; imaging with US, CT, PET, bone scan, MRI optional per NCCN (2014)
What are the 5 regional LN stations in breast cancer?	Regional LN stations in breast cancer: **Level I axillary:** nodes inf/lat to pectoralis minor **Level II axillary:** nodes deep to pectoralis minor **Level III/infraclavicular:** nodes sup/medial to pectoralis minor **Supraclavicular nodes** **Internal mammary (IM) nodes** Rotter's nodes are located in the interpectoral space and are classified as level II axillary nodes.

► **TREATMENT/PROGNOSIS**

What are the most important factors that predict for LRR?	**Increasing number of LNs with Dz and breast tumor size** are the most important factors that predict for LRR.

What are the basic principles of treating LABC?

Inoperable LABC: neoadj chemo is used to shrink the tumor and potentially convert it to be operable.

Operable LABC: Neoadj or adj chemo are used. Modified radical mastectomy (including levels I–II axillary LNs) is the definitive locoregional Tx. Postmastectomy radiation therapy (PMRT) is indicated in all initial stage III Dz. Hormonal therapy and trastuzumab are incorporated as appropriate per receptor status of Dz.

What is a Halsted radical mastectomy?

Halsted radical mastectomy includes **resection of all breast parenchyma with overlying skin and major and minor pectoral muscles en bloc with axillary LNs.**

What is spared with a modified radical mastectomy?

Modified radical mastectomy spares the **pectoralis muscles.**

What is spared with a total or simple mastectomy?

In a total or simple mastectomy, only the breast tissue is removed with overlying skin. **Axillary LNs are not dissected.**

What is considered an "adequate" axillary LND for purposes of staging and clearance?

Oncologic resection of levels I–II is considered standard and adequate. The LNs and axillary fat pad need to be removed en bloc. An axillary LND is considered full if >10 LNs are removed. If suspicious nodes are palpable on intraoperative evaluation of level III, then level III dissection should be performed.

Which major trial demonstrated that not all pts with sentinel LN (SLN) Bx+ Dz need completion axillary LND?

The **American College of Surgeons Oncology Group (ACOSOG) Z11** (*Guiliano AE et al., Ann Surg 2010*) enrolled 856 pts with cN0 T1-2 breast cancer who underwent upfront breast-conserving surgery and SLN Bx. Pts with 1–2+ SLN were randomized to ALND + supine tangent RT vs. RT alone. There was no difference in breast/axillary recurrence.

Do clinically node+ pts always need axillary LND?

Yes—always! Whether the pt receives upfront surgery or neoadj chemo, a full axillary LND is always needed for clinically node+ Dz.

What is standard systemic chemo?

Standard chemo at present includes an **anthracycline- and taxane-based regimen** (e.g., doxorubicin/ cyclophosphamide [AC] and paclitaxel).

Does adding paclitaxel to standard AC chemo improve the outcomes of pts with breast cancer?

Yes. Adding paclitaxel improves response rates, DFS, and OS.

> **NSABP 27** randomized operable pts to preop AC, preop AC + taxol, or preop AC + postop taxol. Here, the addition of taxol did not improve survival outcomes but did improve pCR in the preop group (26% vs. 13%). (*Rastogi P et al., JCO 2008*)

> The **CALGB 9344** study randomized 3,121 operable pts with LN+ Dz and found that adding taxol q3wks × 4 to AC × 4 improved DFS and OS. (*Henderson IC et al., JCO 2003*) In a retrospective study of 1,500 pts on **CALGB 9344**, the benefit of taxol appeared to be in *HER2*+ tumors and not *HER2*–/ER+ tumors. (*Hayes DF et al., NEJM 2007*)

> **ECOG E1199** randomized 4,950 stages II–IIIA breast cancer pts to AC q3wks × 4 → taxol q3wks × 4, AC q3wks × 4 → taxol × 12 weekly, AC q3wks × 4 → Taxotere q3wks × 4, and AC q3wks × 4 → Taxotere × 12 weekly. The weekly taxol arm had improved DFS (HR 1.27) and OS (HR 1.32). The effect was significant in all pts, including those with ER+/*HER2*– tumors. (*Sparano JA et al., NEJM 2008*)

Which meta-analysis showed the benefit of anthracyclines?

The EBCTG/Oxford Overview met-analysis of 18,000 women showed a benefit of anthracyclines over cyclophosphamide/methotrexate/fluorouracil (CMF) (improved DFS and OS), although CMF > no chemo.

What is meant by "dose-dense" chemo?

Dose-dense chemo is **administered q2wks** as opposed to q3wks.

Has dose-dense chemo been demonstrated to be superior in a prospective randomized trial?

Yes. Intergroup trial C9741 randomized 2,005 node+ pts to AC × 4 > taxol × 4 given q3wks vs. q2wks. 4-yr DFS improved from 75% to 82% with the q2wk schedule. The risk ratio for OS was 0.69 in favor of the q2wk schedule. Median follow-up was 36 mos. Severe neutropenia was also less frequent with the dose-dense schedule.

What is the rationale for the use of neoadj chemo for LABC?

Neoadj chemo may convert pts with unresectable LABC to resectability. It may also be used to shrink large breast tumors requiring mastectomy in resectable pts to be managed with breast conservation surgery (BCS). Neoadj trials have the advantage of providing pathologic assessment of chemo response at the time of surgery. If the tumor is not responsive to 1 chemo regimen and progresses clinically, a different chemo regimen can be used.

Which pts have inoperable Dz and definitely need neoadj chemo?

Women with fixed axillary LN (stage N2a), major skin involvement (stage T4b-4d), +/− chest wall (CW) involvement.

What major study determined whether neoadj chemo improves survival compared to adj chemo in LABC?

NSABP B18 was designed to assess whether preop AC resulted in improved DFS and OS compared with postop AC. Secondary aims were to assess response to preop AC and correlate with survival and LR outcomes. Rates of BCS were also assessed. All women were deemed operable at enrollment, and the majority had T2 or smaller primary and clinically node– Dz. At the most recent follow-up (16 yrs) (*Rastogi P et al., JCO 2008*), there has been no significant difference in OS or DFS between the women treated with neoadj vs. adj chemo. There is a trend, however, for women <50 yo for improved DFS and OS when treated preoperatively ($p = 0.09$ and 0.06, respectively). There was a 27% conversion rate from mastectomy to BCS.

What procedures should be done prior to starting neoadj chemo for LABC?

Core Bx and clip localization of the breast tumor (in case the pt has a reaction to chemo). Perform SLN Bx if T3cN0 (but not for T4cN0); if clinically node+, consider FNA to confirm LN involvement.

In NSABP 18 and 27, did pCR at the time of surgery correlate with good OS and DFS outcomes?

Yes. In both **NSABP 18** and **NSABP 27,** pCR at the time of surgery correlated with improved OS and DFS compared with non-pCR pts.

What other seminal neoadj chemo trials addressed neoadj vs. adj chemo and its role regarding BCS?

EORTC 10902 randomized 698 pts with early breast cancer to preop vs. postop chemo (5-FU/epirubicin/cyclophosphamide × 4). Endpoints were BCS, DFS, OS, and tumor response. At 10-yr follow-up, there was no difference in OS or LRR. Neoadj chemo was associated with an improved rate of BCS. (*Van der Hage JA et al., JCO 2001*)

In EORTC 10902, was there a difference in the # of BCS between arms? Was there a difference in outcomes between planned breast-conserved pts and breast-converted pts?

BCS increased from 22%–35% in the preop chemo arm. Although the initial follow-up of **EORTC 10902** indicated that converted breast-conserved pts did worse in terms of OS compared with planned pts—an indication that prechemo staging remains relevant. However, the most recent 10-yr follow-up data indicate that there is no difference in survival outcomes between these 2 groups. (*Van der Hage JA et al., JCO 2001*)

PMRT was the standard of care for many decades. Why did it fall out of favor in the 1980s?

Historically, PMRT was typically offered b/c pts presented at later stages and no chemo was given. **Historical series, while uniformly demonstrating improved LC, did not demonstrate survival benefit.** Meta-analysis by *Cuzick et al.* (9 trials) demonstrated no OS survival benefit with PMRT at 10 yrs. (*Cancer Treat Rep 1987*)

An update by *Cuzick* demonstrated that PMRT increased cardiac mortality and slightly decreased breast cancer mortality. (*JCO 1994*)

What are some criticisms of older PMRT data and meta-analysis?

Criticisms of older PMRT data include the **significant heterogeneity of surgical and RT techniques, old RT techniques with associated cardiac and pulmonary toxicity, and lack of systemic therapy,** implying that clinically undetectable systemic Dz was not well controlled.

What 3 randomized prospective trials are considered to represent the "modern" PMRT experience?

The **Premenopausal Danish Trial (DBCG 82b)** (*Overgaard M et al., NEJM 1997*), the **Postmenopausal Danish Trial (DBCG 82c)** (*Overgaard M et al., Lancet 1999*), and the **British Columbia PMRT Trial** (*Ragaz J et al., JNCI 2005*) represent the "modern" PMRT experience.

What were the design and study outcomes of Premenopausal Danish Trial DBCG 82b?

In **Premenopausal Danish Trial DBCG 82b,** 1,708 women were randomized to mastectomy and adj CMF + chemo (8 cycles) or − RT (9 cycles). Inclusion criteria were +axillary LN, tumor >5 cm, or involvement of skin or pectoral fascia. 10-yr OS was 54% (+ PMRT) and 45% (− PMRT, p <0.001). Crude cumulative LRR was 32% − PMRT and 9% + PMRT. The survival benefit was seen for all pts (N0-3).

What are some criticisms of DBCG 82b trial?

Criticisms of the **DBCG 82b** trial include the inadequate surgical Tx of axilla resulting in a median of 7 nodes removed, an excess of LF occurring in the axilla (44% in the CMF arm), and the use of now-outdated CMF chemo.

What were the design and trial outcomes of Postmenopausal Danish Trial 82c?

In **Postmenopausal Danish Trial 82c,** 1,375 postmenopausal women <70 yo were randomized to postmastectomy tamoxifen × 1 yr vs. tamoxifen + PMRT. Inclusion criteria, surgical characteristics, and RT were as for the Premenopausal Danish Trial 82b. PMRT significantly improved LR (− PMRT 35% vs. + PMRT 8%), DFS (− PMRT 24% vs. + PMRT 36%), and OS (− PMRT 34% vs. + PMRT 45%) at 10-yr follow-up (all significant).

What are some criticisms of Postmenopausal Danish Trial 82c?

In **Postmenopausal Danish Trial 82c,** as in the Premenopausal Danish Trial 82b, inadequate surgical Tx of the axilla resulted in a median of only 7 axillary LNs removed at surgery. A suboptimal duration of tamoxifen was also employed (1 yr vs. the typical 5 yrs).

What was the surgery performed in the Danish 82b and 82c trials?

Pts were surgically managed with total mastectomy + axillary LN sampling (aimed at removing at least 5 LNs, full dissection was not required). A median of 7 nodes were removed. 15% had only 0–3 LNs removed, and 75% had <9 LNs removed. This is significantly less than most centers in the U.S., where >10 LNs represent adequate dissection.

How was the RT given in the Danish 82b and 82c trials?

For 82b, PMRT was given after cycle 1 of CMF and 3–5 wks postop. For 82c, PMRT was given 2–4 wks postop. The RT dose was 48–50 Gy given in 22–25 fx to the CW with ant photon fields to cover supraclavicular, infraclavicular, and axillary nodes and an ant electron field to cover the IM nodes and CW. Posterior axillary boost (PAB) was used for pts with a large AP diameter.

What was the design of the British Columbia Trial?

In the British Columbia Trial, 318 premenopausal, high-risk pts with positive axillary LNs were randomized to CMF chemo × 6–12 mos vs. CMF + RT. Surgery involved total mastectomy + axillary LND (median removal of 11 LNs). RT used Co-60 to 37.5 Gy in 16 fx. A 5-field technique was employed, including an en face photon field to cover bilat IM nodes.

What are the relevant outcomes of the British Columbia Trial?

In the British Columbia Trial, at 20-yr follow-up, adj RT improved LRR before DM (13% vs. 39%), DFS (48% vs. 31%), and OS (47% vs. 37%) (all significant). The benefit was extended to those with 1–3 LN+ Dz as well as those with >4 LN+ Dz.

What are some criticisms of the British Columbia Trial?

In the British Columbia Trial, LRF was high compared with many current series, CMF chemo was employed, and the RT fields included en face photons for IM nodal coverage (though no excessive cardiac deaths were observed).

What was demonstrated by the most recent Early Breast Cancer Trialists' Collaborative Group (EBCTCG) RT meta-analysis?

In the most recent EBCTCG meta-analysis (*EBCTCG collaborators, Lancet 2005*), 78 randomized trials including 42,000 women were included. After BCS, adj RT reduced 5-yr LR from 26% to 7% and increased 15-yr breast cancer mortality from 30.5% to 35.9%. After mastectomy with axillary clearance in node+ pts, PMRT reduced 5-yr LR from 23% to 5% and improved 15-yr breast cancer mortality from 54.7% to 60.1% (both significant); 5.4% in the entire cohort. In pts with node– Dz who had mastectomy with axillary clearance, PMRT reduced 5-yr LR from 6% to 2% ($p = 0.0002$) but caused a 3.6% increase in the 15-yr breast cancer mortality rate. 5-yr tamoxifen use reduced the LR rate by about one-half in pts with ER+ Dz. In all pts, chemo reduced the LR rate by one-third. RT was associated with excess contralat breast cancer, lung cancer, and cardiac mortality. Many "older" trials were included in this analysis.

Similar conclusions were also supported by two other meta-analyses. (*Whelan TJ et al., JCO 2000; Gebski V et al., JNCI 2006*)

Have there been any prospective randomized trials evaluating PMRT in pts treated with neoadj chemo?

No. There have been no prospective randomized trials evaluating PMRT in pts treated with neoadj chemo.

What was demonstrated in the retrospective series from MDACC regarding PMRT in pts treated with neoadj chemo?

Huang E. et al. analyzed the outcomes of 542 pts who had been enrolled in prospective clinical trials and treated with neoadj chemo, mastectomy, and RT. These pts were compared with 134 pts enrolled in the same trials who rcvd no adj RT. Clinical stage, margin status, and hormone receptor status did not favor the adj RT group. CSS was improved with adj RT in pts with clinical stage IIIB or supraclavicular LN+ Dz, clinical T4 tumors, and pathologically ≥4 +nodes. LRR was improved even for those pts with clinical stage III or supraclavicular LN+ Dz who achieved a pCR on neoadj chemo. (*JCO 2004*)

What is the local recurrence rate without radiation for stage III pts who achieve a pCR to neoadj chemo?

33.3%. Retrospective data from MDACC (*McGuire S et al., IJROBP 2007*) show that the 10-yr LRR rate for pts with stage III Dz was significantly improved with RT (7.3% ± 3.5% with vs. 33.3% ± 15.7% without; $p = 0.040$). Within this cohort, use of RT was also associated with improved DFS and OS.

What are the present NCCN guidelines for PMRT?

Per NCCN 2014 guidelines, PMRT is a category 1 recommendation **for pts with ≥4 +LNs. PMRT should be "strongly considered" for 1–3 +LNs.**

What are some arguments for providing PMRT to pts with 1–3 positive axillary LNs?

An argument for treating pts with 1–3 LN Dz with PMRT is that all 3 modern randomized trials (**Danish 82b, Danish 82c, and British Columbia**) showed significant OS benefit with PMRT. This was true in subgroup analysis of this population and even when analysis was restricted to pts who had at least 8 axillary LNs removed in Danish trials. (*Overgaard M et al., Radiother Oncol 2007*)

In EBCTCG meta-analysis, pts with 1–3 LN Dz experienced proportionally similar LR benefit with PMRT as pts with ≥4 +LNs and absolutely similar OS benefit.

Do the LF rates in pts with N1 Dz (1–3 LN+) in the Danish and British Columbia PMRT trials represent the typical experience in this subset of pts in U.S.?

No. The cumulative 10-yr LRR +/– DM for pts with 1–3 LN Dz on retrospective review of pts in prospective trials conducted by the NSABP, the ECOG, and MDACC was 4%–13%. (*Recht A et al., JCO 1999; Katz A et al., JCO 2000; Taghian AG et al., JCO 2004*)

For pts who undergo mastectomy with 1–3 +LNs, what other clinicopathologic factors should be considered when recommending PMRT?

Retrospective studies from the IBCSG, NSABP, and MDACC have suggested that factors such as **+LVI, high grade, younger age, ≤10 LN examined, ≥20% LN+, larger tumor size (T2 or ≥4 cm), and close margins** produce 10-yr LRR >15%.

Under what circumstances should regional LN be treated along with the CW (comprehensive PMRT)?

Comprehensive PMRT (CW + LN) is recommended for most pts who have a LRR risk that warrants PMRT b/c the benefit of RT of regional LN outweighs in most cases the added toxicity. All stage III pts should receive comprehensive PMRT. Consider **CW RT alone** for pts with upfront mastectomy and T3N0. CW RT alone is appropriate for those with T1-2N0 who are being treated for +margin only.

Should the IM nodes be included in all PMRT fields?

This is **controversial.** Some radiation oncologists believe that b/c the IM nodes were treated in the 3 randomized PMRT trials, it should be the gold standard approach. However, others would argue not to include IM nodes routinely b/c 3 randomized trials examining the role of IM nodal dissection did not improve OS for these pts. (*Lacour J et al., Cancer 1976; Meir P et al., Cancer 1989; Veronesi U et al., Eur J Cancer 1999*)

A randomized trial (**EORTC 22922/10925**) testing the effects of IM nodal irradiation on LRC and survival has completed accrual with results pending. Another randomized trial (NCIC-CTG MA-20) showed improved DFS, primarily through reduced DM, with the addition of IM and SCV RT in BCS pts, most of whom had 1–3 +LNs (data not yet published).

NCCN 2014 guidelines state that IM nodal radiation should be given if IM lymph nodes are clinically or pathologically positive. Otherwise, the treatment of IM nodes is at the discretion of the treating physician.

Should pts with T3N0 breast cancer who have had a mastectomy without neoadj chemo be treated with PMRT?

This is **controversial.** Traditionally, pts with T3N0 without other risk factors have been treated with CW-only PMRT or comprehensive PMRT. However, 2 recent retrospective studies have demonstrated that the LF rates are low for T3N0 pts after mastectomy alone with adj chemo, questioning the role of PMRT. This is an evolving area of research, so pts with pT3N0 without other risk factors should be considered for PMRT with appropriate discussion of risk and benefits of RT.

Taghian AG et al. (*JCO 2006*): subset meta-analysis of 5 NSABP postmastectomy chemo trials, with 313 pts with ≥5-cm tumors (N0). The 10-yr isolated LRF was 7.1%, and LRF ± DM was 10%. Almost all LRRs were in the CW. However, the median size of the tumor was 5.5 cm, so the data may not be applicable for very large tumors.

Floyd SR et al. (*IJROBP 2006*): review of a multi-institutional database for ≥5-cm tumors (N0). Of 70 pts, the 5-yr LRF was 7.6%. LVI was a significant prognostic factor for LF.

How should stage II pts with LN+ breast cancer s/p neoadj chemo and modified radical mastectomy (MRM) be managed?

For pts who undergo MRM and achieve a pCR in both LN and breast, the LF rate is 0%–10% without radiation (NSABP B-18, MDACC data) and omission of PMRT can be considered. For pts who undergo MRM and achieve pCR in LN but have persistent Dz in the breast, the LF rate is 10%–13% without radiation (NSABP B-18, MDACC data). These pts can be considered for no radiation, CW radiation only, or CW + regional nodal radiation (RNI). For pts with persistently +LN s/p neoadj chemo, the LF rate is 15%–20% without radiation (NSABP B-18, MDACC data). These pts need comprehensive PMRT.

How should stage II pts with LN+ breast cancer s/p neoadj chemo and BCS be managed?

Pts with pCR in lymph node and breast will still need whole breast irradiation (WBI). For pts with pCR in LN but persistent Dz in the breast, consider RNI if the pt is young (<50 yo). For pts with persistently +LNs after preop chemo, give WBI + RNI.

Which study evaluated the addition of RNI to WBI following BCS?

NCIC-CTG **MA-20** examined 1,832 pts with high-risk node– Dz (T3cN0, T2cN0 w/ ER-/G3/or LVSI), or cN+ Dz treated with BCS and adj chemo +/– endocrine therapy. 85% of pts had 1–3 +nodes, and the majority had axillary LND. Pts were randomized to WBI + RNI vs. WBI alone. The 5-yr LC, 5-yr distant DFS, 5-yr DFS, and 5-yr OS with and without RNI were 96.8% vs. 94.5% ($p = 0.02$), 92.4% vs. 87% ($p = 0.002$), 89.7% vs. 84% ($p = 0.003$), and 92.3% vs. 90.7% ($p = 0.07$), respectively. (*Whelan T et al., ASCO 2011*)

How is IBC managed?

IBC is managed using **combined-modality therapy** with neoadj chemo, modified radical mastectomy, and comprehensive PMRT.

What are 2 acceptable PMRT schedules for IBC?

Conventional: 50 Gy comprehensive RT → 10–16 Gy CW boost.

MDACC: hyperfractionated RT: 1.5 Gy bid to 51 Gy comprehensive RT → 15 Gy boost in 10 fx bid to 66 Gy

In the MDACC retrospective analysis (*Bristol IJ et al., IJROBP 2008*), which IBC pts benefited from escalation of postmastectomy radiation dose from 60 Gy to 66 Gy?

Pts with (a) unknown/close/+ margins, (b) less than partial response to neoadj chemo, and (c) age <45 yrs.

What are the options for a pt with poor response and unresectable Dz after induction chemo for IBC?

Alternative chemo; if there is still no response, can consider preop RT (conventional or hyperfractionated) → consideration for surgery.

For pts who want breast reconstruction after mastectomy, when should the breast reconstruction be done relative to the rest of the adj Tx?

Per NCCN guidelines, if implant reconstruction is planned, breast reconstruction should be performed before RT, b/c successful reconstruction is less likely after RT. However, if autologous reconstruction is planned, this should be performed after RT, b/c cosmesis of the autologous tissue is harmed by RT. In pts with initial T4b-d Dz (i.e., skin involvement), all reconstruction should be delayed to 6–12 mos after RT, b/c skin-sparing mastectomy is contraindicated.

▶ **FOLLOW-UP/TOXICITY**

What is the typical recommended follow-up schedule for pts treated for invasive breast cancer?

IBC recommended follow-up after Tx:
1. Interval H&P q4–6 mos × 5 yrs, then annually
2. Bilat mammogram annually
3. Annual gyn exam for women with intact uterus on tamoxifen
4. Bone health assessment (bone mineral density scan) at baseline and periodically during course of use of AIs

For pts who have large breasts with large medial to lat separation (>22–24 cm), what techniques will improve dose homogeneity?

Photon energy >10 MV to keep max inhomogeneity <10% and field segmentation techniques (IMRT). Avoid medial wedges to reduce scatter to contralat breast in pts <45 yo. Prone treatment can help, but RNI not possible in this position. Breast immobilization with molds (i.e., Aquaplast) can decrease skin toxicity to inframammary fold in the supine position.

What are the acute and late toxicities of whole breast RT?

<u>Acute</u>: RT dermatitis, fatigue, hyperpigmentation, pneumonitis
<u>Late</u>: soft tissue fibrosis, breast size change, telangiectasias, lymphedema, pulmonary fibrosis, precocious cardiovascular Dz, 2nd malignancy

What randomized trials demonstrated the superiority of 3D-IMRT compared to 2D Tx approaches for minimizing cosmetic changes to the breast?

Royal Marsden (*Donovan E et al., Radiother Oncol 2007*) randomized 306 women to 2D-RT or 3D-IMRT. RT was 50 Gy → boost to 11.1 Gy with electrons. There was a significant cosmetic difference in the breast of 2D-RT (58%) vs. 3D-IMRT (40%) pts. Fewer pts in the IMRT group developed palpable induration. There were no differences in the QOL between the groups. A randomized trial (*Pignol JP et al., JCO 2008*) comparing breast IMRT with standard techniques showed IMRT to be superior with respect to moist desquamation (31% vs. 48%) and improved dose distribution.

Are there cosmetic and toxicity differences between 3D-CRT accelerated partial breast irradiation (APBI) (38.5 Gy in 10 fx bid) and WBI (42.5 Gy in 16 fx or 50 Gy in 25 fx +/− boost)?

Yes, APBI yields worse cosmetic results compared with WBI. Early interim results from RAPID, a randomized trial in 2,135 women of APBI vs. WBI (*Olivotto IA et al., JCO 2013*) demonstrated adverse cosmesis at 3 yrs as assessed by nurses (29% vs. 17%, $p <0.001$), by pts (26% vs. 18%, $p = 0.0022$), and by physicians reviewing digital photographs (35% vs. 17%, $p <0.001$). Late grade 1–2 toxicities (telangiectasia, breast induration/fibrosis, and fatty necrosis) were all significantly higher for APBI. Grade 3 toxicities were rare in both groups (1.4% vs. 0%, respectively).

What is the risk of 2ⁿᵈ malignancies in pts treated for early breast cancer with RT?

From the WECARE study (*Stovall M et al., IJROBP 2008*), women <40 yo receiving >1 Gy to the contralat breast had an RR of 3. However, this excessive risk was not seen in pts >40 yo. Sarcomas (mostly angiosarcomas) within the RT field were <1% (~10 cases in 10,000) within 10–30 yrs. (*Taghian A et al., IJROBP 1991; Yap J et al., IJROBP 2002; Kirova YM et al., Cancer 2005*)

What is the risk of lymphedema in pts treated for breast cancer?

The risk of lymphedema is ~5%) after SLN dissection, and 10%–25% after level I–II axillary dissection. Comprehensive nodal RT after axillary dissection further increases the risk to **15%–35%.** (Refer to a review by *Erickson VS et al., JNCI 2001*.)

What is the risk of brachial plexopathy for a pt treated for breast cancer?

Median time to developing brachial plexopathy is ~10–12 mos (range 1.5–77 mos). It is dependent on RT dose and use of chemo. According to JCRT data (*Pierce SM et al., IJROBP 1992*), if the dose is kept at <50 Gy, the risk is <1% without chemo and ~4.5% with chemo. If the dose is above 50 Gy, the risk is 5.6%.

What is the risk of cardiac toxicity, such as ischemic heart Dz after BCT for breast cancer?

According to a population-based case-control study (*Darby SC et al., NEJM 2013*), rates of ischemic heart Dz are proportional to mean heart dose and increase linearly 7.4% per 1 Gy mean heart dose. Risk begins 1–2 years after RT and continues >20 yrs. Mean heart dose should be limited, and other cardiac risk factors should be managed.

What is the risk of pulmonary toxicities, such as lung fibrosis and symptomatic pneumonitis, after BCT for breast cancer?

Pulmonary fibrosis occurs in everyone on imaging in the treated pleura, but clinical pneumonitis is rare (1%–3% after WBI, 3%–5% after comprehensive RT).

46 Esophageal Cancer

Updated by Sonny Batra

▶ **BACKGROUND**

What are the boundaries of the esophagus that divide it into cervical, upper thoracic, midthoracic, and lower thoracic regions?

The esophagus spans from the cricopharyngeus at the cricoid to the gastroesophageal (GE) junction. Relative to the incisors, the **cervical esophagus spans from 15–18 cm,** the **upper thoracic from 18–24 cm,** the **midthoracic from 24–32 cm,** and the **lower thoracic from 32–40 cm.**

Why is esophageal cancer more prone to locoregional spread than other GI cancers?

The esophagus has an adventitial layer but does not have a serosal layer, thus reducing the resistance against local spread of cancer.

What is the incidence and mortality of esophageal cancer in the U.S.?

There are ~18,000 cases diagnosed and ~15,000 deaths per year in the U.S. Males are more commonly affected than females (3:1).

Is there an association between esophageal cancer and HPV infection?

The single largest case-control studies by *Cao B et al.* showed a risk of HPV 2.7-fold greater in cases of esophageal squamous cell cancer (SCC) than in controls. (*Carcinogenesis 2005*)

What are the risk factors for developing esophageal cancer?

Esophageal SCC risk factors: smoking/alcohol tylosis, Plummer-Vinson syndrome, caustic injury to the esophagus, Hx of H&N cancer, and achalasia. HPV infection has been associated in ~20% cases in high-incidence areas (China, Africa, Japan) but none in low-incidence areas (Europe, U.S.).

Esophageal adenocarcinoma risk factors: obesity/ GERD, Barrett esophagus, lack of fruits/ vegetables, low socioeconomic status

What are some protective factors for developing esophageal cancers?

Protective factors for developing esophageal cancer include **fruits/vegetables and *Helicobacter pylori* infection** (possible atrophic gastritis).

How do pts with esophageal cancer typically present?

Dysphagia and weight loss (>90%), odynophagia, pain, cough, dyspnea, and hoarseness

What is the pattern of spread of tumors of the esophagus?

Tumors of the esophagus spread **locoregionally through the extensive submucosal lymphatic plexus or distantly through hematogenous routes.**

What histologies predominate based on the tumor location within the esophagus?

The proximal three-fourths of the esophagus (cervical to midthoracic) are mostly **SCCs** (~40%), whereas **adenocarcinoma** generally is found in the distal esophagus (~60%).

What are some other more uncommon histologies seen for tumors of the esophagus?

Adenocystic, mucoepidermoid, small cell, and sarcomatous (leiomyosarcoma) carcinomas (all typically 1% of cases). Extremely rare types are lymphoma, Kaposi sarcoma, and melanoma.

What are the patterns of failure (locoregional vs. distant) relative to the histology and tumor location of esophageal cancers?

The patterns of recurrence from surgical series suggest that there is **predominant LRF in cancers of the upper and midesophagus** (mostly squamous cell), whereas **distant recurrence is more common in lesions in the distal third of the esophagus** (mostly adenocarcinomas). (*Mariette C et al., Cancer 2003; Katayama A et al., J Am Coll Surg 2003*)

What are the common sites of DM seen for esophageal cancers?

Lung, liver, and bone are the most common sites of distant Dz.

What % of pts with esophageal cancers present with localized Dz vs. distant Dz?

The frequency of distant Dz at presentation depends on the location and size of the tumor. Dz at the middle and lower third of the esophagus tends to present with **localized Dz (25%–50%),** whereas upper thoracic Dz is less commonly localized **(10%–25%).** Tumors >5 cm also tend to have greater **metastatic rate (~75%)** than tumors <5 cm.

What is the most important factor that determines nodal mets and DM?

DOI is the most important factor dictating nodal and distant spread. (*Mariette C et al., Cancer 2003*)

What is the extent of submucosal spread of Dz seen for esophageal cancers, and does it differ by histology?

Gao XS et al. reported the following for SCC: proximal and distal spread 10.5 +/– 13.5 mm and 10.6 +/– 8.5 mm, respectively, with 94% of pts having all tumor contained within a 30-mm margin. For adenocarcinoma, spread of Dz to 10.3 +/– 7.2 mm proximally and 18.3 +/– 16.3 mm distally, with a margin of 50 mm required to encompass all tumor in 94% of cases. (*IJROBP 2007*)

▶ WORKUP/STAGING

What components of the Hx are important in assessing a pt with dysphagia?

Appropriate parts of the Hx in assessing dysphagia Sx include **onset, duration, solids vs. liquids, other Sx of retrosternal pain, bone pain, cough, hoarseness, Hx of smoking/alcohol, GERD, and Hx of prior H&N cancer.**

What should be included in the workup of pts with suspected esophageal cancers?

Suspected esophageal cancer workup: H&P, labs (LFTs, alk phos, Cr), esophagogastroduodenoscopy with Bx. If cancer, then EUS + FNA for nodal sampling for tumor and node staging, CXR, bronchoscopy (for upper/midthoracic lesions to r/o tracheoesophageal fistula), and PET/CT. Laparoscopic staging is done in some institutions, with reports of upstaging and sparing the morbidity of more aggressive Tx in 10%–15% of cases.

To what anatomic extent is esophageal cancer being defined?

Esophageal cancer is defined as **15 cm from the incisors to the GE junction and the proximal 5 cm of the stomach.** A stomach tumor arising ≤5 cm from the GE junction or above is considered esophageal cancer.

What is different about the AJCC 7th edition (2011) of the TNM staging for esophageal cancer?

The AJCC 7th edition **distinguishes the # of nodal mets, subclassifies T4 Dz, expands the Tis definition, and removes the M1a-b designation.**

Tis: high-grade dysplasia and CIS

T1a: involves lamina propria or muscularis mucosae

T1b: involves submucosa

T2: invades muscularis propria

T3: invades adventitia (*Note:* No serosal layer.)

T4a: pleural, pericardial, or diaphragm involvement

T4b: other organs (aorta, vertebral body, trachea)

Nx: regional nodes cannot be assessed

N0: no regional node mets

N1: 1–2 regional LN mets, including nodes previously labeled as M1a*

N2: 3–6 regional LN mets, including nodes previously labeled as M1a*

N3: ≥7 regional LN mets, including nodes previously labeled as M1a*

***M1a** (differ by site): upper thoracic includes cervical LN mets; midthoracic is not applicable; lower thoracic/GE junction includes celiac LN mets. (*Note:* M1a designation is no longer recognized in the 7th edition.)

M1: DM (retroperitoneal, para-aortic LN, lung, liver, bone, etc.)

What are the AJCC 7th edition (2011) stage groupings for esophageal cancer, and what new feature has been added?

Tumor grade (1–3) has been added to the TNM stage groupings, and separate stage groupings are given for SCC and adenocarcinoma:

> **Stage 0:** TisN0M0, G1
> **Stage IA:** T1N0M0, G1-2
> **Stage IB:** T1N0M0, G3; T2N0M0, G1-2
> **Stage IIA:** T2N0M0, G3
> **Stage IIB:** T3N0 or T1-2N1, any G
> **Stage IIIA:** T1-2N2M0, any G; T3N1M0, any G; T4aN0M0, any G
> **Stage IIIB:** T3N2M0, any G
> **Stage IIIC:** T4aN1-2M0, any G; T4b or N3, any G
> **Stage IV:** TXNXM1

Why does SCC have a separate stage grouping from adenocarcinoma in the AJCC 7th edition (2011) staging system?

Tumor location is accounted for in the stage grouping for SCC, with lower regions having a better prognosis compared with upper and middle regions. The only changes compared with adenocarcinoma is in IA, IB, IIA, and IIB stage groupings:

> **Stage IA:** T1N0M0G1, any location
> **Stage IB:** T1N0M0G2-3 any location; T2-3N0M0G1, lower location
> **Stage IIA:** T2-3N0M0G1, upper/middle location; T2-3N0M0G2-3, lower location
> **Stage IIB:** T2-3N0M0G2-3, upper location/middle location; T1-2N1M0 any G, any location

▶ TREATMENT/PROGNOSIS

How are pts with Barrett esophagus and high-grade dysplasia managed?

This is **controversial,** with Tx ranging from esophagectomy to local ablative procedures to active surveillance with acid-suppressive therapies.

What are the pros and cons of doing esophagectomy for pts with high-grade dysplasia?

Pros: prevents progression to invasive carcinoma, removal of unsuspected frank invasive Dz (up to 40% of resected specimens).

Cons: a large morbid procedure for a substantial # of pts with high-grade dysplasia alone, which by itself often does not develop into invasive cancer in the pt's lifetime. Local therapies or surveillance would allow identification of pts with early invasive lesions that are readily curable.

What are the guidelines used for surveillance of high-grade dysplasia of the esophagus?

Serial upper endoscopy at 3- to 6-mo intervals with multiple 4-quadrant Bx at 1- to 2-cm intervals. In a prospective clinical study (*Schnell TG et al., Gastroenterology 2001*), ~16% pts were subsequently identified with invasive cancer with a follow-up of 7.3 yrs. In this study, 11 of 12 pts were found to have early-stage adenocarcinoma, which was managed curatively.

Does the extent of high-grade dysplasia predict for the presence of occult adenocarcinoma?

No. Although ~40%–45% of esophagectomy specimens contain invasive cancers from pts referred for high-grade dysplasia, the extent of high-grade dysplasia in the esophagus does not predict for occult cancer. (*Dar MS et al., Gut 2003*)

What are some local ablative procedures for the management of early-stage esophageal cancers?

Photodynamic therapy, laser ablation, and argon plasma coagulation are some ablative procedures that should be done in a study b/c experience with these is limited.

What is endoscopic mucosal resection (EMR), and what are the criteria for the use of EMR for dysplasia or early-stage (Tis-T1) adenocarcinoma of the esophagus?

EMR involves **submucosal injection of fluid to lift and separate the lesion from the underlying muscular layer,** and resection is carried out by suction to trap the lesion in a cylinder. *Ell C et al.* (*Gastrointest Endosc 2007*) reported in 100 pts a 5-yr survival of 98%, with no deaths from esophageal cancers. Recurrent/metachronous Dz was subsequently detected in 11%, and all were managed with successful repeat EMR. In an earlier report (*Ell C et al., Gastrointest Endosc 2000*), the remission rate was 59% for a less favorable group using less strict criteria.
The criteria to use EMR were **lesions with no ulceration, T1N0, no vascular/lymphatic invasion, <2 cm, and well to moderately differentiated.**

What are the most important features that predict for poor outcomes in pts with T1 esophageal cancers treated with surgical resection alone?

T1b Dz, LVI, and tumor length predict poor outcomes in these pts. (*Cen P et al., Cancer 2008; Bolton WD et al., J Thorac Cardiovasc Surg 2009*)

What are the types of surgical procedures employed for the management of esophageal cancers?

Minimally invasive esophagectomy using laparoscopy, thoracoscopy, or a combination. Traditional surgical approaches include **radical esophagectomy, transhiatal, or transthoracic esophagectomies.**

How do transhiatal and transthoracic esophagectomy procedures compare in terms of dissection extent and location of the Dz?

In general: A transhiatal approach may be less morbid but will have less exposure for tumor clearance and thorough LND compared with a transthoracic approach. Anastomotic leak for the transhiatal approach is easier to manage than the transthoracic approach (cervical vs. intrathoracic leaks).

Transhiatal esophagectomy: Pros: good for distal tumors with possible en bloc resection, laparotomy and a cervical approach (no thoracotomy) with cervical anastomosis, less morbid with less pain, and avoids fatal intrathoracic anastomotic leak. Cons: poor visualization of upper/midthoracic tumors, LND limited to blunt dissection, more anastomotic leaks, and more recurrent laryngeal nerve palsy.

Transthoracic esophagectomy: Pros: Ivor-Lewis (right thoracotomy) is the most common and preferred route and best for exposure for all levels of the esophagus, whereas left thoracotomy provides access to only the distal esophagus. Ivor-Lewis (right thoracotomy and laparotomy) provides direct visualization and exposure with a better radial margin and a more thorough LND. Cons: intrathoracic leak that can lead to fatal mediastinitis. Generally considered to have higher morbidity and mortality than transhiatal.

Does the # of nodes removed from esophagectomy predict for better outcome?

Yes. Data suggest that the # of nodes removed is an independent predictor of survival. In 1 large study, the optimal # was 23. (*Peyre CG et al., Ann Surg 2008*)

Is there evidence to prove that either transhiatal or transthoracic esophagectomy would be superior for Dz control and outcome?

No. There are no data to date showing that 1 approach is superior to the other. Two large meta-analyses comparing transhiatal with transthoracic esophagectomy have shown equivalence. (*Rindani R et al., Aust N Z J Surg 1999; Hulscher JB et al., Ann Thorac Surg 2001*) In general, transthoracic approaches carry greater operative mortality and pulmonary complications, but transhiatal approaches have greater anastomotic leaks and stricture rates as well as recurrent laryngeal nerve injury. 5-yr OS rates are similar between the 2 approaches (20%–25%).

What is the 5-yr OS for pts managed with surgery alone for localized esophageal cancers?

5-yr OS is **20%–25%** for pts managed with surgery alone for localized Dz. This is higher for earlier-stage Dz (T1N0 ~77%) but lower for stage III Dz (~10%–15%).

Is there evidence to support the use of preop chemo (no RT) for Tx of resectable esophageal cancers?

This is **controversial.** Several phase II studies have demonstrated benefit, and 4 randomized studies have reported conflicting results on the benefit of preop chemo.

US Intergroup trial (*Kelsen DP et al., NEJM 1998*): 467 pts (53% adeno, 47% SCC) randomized to 3 × 5-FU/cisplatin preop and 2 × 5-FU/cisplatin postop or immediate surgical resection alone. There were no differences in resectability or survival (4-yr OS 26% vs. 23%, respectively; MS 16 mos vs. 15 mos, respectively). pCR was 2.5%. Pts with complete resection had a 5-yr DFS of 32% vs. 5% with R1-R2 resection.

MRC randomized trial of preop chemo (*MRC, Lancet 2002*): 802 pts (66% adeno, 31% SCC, 3% undifferentiated) randomized to (a) 2 × cisplatin/5-FU preop or (b) immediate surgery. There was a significant benefit of neoadj chemo. MS was 13.3 mos vs. 16.8 mos, respectively, and 2-yr OS was 34% vs. 43%, respectively. The complete resection rate was also improved by chemo (54% vs. 60%, respectively).

MRC Adjuvant Gastric Cancer Infusional Chemo (MAGIC) trial (*Cunningham D et al., Lancet 2008*): pts randomized with gastric, GE junction, and distal esophageal adenocarcinoma (26%) to (a) preop epirubicin/cisplatin/5-FU (ECF) × 3 and postop ECF × 3 or (b) surgery alone showed a survival benefit for chemo. 5-yr OS was 36% vs. 23%, respectively ($p = 0.009$).

German Esophageal Cancer Study Group trial (*Stahl M et al., JCO 2009*): randomized phase III in pts with T3-4NXM0 adenocarcinoma of the GE junction or gastric cardia. The study closed early due to poor accrual (126 of 354 intended). Randomization: (a) induction chemo → surgery or (b) induction chemo → preop CRT → surgery. Chemo was cisplatin/5-FU/leucovorin. RT was 30 Gy in 15 fx. pCR was better in the preop CRT group (15.6% vs. 2%) and in tumor-free LNs (64% vs. 38%). 3-yr OS trended better in the CRT group (47% vs. 28%, $p = 0.07$). Postop mortality was higher in the CRT group (10% vs. 3.8%, $p = 0.26$).

What is the randomized trial evidence to support preop CRT over surgery alone?

This had been controversial until the recent publication of the CROSS trial.

    Urba SG et al. (*JCO 2007*): 100 pts (75% adenocarcinoma, 25% SCC) randomized to cisplatin/vinblastine/5-FU + RT to 45 Gy bid vs. surgery alone. 3-yr OS was 30% vs. 16%, respectively ($p = 0.18$). DM was the same in both arms (60%).

Bosset JF et al. (*NEJM 1997,* EORTC): SCC only, stages I–II. Cisplatin was given 0–2 days prior to RT, and RT was a split course of 18.5 Gy (3.7 Gy × 5) given on days 1 and 22. There was higher postop mortality in the trimodality approach (12% vs. 4%). There was no improvement in DFS or OS.

Burmeister B et al. (*Lancet 2007,* TTROG): 256 pts (67% adenocarcinoma, 33% SCC) randomized to cisplatin + 5-FU with RT to 35 Gy/15 fx. Less intensive chemo (5-FU 800 mg/m^2 vs. 1,000 mg/m^2 in other studies) was used. There was no difference in OS, but there was a trend to improved survival in SCC.

CALGB 9781 (*Tepper J et al., JCO 2008*): 56 pts (75% adenocarcinoma, 25% SCC) randomized (closed due to poor accrual) to cisplatin + 5-FU with RT to 50.4 Gy. pCR rate was 40%. 5-yr OS was 39% vs. 16% ($p = 0.005$). MS was 48 mos vs. 22 mos.

CROSS (*van Hagen P et al., NEJM 2012*): 368 pts (75% adenocarcinoma, 23% SCC, 2% undifferentiated) were randomized to surgery alone or CRT followed by surgery. CRT arm was 41.4 Gy in 23 fx with concurrent carboplatin (AUC 2 mg/mL/min) and paclitaxel (50 mg/m^2) for 5 wks followed by surgery. MS was 49.4 mos with CRT vs. 24.0 mos. Nonhematologic side effects were comparable in the 2 groups.

In the CROSS trial, what % of pts had R0 resection in the CRT arm vs. surgery alone arm and what % had a pCR to CRT?

In the CROSS trial, 92% had an R0 resection in the CRT arm vs. 69% in the surgery alone arm. 29% (23% of adenocarcinoma and **49% of SCC**) had a pCR to CRT (typical CR average of randomized trials 25%–30%). (*van Hagen P et al., NEJM 2012*)

Is there a role for preop RT alone for esophageal cancers?

No. Studies demonstrate no benefit of preop RT alone.

Is there a role for postop RT alone for esophageal cancers?

Postop RT alone has failed to demonstrate a benefit in several randomized trials. Incomplete resection should receive definitive CRT or palliative chemo or RT alone. Completely resected stages II–III adenocarcinoma of the GE junction should receive postop CRT based on the Intergroup gastric trial. (*MacDonald JS et al., NEJM 2001*)

What are the data demonstrating efficacy of definitive CRT vs. RT alone?	**RTOG 85-01** (*Herskovic A et al., NEJM 1992; Cooper JS et al., JAMA 1999*): 130 pts (82% SCC, 18% adenocarcinoma) randomized to 64 Gy RT alone vs. 50 Gy RT + cis/5-FU × 2 during RT and 2 cycles after RT. There was SCC in 88% pts. 5-yr OS was 27% vs. 0% for RT alone. 10-yr OS was 20% for CRT. There was no difference between adenocarcinoma and SCC.
	RT technique used in this trial: initial RT field was the whole esophagus to 50 Gy (RT alone) or 30 Gy (CRT) → CD to 14 Gy (RT) or 20 Gy (CRT) to tumor + 5-cm sup/inf margin.
Is there a benefit of escalating the RT dose during CRT for esophageal cancer?	This is **controversial,** b/c **INT 0123** (*Minsky BD et al., JCO 2002*) is a phase III study that randomized pts to 50.4 Gy vs. 64.8 Gy with cisplatin + 5-FU × 2 → adj cisplatin/5-FU × 2. There was no difference in LC (44% vs. 48%). Excessive deaths in 64.8-Gy arm (11 vs. 2) were seen even before the 50.4-Gy dose (7 of 11 deaths). However, separate analysis excluding the early deaths still did not find a benefit to a higher dose.
Is there evidence to suggest that surgery can be omitted in operable pts with localized esophageal cancer?	**There are no strong data suggesting surgery can be omitted in pts with adenocarcinoma of the esophagus.** However, there are 2 randomized trials examining CRT + surgery vs. CRT alone in pts with SCC that demonstrated a LC benefit of adding surgery but not an OS benefit. This is possibly due to increased postop mortality in pts with SCC.
	Bedenne L et al. (*JCO 2007*): 444 pts enrolled, treated first with CRT (45 Gy or split course 15 Gy × 2); the 230 responding pts (88% SCC) were randomized to surgery or no surgery. LC was better with surgery (66% vs. 57%). There was no difference in survival (34% vs. 40%). The mortality rate was higher in the surgery group (9.3% vs. 0.8%).
	Stahl M et al. (*JCO 2005*): 172 pts with SCC randomized to induction chemo + 40 Gy/chemo + surgery vs. induction chemo + 65 Gy/chemo alone. PFS was better with surgery (64% vs. 41%). Survival was the same between arms, with a trend to better survival with surgery.
Could salvage therapies (surgery or RT) be performed after definitive CRT or surgery for esophageal cancer management?	**Yes.** Salvage surgery can be performed for select pts who recur after definitive CRT but with increased operative morbidity/mortality. (*Tachimori Y et al., J Thorac Cardiovasc Surg 2009*) Salvage RT can be performed for isolated LR after surgery alone, but the dose should be limited to 45 Gy with concurrent chemo because of gastric pull-through.

Can RT be performed in pts with tracheoesophageal fistula?

Yes. Although historically it is contraindicated because of fear that RT may worsen the fistula, available studies demonstrate that RT does not worsen the fistula and may have even caused healing and closure in 1 series. (*Muto M et al., Cancer 1999*)

How are cancers of the cervical esophagus managed in general?

Because of the difficult and morbid surgery (total laryngopharyngoesophagectomy), cancers of the cervical esophagus are managed **like a H&N primary with a nonsurgical approach and definitive CRT.** Case series from MDACC using IMRT + 5-FU/ cisplatin (*Wang SL et al., WJG 2006; Burmeister et al., AOHNS 2000*) show that a high dose toward 70 Gy (60–66 Gy as done for H&N cancers) offers good LC and response (LC 88% and 5-yr OS 55% from the *Burmeister et al.* series). However, late toxicity, such as esophageal stricture, is a problem.

Can definitive RT be used for early-stage (Tis, IA) esophageal cancers?

Yes, for SCC. With doses 60–72 Gy or 55–60 Gy + a brachytherapy boost, the LC and DFS is ~80% in pts with SCC. Tumors >5 cm should rcv CRT because of poorer LC (~50%–60%). (*Hishikawa Y et al., Radiother Oncol 1991*)

What are the radiotherapy doses and techniques for the management of esophageal cancer?

Preop CRT: 41.4–50.4 Gy for adenocarcinoma and SCC

Definitive CRT: 50.4–59.4 Gy for adenocarcinoma and SCC. Even higher doses may be appropriate for SCC of the cervical esophagus.

Field size (to block edge): 5 cm above and below GTV, 1.5–2.5 cm laterally. If escalated above 50 Gy, CD to 2 cm above and below GTV. Consider IMRT technique for cardiac sparing in the gastroesophageal junction region.

▶ TOXICITY

What are the esophageal stricture rates receiving RT alone?

Based on data from *Emami B et al.* (*IJROBP 1991*), a 5% stricture rate occurs when one-third of the esophagus gets 60 Gy, two-thirds get 58 Gy, and 55 Gy for entire esophagus.

What is the dose limitation to the heart?

Dose limitations to the heart are as follows: **whole heart to 30 Gy, two-thirds to 45 Gy, and one-third to 55 Gy.** Try to keep V40 <50% to minimize potential late toxicities.

What are the dose limits for the kidneys, liver, and spinal cord?

Kidneys: keep combined kidneys V18 <30%, or limit one third of 1 kidney to a full dose
Liver: V30 <50%
Spinal cord: no point dose >45 Gy

What types of toxicities are experienced during radiotherapy, and what measures should be taken to help minimize these toxicities?

<u>Acute</u>: esophagitis, skin irritation, fatigue, weight loss
<u>Late</u>: dysphagia, stricture, pneumonitis, laryngeal edema, cardiac injury, renal insufficiency, liver injury
Relief is obtained with **topical anesthesia, narcotics, H2 blockers, feeding tube, and limiting the dose to critical structures.**

Describe an appropriate follow-up schedule for pts after completion of Tx for esophageal cancer?

Follow-up for esophageal cancer after Tx: H&P every 4 mos for 1 yr, every 6 mos for 2 yrs, then annually; at each visit, basic labs such as CBC/chemistry panel +/– endoscopy as clinically indicated; and dilatation for stenosis and nutritional counseling as needed.

Pts with Tis or T1a esophageal cancer who undergo EMR or ablative procedures should have what type of follow-up schedule/procedures?

Tis/T1a esophageal cancer pts with EMR or ablative procedures follow-up: H&P + endoscopy every 3 mos for 1 yr, then annually.

47 Gastric Cancer

Updated by Boris Hristov

▶ BACKGROUND

What is the estimated incidence of gastric cancer in the U.S. and worldwide?

<u>U.S.</u>: 21,600 cases/yr (2013), with 10,990 deaths (7th leading)
<u>Worldwide</u>: ~989,600 new cases/yr; 2nd-leading cause of death (behind lung cancer)

Where are the high-incidence areas in the world?

The highest incidences are found in **East Asia (Japan and China) > South America > Eastern Europe.**

What are some acquired and genetic risk factors for developing gastric cancer?

<u>Acquired factors</u>: *Helicobacter pylori* infection, high intake of smoked and salted foods, nitrates, diet low in fruits/vegetables, smoking, RT exposure, obesity, Barrett esophagus/GERD, prior subtotal gastrectomy
<u>Genetic factors</u>: E-cadherin (*CDH-1* gene) mutation, type A blood group, pernicious anemia, HNPCC, Li-Fraumeni syndrome

How does tumor location relate to the underlying etiology of gastric adenocarcinoma?

Body and antral lesions are associated with *H. pylori* infection and chronic atrophic gastritis, whereas proximal gastric lesions (gastroesophageal [GE] junction, gastric cardia) are associated with obesity, GERD, and smoking.

Which has poorer prognosis: proximal or distal gastric cancer?

Stage for stage, **proximal** gastric cancer has a poorer prognosis.

What are the 2 histologic types of gastric adenocarcinoma? How do these 2 types differ in terms of etiology of the gastric cancer?

Intestinal and diffuse are the 2 histologic types of adenocarcinomas.

Intestinal type: differentiated cancers with a tendency to form glands, occur in the distal stomach, and arise from precursor lesions seen mostly in endemic areas and in older people, more commonly men, suggesting an environmental etiology.

Diffuse type: less differentiated (signet ring cells, mucin producing), have extensive submucosal/distant spread, and tend to be proximal. They do not arise from precancerous lesions, are more common in low-incidence areas, and are more common in women and younger people, suggesting a genetic etiology.

What is the Borrmann classification of gastric cancer?

The Borrmann classification is **based on the gross morphologic appearance.** It is divided into 5 types:

Type I: polypoid/fungating
Type II: ulcerating
Type III: ulcerating/infiltrative
Type IV: diffusely infiltrating (linitis plastica)
Type V: cannot be classified (most aggressive)

What is the Japanese Research Society (JRS) classification of nodal spread?

1st echelon: N1 (stations 1–6)—perigastric nodes (lesser and greater curvature) and periesophageal nodes (proximal gastric)

2nd echelon: N2 (stations 7–11)—celiac axis, common hepatic, splenic

More distant: N3—hepatoduodenal, peripancreatic, mesenteric root; N4—portocaval, PA nodes, middle colic

JRS N1–N4 are not the same as AJCC staging.

What are the patterns of spread for gastric cancer?

Local extension to adjacent organs, lymphatic mets, peritoneal spread, or hematogenous (liver, lung, bone). Liver/lung mets are more common for proximal/GE junction tumors.

What are the anatomic boundaries and organs for the stomach?	<u>Superior</u>: diaphragm, left hepatic lobe <u>Inferior</u>: transverse colon, mesocolon, greater omentum <u>Anterior</u>: abdominal wall <u>Posterior and lateral</u>: spleen, pancreas, left adrenal, left kidney, splenic flexure of colon
What is the most important prognostic factor for gastric cancer?	**TNM stage** is the most important factor, with the histologic grade and Borrmann types not being independently prognostic apart from tumor stage. However, in general, Borrmann types I and II are more favorable compared with type IV.
Is all nodal involvement equally prognostic for gastric cancer?	**No.** The number and location of nodes are important. Minimal LN involvement adjacent to the primary lesion is more favorable.

▶ **WORKUP/STAGING**

How do pts with gastric cancer generally present?	Anorexia, abdominal discomfort, weight loss, fatigue, n/v, melena, and weakness from anemia
What aspects of the physical exam are relevant for evaluating a pt for a possible gastric malignancy?	General physical with focus on abdominal mass (local extension), liver mets, ovarian mets (Krukenberg tumor), distant LN mets (Virchow: left supraclavicular; Irish: left axillary; Sister Mary Joseph: umbilical), ascites, Blumer shelf (rectal peritoneal involvement)
What is important in the workup for gastric cancer?	Gastric cancer workup: H&P (onset, duration, Hx of risk factors), CBC, CMP, esophagogastroduodenoscopy + Bx, EUS +/– FNA of regional LN mets, CT C/A/P, and diagnostic laparoscopy to r/o peritoneal seeding
How many layers are seen on EUS when imaging the GI tract?	**5 layers are seen on EUS:** layers 1, 3, and 5 are hyperechoic (bright), and layers 2 and 4 are hypoechoic (dark). Layer 1 is superficial mucosa, layer 2 is deep mucosa, layer 3 is submucosa, layer 4 is muscularis propria, and layer 5 is subserosa fat and serosa.
What is the rate of upstaging to stage IV using diagnostic laparoscopy?	**35%–40%** of pts are found to have mets using diagnostic laparoscopy.
Why is PET imaging not routinely used in staging gastric cancer?	Only around two thirds of primary tumors are FDG avid (*Shah et al., Proc ASCO 2007*), with GLUT-1 transporter rarely present on the common subtypes of gastric cancer (signet ring and mucinous). Therefore, there are too many false negatives.

What is the AJCC 7th edition (2011) T-staging classification for gastric cancer?

Tis: confined to mucosa without invasion to lamina propria
T1a: invades lamina propria or muscularis mucosae
T1b: invades submucosa
T2: invades muscularis propria
T3*: penetrates subserosa without invasion of visceral peritoneum (serosa)
T4a*: invades serosa
T4b: invades adjacent structures

*Tumor is classified as T3 if it penetrates through the muscularis propria with extension into the gastrocolic or gastrohepatic ligaments or into the greater or lesser omentum without perforation of the visceral peritoneum covering these structures. Tumor is classified as T4 if it penetrates the visceral peritoneum covering the gastric ligaments or the omentum.

What is the AJCC 7th edition (2011) N-staging classification for gastric cancer?

N1: 1–2 LNs
N2: 3–6 LNs
N3: ≥7 LNs
N3a: 7–15 LNs
N3b:>15 LNs

What are the AJCC 7th edition (2011) stage groupings for gastric cancer?

Stage IA: T1N0 (adds to 1)
Stage IB: T1N1, T2a-bN0 (adds to 2)
Stage IIA: T1N2, T2N1, or T3N0 (adds to 3)
Stage IIB: T2N2, T3N1, T4aN0 (adds to 4)
Stage IIIA: T4aN1, T3N2, T2N3 (adds to 5)
Stage IIIB: T4bN0, T4bN1, T4aN2, T3N3 (adds to 6 mostly)
Stage IIIC: T4bN2, T4aN3, T4bN3 (adds to 7 mostly)
Stage IV: TXNXM1

What is the 5-yr OS for the various stages of gastric cancer treated with surgery?

IA: 71%; IB: 57%; IIA: 46%; IIB: 33%; IIIA: 20%; IIIB: 14%; IIIC: 9%; IV: 4% (*SEER 1991–2000*)

► **TREATMENT/PROGNOSIS**

What surgical margin is generally considered adequate in gastric cancer?

≥3 cm proximal and distal margin as long as tumor is well circumscribed and not invading serosa (otherwise ≥5 cm)

For what tumor location is subtotal vs. total gastrectomy indicated? Is there a benefit with total gastrectomy?

Subtotal gastrectomy for **distal tumors** (antrum/body); **total** gastrectomy for **proximal tumors** (cardia, greater curvature)

No. According to the following 2 trials, there is no benefit of advocating total gastrectomy:

Gouzi et al. randomized distal tumors to total gastrectomy vs. subtotal gastrectomy. There were no differences in morbidity/mortality (1.3% vs. 3.2%) or survival outcomes (5-yr OS 48%). (*Ann Surg 1989*)

Italian data from a second randomized trial (*Bozzetti F et al., Ann Surg 1999*) showed no difference in 5-yr survival between subtotal gastrectomy (65%) and total gastrectomy (62%).

Should splenectomy be performed for proximal gastric tumors to get splenic LN clearance?

No, b/c there was no value of splenectomy in a randomized trial (*Csendes A et al., Surgery 2002*). Splenectomy and pancreatectomy had an adverse impact on survival in the Dutch and MRC D1 vs. D2 RCTs (see below).

How are GE junction cancers classified, and how is the classification important therapeutically?

GE junction cancers are classified by the **Siewert classification** as 3 entities:

Type I: adenocarcinoma of distal esophagus, arising from Barrett, that infiltrates GE junction

Type II: adenocarcinoma of cardia portion, arising from cardia and short segment of intestinal metaplasia at GE junction

Type III: adenocarcinoma of subcardial stomach, which may infiltrate GE junction or distal esophagus from below

Type I has lymphatic drainage reminiscent of esophageal primaries (mediastinal and celiac), whereas types II–III drain to celiac, splenic, and para-aortic (P-A) nodes. Esophagectomy is typically recommended for type I tumors, whereas gastrectomy is recommended for types II–III tumors.

What are the types of nodal dissection for gastric cancer?

D0: no nodal dissection

D1: perigastric nodes removed

D2: D1 + periarterial nodes (left gastric, hepatic, celiac, splenic)

D3: D2 + hepatoduodenal, peripancreatic, mesenteric root, portocaval, P-A nodes, middle colic

Is extended lymphadenectomy necessary for surgical cure of gastric cancer?

No. Although results from numerous randomized trials have *not* shown an OS advantage of extended lymphadenectomy, CSS and LRR may be improved with extended dissection in the most recent update of the Dutch trial (see below).

What 4 major trials investigated the extent of lymphadenectomy on outcomes?

Dutch trial (*Bonenkamp JJ et al., NEJM 1999*): 711 pts randomized to D1 vs. D2 dissection. There was greater mortality in the D2 group (10% vs. 4%, *p* = SS), and 5-yr OS was 45% vs. 47% (NSS). In the most recent 15-yr update (*Songun I et al., Lancet Oncol 2010*), the 15-yr OS was 21% in the D1 group and 29% in the D2 group (*p* = 0.34). However, the gastric cancer–related death rate was significantly higher in the D1 group (48%) vs. the D2 group (37%), while deaths from other Dz were similar in the 2 groups. LR was lower in the D2 group (12% vs. 22%) as well as regional recurrence (13% vs. 19%) (all SS).

MRC trial (*Cushieri A et al., Br J Cancer 1999*): 400 pts randomized to D1 vs. D2. There was greater mortality in the D2 group (13% vs. 6.5%), and 5-yr OS was the same (35% vs. 33%).

Japanese trial JCOG9501 (D2 vs. D2 + P-A node dissection [PAND]) (*Sasako M et al., NEJM 2008*) demonstrated that although extended LND does not increase morbidity or mortality, there is also no difference in 5-yr OS (69.2% for D2 vs. 70.3% for D2 + PAND) or for LRR.

An **Italian trial** (D1 vs. D2) (*Degiuli M et al., Br J Surg 2010*) has shown no increased morbidity or mortality with extended lymphadenectomy, but clinical outcomes have not yet been reported.

What is the min number of LNs that should be pathologically assessed in a gastrectomy specimen?

In the U.S., at least **15 LNs** should be assessed by the pathologist, since pt survival improves if >15 LNs are examined.

What are the selection criteria for endoscopic mucosal resection or limited surgical resection (without nodal evaluation) of gastric cancer?

Favorable early-stage gastric cancer: **Tis-T1 (but not involving submucosa), small (≤3 cm), nonulcerated, well differentiated, N0.** In general, these types of tumors have <5% LN met rate.

When is surgery alone adequate for gastric cancer?

T1N0 or T2N0 (but not beyond the muscularis propria). 5-yr OS for favorable early-stage gastric cancer is 80%–90%. For all others, adj Tx is needed (**Ib** [except T2aN0] **to IIIC** [nonmet]).

What is the relapse pattern after "curative" resection of gastric cancer?

Distant Dz (50%) and LRR. LRR is common in the gastric bed, nearby LNs, anastomotic site, gastric remnant, and duodenal stump. In the classic paper of the University of Minnesota reoperative analysis (*Gunderson L et al., IJROBP 1982*), local-only recurrence was seen in 29%, LR and/or regional LN mets in 54%, and LF as any component of failure in 88% of pts.

What is the randomized evidence that demonstrated a benefit of adj CRT after surgical resection for gastric cancer?

INT-0116 (*Macdonald JS et al., NEJM 2001*): 556 pts, stages IB–IV (nonmet) adenocarcinoma of stomach and GE junction (~20%), randomized after en bloc resection to –margin to (a) observation or (b) CRT (1 cycle bolus 5-FU/leucovorin [LV]) before RT, 2 cycles during 45 Gy RT, and 2 cycles after RT. Median follow-up was 5 yrs. CRT was beneficial in all parameters except for DM 3-yr RFS 48% vs. 31%; 3-yr OS 50% vs. 41%; median OS 36 mos vs. 27 mos; and LR 19% vs. 29%. DM 18% surgery vs. 33% CRT (NSS). Toxic deaths of 1% were seen.

What is the major criticism for the benefit of CRT seen in INT-0116?

Suboptimal LND (54% D0, 10% D2) is the major criticism of INT-0116.

How was radiation delivered in INT-0116?

Most pts were treated with **AP:PA fields to 45 Gy**

What does the 10-yr follow-up data from INT-0116 show?

They showed **persistent strong benefit with adj CRT;** hazard ratios were 1.32 (*p* = 0.0046) for OS and 1.51 (*p* <0.001) for RFS favoring CRT; more 2nd malignancies observed in CRT group (21 vs. 8, NS); LF was 2% for CRT arm and 8% for surgery-alone arm and regional relapse rates were 22% and 39%, respectively. (*Smalley SR et al., JCO 2012*)

Is there a benefit to postop CRT for pts with more extensive lymphadenectomy?

Yes. There is a benefit according to a retrospective review from South Korea. (*Kim S et al., IJROBP 2005*) In a series of 990 pts, stages II–IV with D2 resection +/– postop CRT, as done in **INT-0116,** postop CRT benefited all pts regardless of stage. Overall, CRT vs. surgery alone: 5-yr OS 57% vs. 51%, RFS 54.5% vs. 47.9%, and LRF 14.9% vs. 21%, respectively (all SS).

Is there a role for preop CRT for gastric cancer?

Possibly, although no phase III studies have been published to date. However, for GE junction tumors, preop CRT based on randomized data suggests benefit (see Chapter 46 re: CROSS trial, *van Hagen P et al., NEJM 2012*).

A phase II study of neoadj CRT (**RTOG 9904:** *Ajani JA et al., JCO 2006*) using induction chemo × 2 (5-FU/LV/cisplatin) → CRT (continuous infusion [CI] 5-FU/weekly taxol) showed pCR of 26% and R0 resection of 77%.

Is there a role for postop RT alone for resected gastric cancer?

Possibly. Although not standard practice, there are weak data suggesting LC benefit with conflicting results on survival benefit. Most adj RT-alone trials utilized IORT +/– EBRT vs. surgery-alone randomization and found benefit with adj RT.

What is the approach to resectable gastric cancer in Europe and what major RCT is it based on? What is the major weakness of this trial?

Perioperative chemo (without RT) with ECF regimen (epirubicin/cisplatin/5-FU); **MRC Adjuvant Gastric Cancer Infusional Chemo (MAGIC) trial** (*Cunningham D et al., NEJM 2006*): 503 pts with gastric, GE junction, and distal esophageal adenocarcinoma (26%) randomized to (a) preop ECF × 3 and postop ECF × 3 or (b) surgery alone showed a survival benefit for chemo. 5-yr OS was 36% vs. 23%, respectively (*p* = 0.009). The **major weakness of the MAGIC trial is that the pCR rate was 0%.**

What were the arms of CALGB 80101, the U.S. randomized trial for resected high-risk gastric cancer?

CALGB 80101 pts with completely resected, high-risk gastric cancer randomized to (a) the modified Macdonald regimen (5-FU/LV × 1 → CI 5-FU × 2 +RT → 2 cycles 5-FU/LV) or (b) ECF (epirubicin 50 mg/m^2, cisplatin 60 mg/m^2, and CI 5-FU 200 mg/m^2/day × 21 days) × 1 → RT + CI 5-FU × 2 → ECF × 2 cycles.

What did the 3-yr follow-up data from CALGB 80101 show?

The 3-year data show similar OS (50% vs. 52%) and DFS (46% vs. 47%) between the 2 arms. (*ASCO 2011, abstr 4003*)

What is the survival of pts with locally advanced unresectable gastric cancer? How are these pts managed?

5-yr OS is generally **5%–20%.** In most randomized studies of these pts, CRT has benefit over chemo alone (5-yr OS 12%–18% vs. 0%–7%). **GITSG G274** (*Schein PS et al., Cancer 1982*) used CRT (50 Gy) vs. chemo alone (5-FU/1-(2-chloroethyl)-3-(4-methylcyclohexyl)-1-nitrosourea). There was better survival with CRT (18% vs. 7%).

For met gastric cancer pts, what are some palliative Tx options?

Surgical resection for carefully selected pts with good performance status with Sx of obstruction or hemorrhage is better for palliation than stents or bypass. **RT alone or CRT** can be considered for the nonsurgical candidates (short course palliation 30 Gy/10 fx, 37.5 Gy/15 fx). **Endoluminal laser ablation** can be used for proximal lesions with esophageal obstruction → **chemo.** Palliative chemo compared with best supportive care has an overall HR of 0.39, and MS increases from 4.3 mos to 11 mos based on Cochrane meta-analysis. (*Wagner A et al., Cochrane Database Sys Rev 2006*)

What novel targeted therapy may be considered for select pts with met or recurrent gastric cancer?

Trastuzumab (Herceptin); based on the **Trastuzumab for Gastric Cancer (ToGA) randomized trial,** which showed improved median OS (13.5 mos vs. 11.1 mos, $p = 0.0048$) with addition of trastuzumab to chemo (cisplatin/5-FU) vs. chemo alone. (*Bang YJ et al., Lancet 2010*)

What was the *HER2* positive rate in the ToGA trial?

The *HER2+* rate was 22.1%

For the met gastric cancer pt with bleeding or pain from the primary Dz, what are adequate palliative RT doses?

Bleeding: 30 Gy in 10 fx may be sufficient; however, for the initial few doses, a higher fractional dose (4–4.5 Gy) may be better for bleeding control. After 3–4 fx, the practitioner can back down to 3 Gy/fx.

Pain from tumor invasion: 45 Gy may be necessary

What is the irradiation volume and dose of postop CRT after gastric tumor resection?

Tumor bed and nodal volumes constructed with preop/postop imaging and surgical clip placement. In general, node+ Dz requires wide coverage of the tumor bed, remaining stomach, all resection/anastomotic sites, and nodal drainage areas (which is dependent on tumor location). Use 45 Gy to the initial volume as per RTOG 0116. CD to 50.4 Gy to the surgical bed or at-risk areas if margin+ or gross Dz. Pre-Tx J-tube placement (at time of staging laparoscopy) is helpful for nutritional support.

When would it be optional to treat the nodal beds in a resected gastric cancer?

Tx would be optional for pts with –nodes, pts having had adequate surgery and pathologic evaluation for nodes (>10–15 nodes), and wide surgical margins (at least 5 cm).

In general, what are the at-risk regional nodal sites based on anatomic location of the gastric tumor?

1. GE junction: mediastinal, periesophageal, celiac, perigastric
2. Proximal stomach: perigastric, periesophageal, celiac, pancreaticoduodenal, porta hepatis
3. Body: perigastric, splenic, celiac, peripancreatic, porta hepatis
4. Distal stomach: perigastric, periduodenal, peripancreatic, porta hepatis, celiac

How does the target volume differ for proximal vs. distal gastric lesions?

Proximal lesions: include splenic hilum and left medial diaphragm in the target volume, but inf extent does not need to go to L3 (may just go to L1-2 coverage of the superior mesenteric artery/P-A nodes)

Distal lesions: include 1st portion of the duodenal C-loop but not the splenic hilum

For proximal and distal lesions and –nodes with adequate dissection, the remnant of the stomach does not need to be covered. For body lesions, however, the gastric remnant needs to be covered in all cases.

What is the preferred postop radiation planning technique? **3D-CRT (4 field) or IMRT** can spare normal tissues and reduce toxicity better than traditional AP/PA fields, but greater conformality requires a more careful delineation of Tx targets.

What are some long-term complications of gastrectomy? Dumping syndrome (diarrhea, cramping, palpitations, reactive hypoglycemia) and malabsorption (B_{12}, iron, calcium; supplement if necessary)

What is entailed in the follow-up of gastric cancer pts treated with curative intent? H&P q3–6mos × 1–2 yrs, then 6–12 mos × 3–5 yrs, then annually; CBC/CMP, endoscopy, and radiologic imaging as clinically indicated; and monitor for B_{12} and iron deficiency; *HER2*-neu testing if not done previously (*NCCN 2013*)

In treating the postgastrectomy pt with adj CRT, what are the dose-limiting structures and dose limits for these organs? Dose-limiting structures and dose limits:
Remnant of stomach: 45 Gy
Kidney (both): mean <18 Gy, V28 <20%, V23 <30%, V20 <32%, V12 <55%. If the mean kidney dose to 1 kidney >18 Gy, then limit other kidney to V6 <30% (QUANTEC)
Liver: mean liver <32 Gy (QUANTEC)
Heart: one-third <50 Gy
Spinal cord: ≤45 Gy

48 Pancreatic and Periampullary Adenocarcinoma

Updated by Anusha Kalbasi

 BACKGROUND

Approximately how many pancreatic adenocarcinoma (PCA) pts are diagnosed per yr in the U.S.? As of 2013, the incidence of PCA is **~45,000 cases/yr** in the U.S., with ~35,000 deaths. Its incidence is higher in developed countries.

Where does PCA rank in cancer incidence in the U.S.? Cancer mortality?

As of 2009, PCA is the 10th most common cancer Dx but the **4th most common cause of cancer death in the U.S.**

Is there a racial or sex predilection for PCA?

Yes. Blacks are more commonly affected than whites; however, the incidence is similar among males and females.

In what decades of life does PCA incidence peak?

The peak age of PCA is in the **6th–7th decades** of life.

What are 3 environmental exposures associated with PCA?

Most common environmental risk factors for PCA:
1. Tobacco smoking
2. 2-naphthylamine
3. Benzidine

What % of PCA is familial?

~5% of PCA is familial.

What 2 genetic mutations have most frequently been associated with familial PCA?

p16 and *BRCA2* are the 2 most common familial associated genetic changes found in PCA.

Is chronic pancreatitis associated with increased risk of PCA?

No. Chronic pancreatitis is not associated with risk of PCA. Historically, there appeared to be an association, but this can be explained by confounding factors.

Approximately at what vertebral bodies are the pancreas, celiac axis, and superior mesenteric artery (SMA) located?

<u>Pancreas</u>: L1-2
<u>Celiac axis</u>: T12
<u>SMA</u>: L1

What % of PCA arise in the head, body, and tail of the pancreas?

Common PCA sites are **75% in the head, 15% in the body, and 10% in the tail.**

What is the distribution of local, regional, and metastatic disease at Dx?

~10% of PCA pts have local disease at diagnosis
~25% of PCA pts have regional node+ disease at diagnosis
~50% of PCA pts have DM at diagnosis

For PCA, what are the 3 most common sites of DM?

Common sites of DM for PCA include the **liver, peritoneum, and lungs.**

Is there a role for screening in PCA?

No. There is no current role for PCA screening. There are studies evaluating the role of screening 1st-degree relatives of PCA with EUS, but this is still experimental.

What % of pancreatic tumors are from the exocrine pancreas?

~95% of PCA are from the exocrine pancreas.

What are the 4 most common pathologic subtypes of exocrine pancreatic tumors?	Most common subtypes of exocrine pancreatic tumors: 1. Ductal adenocarcinoma (80%) 2. Mucinous cystadenocarcinoma 3. Acinar cell carcinoma 4. Adenosquamous carcinoma
What are the most common oncogenes in PCA?	**K-ras oncogene** is present in ~95% of PCA. p16 mutations are seen in ~90% of PCA. p53 mutations occur in 55%–75% of PCA. DPC4 mutations occur in ~50% of PCA.
What are the most common presenting Sx of PCA?	Common presenting Sx of PCA are **pancreatic/biliary duct obstruction, jaundice, and abdominal pain.**
What Dz is commonly diagnosed 1–2 yrs prior to a PCA Dx?	60%–80% of PCA pts are diagnosed with diabetes 1–2 yrs prior to Dx. However, only a small proportion of diabetic pts develop PCA.
Periampullary cancers refer to tumors arising from what 4 structures?	Periampullary tumors are those arising from the **ampulla of Vater, distal common bile duct (CBD), head of the pancreas, and adjacent duodenum.**

▶ WORKUP/STAGING

What is the DDx of a pancreatic mass?	The DDx of a pancreatic mass includes exocrine cancer, islet cell/neuroendocrine cancer, cystic adenomas, papillary cystic neoplasms (e.g., intraductal papillary mucinous tumor), lymphoma, acinar cell carcinoma, and metastatic cancer.
What is the initial workup for suspected PCA?	Suspected PCA workup includes a focused H&P, labs including CBC, CMP, and CA19-9, and abdominal CT scan.
In what circumstance will a PCA pt not excrete any CA19-9?	**If a pt is red cell Lewis antigen A–B negative,** then the pt cannot excrete CA19-9. The Lewis antigen–phenotype is present in 5%–10% of the population.
What is the appropriate imaging for suspected PCA?	Triphasic thin-sliced CT abdomen. The 3 phases include arterial, portal venous, and parenchymal phases of enhancement.
Name 4 appropriate procedures for obtaining tissue from a suspicious pancreatic mass.	Procedures to obtain tissue from a suspicious pancreatic mass: 1. EUS-guided FNA 2. CT-guided FNA 3. Endoscopic retrograde cholangiopancreatography (ERCP) 4. Pancreatic resection (i.e., histologic Dx is not required before surgery)

When is it appropriate to obtain tissue prior to surgery for lesions suspicious on imaging?

Tissue diagnosis prior to surgery is not routinely necessary, except for: (1) clinical trial enrollment, (2) prior to neoadjuvant therapy, or (3) prior to chemo/CRT in unresectable patients.

What is the major advantage of EUS-guided FNA over CT-guided FNA of a pancreatic mass?

EUS-guided FNA is associated with **lower risk of peritoneal seeding** (2% vs. 16%).

When is ERCP indicated instead of EUS?

ERCP carries a higher risk of iatrogenic pancreatitis, so it is reserved for cases where PCA is causing biliary obstruction and cholangitis requiring stenting.

What is the NCCN 2014 classification scheme for PCA?

PCA are classified into 4 categories (and per AJCC 7th edition [2011] staging):
1. Resectable (T1-3N0 or N+) (stages I–II)
2. Borderline resectable (T4NX) (stage III)
3. Locally advanced (T4NX) (stage III)
4. Metastatic (TXNXM1) (stage IV)

What 3 criteria are necessary for a primary pancreatic tumor to be resectable (per NCCN)?

NCCN resectability for PCA is defined as:
1. No distortion of SMV or portal vein
2. Clear fat plane around celiac artery, SMA, and hepatic artery
3. No distant mets or mets to nodes beyond field of resection

What characteristics make a primary pancreatic tumor unresectable (per NCCN)?

Unresectable characteristics include:
1. >180-degree encasement of SMA
2. Any celiac abutment for head lesions; >180-degree encasement for body/tail lesions
3. Unreconstructable SMV/PV occlusion
4. Aortic invasion/encasement

What are the characteristics of borderline resectable pancreatic head/body tumors (per NCCN)?

The definitions vary, but NCCN definition of borderline resectability for PCA are:
1. SMV/PV involvement (distortion, narrowing or occlusion) that can be resected and reconstructed using nearby vessels.
2. Tumor abutment on SMA ≥180-degrees
3. Gastroduodenal artery encasement up to the hepatic artery, including up to short segment encasement or direct abutment of the hepatic artery, without celiac axis involvement.

What pancreatic tail lesions are considered "borderline resectable"?

Invasion into the adrenal gland, colon, mesocolon, or kidney are considered borderline resectable for PCA tail lesions.

What location of PCA is associated with higher rates of resectability: head, body, or tail?

PCA **head** tumors are more resectable b/c they cause Sx early (and therefore present with earlier-stage Dz).

At presentation, what % of PCA pts is resectable?	10%–20% of PCA pts are potentially resectable at presentation.
What % of pts with resectable PCA tumors by CT imaging will be resectable at the time of surgery?	~65%–80% of PCA pts deemed resectable by CT are resectable at the time of surgery.
What is the role of staging laparoscopy?	Staging laparoscopy at the time of surgery is not routinely warranted. Select pts with tumors >3 cm, tumors in the body/tail, equivocal CT findings of metastasis, or CA19-9 >100 U/mL may benefit.
What imaging is indicated to assess for metastatic disease?	CT chest is routinely performed for mets workup of PCA. PET-CT may be more sensitive for systemic disease, but is not yet standard.
What is the significance of a postresection CA19-9 >90 U/mL?	In **RTOG 9704,** 53 pts (14%) had CA19-9 >90 U/mL, and only 2 of these pts survived up to 3 yrs.
What is the AJCC 7th edition (2011) T and N staging for PCA?	**T1:** limited to pancreas and ≤2 cm **T2:** limited to pancreas and >2 cm **T3:** extends beyond pancreas but without celiac axis or SMA involvement **T4:** celiac axis or SMA involvement **N1:** regional node involvement
What are the AJCC 7th edition (2011) stage groupings for PCA?	**Stage 0:** Tis **Stage IA:** T1N0M0 **Stage IB:** T2N0M0 **Stage IIA:** T3N0M0 **Stage IIB:** T1-3N1M0 **Stage III:** T4NXM0 **Stage IV:** TXNXM1
What is the stage of a PCA pt with positive cytology at time of laparoscopy?	Positive cytology is **stage IV** (M1).
Does the AJCC 7th edition (2011) TNM staging for ampullary, bile duct, and duodenal cancer differ from PCA?	**Yes.**

▶ TREATMENT/PROGNOSIS

What is the 5-yr OS for all stages of PCA?	5-yr OS is 5% for all stages of disease.
What surgical procedure is required to resect a pancreatic head lesion?	Surgery utilized for pancreatic head resection includes **pylorus-preserving pancreaticoduodenectomy** (PPPD) or **classic pancreaticoduodenectomy** (Whipple procedure).

What anastomoses are performed in the classic pancreaticoduodenectomy (Whipple)?	There are 3 anastomoses performed for the Whipple procedure: 1. Pancreaticojejunostomy 2. Choledochojejunostomy (hepaticojejunostomy) 3. Gastrojejunostomy
What are the 4 most favorable prognostic factors after resection?	Most favorable prognostic factors after resection of PCA: 1. Negative margins (R0) 2. Low grade (G1) 3. Small tumor size (<3 cm) 4. N0 status
What is the modern MS for unresectable, margin-negative resected, and margin-positive resected PCA pts?	The MS for PCA patients with the following surgeries in the era of adjuvant and definitive CRT is: 1. Unresectable ~11 mos 2. Margin+ resection ~16–18 mos 3. Margin– resection ~25 mos
What is the current mortality rate for pancreaticoduodenectomy?	At tertiary care centers with high throughput, the mortality rate for pancreaticoduodenectomy is <4%.
What is the most feared complication for pancreaticoduodenectomy?	Anastamotic leaks are the most important complications after pancreaticoduodenectomy and can lead to peritonitis, abscess, autodigestion, hemorrhage, and delayed gastric emptying.
Is there a benefit to R1 or R2 resection over definitive CRT for PCA?	**No.** Retrospective evidence suggests that survival is similar between PCA pts who had R1 or R2 resection and definitive CRT. Therefore, planned resections should be done in pts where R0 resections are likely. Debulking surgery does not improve outcome over definitive CRT.
Should pts with resectable PCA undergo extended retroperitoneal lymphadenectomy?	**No.** Resectable PCA pts should not undergo an extended retroperitoneal lymphadenectomy. There is no survival benefit to extended lymphadenectomy by an RCT (5-yr 25% vs. 31%, NSS). (*Riall TS et al., J Gastrointest Surg 2005*)
Can definitive CRT replace surgical resection for resectable PCA?	**No.** Surgery alone is superior to CRT alone for pts with resectable PCA per the Japanese PCA Study Group in an RCT of surgery alone vs. definitive CRT (50.4 Gy with continuous infusion [CI] 5-FU). The trial was stopped early due to the benefit of surgery: MS was 12 mos vs. 9 mos, and 5-yr OS was 10% vs. 0%. (*Doi R et al., Surg Today 2008*)
What are the adj Tx options for a PCA pt s/p resection?	Adj Tx options after a pancreaticoduodenectomy: 1. Adj gemcitabine (**CONKO-001**) 2. Adj gemcitabine alone → 5-FU/RT→ gemcitabine alone (**RTOG 9704**) 3. Adj 5-FU/RT (**GITSG 91-73**); consider maintenance gemcitabine afterward

4. Adj 5-FU → 5-FU/RT → 5-FU (**RTOG 9704**)

5. Observation alone

What is the standard postop radiation Tx volume, dose, and fractionation for PCA?

Standard adj RT volume includes tumor bed, anastomoses (pancreaticojejunostomy and choledochojejunostomy), and LN basin (peripancreatic, celiac, superior mesenteric artery, porta hepatis, and aortocaval). The initial volume is treated to 45 Gy in 1.8 Gy/fx with a cone down to 50.4–59.4 Gy to the surgical bed depending on extent of resection. Small bowel should be excluded after 50.4 Gy.

For pts with resected PCA, LF is the site of 1st failure for what % of pts treated with adj CRT? Distant failure as the 1st site?

Based on **RTOG 9704,** LF was site of 1st failure in 23%–28% of PCA and distant failure was 1st site in 71%–77%.

What U.S. study 1st reported a benefit of adj CRT vs. no additional Tx for resected PCA? Describe the arms of this study and the major results.

The **Gastrointestinal Tumor Study Group (GITSG 91-73)** trial 1st reported benefit to adj CRT for PCA in 1985. All pts had R0 resections.

Standard arm: postop observation

Experimental arm: adj CRT using split-course RT to 40 Gy (2-wk break after 20 Gy) with intermittent bolus 5-FU → 2 full yrs of adj 5-FU alone

Improved MS (20 mos vs. 11 mos) and 2-yr OS (42% vs. 15%) in the adj CRT arm (*Kalser MH et al., Arch Surg 1985*)

Did the EORTC 40891 study on PCA support or contest the benefit of adj CRT?

Support. The **EORTC 40891** trial used the same randomization as GITSG 91-73, except the Tx arm did *not* rcv maintenance adj 5-FU for 2 yrs. Median PFS was 17 mos (CRT) vs. 16 mos (observation), NSS; MS was 24 mos (CRT) vs. 19 mos (observation), NSS. For the subset of PCA pts, 5-yr OS was 20% (CRT) vs. 10% (observation) (*p* = 0.09). (*Klinkenbijl JH et al., Ann Surg 1999*) Of note, in addition to T1-2N0-1 PCA, 45% of pts had periampullary adenocarcinoma, which were excluded in GITSG 91-73, and generally have better prognosis. Authors concluded that routine adj CRT was not warranted, although statistical reanalysis of this study found a significant survival benefit with adj therapy. (*Garofalo MC et al., Ann Surg 2006*)

Did the European Study Group for Pancreatic Cancer-1 (ESPAC-1) study on PCA support or contest the benefit of adj CRT?

Contest. ESPAC-1 included pts with grossly resected adenocarcinoma of the pancreas. The study used a 2 × 2 factorial design; surgery +/– CRT and +/– adj chemo. Adj CRT was similar to GITSG. Adj chemo was 6 mos of 5-FU. MS was 15 mos (CRT) vs. 16 mos (no CRT), NSS; OS was 20 mos (chemo) vs. 14 mos (no chemo) (*p* = 0.0005).

Criticisms: Physicians could randomize pts into 2×2 or directly into 1 of the 2 randomizations. "Background Tx" was allowed (i.e., observed pts may have rcvd chemo +/− RT). There was no central RT QA. (*Neoptolemos JP et al., Lancet 2001*) *Note:* Analysis of 2×2 subset suggests that CRT had a deleterious effect; 5-yr OS was 10% (CRT) vs. 20% (no CRT) ($p = 0.05$).

How does the presence of a +margin after resection for PCA influence the decision for adj CRT?

UK Clinical Trials Unit meta-analysis of 5 RCTs, including individual data from 4 RCTs, found that the benefit of adj CRT was greater in R1 pts compared to R0 pts, although the difference was not SS. Also, the benefit of adj chemo alone decreased in R1 pts compared to R0 pts, suggesting that CRT may have a more important role in R1 pts. (*Butturini G et al., Arch Surg 2008*)

Which study supports the role for adj gemcitabine for resected PCA over best supportive care? What subset of pts were excluded from this trial?

CONKO-001 included T1-T4, N0-N1 pts in a RCT of observation vs. adj gemcitabine. Outcomes favored adj Tx: median DFS was 13 mos vs. 7 mos (SS). MS was 23 mos vs. 20 mos (SS), and 5-yr OS was 21% vs. 10% (SS), 10-yr OS was 12.2% vs. 7.7%. (*Oettle H et al., JAMA 2013*) *Note:* Pts with CA19-9 >90 were excluded from this trial.

What study compared adj 5-FU to gemcitabine following surgical resection?

ESPAC-3 showed a MS of 23 mos for pts treated with 5-FU (and folinic acid) vs. 23.6 mos for pts treated with gemcitabine (NSS). (*Neoptolemos JP et al., JAMA 2010*)

Did the study RTOG 9704 on PCA support or contest a benefit of gemcitabine-based adj CRT?

This is **controversial. RTOG 9704** randomized R0 and R1 PCA pts to CI 5-FU (250 mg/m^2/d) CRT (50.4 Gy) and pre- and post-CRT with either additional 5-FU or gemcitabine. Among all eligible pts, there were no differences. In a preplanned subset analysis of pts with pancreatic head tumors, trends favored gemcitabine: MS was 20.5 mos vs. 16.7 mos, and 3-yr OS was 31% vs. 22%, but results were NSS ($p = 0.09$). The 3-yr LR was significantly better for the gemcitabine arm (23% vs. 28%). Updated 2012 results showed significantly worse survival in pts with CA19-9 >90 U/mL. (*Regine W et al., JAMA 2008; Berger AC et al., IJROBP 2012*)

What is the Picozzi regimen for pts with PCA?

The Picozzi regimen is **adj CRT with interferon-alfa, 5-FU, cisplatin, and RT** (45—54 Gy). 42% of pts were admitted during CRT and 95% of pts had ≥G3 toxicity; however, outcomes were very promising: 5-yr OS was 55%, and MS was 25.4 mos. (*Picozzi VJ et al., Am J Surg 2003, Ann Oncol 2011*)

What is the Tx paradigm for borderline resectable PCA?

Borderline resectable PCA Tx paradigm: consider staging laparoscopy, stent placement if jaundice, and neoadj CRT → resection.

What neoadj CRT regimen should be used for borderline resectable PCA?

There is **no standard neoadj Tx for PCA.** Use similar paradigms as for locally advanced cases: (1) 5-FU/RT, (2) gemcitabine/RT, (3) gemcitabine/ Abraxane or FOLFIRINOX (leucovorin, fluorouracil, irinotecan, and oxaliplatin) followed by 5-FU/RT or (4) induction gemcitabine/Taxotere/ Xeloda (GTX) → 5-FU/RT, with RT to 45–50.4 Gy in 1.8–2 Gy/fx or 30 Gy in 3 Gy/fx per the MDACC paradigm. (*Breslin TM et al., Ann Surg Oncol 2001*)

What is the Tx paradigm for locally advanced PCA?

Locally advanced unresectable PCA Tx paradigm: biliary stent (if jaundice) can be done 1st → (1) definitive CRT, (2) induction chemo → restage → CRT, or (3) chemo alone. CRT regimens typically involve 5-FU or gemcitabine. Chemo alone or induction chemo involves gemcitabine, gemcitabine + Abraxane, FOLFIRINOX, or other combination in clinical study.

What is the role of regional LN radiation with neoadj or definitive CRT for borderline resectable or locally advanced PCA?

LN irradiation is controversial in the neoadj or definitive setting. In this setting, some institutions trend toward using smaller fields that treat gross tumor plus a small margin (*McGinn CJ et al., JCO 2001*), with others have continued to treat LN in the definitive setting. (*Ben-Josef E et al., IJROBP 2004*)

What is the evidence to support induction chemo prior to CRT in locally advanced PCA?

In a retrospective study of locally advanced PCA pts from MDACC, pts who received induction gemcitabine followed by CRT had longer MS than pts that had initial CRT (12 mos vs. 8 mos). They hypothesize that induction chemo may select for pts that benefit from CRT. (*Krishnan S et al., Cancer 2007*)

What definitive CRT regimen should be used for locally advanced PCA?

Standard regimen for definitive CRT: 5-FU (CI 250 mg/m^2/d) + RT, with RT to 50–60 Gy in 1.8 Gy/fx or 30 Gy in 3 Gy/fx.

What study established the role of definitive CRT vs. RT alone in locally advanced PCA? What were the study arms and survival outcomes?

The **GITSG 9273** trial (pts enrolled in the 1970 s). Arm 1: RT alone, split-course 60 Gy in 2 Gy/fx; arm 2: 5-FU + RT, split-course RT to 40 Gy in 2 Gy/ fx; arm 3: 5-FU + RT, split-course RT to 60 Gy in 2 Gy/fx. All arms rcvd maintenance 5-FU × 2 yrs. MS favored the CRT arms: 5.3 mos (arm 1) vs. 9.7 mos (arm 2) vs. 9.3 mos (arm 3). 1-yr OS favored the CRT arms: 10% (arm 1) vs. 35% (arm 2) vs. 46% (arm 3). There were no statistical differences between the CRT arms. (*Moertel CG et al., Cancer 1981*)

What study suggests that gemcitabine alone may be superior to 5-FU–based CRT in locally advanced PCA? What were the study arms and survival outcomes?

FFCD/SFRO study (French). Arm 1: RT (60 Gy) + CI 5-FU + intermittent cisplatin → maintenance gemcitabine; arm 2: induction gemcitabine → maintenance gemcitabine. Upfront CRT was more toxic and had worse survival outcomes. MS was 8.6 mos vs. 13 mos, and 1-yr OS was 32% vs. 53%. *Criticism:* The upfront CRT was not standard and was very poorly tolerated. (*Chauffert B et al., Ann Oncol 2008*)

What study suggests that concurrent gemcitabine-based CRT is superior to gemcitabine alone for locally advanced PCA?

ECOG 4201, which closed early due to slow accrual. 71 pts (69 evaluable). Arm 1: gemcitabine alone; arm 2: gemcitabine + RT, then gemcitabine alone. MS and 2-yr OS were better with CRT (11.1 mos vs. 9.2 mos and 12% vs. 4%, respectively). There were higher G4/5 toxicities with arm 2, but G3/4 toxicities were similar. (*Loehrer PJ et al., JCO 2011*)

What 2 regimens may have greater activity than gemcitabine alone in metastatic PCA?

FOLFIRINOX and **gemcitabine + Abraxane** both were superior to gemcitabine alone in 2 separate phase III RCTs in metastatic PCA. In a French study of 342 pts, FOLFIRINOX had an MS of 11.1 mos vs. 6.8 mos for gemcitabine and increased QOL despite increased G3/4 toxicities. (*Conroy T et al., NEJM 2011*) The Metastatic Pancreatic Adenocarcinoma Clinical Trial (MPACT) international study of 861 pts showed gemcitabine + Abraxane had MS of 8.5 mos vs. 6.7 mos for gemcitabine alone. (*Von Hoff DD et al., NEJM 2013*)

Estimate the MS and 3-yr OS for pts with resectable PCA at Dx, based on RTOG 9704.

Outcomes for resected PCA, if treated with adj CRT: **MS was ~20 mos and 3-yr OS was ~30%** based on **RTOG 9704;** if untreated, MS was 11–12 mos.

Estimate the MS and 1-yr OS for pts with locally advanced PCA at Dx, based on GITSG 9273.

Outcomes for locally advanced PCA: **MS was ~9 mos and 1-yr OS was ~35%** based on **GITSG 9273.**

Estimate the MS and 1-yr OS for pts with metastatic PCA at Dx.

Outcomes for metastatic PCA: **MS was ~6 mos, and 1-yr OS was ~20%** based on an NCIC study.

In PCA pts, what are 3 Tx options for tumor-associated biliary obstruction?

Tx options for tumor-associated biliary obstruction:
1. Endoscopic biliary stent
2. Percutaneous biliary drainage with subsequent internalization
3. Open biliary-enteric bypass

In PCA pts, what are 3 Tx options for tumor-associated gastric outlet obstruction?

Tx options for tumor-associated outlet obstruction:
1. Gastrojejunostomy
2. Enteral stent
3. PEG tube

In PCA pts, what Tx should be considered for tumor-associated severe abdominal pain refractory to analgesic medications?

Celiac plexus neurolysis is an effective option for Tx-refractory pain.

In the absence of 3D planning, what are the borders for the initial AP and lat RT fields for PCA of the head?

Classic pancreatic head fields rcvd 45 Gy in 1.8 Gy/fx.

AP superior: T10-11 interspace
AP inferior: L3-4 interspace
AP left: 2 cm from left border of vertebral body
AP right: 2 cm to right of preop duodenum
Lateral superior-inferior: same as AP
Lateral posterior: 2 cm into vertebral body
Lateral anterior: 2 cm ant to preop gross Dz or duodenum

Are there any data on stereotactic body radiation therapy (SBRT) for pancreatic cancer?

Several studies have evaluated SBRT for unresectable PCA. Early reports suggest excellent LC; however, a significant proportion of pts experience duodenal toxicity.

Stanford (*Chang DT et al., Cancer 2009*): 77 pts with unresectable PCA rcvd 25 Gy × 1 with CyberKnife SBRT. The 6- and 12-mo isolated LR rate was 5% and 5%, respectively. The PFS at 6 and 12 mos were 26% and 9%, respectively. The 1-yr OS was 21%. At 12 mos, the ≥G2 late toxicity was 25%, including 1 small bowel perforation (G4), 1 duodenal stricture (G3), and 3 gastric ulcers (G3).

Beth Israel Deaconess (*Mahadevan A et al., IJROBP 2010*): 36 pts with unresectable PCA rcvd 24–36 Gy CyberKnife SBRT in 3 fx. Gemcitabine was given after SBRT. LC rate was 78%, and MS was 14.3 mos. 39% developed ≥G2 toxicity (25% G2, 14% G3), including 3 pts with vomiting and dehydration (G3) and 2 pts with GI bleed (G3).

Is there a potential for dose escalation with the use of IMRT in pancreatic cancer?

Yes. A phase I–II trial of IMRT dose-escalation (50 to 60 Gy) **with concurrent gemcitabine** in 50 pts with unresectable PCA found dose-limiting toxicities in 11 pts, including duodenal bleed (3 pts) and perforation (1 pt). The recommended dose was 55 Gy, with an estimated 24% rate of dose-limiting toxicity. (*Ben-Josef E et al., IJROBP 2012*)

Do Tx paradigms differ between pancreatic and periampullary adenocarcinoma?	**Yes.** Tx paradigms can differ between pancreatic vs. periampullary cancers. Consider observation for completely resected T1-T2, N0 ampulla of Vater carcinoma. Retrospective reviews suggest high OS (5-yr OS ~80%) with observation alone. (*Willett C et al., Surg Gynecol Obstet 1993*) Otherwise, periampullary adenocarcinoma generally follows PCA paradigms, especially for T3-T4, poor histologic grade, LVSI/PNI, (*Krishnan S et al., IJROBP 2008*), or node+ pts. (*Zhou J et al., Radiother Oncol 2009*)

▶ TOXICITY

What are the expected acute and late RT toxicities associated with Tx of resected and unresectable PCA?	Acute toxicities: nausea, diarrhea, small bowel obstruction, weight loss, anorexia, abdominal pain Late toxicities: small bowel obstruction/stenosis/perforation, gastric/small bowel ulceration and/or bleeding, biliary stenosis obstruction, 2nd malignancies
What are the standard dose limitations for the liver, kidneys, spinal cord, and stomach and small bowel for pancreatic RT?	Standard dose limits for normal structures during pancreatic cancer RT: Liver: mean <30 Gy Kidneys: mean <15–18 Gy for each kidney Spinal cord: ≤45–50 Gy Stomach and small bowel: V15 <120 cc (if contouring individual loops); V45 <195 cc (if contouring peritoneal space)
What are duodenal toxicities related to fractionated RT or SBRT for PCA?	Radiation can induce duodenal injury: ulceration, bleeding, perforation, and fistula formation. These mostly occur in the 1st 12 mos after completing RT.
What are duodenal constraints for fractionated RT?	For fractionated RT, duodenum **V55 Gy <1 cm^3**, and maximum **point dose <60 Gy** was associated with decreased G2 or higher toxicity. (*Kelly P et al., IJROBP 2013*)
What is the typical follow-up schedule after Tx of pancreatic cancer?	Pancreatic cancer follow-up schedule after Tx: surveillance every 3–6 mos × 2 yrs, then annually. At each visit, perform full H&P for Sx assessment, and consider CA19-9 levels, LFTs, and contrast CT scan chest/abdomen.

Hepatocellular Carcinoma

Updated by Richard Tuli

▶ BACKGROUND

What liver Dz is associated with hepatocellular carcinoma (HCC)?

Most HCCs develop in pts with cirrhosis from **liver parenchymal Dz.** Exposures and Dz that cause chronic hepatitis and cirrhosis are almost uniformly associated with HCC.

HCC is most common in what 2 regions in the world?

Most common regions for HCC:
1. Asia (East > Southeast)
2. Africa (middle > East > West)

Name 2 viruses associated with HCC.

Most important viral causes of HCC:
1. Hepatitis B virus (HBV; carrier state without associated cirrhosis is also a cause)
2. Hepatitis C virus (HCV)

Name the 2 most important environmental exposures associated with HCC.

Environmental exposures associated with HCC:
1. Heavy ethanol consumption, which leads to cirrhosis
2. Aflatoxin B, a mycotoxin that contaminates corn, soybeans, and peanuts, generally in sub-Saharan Africa and East and Southeast Asia

Name 3 hereditary conditions associated with HCC.

Relatively common hereditary conditions associated with HCC:
1. Hemochromatosis
2. α1-antitrypsin deficiency
3. Wilson Dz

Is there a sex predilection for HCC?

Yes. Males are 3 times more likely to develop HCC.

Worldwide, where does HCC rank as a cause of cancer death?

Worldwide, HCC is the **4th leading cause of cancer death** (3rd for men), but rates vary dramatically by region.

HCC incidence peaks in what decade of life?

HCC incidence peaks in the **6th decade** of life.

What is the most common clinical presentation of HCC?

The most common clinical presentation of HCC is **rising AFP in the setting of worsening pre-existing liver Dz.**

Who should be screened for HCC and how?

Pts with cirrhosis, hepatitis B carrier state, or nonalcoholic steatohepatitis should be screened for HCC. Screen with **AFP and liver US** every 6–12 mos.

Do most pts with HCC present with localized or metastatic Dz?	90% of HCC pts present with **localized Dz.**
In HCC, what are the most common sites of met spread?	HCC most commonly metastasizes to **intra-abdominal LNs and lungs.** Less common sites of mets include bone, brain, and adrenal glands.

▶ **WORKUP/STAGING**

What is the workup of suspected HCC?	Suspected HCC workup: H&P, AFP, CBC, CMP with LDH, LFTs, PT/INR, hepatitis panel (HBV/HCV studies), triphasic CT abdomen or MRI liver, chest imaging, and percutaneous Bx if necessary
For a pt with suspected HCC, when is a Bx unnecessary to establish the Dx?	In HCC, a Bx is not necessary to establish Dx if: 1. A liver lesion is >2 cm, has classic appearance by 1 imaging modality (CT, US, MRI, angiography) and is associated with AFP >200 ng/mL 2. A liver lesion is 1–2 cm and has classic appearance by 2 imaging modalities *Note:* If a liver lesion is <1 cm, then the pt should be followed with serial imaging.
In what HCC variant is the AFP level often normal?	AFP levels are normal in the majority of pts with **fibrolamellar carcinoma** (FLC), a variant of HCC. It is found commonly in females and has a good prognosis. Note that some authors argue that FLC is not truly a variant of HCC b/c it usually occurs in the absence of cirrhosis.
What are the characteristic triphasic CT and MRI findings of an HCC liver lesion?	<u>On dynamic CT</u>: early phase, tumor is seen as hyperintense b/c of increased vascularity. In the delayed phase, the tumor is hypodense.
What is the AJCC 7th edition (2011) TNM staging for HCC?	<u>On MRI T_1-weighted images</u>: low signal intensity and intermediate signal intensity on T_2; HCC appears hypervascular, has increased T_2 signal, and shows venous invasion
What are the AJCC 7th edition (2011) stage groupings for HCC?	*Note:* Bold text highlights 7th edition changes. **T1:** solitary tumor without vascular invasion **T2:** solitary tumor with vascular invasion or multiple tumors ≤5 cm **T3a: multiple tumors >5 cm** **T3b: single tumor or multiple tumors of any size involving major branch of portal or hepatic veins** **T4:** tumor with direct invasion of adjacent organs other than gallbladder or with perforation of visceral peritoneum **N1:** regional LN mets (hilar, hepatoduodenal ligament, **inf phrenic LN** [no longer classified as M1], and caval LNs) **M1:** DMs

What are the AJCC 7th edition (2011) stage groupings for HCC?

Note: Bold text highlights 7th edition changes.
Stage I: T1N0
Stage II: T2N0
Stage IIIA: T3aN0
Stage IIIB: T3bN0
Stage IIIC: T4N0
Stage IVA: TXN1M0
Stage IVB: TXNXM1

Name 3 systems (other than AJCC) used to stage HCC internationally.

Staging systems for HCC commonly used outside the U.S.:
1. BCLC (Barcelona Clinic Liver Cancer)
2. CLIP (Cancer of the Liver Italian Program)
3. JIS score (Japanese Integrated Staging)
Applicability of each of these staging systems appears to depend on the Tx method.

What does a Child-Pugh score predict in pts with chronic liver Dz?

The Child-Pugh score was originally used to estimate operative mortality risk but is currently used to **assess OS prognosis** for pts with liver failure. Based on cumulative scores, pts are divided into class A, B, or C, with C being the poorest risk.

What are the 5 components of the Child-Pugh score in chronic liver Dz?

Components of the Child-Pugh score include **total bilirubin, serum albumin, INR, degree of ascites, and degree of hepatic encephalopathy.**

What does the acronym MELD represent, and what does the MELD score predict in chronic liver Dz?

MELD stands for **M**odel for **E**nd-Stage **L**iver **D**isease, initially developed to predict the 3-mo mortality after a transjugular intrahepatic portosystemic shunt procedure. Now, it is **used to assess severity of chronic liver Dz and the 3-mo OS without a liver transplant.** The MELD score is highly correlated with the Child-Pugh score.

What are the 3 components of the MELD score in chronic liver Dz?

Components of the MELD score include **total bilirubin, INR, and Cr.**

▶ TREATMENT/PROGNOSIS

What 3 features of the HCC pt and the pt's tumors define the appropriate Tx paradigm?

The 3 features that define the Tx options for a pt with HCC are whether the pt (a) has metastatic Dz, (b) has resectable localized tumor, and (c) is medically fit for major surgery.

What are the only 2 curative Tx options for HCC?

The only 2 established curative Tx options for HCC are **partial hepatectomy to −margins and liver transplantation.** Potentially curative RT Tx with hypofractionated photons and proton therapy are being explored.

Partial hepatectomy is an option in which HCC pts?

Partial hepatectomy is a potentially curative option in HCC pts who are medically fit for surgery, have a solitary mass without major vascular involvement, are Child-Turcotte-Pugh class A with mild or moderate portal hypertension, and have adequate future liver remnant (if no cirrhosis, require >20% of liver; if Child-Pugh A cirrhosis, require >30% of liver). Attempt at curative resection in HCC pts with multifocal tumors and major vascular invasion is controversial.

What % of HCC pts will have an LR after partial hepatectomy after 5 yrs?

~**75%** of pts with HCC will have an LR after 5 yrs (new primary or local spread). (*Mathurin P et al., Aliment Pharmacal Ther 2003*)

In pts with localized resectable HCC, what adj Tx improves LC and survival after partial hepatectomy?

A study from China found that in pts with HCC s/p partial hepatectomy, **adj intra-arterial lipiodol I-131** improved LC and possibly OS. (*Lau WY et al., Ann Surg 2008*) Confirmatory studies are under way.

What criteria are used to determine if liver transplant is an option for a pt with HCC?

The **United Network for Organ Sharing (UNOS) criteria** are used to determine if liver transplantation is appropriate in a pt with HCC. Per the UNOS criteria, transplantation is an option for medically fit pts with a **single tumor ≤5 cm** or **2–3 tumors ≤3 cm.**

What are the Tx options for an HCC pt with localized Dz who is medically unfit for major surgery?

Tx options for an HCC pt with localized Dz but who is unfit for major surgery include:
1. Sorafenib for Child-Pugh A or B pt
2. Tumor ablation procedure (radio frequency, cryoablation, microwave, percutaneous alcohol injection)
3. Tumor embolization procedure (chemoembolization [aka transarterial chemoembolization], bland embolization, radioembolization)
4. EBRT, including stereotactic body radiation therapy (SBRT) and proton therapy techniques

In the U.S., what isotope is most commonly used for radioembolization for HCC pts?

In the U.S., the most commonly used isotope for radioembolization in HCC pts is **yttrium-90,** a pure β emitter.

What are the 2 forms of microspheres used for radioembolization in HCC pts, and what is the difference between them?

Microspheres used for radioembolization in HCC pts:
1. TheraSphere (glass microspheres)
2. SIR-Spheres (resin microspheres)

Estimate the response rate of HCC to yttrium-90–labeled microspheres.

The response rate of HCC to yttrium-90–labeled microspheres **varies from 50%–80%** depending on the definition of response used.

What are the EB Tx options with either medically inoperable or technically unresectable HCC?

A number of methods of externally irradiating pts with HCC have been explored:

1. Whole liver RT for palliation (21 Gy in 7 fx)
2. High-dose RT (>50 Gy) with standard fractionation
3. Hyperfractionated RT with chemosensitization
4. Hypofractionated stereotactic RT
5. Proton therapy

Currently, there is no standard EB technique for unresectable or medically inoperable HCC pts.

What are the Tx options for an HCC pt with metastatic Dz?

The only standard active Tx option for metastatic HCC is **sorafenib, a small molecule tyrosine-kinase inhibitor that acts against c-raf and PDGF-α.** HCC typically does not respond to traditional cytotoxic chemo.

What is the MS in metastatic or inoperable HCC pts treated with sorafenib alone?

The MS of metastatic or inoperable HCC pts treated with sorafenib alone is **10.7 mos vs. 7.9 mos** ($p = 0.0058$) **in pts treated with placebo.** (*Llovet JM et al., NEJM 2008*)

What are the dose and results of SBRT for HCC?

In a sequential phases I–II trial of SBRT for HCC, 102 pts with Child-Turcotte-Pugh class A Dz with at least 700 cc of non-HCC liver were treated with SBRT (24–54 Gy in 6 fx; median 36 Gy). Median OS was 17 mos with 87% local control at 1 yr. 30% experienced grade ≥3 toxicity. (*Bujold A et al., JCO 2013*)

Another single institutional experience utilized 12.5 Gy × 3 (<4 cm and no cirrhosis) or 5 Gy × 5 or 10 Gy × 5 (≥4 cm with cirrhosis) with LC rates of 94% and 82% in 1 and 2 yrs, respectively. (*Mendez Romero A et al., Acta Oncol 2006*)

Is there a role for sorafenib with radiotherapy?

Phase I data exist regarding the safety and tolerability of sorafenib with RT and suggests that sorafenib exacerbates RT toxicity. (*Dawson LA et al., ASTRO 2012*) RTOG 1112 is a phase III study currently randomizing pts with Child-Turcotte-Pugh class A and BCLC B/C HCC to sorafenib alone vs. sequential SBRT followed by sorafenib.

What is the role for proton beam in the management of unresectable HCC?

A Japanese prospective study enrolled 51 pts with tumors >2 cm from the porta hepatis and GI tract and treated them with 66 cobalt Gray equivalents in 10 fx. LC was 94.5% at 3 yrs and 87.8% at 5 yrs. There were minor grade 1 acute adverse events, and only 3 pts were rated higher than grade 2. (*Fukumitsu N et al., IJROBP 2009*)

Is there a QOL benefit to palliative radiotherapy for HCC?

A phase II study assessed the benefit of 8 Gy × 1 for pts with HCC or liver mets unsuitable for or refractor to standard therapies. At 1 mo, 48% were noted to have an improvement in symptoms (FACT-Hep 29%, EORTC QLQ-C30 functional 11%–21%, symptom 11%–50%) (*Soliman H et al., JCO 2013*)

▶ **TOXICITY**

What are the components of the clinical syndrome of radiation-induced liver Dz (RILD)?

Signs and Sx of RILD include fatigue, RUQ pain, ascites, anicteric hepatomegaly, and elevated liver enzymes (esp alk phos which occurs 3 mos to 2 wks following completion of RT).

What is the histologic hallmark of RILD?

The pathologic hallmark of RILD is **veno-occlusive Dz with venous congestion of the central portion of the liver lobule.** Hepatocyte atrophy and fibrosis eventually develop.

What is the Emami RILD TD 5/5 for whole liver RT in 2 Gy/fx?

The Emami RILD TD 5/5 for whole liver RT in 2 Gy/fx is **30 Gy.**

What is the Emami RILD TD 50/5 for whole liver RT in 2 Gy/fx?

The Emami RILD TD 50/5 for whole liver RT in 2 Gy/fx is **42 Gy.**

What is the RILD TD 5/5 for whole liver RT in 6 fx?

The RILD TD 5/5 for whole liver RT in 6 fx is **~21 Gy.**

What is the RILD TD 5/5 for RT to more than one third of the liver in 1.8 Gy/fx?

The RILD TD 5/5 for RT to more than one-third of the liver in 1.8 Gy/fx is **~68.4 Gy.**

50 Biliary Tree and Gallbladder Cancer

Updated by Anusha Kalbasi

▶ BACKGROUND

What are the 3 anatomic subtypes of biliary cancer (cholangiocarcinoma [CC])?

CC is grouped into **intrahepatic** (~10%), **perihilar/Klatskin** (~60%), and **extrahepatic** (~30%) subtypes. Klatskin tumors involve the hepatic duct bifurcation.

How is gallbladder (GB) cancer distinct from CC?

GB cancer has unique epidemiology, presentation, staging, and surgical treatment.

What are major risk factors for CC?

Liver flukes (especially in Southeast Asia), **primary sclerosing cholangitis,** and **choledochal cysts,** all of which cause bile duct inflammation, are risk factors for CC.

What is the major risk factor for GB cancer?

Cholelithiasis increases the risk for GB cancer (presumably via chronic inflammation).

What is the annual incidence/mortality of CC and GB cancer in the U.S.?

There are **~10,000/yr new cases** of CC and GB cancer in U.S. and **~3,500/yr deaths.**

What is the histology of most CC and GB cancer?

Most CC and GB cancers are **adenocarcinomas.** They are difficult to distinguish from pancreatic adenocarcinoma on histopathology alone.

What less common pathologic subtype of GB cancer and CC has better prognosis?

Papillary adenocarcinoma is associated with improved prognosis compared with other adenocarcinomas of the biliary tree and GB.

What are the incidence and major sites of DM for CC and GB cancer?

30%–50% of CC and 40%–50% of GB cancer present with DM, most commonly **to liver, peritoneum, and lung.**

What is the MS for unresectable or MD?

MS is <6 mos for unresectable or metastatic CC and GB cancer.

What is the incidence of LN mets in resectable CC and GB cancer?

30%–50% of hilar and extrahepatic CC have LN mets at resection, but lower for intrahepatic CC. 40%–50% of GB cancer have LN mets at resection.

What is the LN drainage for hilar or extrahepatic CC?	Pericholedochal → portal vein LNs → common hepatic artery LNs → pancreaticoduodenal LNs → celiac axis/superior mesenteric artery (SMA) LNs → aortocaval LNs. Drainage does not ascend toward hepatic hilum.
How are LN mets different for intrahepatic CC?	Intrahepatic CC has a lower rate of LN mets than hilar or extrahepatic CC.
What is the most common route of spread for GB cancer and CC?	GB cancer and CC most commonly spread by **direct extension** (to the liver for GB cancer and along the biliary tree for CC).
What is the most common presenting symptom for CC? GB cancer?	**Painless jaundice** is the most common presenting symptom of CC. **Biliary colic** and chronic cholecystitis are the most common presenting symptoms of GB cancer.
How is GB cancer most commonly diagnosed?	GB cancer is most often incidentally diagnosed at **cholecystectomy** for presumed benign Dz.
What is a common and deadly complication of locally advanced Dz?	Biliary obstruction and sepsis is a common complication of poorly controlled locoregional Dz.

▶ WORKUP/STAGING

What initial labs should be sent if suspecting CC or GB cancer?	Bilirubin, alk phos, aspartate, and alanine aminotransferases (can often be normal), γ-glutamyl transpeptidase, CEA, and CA19-9 are particularly helpful in CC or GB cancer.
In what patients is CA19-9 less reliable?	**Pts without Lewis blood group antigen** (10% of population) do not have CA19-9. **Hyperbilirubinemia** can decrease specificity and accuracy of CA19-9.
What initial imaging is used for suspected CC and GB cancer?	**RUQ US, contrast-enhanced CT (preferably multiphase), and magnetic resonance cholangiopancreatography** (MRCP) are typically performed for pts with suspected CC or GB cancer.
On contrast-enhanced CT, how can hepatocellular carcinoma and intrahepatic CC be distinguished?	On contrast-enhanced CT of the liver, hepatocellular carcinoma usually enhances during the arterial phase, while intrahepatic CC may show **delayed enhancement.**
What is the imaging study of choice for extrahepatic CC?	**MRCP** is the imaging study of choice for extrahepatic CC, as it has improved the ability to define tumor extent and LN involvement.
What invasive imaging strategies are available?	Endoscopic retrograde cholangiopancreatography (ERCP) and percutaneous transhepatic cholangiography (PTC) can help image obstruction, but MRCP/CT are preferred.

How is a pathologic diagnosis obtained for CC?

For resectable pts without obstruction, pathology can be obtained at surgery. For unresectable pts or pts with obstruction requiring stenting, **duct brushings** can be obtained at ERCP, or **biopsy** can be done at time of PTC or EUS.

How is a pathologic diagnosis obtained for GB cancer?

Definitive resection is the diagnostic approach if GB cancer is suspected. **Bile cytology (low yield) or percutaneous biopsy** can be performed in unresectable pts.

When is ERCP- or PTC-based stenting indicated prior to surgery?

If bilirubin is elevated (i.e., >10–15), ERCP- or PTC-guided stents are placed to decompress obstruction and allow liver recovery prior to surgery.

In addition to locoregional imaging, what staging imaging is recommended for GB cancer and CC?

In addition to locoregional imaging, staging for GB cancer and CC should include **chest imaging.**

What staging procedure is recommended at the beginning of surgery for GB cancer or CC?

Staging laparoscopy is generally recommended at the beginning of surgery for GB cancer or CC to r/o peritoneal dissemination.

How does the AJCC 7th edition (2011) staging organize different sites of biliary cancers?

There is a different staging system for GB cancer, intrahepatic CC, perihilar CC, and distal extrahepatic CC. Of note, the AJCC staging for intrahepatic CC is no longer the same as primary liver tumors.

How should tumors arising from the middle of the common bile duct be staged?

These extrahepatic CCs are exceedingly rare, but they are **staged according to how they are managed,** either as a proximal lesion (by combined hepatic and hilar resection) or as distal lesions (by pancreaticoduodenectomy).

What is the AJCC 7th edition (2011) T staging for intrahepatic CC?

Tis: CIS
T1: solitary tumor without vascular invasion
T2a: solitary tumor with vascular invasion
T2b: multiple tumors +/– vascular invasion
T3: tumor perforating visceral peritoneum or directly invading local extra hepatic structures
T4: periductal invasion

What is the AJCC 7th edition (2011) T staging for perihilar CC?

Tis: CIS
T1: tumor confined to bile duct, with extension up to muscle layer or fibrous tissue
T2a: tumor invades beyond bile duct wall to surrounding fat
T2b: tumor invades liver
T3: tumor invades unilat branches of portal vein (right or left) or hepatic artery (right or left)

T4: tumor invades any of the following: main portal vein or bilat branches, common hepatic artery, 2nd-order biliary radicals bilaterally; or unilat 2nd-order biliary radicals with contralat portal vein or hepatic artery involvement

What is the AJCC 7th edition (2011) T staging for distal bile duct CC?

Tis: CIS
T1: tumor confined to bile duct histologically
T2: tumor invades beyond bile duct wall
T3: tumor invades liver, gallbladder, pancreas, and/ or unilat branches of the portal vein (right or left) or hepatic vein (right or left)
T4: tumor invades celiac axis or SMA

What is the AJCC 7th edition (2011) T staging for GB cancer?

The GB and cystic duct are included in this current classification:
Tis: CIS
T1: tumor invades **lamina propria (T1a)** or muscle layer (T1b)
T2: tumor invades perimuscular connective tissue but not into liver or beyond serosa
T3: tumor perforates serosa and/or directly invades liver and/or invades 1 adjacent organ/structure (stomach, duodenum, colon, pancreas, omentum, or extrahepatic bile ducts)
T4: tumor invades main portal vein, hepatic artery, or multiple extrahepatic organs/structures

What is the AJCC 7th edition (2011) N classification for perihilar CC and GB cancer?

Hilar LNs are distinguished separately from other regional LN mets:
N1 (mets to hilar nodes): nodes of cystic duct, common bile duct (CBD), hepatic artery, and/or portal vein
N2 (mets to regional nodes): periaortic, aortocaval, SMA, and/or celiac

What is the AJCC 7th edition (2011) N classification for intrahepatic CC and distal extrahepatic CC?

Any regional lymph node metastasis is classified as N1.
N0: no regional LNs
N2: regional LN mets present

What are the AJCC 7th edition (2011) groupings for biliary cancers (GB and perihilar)?

Stage 0: TisN0
Stage I: T1N0M0
Stage II: T2N0M0
Stage IIIA: T3N0M0
Stage IIIB: T1-3N1M0
Stage IVA: T4N0-1M0
Stage IVB: Any N2 or M1

What are the AJCC 7th edition (2011) groupings for intrahepatic CC?	**Stage 0:** TisN0 **Stage I:** T1N0M0 **Stage II:** T2N0M0 **Stage III:** T3N0M0 **Stage IV:** T4N0M0 **Stage IVA:** T4N0M0 or TxN1M0 **Stage IVB:** Any M1
What AJCC stage grouping do distal extrahepatic CC have in common?	**Pancreatic cancer, including N staging** (N0 or N1), since it is managed with similar approaches.

▶ TREATMENT/PROGNOSIS

What % of CC and GB cancer pts have potentially resectable Dz at presentation?	Resectability varies widely depending on site <u>Intrahepatic</u>: 30%–90% <u>Hilar</u>: ~50% <u>Distal extrahepatic</u>: 80%–90% <u>GB cancer</u>: 10%–30%
What is the classification system used to determine resectability of hilar CC?	Bismuth classification; **type IV is unresectable** **Type I/II:** involving CBD without involving left/right hepatic ducts **Type III:** involving either left or right hepatic duct in addition to CBD **Type IV:** involves both left and right hepatic ducts
What is the surgical approach for each subtype of CC and GB cancer?	The surgical approach depends on site: **Intrahepatic:** usually requires a lobectomy. **Hilar:** at least lobectomy, resection of extrahepatic bile duct, roux-en-Y hepaticojejunostomy, and LN staging. **Distal extrahepatic:** pancreaticoduodenectomy (Whipple) with LN staging **GB cancer:** extended cholecystectomy with LN staging
When is a routine cholecystectomy sufficient surgery for an incidentally diagnosed GB cancer?	Following cholecystectomy for presumed benign Dz, **pts with ≤T1a** (not beyond the lamina propria) GB cancer do not require a 2nd oncologic resection. 5-yr survival rates approach 100%.
How is an extended cholecystectomy different from a routine cholecystectomy?	Extended cholecystectomy should include en bloc resection of GB, segments IVb and V of liver, and regional LN dissection.
What 2nd surgery should be performed after ≥T1b GB cancer is discovered on cholecystectomy?	Following cholecystectomy for presumed benign Dz, pts with incidentally discovered ≥T1b GB cancer require **radical re-resection of the GB bed (2-cm margins), regional nodal dissection, and resection of the port sites.**

What is the 5-yr survival for patients after resection for CC?

Based on numerous retrospective studies, the MS based on site:
Intrahepatic: 17%–40% (MS 26–37 mos)
Hilar: 10%–35% (MS 14–37 mos)
Distal extrahepatic: 23%–50% (MS 18–36 mos)
GB cancer (T3-T4): 0%–45%

What are the prospective data supporting adjuvant chemo, RT, or CRT in CC or GB cancer?

Gemcitabine + cisplatin has been shown to be superior to gemcitabine alone in a phase III RCT of locally advanced or metastatic CC or GB cancer (*Valle J et al., NEJM 2010*), with MS 11.7 mos vs. 8.2 mos. **There are no prospective data for RT alone or CRT.**

What is the recommended adj Tx for localized (but >T1a) GB cancer?

Single-institution retrospective series suggest that **adj 5-FU–based CRT** may benefit resected GB cancer pts. (*Kresl JJ et al., IJROBP 2002; Ben-David MA et al., IJROBP 2006; Czito BG et al., IJROBP 2005; Yu JB et al., JCO 2008; Gold DJ et al., IJROBP 2009*)

What is the range of MS in studies of adj RT or CRT for GB cancer?

MS ranges from 23–58 mos in retrospective studies of adj treatment in resected GB cancer.

What is the treatment approach for localized, unresectable GB cancer?

The approach is similar to unresectable pancreatic cancer: a combination of systemic chemo alone and/or CRT. Gemcitabine and cisplatin is the reference systemic regimen.

What is the recommended adj Tx for localized, resectable CC with good PS?

Single-institution series suggest that **5-FU or gemcitabine based CRT** is an appropriate adj Tx for localized resectable CC (*Hughes MA et al., IJROBP 2007; Nelson JW et al., IJROBP 2009; Shinohara T et al., IJROBP 2008; Kim TH et al., IJROBP 2011*). This is also appropriate for unresectable CC. (*Pitt HA et al., Ann Surg 1995*)

What is the recommended Tx for localized, unresectable CC?

A combination of chemo alone and CRT is recommended for definitive treatment of unresectable CC. (*Urego M et al., IJROBP 1999; Leong E et al., J GI Cancer 2012; Morganti AG et al., IJROBP 2000; Crane CH et al., IJROBP 2002; Ben-David MA et al., IJROBP 2006*)

What is the range of MS in studies of adj RT or CRT for hilar or extrahepatic CC?

MS ranges from 20–37 mos in studies of adj Tx in resected hilar and extrahepatic CC.

What RT approaches have been used for adj and definitive treatment of CC?

EBRT (most common), intraoperative RT, intraluminal brachytherapy, combination brachytherapy and EBRT, and more recently hypofractionated RT and SBRT.

Define target structures and doses for adjuvant treatment for hilar/extrahepatic CC.

The CTV is defined by the **LN basin** (initial volume, **45 Gy** in 1.8 Gy/fx) and **surgical bed** (boost volume, **5–15 Gy,** depending on extent of resection). LN basin includes porta hepatis, hepatic artery, pancreaticoduodenal, celiac, and superior mesenteric artery LNs. Inferior aortocaval nodes are often omitted.

Define target structures and doses for adj Tx for intrahepatic CC and GB cancer.

Same as above, except for GB cancer and intrahepatic CC, and LN basin **includes pericholedochal LNs.** For intrahepatic CC, LN basin may be limited to pericholedochal LNs if LN dissection was negative at surgery.

What is the appropriate target and dose for definitive RT of CC and GB cancer?

For hilar/extrahepatic CC, the CTV includes the gross Dz + margin and the LN basin (controversial). For intrahepatic CC and GB cancer, the CTV includes the gross Dz + margin only. Gross Dz is treated to the highest dose possible, considering organs at risk, usually ~60 Gy in 1.8–2 Gy/fx.

Is liver transplantation more appropriate for intrahepatic CC or for extrahepatic CC?

Although liver transplantation is generally considered to be contraindicated for intrahepatic CC (due to poor outcomes), single-institution studies show promising results for transplantation in well-selected, early-stage, hilar/**extrahepatic** Dz. (*Rea DJ et al., Ann Surg 2005*)

Describe the clinical scenarios for consideration of SBRT.

Safety and efficacy of SBRT for liver lesions has been shown in mets and hepatic CC. Retrospective studies have reported feasibility of SBRT for hilar CC, and some intrahepatic CC, +/– concurrent gemcitabine or FU-based chemo. Dose and fractionation were 30 Gy in 3 fx (with gemcitabine) to 45 Gy in 3 fx (no chemo). (*Polistina FA et al., Radiother Oncol 2011; Kopek N et al., Radiother Oncol 2010*)

What are the transarterial treatment approaches for CC and in which Dz subset have they been utilized?

Transarterial embolization, chemoembolization, and radioembolization have been studied in unresectable intrahepatic CC. A large retrospective study examined each of these modalities in 198 pts with unresectable intrahepatic CC. (*Hyder O et al., Ann Surg Oncol 2013*) MS was 13.2 mos.

Which vessel is used to radioembolize liver tumors and why?

The **hepatic artery** is used for embolization because it is the major blood supply to liver tumors, unlike normal liver tissue, which derives its blood supply primarily from the portal vein.

What is the most used radioisotope for radioembolization in CC? What are its properties?

Yttrium-90 labeled spheres made of glass or resin are used for radioembolization. Yttrium-90 undergoes β-**decay,** with a half-life of 64 hrs (2.7 days).

 TOXICITY

For issues related to toxicity, please refer to the Hepatocellular Carcinoma section.

51 Colorectal and Small Bowel Cancer

Updated by Richard Tuli

What is the incidence of rectal cancer in the U.S.?

34,000 cases/yr of rectal cancer in the U.S.

What is the median age for rectal cancer?

The median age for rectal cancer is the **7th decade** of life.

What is the incidence of colon cancer in the U.S.?

The incidence of colon cancer in the U.S. is 180,000 cases/yr and is the **# 2 cause of cancer deaths in the U.S.** after lung cancer.

What is the median age for sporadic colon cancer?

The median age for sporadic colon cancer is **63 yrs.**

What is the sup/cranial extent of the rectum, and how long is it?

The rectum begins at **S3** and is **~15 cm** long.

What are the most common sites of mets in rectal cancer?

Rectal cancer metastasizes mostly to the **liver** (via the sup rectal vein) → and the lung.

Where in the GI tract does small bowel cancer most frequently arise?

Small bowel cancer arises most frequently in the **duodenum** (duodenum > jejunum > ileum).

What type of adenomas are more likely to progress to invasive rectal cancer?

Villous adenomas are more likely to progress to invasive rectal cancer (than tubular adenomas).

How are average-risk individuals defined as far as colorectal cancer is concerned?

Average-risk colorectal individuals are **≥50 yo asymptomatic pts without a family Hx** of colorectal cancer.

What are the colorectal cancer screening options for average-risk individuals?

Colonoscopy (q10yrs), fecal occult blood test (q1yr), and sigmoidoscopy (q5yrs) or double-contrast barium enema (q5yrs) are the colorectal screening options for average-risk individuals.

How frequently should individuals with inflammatory bowel Dz (IBD) have a screening colonoscopy?

Individuals with IBD should undergo a screening colonoscopy **every 1–2 yrs.**

How frequently should individuals with a family Hx of colorectal cancer have a screening colonoscopy? When should screening begin for such individuals?

Individuals with a family Hx of colorectal cancer should have a colonoscopy **every 1–5 yrs** and should begin screening at **age 40 yrs or 10 yrs prior to the earliest cancer Dx in the family.**

What are the dietary risk factors for developing colorectal cancer?

Risk factors for colorectal cancer include a diet **rich in fat and low in fiber and antioxidants.**

Is smoking a risk factor for colorectal cancer?

Yes. Smoking is a risk factor for colorectal cancer. (*Stürmer T et al., J Natl Cancer Inst 2000*)

Which supplements and which drug have shown promise as chemopreventative agents in colorectal cancer?

Calcium, vitamin D, and folic acid supplementation have shown some benefit in preventing colorectal cancer, while **aspirin** administration has been associated with a lower risk of developing colorectal polyps.

What are 2 common familial/heritable risk factors for developing colorectal cancer?

The 2 most common familial conditions associated with colorectal cancer are **familial adenomatous polyposis** (FAP) and **HNPCC** (aka Lynch syndrome).

What % of colorectal cancer cases are attributable to HNPCC?

5% of colorectal cancer cases are attributable to HNPCC.

What 2 familial syndromes, other than FAP and HNPCC, have been associated with a higher risk for developing colon cancer?

Cowden syndrome and **Gardner syndrome** predispose pts to developing colon cancer (in addition to other cancers).

Initial mutation of what tumor suppressor gene leads to a greater chance for developing colorectal cancer? With what familial condition is this mutation associated?

Initial mutation in the adenomatous polyposis coli (*APC*) tumor suppressor gene leads to a higher chance for developing colorectal cancer; this mutation is also associated with **FAP.**

Mutation of what oncogene leads to a greater chance for developing colorectal cancer?

Initial mutation in the **K-ras** oncogene leads to a higher chance for developing colorectal cancer.

Most familial HNPCC cases have been associated with mutations in what genes? What do these genes regulate?

Most familial cases identified as HNPCC have been associated with mutations in the *hMLH1* or *hMSH2* gene, which **regulate mismatch repair.**

Pts with what chronic inflammatory condition are at an ~20-fold increased risk for developing colorectal cancer?

Pts with **ulcerative colitis** are at an ~20-fold increased risk for developing colorectal cancer.

▶ **WORKUP/STAGING**

What is the most common presenting Sx in rectal cancer?

Hematochezia is the most common presenting Sx in rectal cancer.

What must the physical exam include for pts with suspected rectal cancer?

The physical must include DRE and pelvic exam for women.

How is the Dx of rectal cancer typically established?

Endoscopic Bx is a typical way of establishing the Dx. A full colonoscopy should be performed to r/o more proximal lesions.

What studies are performed in the workup of rectal cancer pts, and what is the purpose of each modality?

For staging purposes, EUS or pelvic MRI must be performed in rectal cancer pts for T and N staging. **To r/o met Dz, CT C/A/P** with IV and oral contrast is performed.

What labs are collected as part of the staging workup for colorectal cancers?

Labs for the workup of colorectal cancer: **CBC, chem 7, LFTs, CEA**

Is a PET scan routinely indicated for pts with rectal cancer?

No. A PET scan is not routinely indicated in pts with localized rectal cancer.

What is the AJCC 7th edition (2011) T staging for colorectal cancer?

The T staging for rectal cancer is based on the DOI:
Tis: CIS or invasion into lamina propria
T1: invades submucosa
T2: invades muscularis propria
T3: invades through muscularis and into pericolorectal tissues
T4a: penetrates surface of visceral peritoneum
T4b: invades or adheres to adjacent organs

What is the AJCC 7th edition (2011) N staging for colorectal cancer?

In the 2002 edition of AJCC, N1 designated involvement of 1–3 regional LNs, whereas N2 designated involvement of ≥4 LNs.
In the **AJCC 7th edition,** N1 and N2 are further broken down:
N1a: mets to 1 regional LN
N1b: mets to 2–3 regional LNs

N1c: tumor deposits in subserosa, mesentery, or nonperitonealized pericolic or perirectal tissues *without* regional LN mets

N2a: mets to 4–6 LNs

N2b: mets to ≥7 LNs

What is the AJCC 7th edition (2011) breakdown of M staging for colorectal cancer?

M1a: DMs to a single organ or site (e.g., liver, lung, ovary, nonregional LNs)

M1b: mets >1 organ/site or deposits in peritoneum

What are the AJCC 7th edition (2011) TNM stage groupings for colorectal cancer?

Stage I: T1-2N0

Stage IIA: T3N0

Stage IIB: T4aN0

Stage IIC: T4bN0

Stage IIIA: T1-2N1 or N1c; T1N2a

Stage IIIB: T3-4aN1 or N1c; T2-3N2a; T1-2N2b

Stage IIIC: T4aN2a; T3-4aN2b; T4bN1-2

Stage IVA: TXNXM1a

Stage IVB: TXNXM1b

How does the old Dukes staging for colorectal cancers correspond to the current AJCC staging system?

Dukes A: stage I

Dukes B: stage II

Dukes C: any nodal involvement (or stage III)

What is the AJCC 7th edition (2011) T staging for small intestine cancers?

Tis: CIS

T1a: invades lamina propria

T1b: invades through mucosa into submucosa

T2: invades into muscularis propria

T3: invades through muscularis propria into subserosa or into mesentery/retroperitoneum ≤2 cm

T4*: perforates visceral peritoneum or invades adjacent organs (including other loops of small bowel, mesentery or retroperitoneum >2 cm, and abdominal wall (extension from serosa)

Note: For the duodenum, invasion into pancreas or bile duct constitutes T4.

What are the AJCC 7th edition (2011) N and M staging for small intestine cancers?

N0: no regional LNs

N1: mets to 1–3 LNs

N2: ≥4 LNs

M0: no DM

M1: DMs

What are the AJCC 7th edition (2011) stage groupings for small intestine cancers?

Stage 0: Tis

Stage I: T1-2N0

Stage IIA: T3N0

Stage IIB: T4N0

Stage IIIA: TxN1

Stage IIIB: TXN2

Stage IV: TXNXM1

What special laboratory test is routinely performed for colorectal cancer pts? Why?

CEA is routinely ordered for pts with colorectal cancer b/c it may help monitor response to therapy and Dz progression.

Describe the CEA trends for colorectal cancer pts after surgery and in the setting of a relapse.

Postresection for colorectal cancer, CEA levels should return to reference range in 4–6 wks. CEA increases 4–6 mos before a recurrence are clinically apparent (a rapid rise suggests hepatic or bony mets, while a slow rise suggests LR).

What is the most powerful predictor of LN involvement in rectal cancer?

The most powerful predictor of LN involvement in rectal cancer is **DOI.**

What % of T1 rectal cancer pts have micrometastatic Dz in the LNs that is undetectable by current imaging techniques?

Up to 15% of T1 rectal cancer pts have micrometastatic Dz in the LNs undetectable by imaging.

▶ **TREATMENT/PROGNOSIS**

What is the Tx paradigm for nonmet rectal cancer?

Nonmet rectal cancer Tx paradigm: in general, T1-2N0 rectal cancer pts get upfront surgery +/– adj CRT, whereas T3-4 or N+ pts should rcv neoadj CRT → surgery and adj 5-FU/leucovorin or FOLFOX.

What are the surgical options for rectal cancer pts?

The surgical options for rectal cancer include **transanal excision** (local excision), or transabdominal resection (abdominoperineal resection [**APR**] for low-lying lesions, or low anterior resection [**LAR**] for mid/upper-lying lesions).

What are the criteria for transanal excision alone in rectal cancer? On what 2 studies is this based?

The criteria for transanal excision alone in rectal cancer include T1 lesion, ≤3-cm tumor that is superficial (<3 mm submucosal depth), lesion involving less than or equal to one-third of rectal circumference, N0 by EUS or MRI, low-grade tumor/no LVI, negative margins, and reliable pt.

CALGB 89-84 (*Steel GD et al., Ann Surg Oncol 1999*): phases I–II intergroup trial that treated all T1 or T2 Dz with local excision. Eligibility were tumor ≤4 cm, <10 cm from anal verge, <40% bowel circumference, and at least 2-mm-deep margin. T1 Dz had surgery alone, and T2 Dz all rcvd adj CRT. 6-yr OS was 85%–87%, and the LF rates were 4% (T1) and 14% (T2).

RTOG 82-02 (*Russell AH et al., IJROBP 2000*): same eligibility criteria as CALGB 89-84, phase II, all transanal excision. T1 lesions ≤3 cm, >3-mm margins, well to moderately differentiated tumors, no LVI; normal CEA levels were observed after surgery. Pts with T1 with poor risk features and all T2-3N0 pts rcvd adj CRT (5-FU). 5-yr OS was 78%, with LF rates of 4% (T1), 16% (T2), and 23% (T3).

For pts who cannot have a definitive transabdominal resection, what are the indications for adj CRT after transanal excision of rectal cancer?

For pts who cannot have a definitive transabdominal resection, adj CRT alone should be administered to pts with a poor-risk T1 lesion after local excision (poorly differentiated, with bad histologies, margins <3 mm, >3-cm size, and +LVSI); all T2 cancer after local excision; and for all T3-4 or N+ cancers after LAR or APR. Low-risk T1 tumors after local excision do not need adj therapy.

What definitive transabdominal surgical approach for rectal cancer permits sphincter preservation?

LAR spares the sphincter and is therefore a preferred surgical option (if feasible) for rectal cancer pts; in contrast, APR requires a colostomy.

What is the pattern of failure for rectal cancer historically after surgery alone?

For rectal cancer, the pattern of failure after surgery is primarily **locoregional.**

What is the approximate LR rate for T3-4 or N1 rectal cancer after surgery alone?

The historic LR rate for T3-4 or N1 rectal cancer is ~25%. This is improved with better surgery (i.e., total mesorectal excision [TME], LR 11% [Dutch TME study]).

What is the significance of a positive circumferential margin at the time of surgery for rectal cancer?

A positive circumferential margin predicts for inferior LC, DM, and OS rates after surgery for rectal cancer based on meta-analysis. (*Nagtegaal ID et al., JCO 2008*)

What kind of surgical technique is currently standard in the surgical management of rectal cancer? Why is this important?

TME is a standard surgical technique in the operative management of rectal cancer and is carried out with LAR or APR. It **helps reduce the rate of positive radial margins and improves LC.**

What are the indications for adj CRT after definitive transabdominal resection for rectal cancer?

After a definitive transabdominal resection (LAR or APR—TME or non-TME based) for rectal cancer, adj CRT is indicated **if the pathology is node+ or ≥T3.**

What are some options for rectal cancer pts with solitary or oligometastatic Dz to the liver that is resectable?

Surgical resection of the metastatic site is the only modality with proven survival benefit. How these cases should be managed needs to be determined on a case-by-case basis in a multidisciplinary setting. Some options for oligometastatic (resectable) rectal cancer include:

1. Induction chemo → restaging → resection of the mets → CRT to primary → LAR if possible +/− additional chemo
2. If the pt is symptomatic, consider preop CRT or short-course RT (5 Gy × 5) as done in Europe → surgery of both primary and metastatic site → adj chemo (FOLFOX/Avastin)

What % of rectal cancer pts are technically resectable at presentation?

80% of rectal cancer pts are technically resectable at presentation.

What are the most commonly used sensitizing chemo regimens given with RT for rectal cancer?

Continuous infusion 5-FU (225–250 mg/m^2/day) or capecitabine (Xeloda) 825 mg/m^2 bid 5–7 days/wk are commonly used sensitizing chemo regimens.

What are the data addressing adj RT alone in rectal cancer, and what do they show?

There are many RCTs (e.g., MRC **3, NSABP R-01**) that investigated adj RT alone, showing **improvement in LC only** but **no** improvement in OS, DFS, or MFS); this was confirmed by a meta-analysis. (*CCCG, Lancet 2001*)

What major studies established a role for adj CRT in rectal cancer?

Gastro-Intestinal Study Group **GITSG 7175** (*GITSG collaborators, NEJM 1985; Thomas PR et al., Radiother Oncol 1988*) randomized pts after surgery to observation, chemo alone, RT alone, or CRT and found that adj CRT in rectal cancer significantly improved OS (45% vs. 27% at 10 yrs) and LF rates (10% vs. 25%) when compared with surgery alone.

Intergroup/NCCTG 79-47-51 (*Krook JE et al., NEJM 1991*) randomized stages II–III rectal cancer pts to RT alone or CRT (5-FU × 2 > 5-FU + RT > 5-FU × 2) after surgery (50% APR). 5-yr LR, DM, and OS were better for CRT (LR: 14% vs. 25%; DM: 29% vs. 46%; OS: 55% vs. 45%). There was worse acute grades 3–4 diarrhea (20% vs. 5%) but no late complications for the CRT arm.

What are some major criticisms of the rectal cancer trial GITSG 7175?

GITSG 7175 is criticized b/c it was underpowered, 5-FU was given by bolus with semustine (which causes leukemias), randomization was unequal, and there was no intention-to-treat analysis.

Which studies demonstrated that semustine is not a necessary component of CRT in rectal cancer?

GITSG 7180 and **NCCTG 86-47-51** demonstrated that semustine is not a necessary component of CRT in rectal cancer.

Which study compared preop RT with postop RT (without chemo) in rectal cancer?

The **Swedish Uppsala trial** (*Frykholm GJ et al., Dis Colon Rectum 1993*) compared adj to neoadj RT in rectal cancer and found no OS benefit but improved LR rates (13% vs. 22%) and lower SBO rates (5% vs. 11%) with preop RT.

Which study compared surgery alone with preop RT in rectal cancer? What did it find, and what were its limitations?

The **Swedish Rectal Cancer trial** (*NEJM 1997*) compared neoadj RT (25 Gy in 5 fx) to surgery alone in rectal cancer and found a significant **improvement in OS** (38% vs. 30%) and LR (9% vs. 26%) at 13 yrs with neoadj RT. The trial is often criticized b/c TME was not used and there was a high recurrence rate for the surgery-alone arm (26%).

Can the use of TME obviate the need for neoadj RT for rectal cancer?

No. TME does not offset the benefit of neoadj RT based on the Dutch TME study. (*Peeters KC et al., Ann Surg 2007*) The study compared TME alone to neoadj RT and TME and found no OS benefit, but there was an improved LR rate (6% vs. 11%) with the addition of neoadj RT.

What was the RT dose/fx scheme in the Dutch and Swedish rectal cancer studies? How long after the completion of RT do pts go to surgery?

Both the Dutch and Swedish rectal cancer studies used neoadj RT in **25 Gy in 5 fx** (5 Gy × 5). Pts typically underwent surgical resection **within 1 wk** of RT completion.

What were the arms in the MRC CR07/NCIC C016 rectal cancer study, and what were its main findings?

The **MRC CR07/NCIC C016** rectal cancer study (*Sebag-Montefiore D et al., Lancet 2009*) randomized pts to preop RT (25 Gy in 5 fx) vs. selective postop CRT (45 Gy in 25 fx) and found better outcomes with preop RT in terms of LR (4% vs. 11%, SS) and DFS (77% vs. 71%, SS). OS was similar at 4-yr follow-up. A short neoadj RT course is an acceptable option.

Is neoadjuvant short course RT an acceptable alternative to standard CRT for locally advanced rectal cancer?

The Trans-Tasman Radiation Oncology Group TROG 01.04 randomized locally advanced rectal cancer pts to neoadjuvant short course (SC) RT (5 Gy × 5) and early surgery vs. standard CRT (50.4 Gy + 5-FU 225 mg/m^2/d) and surgery in 4–6 wks. 3-yr LRR were 7.5% SC and 4.4% CRT (= 0.24), 5-yr OS was 74% SC and 70% CRT, and late toxicity rates were not different.

Which major European rectal cancer study compared neoadj CRT to adj CRT and what were its findings?

The **German Rectal Cancer trial** (*Sauer R et al., NEJM 2004*) compared preop to postop CRT in T3-4 or node+ rectal cancer (RT was to 50.4 Gy for the neoadj arm and 55.8 Gy for the postop arm with 5-FU chemo (CI 5-FU days 1–5 at 1000 mg/day, wks 1 and 5). All pts rcvd 4 additional cycles of bolus 5-FU (500 mg/m^2/day, days 1–5, q4wks) at 4 wks after completion of initial therapy. The study found a similar 5-yr OS and DFS between the 2 arms but better LR rates (6% vs. 13%), fewer acute (27% vs. 40%) and late toxicities (14% vs. 24%), and better sphincter-preservation rates (39% vs. 19%) in the preop CRT arm. Most of the acute and late toxicities were esp b/c of acute/chronic diarrhea and anastomotic stricture. A recent update confirmed persistent benefit in LRR (7.1% vs. 10.1%, $p = 0.05$) with no significant differences in DM rates and DFS. (*Sauer R et al., JCO 2012*)

What is the pathologic CR rate for preop CRT for rectal cancer?

According to the German Rectal Cancer trial, the **pCR rate is 8%.**

What % of pts receiving neoadj CRT will be overtreated b/c of having stage I Dz instead of the presumed more advanced Dz?

~18% of pts will be overtreated with neoadj CRT b/c of an apparent stage I Dz. This is based on the results of the postop arm of the German Rectal Cancer trial, where 18% of the pts did not rcv postop CRT b/c of T1-2N0 Dz found at resection. All of these pts were thought to have T3-4 or node+ Dz based on EUS.

What was a major criticism of the German Rectal Cancer trial (*Sauer R et al., NEJM 2004*)?

A major criticism of the German Rectal Cancer trial (*Sauer R et al., NEJM 2004*) was that **only 54% of adj pts rcvd a full RT dose** (vs. 92% in the neoadj arm).

Did pts in the German Rectal Cancer trial have TME as part of their surgery?

Yes. All pts in the German Rectal Cancer trial (*Sauer R et al., NEJM 2004*) had TME at the time of surgery.

What was the sphincter-preservation rate in the neoadj CRT arm in the German Rectal Cancer trial (*Sauer R et al., NEJM 2004*)?

The sphincter-preservation rate in the neoadj CRT arm in the German Rectal Cancer trial (*Sauer R et al., NEJM 2004*) was **39% at 5 yrs** (compared with 19% in the postop CRT arm).

How long after neoadj CRT should surgery be performed for rectal cancer? Why is this done?

Surgery should be performed **~6–8 wks** after neoadj CRT for rectal cancer to allow for adequate **downstaging.**

How long after surgery should adj CRT be initiated for rectal cancer?

Adj CRT for rectal cancer should begin **4–6 wks** after surgery.

What did all pts in the German Rectal Cancer trial (*Sauer R et al., NEJM 2004*) rcv after either surgery (neoadj CRT arm) or CRT (adj arm)?

All pts in the German Rectal Cancer trial (*Sauer R et al., NEJM 2004*) rcvd 4–5 cycles of **bolus 5-FU** (500 mg/m^2/day, days 1–5, q4wks) 4 wks after either surgery (neoadj CRT arm) or CRT (adj arm).

Which 2 major randomized studies compared neoadj RT to neoadj CRT in rectal cancer, and what did they find? How was CRT delivered in both studies? What was a major limitation of these trials?

The **French FFCD 9203** (*Gerard JP et al., JCO 2006*) and **EORTC 22921** (*Bosset JF et al., NEJM 2006*) compared neoadj RT with neoadj CRT in rectal cancer. The French study found no OS difference but did find improved LR with neoadj CRT at 5 yrs (8% vs. 16%, SS). The EORTC study also found no OS difference and improved LR with neoadj CRT at 5 yrs (9% vs. 17%). Grades 3–4 acute toxicity was higher in the CRT vs. RT arms. Both trials used neoadj CRT with 45 Gy (1.8) and 5-FU (350 mg/m^2/day, wks 1 and 5 of RT). A small% of pts actually rcvd adj CT (EORTC: 43%).

How should rectal cancer pts be simulated in preparation for RT?

Rectal cancer pts should undergo CT simulation **in the prone position, on a belly board, and with a full bladder** (with optional placement of anal/vaginal markers and/or rectal contrast).

What structures should be encompassed within the RT field for rectal cancer?

For rectal cancer, the **tumor bed** (+ 2–5-cm margin) and **presacral/internal iliac nodes** should be included in the RT fields.

What additional nodal chain needs to be covered in the RT fields with T4 rectal cancer?

The **external iliac nodes** need to be encompassed for T4 rectal lesions (invasion of bladder, vagina, uterus, but may not be necessary for bony sacrum invasion).

What RT fields are generally employed for rectal cancer?

Whole pelvis fields (3 fields) with a PA field and 2 opposed lat fields are typically employed for rectal cancer.

What are the RT doses for rectal cancer?

RT doses for rectal cancer:
Neoadj/postop: initial whole pelvis (3 field) to 45 Gy in 1.8 Gy/fx; CD to tumor bed +2–3 cm (opposed lats only, or 3D-CRT) to **50.4 Gy (preop)** (or **55.8 Gy (postop)** if the small bowel is out of the way)
Definitive/unresectable: initial to 45 Gy, CD1 to 50.4 Gy; consider CD2 with conformal RT to **54–59.4 Gy** (if dose to the small bowel is limited)

Describe the anatomic boundaries of the RT fields for rectal cancer.

Anatomic boundaries for the RT fields in rectal cancer:

Posterior-anterior: sup at L5-S1, inf at bottom of ischial tuberosity or 3 cm below tumor volume, lat at 1.5 cm from pelvic inlet

Laterals: 1 cm post behind entire bony sacrum, ant behind pubic symphysis for T3 (in front if T4), sup-inf same as PA; blocks applied to spare small bowel

Which border is not altered for the CD fields in the Tx of rectal cancer?

The **post border on the lat fields** usually stays the same (behind the bony sacrum) for the CD portion of the RT for rectal cancer given the high rate of LR in this region.

When is IORT indicated for rectal cancer, and what is the dose?

IORT should be considered in rectal cancer for **close/+margins or as an additional boost,** esp with T4 tumors or with recurrent tumors. The typical dose is **10–15 Gy** to the 90% IDL.

What study showed a benefit with IORT in colorectal cancer?

A retrospective study from Mayo by *Gunderson et al.* evaluated IORT in addition to EBRT and found improved OS and LR rates with addition of IORT (10–20 Gy) when compared with historical controls. (*IJROBP 1997*)

When can RT be considered in colon cancer? When is it given in relation to surgery and to what dose?

RT can be considered **for fixed T4 colon cancer lesions or with a close/+margin.** RT is typically **given after resection/debulking to a dose of 45–50.4 Gy.**

What major study investigated the role of adj RT in colon cancer? What did it find? What was the limitation of this study?

The **Intergroup 0130** study (*Martenson JA Jr et al., JCO 2004*) compared adj chemo to adj CRT in colon cancer and found no difference in OS or LC with addition of RT. This study was underpowered to show a difference between groups.

Which randomized study investigated the role of elective para-aortic (P-A) RT in rectal cancer? What did it conclude?

The **EORTC trial by** *Bosset et al.* evaluated the role of elective P-A RT in rectal cancer (25 Gy to LNs and liver) and found no benefit in terms of OS, DFS, or LC. (*Radiother Oncol 2001*)

What is the Tx paradigm for small bowel cancer, and what is the role of adj chemo and/or RT?

Small bowel cancer Tx paradigm: resection → 5-FU–based chemo. CRT is considered in cases of close/+margins, but retrospective studies have found no convincing benefit. (e.g., *Kelsey CR et al., IJROBP 2007*)

Why did NSABP R-03 (*Roh MS et al., JCO 2009*) close prematurely, and what were its findings?

NSABP R-03 closed prematurely b/c of poor accrual. It randomized T3-4 or node+ rectal cancer pts to neoadj CRT vs. postop CRT (5-FU based). There was improved 5-yr DFS (65% vs. 53%, SS) with neoadj CRT but no difference in LR or OS. The pCR rate was 15%.

Is there a role for IMRT in the treatment for rectal cancer?

RTOG 0822, a single arm phase II study, investigated neoadjuvant XELOX (capecitabine plus oxaliplatin) with IMRT for pts with locally advanced rectal cancer with a primary endpoint of grade ≥2 GI toxicity using RTOG 0247 for historical comparison. Preliminary data reported at ASTRO 2011 showed no statistically significant benefit (51% vs. 58%, $p = 0.3$). *Zhu et al.* utilized a similar regimen (XELOX plus IMRT) in a single arm prospective study of 42 pts and noted grade 3 hematologic, GI, and skin toxicities of 4.7%, 14.3%, and 26.2%, respectively. Grade 4 toxicity was not observed.

▶ TOXICITY

How does the toxicity of CI 5-FU differ from that of bolus administration?

Bolus administration of **5-FU confers greater hematologic toxicity,** whereas **CI confers greater GI toxicity.** (*Smalley SR et al., JCO 2006*)

What was a major late complication of neoadj RT in the Swedish Rectal Cancer trial?

SBO was more likely in the neoadj RT arm in the Swedish Rectal Cancer trial (RR 2.5) (*Birgisson H et al., Br J Surg 2008*), and may be a limitation of a hypofractionated regimen (5 Gy × 5).

What 3 toxicities were worse with neoadj RT in the Swedish Rectal Cancer trial?

Median bowel movement frequency (20 movements/wk vs. 10 movements/wk, SS), fecal incontinence (62% vs. 27%, SS), and impaired social life (30% vs. 10%, SS) were worse in the neoadj RT arm when compared with surgery alone in the Swedish Rectal Cancer trial.

What should the small bowel RT dose be limited to in rectal cancer?

The small bowel dose should be limited to **45 Gy** in the Tx of rectal cancer.

What does the post-Tx surveillance include for colorectal cancer?

Post-Tx rectal cancer surveillance: H&P q3–6 mos for 2 yrs (then q6 mos for 5 yrs) and CEA on same schedule for ≥T2 lesions. CT C/A/P is performed q1yr for 3 yrs and colonoscopy at 1 yr (then in 3 yrs, then every 5 yrs if normal vs. annually if abnl/suspicious).

Which retrospective study found comparable Tx results/toxicity with RT in rectal cancer pts with IBD?

A **Mt. Sinai study by *Green et al.*** found comparable Tx results/toxicity with RT in rectal cancer pts with IBD. (*IJROBP 1999*)

| How long after conventional RT can side effects develop, and what are some common side effects of RT? | Signs and Sx can occur as early as **6–18 mos** following RT. Frequent Sx include diarrhea (bloody), colicky abdominal pain, and n/v. Less common are SBO, fistulas, bowel perforation, and severe bleeding. Bowel malabsorption may occur with weight loss. Damage to the ileum can impair resorption of vitamin B_{12} and bile acid with steatorrhea as a consequence. (*Guckenberger et al., Int J Colorectal Dis 2006*) |
| What are some dose limiting structures? | Small bowel: ≤45 Gy, small volume can go to 50.4 Gy
 Femoral heads: ≤45 Gy |

52 Anal Cancer
Updated by Richard Tuli

▶ BACKGROUND

What is the incidence of anal cancer in the U.S.?	**~7,000 cases/yr** in the U.S.
Is there a sex predilection for anal cancer?	**Yes.** Anal cancer is more common in **females** than males (2:1).
What are some risk factors for anal cancer?	Hx of STDs/anal warts; multiple sexual partners (>10); anal-receptive intercourse; immunodeficiency (HIV, solid organ transplantation); smoking; Hx of cervical, vulvar, or vaginal cancer (HPV)
Is anal cancer an AIDS-defining illness?	**No.** However, the demographically adjusted rate ratio for HIV infected men and women relative to uninfected cohorts is 80 and 30, respectively. Cervical cancer is an AIDS-defining illness.
What is the predominant histology of anal cancer?	**Squamous cell carcinoma** (75%–80%) is the predominant histology.
What virus strains are strongly associated with anal cancer?	HPV strains **16, 18, 31, 33, and 35** are strongly associated with anal cancer. Anal cancers are associated with HPV infection in 75%–90% of cases, with HPV16 the most common subtype.

How long is the anal canal, and where does it extend?

The anal canal is **4-cm long,** extending distally from the anal verge (palpable junction between the internal sphincter and subcutaneous part of the external sphincter, aka the intersphincteric groove) to the anorectal ring (where the rectum enters the puborectalis sling) proximally.

What is the histopathologic significance of the dentate line (aka pectinate line)?

The dentate line is the anatomic site where mucosa changes from nonkeratinized squamous epithelium distally to colorectal-type columnar mucosa proximally (dividing the upper from the lower anal canal).

Describe the anatomic location of the anal verge.

The anal verge is located at the junction of nonkeratinized squamous epithelium of the anal canal and keratinized squamous epithelium (true epidermis) of perianal skin.

Which site carries a better prognosis: the anal margin or anal canal?

The **anal margin** carries a better prognosis.

Which pathology carries a higher risk for local and distant recurrence?

Adenocarcinoma carries a higher risk.

What is the significance of the dentate line in terms of LN drainage?

Above dentate line: drains to pudendal/hypogastric/obturator/hemorrhoidal → internal iliac nodes

Below dentate line: drains to inguinal/femoral nodes → external iliacs

What % of anal cancer pts present with +LNs?

25%–35% of these pts present with +LNs.

What are the 2 most common sites of DM?

Liver and lung

What is the occult positivity rate for inguinal nodes (i.e., if clinically–) in anal cancer?

For inguinal nodes, the occult positivity rate is **10%–15%.**

What is the rate of extrapelvic visceral mets at presentation for anal cancer?

Extrapelvic visceral mets are present in **5%–10%** of pts.

In anal cancer, what % of clinically palpable LNs are actually involved by cancer?

50% of clinically palpable LNs involve cancer, while the other 50% are usually reactive hyperplasia.

In anal cancers, what are the most important prognostic factors for LC and survival?

Tumor size and DOI predict for LC. The **extent of inguinal or pelvic LN involvement** predicts for survival.

▶ **WORKUP/STAGING**

What are 4 common presenting Sx in anal cancer?

Bleeding, pain/sensation of mass, rectal urgency, and pruritus

What does the workup for anal cancer pts include?

Anal cancer workup: H&P (including gyn exam for women with cervical cancer screening), labs (HIV if risk factors), imaging, Bx of lesion, and FNA of suspicious LN

What imaging studies are typically done for anal cancer pts?

Transanal US (to assess for perirectal nodes/assess invasion), CXR or CT chest with IV contrast, CT abdomen/pelvis with IV and oral contrast, and PET/CT

Is PET/CT more or less sensitive than diagnostic CT alone for detecting locoregional and met Dz?

Mistrangelo M et al. (*IJROBP 2012*) found PET/CT to be superior to CT in detecting the primary tumor (89% vs. 75%); *Bhuva NJ et al.* also found PET/CT diagnosed occult metastatic Dz following CT imaging in 5% of pts and changed staging in 42% of pts, with the majority being upstaged. (*Ann Oncol 2012*)

What features of anal lesions need to be appreciated on physical exam? Why?

The **degree of circumferential involvement and anal sphincter tone** should be appreciated, b/c these **may dictate Tx.**

What is the approach to suspicious inguinal LNs in anal cancer pts?

FNA Bx should be performed for suspicious inguinal LNs.

On what is the T staging for anal cancer based? Define T1-T4.

T staging as per AJCC 7th edition for anal cancer is based on the **size of the lesion.**
  T1: ≤2 cm
  T2: >2–5 cm
  T3: >5 cm
  T4: invasion of adjacent organs (vagina, urethra, bladder)

Does tumor invasion of sphincter muscle by anal cancer constitute a T4 lesion?

No. Direct invasion of the rectal wall, perirectal skin, subcutaneous tissue, or sphincter muscle are *not* classified as T4.

Most pts with anal cancer present with what T stage?

Most anal cancer pts present at stage **T2 or T3.**

What is the N staging of isolated perirectal nodal involvement in anal cancer?

Isolated perirectal nodal involvement is staged as **N1.**

What is the N staging of unilat inguinal or internal iliac LNs in anal cancer?	Unilat inguinal or internal iliac LNs are staged as **N2.**
What N stage is an anal cancer pt with both perirectal and inguinal LNs?	Perirectal and inguinal LNs reflect stage **N3.**
What N stage is an anal cancer pt with bilat inguinal or internal iliac LNs?	Bilat inguinal or internal iliac LNs reflect stage **N3.**
What anal cancer pts have AJCC stage III Dz?	**Node+ or T4 pts** have AJCC stage III Dz.
What is the AJCC 7th edition (2011) stage grouping for anal cancer?	**Stage I:** T1N0 **Stage II:** T2N0 or T3N0 **Stage IIIA:** T1-3N1 or T4N0 **Stage IIIB:** T4N1 or TXN2 or N3 **Stage IV:** TXNXM1
What are the 5-yr OS and LR rates after surgical resection alone for anal cancer?	The 5-yr OS rate after complete surgical resection is **~70%,** and the LR rate is **~40%.** (Mayo review of 118 pts: *Boman BM et al., Cancer 1984*)
What % of pts who relapse develop local recurrent Dz as part of the total failure pattern?	~80% develop local recurrent Dz. (*Boman BM et al., Cancer 1984. Note:* This was also a surgical series.)
What are the OS and sphincter preservation rates for all-comers with anal cancer at 5 yrs after definitive CRT?	**OS is ~70%** (**RTOG 9811**) and **sphincter preservation rate is 65%–75%** after CRT alone.

▶ TREATMENT/PROGNOSIS

What are the criteria for local excision alone in anal cancer? What are the LC rates in such carefully selected pts?	Small T1 lesion (<2 cm), well differentiated, –margins, <40% circumferential involvement, no sphincter involvement, compliant pts. For these well-selected pts, there is **>90% LC.** (*Boman BM et al., Cancer 1984*)
Can radiotherapy alone be employed for early-stage anal cancer?	**Yes.** However, it can be employed only for **T1N0** lesions. There were excellent LC rates of 100% and CR rates of 96% in 1 series. (*Deniaud-Alexandre E et al., IJROBP 2003*)

What was the standard surgical procedure for anal cancer before the advent of CRT? What was the disadvantage of this approach?

Abdominoperineal resection (APR) is the standard surgical procedure, but the disadvantage is that it **requires permanent colostomy.**

Currently, when should surgery alone be considered sufficient for management of anal cancer?

Surgery is sufficient **with anal margin cancers in which the sphincter can be spared.**

Historically, what has been the sphincter preservation approach for the Tx of anal cancers?

Radiotherapy alone was employed in Europe since the early 1900s, whereas surgical resection was standard in the U.S. Radiotherapy alone produced similar survival and control rates as surgery but allowed sphincter preservation. These results were better for less advanced tumors. *Papillon and Montbarbon* (*Dis Colon Rectum 1987*) reported (in the largest series of 159 pts with the use of EBRT and interstitial brachytherapy [30–42 Gy EBRT → implant 15–20 Gy]) a 5-yr OS of 65% and a sphincter preservation rate of 70%–82% (>4-cm tumor vs. <4-cm tumor).

What 2 seminal studies from the 1970s and 1980s in the U.S. demonstrated that surgical resection may not be needed after CRT, even after a short course of Tx?

The **Wayne State** experience (*Nigro ND et al., Dis Colon Rectum 1974, 1983*): preop regimen of **30 Gy/15 fx** with continuous infusion 5-FU (1000 mg/m^2 × 4 days) and mitomycin-C (MMC; 15 mg/m^2 bolus), with APR scheduled 6 wks after the regimen. 31 pts had completion surgery vs. 73 had definitive CRT alone. 71% pts had pCR in the surgical specimen. In the surgery arm, the follow-up NED rate was 79%. In the definitive CRT arm, the follow-up NED rate was 82%.
Princess Margaret Hospital (*Cummings BM et al., IJROBP 1991*): prospective nonrandomized studies comparing RT alone, 5-FU + RT, or 5-FU/MMC + RT. OS was 70% in all groups, with LC best in the 5-FU/MMC arm of 93% compared with 60% in the RT-alone arm.

What was the chemo regimen and RT dose delivered in the original anal cancer studies by *Nigro ND et al.*?

In *Nigro ND et al.*, the regimen was 5-FU (1,000 mg/m^2 × 4 days)/MMC (15 mg/m^2 bolus) with an RT dose of 30 Gy (2 Gy per fx). (*Dis Colon Rectum 1974, 1983*)

Anal margin tumors are treated like what other cancer?

Anal margin tumors are treated in the same manner as **skin cancer.**

What is the current Tx paradigm for anal canal cancer?

Anal cancer Tx paradigm: definitive CRT

What chemo doses are used in anal cancer, and what is the scheduling?

Anal cancer doses/scheduling: 5-FU 1000 mg/m^2/day intravenously on days 1–4 and 29–32; MMC 10 mg/m^2 intravenous bolus on days 1 and 29

What is the main radiobiologic advantage of MMC?

MMC is a **hypoxic cell radiosensitizer.**

For which pts is APR currently reserved?

APR is reserved as **salvage for pts who fail RT or those who have had prior pelvic RT.**

Are there data directly comparing surgery with CRT in anal cancer?

No. There is no randomized evidence. However, 1 retrospective analysis from Sweden showed better 5-yr OS in pts who rcvd RT ± chemo, supporting CRT as a better initial Tx option. (*Goldman S et al., Int J Colorectal Dis 1989*)

What 2 major European randomized studies in anal cancer demonstrated the inferiority of definitive RT compared to combined CRT?

UK Coordinating Committee on Cancer Research (UKCCCR) (ACT I) (*Lancet 1996*): 585 pts, any stage, randomized to RT vs. RT + 5-FU/MMC. RT was 45 Gy to the pelvis → 15–25 Gy with >50% response. If there was <50% response, then surgery was performed. Response was measured 6 wks after completion of *induction* therapy. The CR rate trended better in CRT (39% vs. 30%, $p = 0.08$), with 3-yr LC of 64% vs. 41% ($p < 0.0001$). The risk of death from anal cancer was also reduced in the CRT arm (HR 0.71, $p = 0.02$), but there was a nonsignificant benefit of 3-yr OS of 65% vs. 58% ($p = 0.25$).

13-yr update (*Northover J et al., Br J Cancer 2010*): The absolute risk of LRR was reduced by 25% and remained stable after 5 yrs. The risk of death was reduced by 12%, and absolute reduction in the colostomy rates remained at 10%, favoring CRT (all SS).

EORTC (*Bartelink H et al., JCO 1997*): 577 pts, T3-4 or node+, RT vs. RT + 5-FU/MMC. Boost was given based on the response assessed at 6 wks: 20 Gy to CR and 15 Gy to PR. The CR rate was measured after completion of the *entire course* of therapy. The CR rate was superior in the CRT arm (80% vs. 54%, $p = 0.02$), as well as 3-yr LC (69% vs. 55%, $p = 0.02$), but not 3-yr OS (69% vs. 64%).

What is 1 explanation why the UKCCCR study had substantially inferior rates of CR and LC compared with the EORTC study in anal cancer?

1. The CR rate was measured 6 wks after induction therapy in the UKCCCR, whereas it was measured 6 wks after completion of *all* therapy in the EORTC study (which had a longer course of Tx b/c boost was not delivered until after 6 wks of initial therapy).
2. The definition of LC is different between the 2 studies. In the UKCCCR study, the definition was more strict, with failure defined as <50% tumor reduction after just 6 wks of 45 Gy to the pelvis.

Can MMC be removed from the standard regimen of 5-FU/MMC for the Tx of anal cancer? What major study addressed this question?

No. MMC cannot be deleted from the standard regimen.

RTOG 87-04 (*Flam M et al., JCO 1996*): 291 pts, MMC/5-FU + RT vs. 5-FU + RT. RT was 45–50.4 Gy. There was no difference in OS (76% vs. 67%, $p = 0.31$), but MMC improved the CR rate (92% vs. 22%) and colostomy rate (9% vs. 22%) at 4 yrs. Grade 4 or 5 heme toxicity was worse (26% vs. 7%).

Can cisplatin be substituted for MMC in the Tx of anal cancer? What 2 major studies addressed this question?

2 RCTs suggest that substituting cisplatin for MMC does not improve and possibly worsens outcomes:

RTOG 98-11 (*Gunderson LL et al., JCO 2012*): 649 pts, all stages except T1 or M1; excluded AIDS or prior cancers; randomized to standard MMC-based therapy vs. 2 cycles of cisplatin/5-FU → cisplatin/5-FU × 2 with RT. RT was 45 Gy to the pelvis, with boost for T2 residual to 10–14 Gy. **DFS and OS were significantly superior in MMC-arm.** 5-yr DFS: 67.8% vs. 57.8%, $p = 0.006$; 5-yr OS: 78.3% vs. 70.7%, $p = 0.026$. There was a trend toward statistical superiority of MMC arm for colostomy-free survival, locoregional failure, and colostomy failure. Acute grade 3–4 severe heme toxicity was significantly worse in the MMC arm (61.8% vs. 42.0%, $p < 0.001$) but not in long-term toxicities (13.1% vs. 10.7%). *Major criticism:* Neoadj chemo on the experimental arm may have confounded the results.

ACTII (*James R et al., Lancet Oncol 2013*): 2×2 design, 940 pts (T1-2 [50%], T3-4 (43%), 30% N+, 85% anal canal, 15% anal margin) treated with 5-FU (1000 mg/m^2/day, days 1–4, days 29–32) and RT (50.4 Gy) and randomized to concurrent MMC (12 mg/m^2, day 1) or CDDP (cis-diamminedichloroplatinum) (60 mg/m^2, days 1 and 29). 2nd randomization involved adding maintenance therapy (4 wks after CRT) to 2 cycles 5-FU/CDDP or no maintenance. Median follow-up was 5.1 yrs. *Results:* No difference in CR rate at 26 wks (90.5% MMC vs. 89.6% cis). Hematologic grade three-quarters side effects occurred in 26% cis vs. 16% MMC. 3-yr PFS, OS, and colostomy-free survival did not differ significantly between groups. The authors concluded that 5-FU/MMC/RT without maintenance chemo remain the standard of care.

What is the role of brachytherapy in anal cancer?

Brachytherapy is **generally not done** in the U.S. due to poor LC (<30% for large lesions) and higher complication rates. An older French experience showed favorable results with combined interstitial (Ir-192) and EBRT. (*Papillon J & Montbarbon JF, Dis Colon Rectum 1987*)

What is the recurrence rate after definitive CRT for anal cancer, and what are the salvage rates at 5 yrs?

The recurrence rate is **30%,** and the salvage rate at 5 yrs is **40%–60%.**

Describe the RTOG AP/PA technique for anal cancer and the corresponding doses.

The initial AP/PA from L5-S1 is 30.6 Gy (at 1.8 Gy/fx), then reduced AP/PA from the bottom of the sacroiliac joints (and off inguinals after 36 Gy if node–) to 45 Gy, then conformal CD to tumor + 2–2.5-cm margin (and electron boost if node+) to 55–59.4 Gy. The dose to the inguinals is supplemented by bilat electron fields that make up for lack of dose contribution from the PA field to the appropriate doses (to 36 Gy or to the final boost volume for node+ Dz).

How is the anal cancer pt simulated for the AP/PA RTOG technique?

Pt is simulated supine with full bladder and oral contrast and with hips in frog-leg position immobilized with vac-lock cradle, with placement of rectal tube, anal BB, and bolus over inguinal nodes.

How is the AP field different from the PA field for the AP/PA RTOG technique in anal cancer?

The AP field is wider (to the edge of the greater trochanter) than the PA field. As well, the PA field is typically of lower energy (6 MV) than the AP field (18 MV). This technique spares the dose to the femoral head and neck.

Per RTOG 98-11, which anal cancer pts need to receive a boost beyond 45 Gy?

Pts with **T3, T4, or node+ lesions or T2 lesions with residual Dz after 45 Gy** need a boost >45 Gy.

What is the dose per fx for anal cancer per RTOG 98-11?

Per **RTOG 98-11,** the dose per fx for anal cancer is **1.8 Gy/fx to 45 Gy initially, then 2 Gy/fx to 55–59 Gy total for the CD portion.**

What is the min Rx depth for adequate inguinal node coverage in anal cancer?

The min Rx depth is **3 cm.**

How far caudally should inguinal nodes be covered in anal cancer?

Inguinal nodes should be covered to the **inf border of the lesser trochanter.**

What is the MDACC technique for the Tx of anal cancer?

Field setup is similar as in the RTOG technique for the 1st 30.6 Gy. After this dose, the pt is placed prone on a belly board and a 3-field technique is employed, with portal weighted 2 (PA): 1 (right lat): 1 (left lat), energy is 15–18 MV, prescribed to 95% IDL, with the sup border reduced to bottom of the sacroiliac joint. This 3-field plan treats the mini-pelvis to 50.4 Gy. A boost is given to the primary and involved nodes to 55 Gy. The contribution to the inguinals from the 3-field approach is 5–7 Gy. Daily electron boost supplements the needed dose for the involved inguinal area.

What is the standard CRT regimen for anal cancer pts who are HIV+?

HIV+ pts can typically be treated with the same RT + 5-FU/MMC regimen as HIV– pts. HIV+ pts with CD4 counts <200/mm^3 or other complications of HIV may require chemo and/or RT dose adjustments.

What is the role/evidence for IMRT in anal cancer?

RTOG 0529, a phase II single arm study, assessed the utility of 5-FU/MMC and dose-painted IMRT in reducing grade 2+ GI/GU toxicities compared with the conventional arm from RTOG 9811. Of 52 evaluable pts, a significant reduction was noted in acute grade 2+ hematologic (73% vs. 85%, $p = 0.03$), grade 3+ GI (21% vs. 36%, $p = 0.008$) and grade 3+ dermatologic adverse events (23% vs. 49%, $p < 0.0001$). Of note, 81% required dose-painted IMRT replanning on central review. (*Kachnic LA et al., IJROBP 2013*) Preliminary cancer control outcomes appear similar to those in RTOG 9811. In addition, numerous retrospective studies suggest decreased toxicity and comparable efficacy. (*Milano MT et al., IJROBP 2000; Menkarios C et al., Radiat Oncol 2007*)

What RT dose should the bowel be kept under in anal cancer pts?

The bowel should be kept to a dose **<45–50.4 Gy.**

What is the main toxicity of MMC?

MMC has **acute hematologic toxicities** but does not contribute to late toxicities.

Most anal cancer recurrences are within what timeframe?

Most anal cancers recur within **2 yrs.**

According to the NCCN guidelines (2014), what is the post-Tx follow-up for anal cancer?

Post-Tx anal cancer follow-up: Evaluate in 8–12 wks after Tx with DRE. Bx only if there is suspicious persistent Dz, progressive Dz, or new Sx (e.g., pain, bleeding). If there is complete remission, perform exam q3–6mos for 5 yrs with inguinal nodal evaluation, DRE, and anoscopy. Perform pelvic CT annually × 3 yrs (optional if T3-4 or node+ Dz).

What is the mean time to tumor regression after CRT?

The mean time to tumor regression after CRT is **3 mos (but can be up to 12 mos);** therefore, there is no benefit to routine post-Tx Bx. (*Cummings BJ et al., IJROBP 1991*)

If a pt has Bx-proven persistent Dz 3 mos after completing Tx, should the pt be referred immediately for salvage surgery?

No. Pts may be re-evaluated again after 4 wks. If there is still no regression, or if there is progression, consider Bx again and restage if necessary. If there is evidence of regression, continue observation and evaluation in 3 mos.

Part VIII Genitourinary

53 Low-Risk Prostate Cancer

Updated by Anand Shah

▶ BACKGROUND

What is the annual incidence and mortality of prostate cancer in the U.S.?	**~24,0000 Dx** of and **~30,000 deaths** from prostate cancer annually in the U.S.
Approximately how many U.S. men will develop prostate cancer during their lifetime?	**~1 in 6** U.S. men will be diagnosed with prostate cancer during their lifetime.
What are the 4 zones of the prostate?	Zones of the prostate: 1. Peripheral zone 2. Central zone 3. Transitional zone 4. Anterior fibromuscular stroma
Prostate cancers develop most commonly in which zone?	Two-thirds of prostate cancers arise in the **peripheral zone.**
Benign prostatic hypertrophy (BPH) develops in which zone?	BPH develops in the **transitional zone.**
What is median lobe hypertrophy?	Median lobe hypertrophy refers to a characteristic transitional zone hypertrophy (BPH) that mushrooms superiorly into the rest of the prostate and bladder. The term does not refer to enlargement of the central zone, which is typically small and compressed in older men.
What is the name for the nerves responsible for penile erections, and where are these nerves located with respect to the prostate?	The **neurovascular bundles** are paired nerves **located along the posterolat edge of the prostate** and are responsible for penile erection.

Name the 3 histologic cell types seen in the normal prostate.

Histologic cell types seen in the normal prostate:
1. Secretory cells (produce PSA and involute with hormonal deprivation)
2. Basal cells (flattened basement membrane where stem cells that repopulate the secretory layers reside)
3. Neuroendocrine cells

Describe the Gleason score and what it represents.

The Gleason score is a grade assigned to prostate cancer specimens that reflects the degree of aggressiveness based on the tumor's resemblance to normal glandular tissue. A primary (or predominant) pattern is recorded followed by a secondary or lesser pattern. The Gleason score is the sum of the primary and secondary pattern values and can be between 2 and 10.

Grade 1: small, well-formed glands, closely packed
Grade 2: well-formed glands, but more tissue between them
Grade 3: darker cells, some of which have left the gland and are invading the surrounding tissue
Grade 4: few recognizable glands with many cells invading the surrounding tissue
Grade 5: no recognizable glands; sheets of cells throughout the surrounding tissue

How often is higher-grade Dz diagnosed in a radical prostatectomy specimen (upstaging) than that seen in Bx specimens?

One-third of cases are higher grade in postprostatectomy specimens than that diagnosed in Bx specimens.

What racial groups are associated with the highest and lowest risks for prostate cancer?

Black men are at highest risk for the development of prostate cancer (and their Dz presents more aggressively [higher Gleason score, more advanced stage]). **Asians are at the lowest risk** for the development of prostate cancer. A 30- to 50-fold difference in the incidence of the Dz is observed between native Asians and black men. (*Ross R et al., Cancer 1995*)

Describe 5 clinical factors associated with the Dx of prostate cancer.

Clinical factors associated with the Dx of prostate cancer:
1. Advanced age
2. African American race
3. Past prostate Bx showing prostatic intraepithelial neoplasia (PIN; especially high-grade PIN)
4. Obesity
5. High dietary intake of fats

Is there a causative relationship between vasectomy and subsequent development of prostate cancer?

No. Studies show no consistent trend between vasectomy and subsequent development of prostate cancer. The National Institutes of Health has concluded that information regarding a relationship between them is not convincing and that a causative relationship has not been established. (*Healy B et al., JAMA 1993*)

Define the incidence of high-grade PIN or adenocarcinoma of the prostate on autopsy studies as a function of age.

Incidental finding of prostate adenocarcinoma on autopsy studies increases with age, with the avg Gleason score between 6 and 7. In 1 study, the following incidence of either high-grade PIN or prostate cancer was found:

Age ≤39: 0.6% (cancer: 0.6%)
Age 40–49: 19.2% (cancer: 0%)
Age 50–59: 40.3% (cancer: 23.4%)
Age 60–69: 61.2% (cancer: 34.7%)
Age 70–81: 45.5% (cancer: 45.5%)

(*Ming Y et al., J Urol 2008*)

Does finasteride decrease the incidence of prostate cancer?

Yes. In a phase III trial comparing finasteride vs. placebo given for 7 yrs to test the role of finasteride as a chemoprevention agent in men age ≥55 yrs (without evidence of prostate cancer), finasteride reduced the incidence of prostate cancer by 25% (30.6% vs. 18.6%) but increased the risk of more aggressive (Gleason 7–10) tumors (37% of tumors on the finasteride arm vs. 22% of tumors on the placebo arm). (*Thompson IM et al., NEJM 2003*) Follow-up studies suggest that finasteride likely does not affect grade but rather shrinks the prostate, making high-grade Dz more easily detected on subsequent Bx. (*Lucia MS et al., JNCI 2007*)

Describe 5 factors that can increase the level of PSA.

Factors that can increase PSA levels in the body:
1. Prostate cancer
2. Prostate manipulation (prostate Bx or DRE)
3. Infection (prostatitis)
4. Ejaculation shortly before PSA testing
5. BPH

Define the risk of prostate cancer as a function of total PSA level.

Prostate cancer risk increases as the total PSA level increases:
PSA ≤4: 5%–25%
PSA 4–10: 15%–25%
PSA >10: 50%–67%

Screening programs for prostate cancer include what 2 clinical assessments?

Screening for prostate cancer includes **DRE and a serum PSA.**

Describe 4 variants of absolute PSA that can be helpful in assessing a man's risk of prostate cancer.

Variants of absolute PSA that identify prostate cancer risk:
1. PSA as a function of age
2. PSA velocity
3. PSA density
4. Ratio of free to total PSA

Describe the upper limits of normal PSA values as a function of age.

Normal PSA values in men (without prostate cancer) will increase with age.
Upper-limit normal PSA values by age:
<u>40–49 yrs</u>: 1.5–2.5
<u>50–59 yrs</u>: 2.5–4
<u>60–69 yrs</u>: 4–5.5
<u>70–79 yrs</u>: 5.5–7

What is prostate-specific antigen velocity (PSAV), and how is it used in prostate cancer screening?

PSAV is a measure of the rate of change of the total PSA annually. A **PSA velocity ≥2 ng/mL/yr is associated with a higher risk of finding Gleason ≥7 prostate cancer on prostatectomy.** (*Loeb S et al., Urology 2008*)

What is prostate-specific antigen density (PSAD), and how is it used in prostate cancer screening?

PSAD is the **total serum PSA value divided by the volume of the prostate gland** (ellipsoid volume = length × width × height × 0.52). A PSAD of ≥0.15 ng/mL/cm^3 identifies men with a higher risk of detecting prostate cancer on a screening Bx.

What is the relationship between prostate cancer and the ratio of serum free-to-total PSA?

The end product of normal PSA biosynthesis within the prostate epithelium and ducts is inactive "free PSA," a fraction of which diffuses into the circulation. In prostate cancer, tumors disrupt the prostate basement membrane and allow precursor forms of PSA to leak into the circulation, which decreases the relative proportion of free PSA. Hence, the ratio of free-to-total PSA will be lower in men with prostate cancer. **A ratio of <7% is highly suspicious for prostate cancer,** whereas a ratio of >25% is rarely associated with malignancy.

What are population-based screening recommendations by the American Cancer Society (ACS) for prostate cancer? U.S. Preventive Services Task Force (USPSTF)?

The ACS recommends that asymptomatic men who have a ≥10-yr life expectancy have an opportunity to make an informed decision about screening. Men at average risk should receive information at age 50 yrs, and men at higher risk should receive information before age 50 yrs. Consider the Prostate Cancer Prevention Trial's Prostate Cancer Risk Calculator. The USPSTF recommends against PSA-based screening for prostate cancer.

In a recent European-based study, PSA screening has shown what in terms of prostate cancer Dx and deaths?	In a randomized European study comparing PSA screening to no screening, 182,160 men were enrolled. With a median follow-up of 11 yrs, the cumulative incidence of prostate cancer was 9.6% in the screened group and 6.0% in the control group. The rate ratio for death from prostate cancer in the screening group vs. control group was 0.79 (p <0.01). **1,055 men need to be invited to undergo screening and 37 prostate cancers need to be detected to prevent 1 death from prostate cancer.** (*Schroder FH et al., NEJM 2012*)
Annual DRE and PSA screening in the U.S. population has shown what in terms of prostate cancer Dx and deaths?	In phase III of the U.S. Prostate, Lung, Colorectal, and Ovarian Cancer (PLCO) screening trial, ~76,700 men were randomized to (1) intervention (organized screening with annual PSA × 6 yrs + annual DRE × 4 yrs) or (2) control (usual care in which opportunistic screening with PSA or DRE was allowed). After 13 yrs of follow-up, the incidence of prostate cancer was higher in the intervention vs. control group (108 vs. 97 cases/10,000 person-yrs). The incidence of death was similar between the groups (3.7 vs. 3.4 cases/10,000 person-yrs). The authors concluded there was no mortality benefit for organized vs. opportunistic screening. (*Andriole GL et al., JNCI 2012*)
What is the most common presentation of prostate cancer?	In the PSA era, most pts present with an **abnl PSA and no associated Sx.**
In men with symptomatic prostate cancer, what local Sx may arise at Dx?	Local Sx that may arise at Dx in men with prostate cancer Sx: 1. Lower tract Sx such as urgency, frequency, nocturia, dysuria 2. Hematuria 3. Sx of rectal involvement, such as hematochezia, constipation, intermittent diarrhea, reduced stool caliber 4. Renal impairment from bladder outlet obstruction
What is the most common site of metastatic spread of prostate cancer?	**Bone** is the most common site of metastatic spread. Blastic > lytic lesions.
What organ is frequently the site of metastatic Dz in other tumors yet almost never harbors metastatic Dz in prostate cancer?	The **brain** is a frequent site of metastatic Dz in nonprostate carcinoma but almost never is a site of mets in prostate cancer.

▶ **WORKUP/STAGING**

Name 4 important aspects of a focused Hx to include in a pt with newly diagnosed prostate cancer.

Important aspects of a focused Hx to include in a pt with newly diagnosed prostate cancer:

GI/GU Sx: may be a clinical presentation of the cancer itself but also may inform the most appropriate type of therapy given the baseline GI/GU function

Comorbid illnesses: such information may inform appropriate types of therapies for the pt; specifically and ascertain a Hx of inflammatory bowel Dz, hernia repair, or previous bowel surgeries (is the pt a surgical candidate; hormone suppression candidate?)

Medications: ask about current use of α-blockers or androgen suppression

New-onset bone pain: should result in a thorough evaluation for bone mets

The lab workup for prostate cancer includes what tests?

Prostate cancer lab workup: PSA, CBC, and BMP. Consider free PSA (if cancer Dx uncertain), alk phos (to assess for bone mets), or LFTS (if androgen receptor blockers will be used, as these are associated with hepatotoxicity).

Describe the AJCC 7ᵗʰ edition (2011) clinical TNM staging of prostate cancer.

Note: Per the AJCC, clinical T staging *may* use imaging. However, for research purposes, investigators should specify that the staging was based on DRE only or on DRE and imaging.

cT1: clinically inapparent tumor not palpable or visible by imaging

cT1a: incidental histologic finding in ≤5% of tumor resected

cT1b: incidental histologic finding in >5% of tissue resected

cT1 c: tumor identified by needle Bx

cT2: organ-confined Dz

cT2 a: tumor involves less than or equal to one half of 1 lobe

cT2b: tumor involves more than one half of 1 lobe (but not both lobes)

cT2 c: tumor involves both lobes of prostate

cT3: tumor extends through prostatic capsule

cT3 a: ECE

cT3b: seminal vesicle involvement

cT4: adjacent organ involvement (bladder neck, external sphincter, rectum, pelvic wall, or levator muscles

N1: regional LN mets

M1: DMs

M1 a: nonregional LNs

M1b: bone(s)

M1 c: other sites

Describe the AJCC 7th edition (2011) pathologic TNM staging of prostate cancer.

pT2: organ-confined Dz

pT2 a: tumor involves one half of 1 side or less

pT2b: tumor involves more than one half of 1 side (but not both sides)

pT2 c: tumor involves both sides

pT3: tumor extends through prostatic capsule

pT3 a: ECE or microscopic invasion of bladder neck

pT3b: seminal vesicle involvement

pT4: involvement of rectum, levator muscles, and/or pelvic wall

Note: Per the AJCC, pathologic assessment is based on evaluation of a prostatectomy specimen, unless a Bx shows involvement of the rectum, seminal vesicles, or extraprostatic tissues.

N1: regional LN mets

M1: DMs

M1 a: nonregional LNs

M1b: bone(s)

M1 c: other sites

What are the 3 most important clinical and pathologic factors for risk stratifying men with locally confined prostate cancer?

Most important clinical and pathologic factors used to risk stratify men with locally confined prostate cancer:

1. Pre-Tx PSA
2. DRE-defined clinical T stage
3. Gleason score

Define the low-, intermediate-, and high-risk groupings according to the D'Amico criteria, and estimate the 10-yr PSA FFS after radical prostatectomy for each group.

Definitions of risk groups and associated 10-yr PSA PFS after prostatectomy (according to D'Amico criteria):

Low risk: T1 c-T2 a, PSA ≤10, Gleason ≤6 (10-yr PSA FFS: 83%)

Intermediate risk: T2b, PSA >10 but ≤20, Gleason 7 (10-yr PSA FFS: 46%)

High risk: T2 c, PSA >20, Gleason ≥8 (10-yr PSA FFS: 29%)

(*D'Amico AV et al., J Urol 2001*)

Describe the recommended procedure for Bx of the prostate.

Prostate Bx should be performed using a transrectal approach with a 5- to 7.5-MHz transducer in the rectum. A **sextant Bx** directed at the peripheral zone should result in 12 cores of prostate tissue for Bx.

Describe the appearance of prostate cancer on TRUS.

Prostate cancer on TRUS is usually **hypoechoic.**

What imaging studies are recommended in the workup of low-risk prostate cancer?

Unless concerning local Sx are present on evaluation of the pt with newly diagnosed low-risk prostate cancer, such as pelvic pain or focal bony pain, **no imaging studies are recommended for staging a man with low-risk prostate cancer.**

▶ **TREATMENT/PROGNOSIS**

Define the difference between watchful waiting and active surveillance.

Active surveillance is the *postponement* of immediate therapy, with definitive Tx given if Dz progresses. The goal of care is to cure those with progressive Dz while avoiding unnecessary Tx in pts with clinically insignificant Dz. **Watchful waiting *forgoes* definitive Tx at Dx with the goal of care to provide palliative Tx for symptomatic progression.** Watchful waiting is reserved for elderly men or those with substantial comorbidity. (*Dall'Era M et al., Curr Urol Rep 2008; NIH Consensus Statement 2011*)

In men with early-stage prostate cancer, what is the benefit in terms of upfront surgical management vs. watchful waiting? Are there randomized data to support an approach?

The role of definitive Tx in men with early-stage prostate cancer is controversial. A Swedish study, **SPCG-4,** randomized 695 men with T1-T2 prostate cancer (all grades) to radical prostatectomy vs. watchful waiting. **Surgery improved 18-yr incidence of cause-specific death (17.7% vs. 28.7%) and DM (26.1% vs. 38.3%).** Results should be interpreted with caution, as the study was conducted in a pre-PSA screening era and included pts with Gleason scores 7–10. (*Bill-Axelson A et al., NEJM 2014*)

What is the premise underlying active surveillance in prostate cancer care?

A majority of men with low-risk prostate cancer would not have any adverse clinical consequences if their Dz was left untreated. Active surveillance delays definitive Tx for the majority of these men while reserving curative Tx until it is justified based on defined clinical markers of Dx progression. (*NIH Consensus Statement 2011*)

What follow-up procedures are involved in active surveillance? For watchful waiting?

Active surveillance commonly includes biannual DRE and PSA test with annual prostate Bx. It is unclear when the interval should increase between biopsies or to discontinue screening altogether. Pts are referred for definitive management for increasing **Gleason score,** increasing **volume** (as estimated by # of cores and % of cores involved), or **pt preference. In watchful waiting treatment is reserved only for symptomatic disease progression and thus follow-up is minimal.**

What group of pts may be most appropriate for watchful waiting?

The pts most appropriate for watchful waiting include those too old or too ill to benefit from Tx or those with asymptomatic metastatic Dz.

What 5 criteria are needed for a pt best suited for active surveillance in early-stage, small-volume Dz?

Although there is no consensus on what group of men, if any, may be appropriate for expectant management in early-stage Dz, in general they should meet the following criteria:

1. Older age (age >65 yrs) or with comorbid Dz
2. Clinical T1 or T2 a Dz

3. PSAD ≤0.1
4. Combined Gleason grade ≤6
5. ≤50% involvement of ≤2 cores of 12

What % of men with low-grade, early-stage Dz will eventually need definitive management with curative intent b/c of progressive Dz?

In a prospective cohort study at the Johns Hopkins Hospital of men undergoing active surveillance, after median follow-up of 3 yrs, **25% of men underwent definitive management based on Dz progression on Bx or pt preference.** Of these men with progressive Dz on Bx, those who opted for surgical management at the time of follow-up had a proportion with curable Dz that was similar to those men who would be qualified for expectant management upfront but instead chose to undergo upfront surgery. (*Carter HB et al., J Urol 2007*) In a prospective, single-arm cohort of 450 men undergoing active surveillance, the 10-yr prostate cancer actuarial survival was 97.2%. Overall, **30%** of men were found to have progressive Dz and were offered definitive therapy. (*Klotz L et al., JCO 2009*)

What 3 standard Tx options are available to an otherwise healthy man with no adverse GI/GU Sx and low-risk Dz by D'Amico criteria?

Standard Tx options available to an otherwise healthy man with no adverse GI/GU Sx and low-risk Dz (by D'Amico criteria):
1. Active surveillance (in carefully selected pts)
2. Radical surgery
3. RT (brachytherapy [brachy] or EBRT alone)

Does dose escalation improve outcomes in men with low-risk prostate cancer?

Yes. Dose escalation improves biochemical FFS in men with low-risk prostate cancer. This has been seen in at least 2 randomized trials that included men with low-risk Dz: **PROG 9509** (*Zietman AL et al., JCO 2010*) and the **MDACC RCT** (*Kuban D et al., IJROBP 2008*).

Describe the design and outcomes of PROG 9509, which evaluated dose escalation in prostate cancer.

PROG 9509 included 392 men with low-risk prostate cancer (cT1b-T2b, PSA <15 ng/mL, Gleason <7). All men were treated with 50.4 Gy using photon RT and then were randomized to a proton boost to a total dose of 70.2 GyE (gray equivalent) vs. 79.2 GyE. **Dose escalation improved 10-yr biochemical failure (32.2% vs. 16.7%).**

Describe the design and outcomes of the MDACC trial that evaluated dose escalation in prostate cancer.

The MDACC dose escalation trial enrolled 301 pts with cT1b-T3 prostate cancer: 21% were low risk, 47% were intermediate risk, and 32% were high risk. Pts were randomized to 70 Gy vs. 78 Gy. **Dose escalation improved 8-yr freedom from failure (78% vs. 59%).** This improvement was seen in the low- and high-risk subsets but not in the intermediate-risk subset. 8-yr CSS was not significantly different (99% vs. 95%), nor was 8-yr OS (78% vs. 79%). (*Kuban D et al., IJROBP 2008*)

What RCTs have compared surgery, EBRT, and brachy for low-risk prostate cancer?

Currently, no RCTs have compared surgery, EBRT, and/or brachy for low-risk prostate cancer. Multiple trials comparing definitive modalities for low-risk pts have been attempted, but all have failed due to inadequate accrual. ProtecT is a large U.K.-based trial designed to address this question and has closed to accrual.

What data support the use of prostatectomy, EBRT, or LDR brachy alone for low-risk prostate cancer?

Numerous retrospective studies suggest similar outcomes for low-risk prostate cancer pts treated with prostatectomy, EBRT, or LDR brachy. *D'Amico AV et al.* reviewed low-risk pts treated at the University of Pennsylvania or the Joint Center in Boston and found **no difference in 5-yr biochemical FFS (~88%)** in men treated with prostatectomy, EBRT, or brachy alone. (*JAMA 1998*) *Kupelian P et al.* reviewed low-risk pts from the Cleveland Clinic and Memorial Sloan Kettering and found **similar 5-yr biochemical FFS (~81%–83%)** for men treated with prostatectomy, LDR brachy, and EBRT (to total doses >72 Gy). However, in a subset of men treated with EBRT to <72 Gy, 5-yr biochemical FFS was significantly worse (51%). (*IJROBP 2004*)

What data support the use of hypofractionation for localized prostate cancer?

Recent studies have examined moderate (2.4–4 Gy/fx) and extreme hypofractionation (6.5–10 Gy/fx) in prostate cancer. Results of moderate hypofractionation RCTs are inconclusive to date. (*Cabrera AR et al., Sem Rad Oncol 2013*) No RCTs of extreme vs. conventional fractionation have been published. *Maden BL et al.* (*IJROBP 2007*) enrolled 40 pts in a phase I/II trial for localized Dz using 33.5 Gy in 5 fx. 4-yr actuarial biochemical FFR was 70% (by ASTRO failure definition) and 90% (alternative nadir +2 ng/mL definition) with no reported late ≥grade 3 GU/GI toxicity. *Wiegner EA et al.* (*IJROBP 2010*) reported erectile dysfunction rates following SBRT to be comparable to other forms of RT.

Describe the setup of a pt with prostate cancer undergoing CT imaging to plan RT Tx.

A pt undergoing CT imaging to plan RT Tx can be simulated in the prone or supine position. Some institutions use a pelvic MRI or a urethrogram to locate the urogenital diaphragm and, hence, the apex of the prostate. The pt is often instructed to have a full bladder and an empty rectum, although techniques vary at institutions. A rectal balloon may be used to reduce prostate motion and decrease integral dose to the rectum.

Describe 4 techniques to verify prostate position in daily RT Tx.	Techniques to verify prostate position in daily RT Tx: 1. 2D-IGRT + fiducials 2. 3D-IGRT +/– fiducials 3. Implantable radiofrequency transponder 4. BAT US

▶ **TOXICITY**

What are the most common side effects after radical prostatectomy?	The most common significant side effects after radical prostatectomy are **erectile dysfunction, urinary incontinence, and urethral stricture.**
In men with intact erectile function prior to radical prostatectomy, what % retain erectile function after a nerve-sparing procedure?	In men with intact erectile function prior to surgery, at least **50%** will retain erectile function after a nerve-sparing prostatectomy, depending on surgeon volume.
What % of men who undergo a radical prostatectomy have significant postop urinary incontinence?	~33% of men who undergo a radical prostatectomy have significant postop urinary incontinence. (*Gunderson LL et al., Clin Radiat Oncol, 3rd ed. 2010*) The severity of incontinence after surgery peaks immediately and improves over mos.
What are the most common acute and late side effects of EBRT and brachy?	Most common acute side effects: fatigue, urinary urgency/frequency, proctitis/diarrhea. Most common late side effects: erectile dysfunction (inability to maintain an erection for intercourse), cystitis, proctitis (frequency/bleeding)
Estimate the rate of grade 3 or higher late GU or GI RT toxicity with IMRT for prostate cancer.	Numerous retrospective studies suggest that **grade 3 or higher late GU or GI RT toxicity with IMRT for prostate cancer is rare** (≤1%).
Estimate the rate of erectile dysfunction in previously potent men 2+ yrs after Tx with definitive prostate RT.	~50% of men who were previously potent will no longer be able to maintain erections for intercourse 2+ yrs after definitive prostate RT. (*Robinson JW et al., IJROBP 2002*)
What are the current RTOG rectal DVH constraints for RT Tx to the prostate?	For prostate cancer pts being treated in 1.8 Gy/fx, appropriate dose constraints for the **rectum** (per an RTOG consensus statement): V70 ≤20% V50 ≤50% (*Lawton CA et al., IJROBP 2009*)

| What are the current RTOG bladder DVH constraints for RT Tx to the prostate? | For prostate cancer pts being treated in 1.8 Gy/fx, appropriate dose constraints for the **bladder** (per an RTOG consensus statement):
    V70 ≤30%
    V55 ≤50%

(*Lawton CA et al., IJROBP 2009*) |

54 Intermediate- and High-Risk Prostate Cancer

Updated by Abigail T. Berman and John P. Christodouleas

▶ BACKGROUND

Estimate the annual incidence and mortality of prostate cancer in the U.S.	**~25,0000 Dx** of and **~27,000 deaths** from prostate cancer annually in the U.S.
Where does prostate cancer rank as a cause of cancer death in men in the U.S.? Has this increased or decreased?	Prostate cancer is essentially tied with colorectal cancer as the **2nd most common cause of cancer death** behind lung cancer. There has been a 36% decrease in the death rate from prostate cancer since 1990.
What % of newly diagnosed prostate cancer is cT3 Dz or higher?	**12%–28%** of men with newly diagnosed prostate cancer have cT3 Dz or higher.
What % of newly diagnosed prostate cancer is Gleason ≥7 on Bx?	In the U.S., **~1 in 3** of all newly diagnosed prostate cancer in a screened population is Gleason ≥7. (*Andriole GL et al., NEJM 2009*)
What % of newly diagnosed prostate cancer are Gleason ≥8 on Bx?	In the U.S., **~1 in 10** of all newly diagnosed prostate cancer in a screened population is Gleason ≥8. (*Andriole GL et al., NEJM 2009*)

Estimate the risk of Gleason ≥7 prostate cancer in a man who has pre-Bx PSA of <4 ng/mL.	In a man with a pre-Bx PSA <4 ng/mL, the risk of Gleason ≥7 is **~PSA × 2.**
In which portion of the prostate is the prostatic capsule not clearly defined?	**At the apex of the prostate,** the prostatic capsule is not clearly identifiable. Some authors argue that the prostate does not have a true capsule but rather simply has an outer fibromuscular band that continuously transitions to periprostatic tissues and organs. The transition at the apex is particularly difficult to identify. (*Ayala AG et al., Am J Surg Pathol 1989*)
In which portion of the prostate is ECE most commonly found?	ECE is most commonly found in the posterolat portion of the prostate **at the prostatic neurovascular bundle.**

▶ **WORKUP/STAGING**

By the D'Amico criteria, which localized prostate cancer pts are considered to have intermediate-risk Dz?	A pt has intermediate-risk prostate cancer if he has any or all of the following 3 risk factors (but no high-risk factors): **stage T2b, Gleason 7, and pre-Tx PSA 10.1–20 ng/mL.** (*D'Amico A et al., J Urol 2001*) The NCCN guidelines 2014 allow but do not require that patients with >1 intermediate risk factor may be considered high risk.
By the D'Amico criteria, which localized prostate cancer pts are considered to have high-risk Dz?	A pt has high-risk prostate cancer if he has any or all of the following 3 risk factors: **stage ≥T2c, Gleason ≥8, and pre-Tx PSA >20 ng/mL.** (*D'Amico A et al., J Urol 2001*)
What is the sensitivity and specificity of endorectal coil MRI for determining the presence of prostatic ECE and seminal vesicle invasion (SVI)?	The estimates for the sensitivity and specificity of endorectal coil MRI as a predictor of prostatic ECE and SVI vary widely, between **13%–95% and 23%–80% (sensitivity)** and **49%–97% and 81%–99% (specificity), respectively.** The experience of the radiologist appears to play an important role in the accuracy of the tool.
If an endorectal coil MRI is ordered as part of the workup for prostate cancer, how long after Bx should it take place?	There is no consensus on the role of endorectal coil MRI as part of the workup for prostate cancer. However, if an MRI is ordered, wait **6–8 wks after Bx to avoid artifact** caused by post-Bx hemorrhage.

▶ **TREATMENT/PROGNOSIS**

What are the Tx options for a man with localized intermediate-risk prostate cancer?

Tx options for a man with intermediate-risk prostate cancer:
1. EBRT +/– short-term androgen suppression (AS) (4–6 mos) +/– brachytherapy (brachy) boost
2. Brachy +/– AS
3. Prostatectomy (less ideal for pt with >1 intermediate risk factor).

If he has a life expectancy <10 yrs, also consider active surveillance.

What are the Tx options for a man with localized high-risk prostate cancer?

Tx options for a man with high-risk prostate cancer:
1. EBRT + long-term AS (2–3 yrs) +/– pelvic node RT +/– brachy boost
2. Prostatectomy (less ideal for high-risk pts)

Estimate the 5-yr biochemical failure-free survival (bFS) for D'Amico intermediate- and high-risk prostate cancer pts treated with prostatectomy alone.

After prostatectomy alone, 5-yr bFS is **~65% for intermediate-risk** and **~35% for high-risk prostate cancer pts.** (*D'Amico A et al., J Urol 2001*)

Estimate the 10-yr bFS for prostate cancer pts with cT2b and ≥cT2c Dz treated with prostatectomy alone.

After prostatectomy alone, 10-yr bFS is **~62% for cT2b, and ~57% for ≥cT2c.** (*Han M et al., Urol Clin N Am 2001*)

Estimate the 10-yr bFS for prostate cancer pts with Gleason 3 + 4 = 7, 4 + 3 = 7, and Gleason 8–10 Dz treated with prostatectomy alone.

After prostatectomy alone, 10-yr bFS is **~60% with Gleason 3 + 4 = 7, ~33% with 4 + 3 = 7, and ~29% with Gleason 8–10.** (*Han M et al., Urol Clin N Am 2001*)

Estimate the 10-yr bFS for prostate cancer pts with a pretreatment prostate-specific antigen (pPSA) from 10–20 and >20 ng/mL treated with prostatectomy alone.

After prostatectomy alone, 10-yr bFS ~57% with pPSA 10–20 ng/mL and 48% with pPSA >20 ng/mL are **57% and 48%,** respectively. (*Han M et al., Urol Clin N Am 2001*)

What classifies patients as unfavorable vs. favorable intermediate risk?

Factors that may identify an unfavorable intermediate risk subgroup include primary Gleason 4 Dz, >50% positive cores, or 2 intermediate risk factors (*Zumsteg ZS et al., Eur Urol 2013*).

What are the benefits of neoadj AS prior to radical prostatectomy?

The benefits of neoadj AS prior to prostatectomy include **decreased +margin and LN positivity rates.** This has been shown in multiple randomized trials. In addition, a longer duration of neoadj therapy (6–8 mos vs. 3 mos) is associated with improvements in these pathologic outcomes. (*Kumar S et al., Cochrane Database Syst Rev 2006*)

Why is neoadj AS prior to radical prostatectomy not commonly used?

Despite improvement in pathologic outcomes with neoadj AS prior to prostatectomy, **long-term bFS rates do not appear to be improved.** This negative result has been found in multiple randomized studies. (*Kumar S et al., Cochrane Database Syst Rev 2006*)

What is the role of adj AS therapy after prostatectomy?

In prostate cancer pts found to have **node+ Dz after prostatectomy, immediate adj AS is indicated** and improves OS. (*Messing EM et al., Lancet Oncol 2006*) There appears to be no OS or CSS in node– men after prostatectomy (*Wirth MP et al., Euro Urol 2004*), although the RCT evaluating this question used only an antiandrogen instead of a gonadotropin-releasing hormone (GnRH) agonist or total AS with both.

What study established the role of adj AS for node+ pts after prostatectomy? What is the main criticism of this study?

Messing EM et al. showed an OS benefit of immediate adj AS vs. observation for node+ prostate cancer pts after prostatectomy (MS 13.9 yrs vs. 11.3 yrs, respectively). The main criticism of this study is that **AS was not initiated in the observation arm until clinical Dz progression rather than an elevated absolute PSA or PSA velocity.** (*Lancet Oncol 2006*)

Is active surveillance a reasonable approach in intermediate-risk Dz?

Per the NCCN guidelines 2014, active surveillance is an option for men with <10-yr life expectancy. Longer follow-up is needed, but studies show ~50% of men receive definitive treatment. (*Bul et al., BJU Int 2012; Godman et al., Eur Urol 2012*)

Is LDR brachy alone appropriate for intermediate- or high-risk Dz? Describe 1 study that argues against LDR brachy.

Per the American Brachytherapy Society guidelines, LDR brachy alone is not appropriate for high-risk Dz but may be considered for highly selected pts with intermediate-risk Dz. (*Davis BJ et al., Brachytherapy 2012*) A retrospective study by *D'Amico A et al.* (*JAMA 1998*) found that LDR brachy alone was associated with worse 5-yr biochemical progression-free survival (bPFS) compared to prostatectomy and EBRT alone in both intermediate- and high-risk subgroups. However, several single-institution series suggest that well-selected intermediate-risk pts receiving a high-quality implant have excellent outcomes after LDR brachy alone (5-yr bPFS >95%). (*Taira AV et al., IJROBP 2009*)

What is the role of neoadj AS and LDR brachy for pts with intermediate- or high-risk prostate cancer?

Neoadj AS may be used **to cytoreduce large prostates.** (*Nag S et al., IJROBP 1999*) However, several large retrospective studies have failed to show that AS improves cancer control outcomes in combination with LDR brachy.

What is the role of EBRT + LDR brachy for intermediate- and high-risk prostate cancer?

EBRT + LDR brachy without AS is not commonly used in pts with high-risk Dz. However, multiple institutional series have shown good long-term outcomes in intermediate-risk pts (10-yr bPFS 79%–90%). (*Ragde H et al., Cancer 2000; Sylvester JE et al., IJROBP 2003*) There has been 1 RCT of combination EBRT +/– LDR brachy boost in pts with intermediate- and high-risk Dz. (*Sathya JR et al., JCO 2005*) This study compared iridium implant (35 Gy over 48 hrs) + EBRT (40 Gy) vs. EBRT alone (66 Gy) and found that the combined Tx improved biochemical/clinical failure rates (29% vs. 61%) and 2-yr post-RT positive prostate Bx rates (24% vs. 51%), suggesting that LDR brachy may be a reasonable way to dose escalate in these pts. The major weakness of this RCT is the relatively low dose and the lack of AS in the control arm.

What is the role of EBRT + HDR brachy for localized intermediate- and high-risk prostate cancer?

Long-term data from *Demanes DJ et al.* and other authors have shown good long-term results with EBRT + HDR brachy in both intermediate- and high-risk pts (10-yr bPFS of 87% and 63%, respectively). (*Am J Clin Oncol 2009*) There has been 1 RCT of EBRT +/– HDR brachy boost: *Hoskin P et al. (Radioth Oncol 2012)* This study included low-, intermediate-, and high-risk pts, comparing EBRT (37.75 Gy in 2.75 Gy) + HDR (17 Gy in 8.5 Gy) vs. EBRT alone (55 Gy in 2.75 Gy), and found improved biochemical relapse-free survival in the combo arm (median time to relapse 9.7 yrs vs. 6.2 yrs) without excess toxicity. No difference in OS. Most pts in both arms (~75%) had neoadj AS. The major weakness of this RCT is the relatively low biologically effective dose in the control arm.

What studies support the use of short-course (4–6 mos) AS with EBRT in localized intermediate-risk prostate cancer?

The 1st study to show a benefit to short-course AS in locally advanced prostate cancer was **RTOG 8610,** although all of these pts were high risk as defined by the D'Amico criteria. None of the published studies of short-course AS specifically studied intermediate-risk pts. **RTOG 9408** enrolled all risk group pts (but mainly intermediate risk) and found a 10-yr OS benefit to the addition of short-course AS. (*Jones CU et al., NEJM 2011*) In addition, intermediate-risk pts were included in *D'Amico A et al.* (*JAMA 2004*), *Laverdiere J et al.* (*J Urol 2004*), and *Denham JW et al.* (*Lancet Oncol 2005;* **TROG 96.01**), all of which showed improved Dz-specific outcomes with the addition of short-course AS to EBRT. It is unclear whether dose escalation mitigates the benefit of short-course AS in intermediate-risk pts.

Describe the study design and results of RTOG 8610, which studied the benefit of short-course AS in locally advanced prostate cancer.

RTOG 8610 enrolled 456 men with cT2-T4 (bulky) prostate cancer. N1 pts were eligible if below the common iliac. All were treated with EBRT (65–70 Gy) and randomized to 4 mos of AS (beginning 2 mos prior to EBRT) or observation with AS at relapse. **10-yr OS and MS favored the short-course AS arm (43% vs. 34% and 8.7 yrs vs. 7.3 yrs, respectively) although the difference was NSS.** Short-course AS improved 10-yr CSM (23% vs. 36%) and distant failure (35% vs. 47%). (*Roach M et al., JCO 2008*)

Describe the study design and results of RTOG 9408, which studied the benefit of short-course AS in locally confined prostate cancer.

RTOG 9408 enrolled 1979 pts with T1b-T2b, PSA ≤20, prostate cancer (54% were intermediate risk). Pts were randomized to EBRT alone (66.6 Gy) +/- 4-mo AS (flutamide and LHRH agonist) beginning 2 mos prior to EBRT. **12-yr OS favored the short-course AS arm (54% vs. 61%).** AS also reduced the rates of +prostate biopsy at 2 years (39% vs. 20%). (*Jones CU et al., NEJM 2011*)

Describe the study design and results of TROG 96.01, which studied the benefit of short-course AS in locally advanced prostate cancer.

TROG 96.01 enrolled 818 pts with T2b-T4 prostate cancer treated with EBRT (66 Gy in 2 Gy). Pts were randomized to 0, 3, or 6 mos of AS starting 2 mos prior to EBRT. With only a median follow-up of 5.9 yrs, the 3- and 6-mo AS arms had improved LF, biochemical failure, and freedom from salvage Tx compared to the no-AS arm. The 6-mo arm also had improved distant failure and prostate cancer–specific survival (PCSS) compared to the no AS arm. As of yet, there are no OS differences among any of the 3 arms and no consistent cancer control differences between 3- and 6-mo arms. (*Denham JW et al., Lancet Oncol 2005*)

Describe the study design and results of the RCT by D'Amico et al., which studied the benefit of short-course AS in locally advanced prostate cancer.

D'Amico A et al. (DFCI trial) enrolled 206 men with cT1b-T2b and 1 of the following: PSA 10–40 ng/mL or Gleason 7–10 or ECE/SVI by MRI. 74% were intermediate risk. Pts were randomized to EBRT alone (70 Gy) +/– 6 mos of AS (flutamide and LHRH agonist) beginning 2 mos prior to EBRT. **The AS arm had improved 8-yr OS (74% vs. 61%).** Unplanned subset analysis suggested that benefit may be limited to men without significant comorbidities. (*Nguyen PL et al., IJROBP 2010*)

Is AS still beneficial with dose-escalated RT?

Retrospective analysis of 710 intermediate-risk pts treated with ≥81 Gy indicates that AS is still beneficial with an adjusted HR of 0.297. (*Zumsteg ZS et al., IJROBP 2012*)

When should AS be started in a prostate cancer pt being treated with EBRT and AS?

In prostate cancer pts being treated with EBRT + AS, **AS is usually started 2 mos prior to the start of EBRT.** Preclinical experiments suggest that neoadj AS may improve prostate cancer RT sensitivity compared to concurrent AS, possibly due to improved tumor oxygenation with neoadj AS. Furthermore, the RCTs that established the role of short-course AS started it neoadjuvantly (**RTOG 8610, D'Amico trial, TROG 96.01**). However, **RTOG 9413,** which compared neoadj/concurrent vs. adj short-course AS, showed no bPFS benefit (or detriment) to neoadj AS.

Describe the study design and results of RTOG 9413, which studied the benefit of the sequence of short-course AS and pelvic node RT in locally advanced prostate cancer.

RTOG 9413 had a 2 × 2 factorial design. It randomized 1323 intermediate- and high-risk pts to 4 mos of AS beginning 2 mos prior to or immediately following EBRT. The 2nd randomization was regarding RT field size: whole pelvis (WP) RT vs. prostate and seminal vesicles only (PSVO). After a median follow-up of 7 yrs, there was **no difference in PFS in the neoadj vs. adj AS arms and no difference in PFS in the WP and PSVO arms.** Interpretation of this trial is limited by the fact that there was an unexpected interaction between the 2 randomizations of this study. (*Lawton C et al., IJROBP 2007*)

What is the appropriate duration of neoadj AS prior to EBRT in prostate cancer pts?

Prostate cancer pts who are treated with neoadj AS usually rcv 2 mos of AS prior to EBRT. 1 RCT enrolled 378 men with localized prostate cancer of any risk group, and all were treated with EBRT (66–67 Gy) without concurrent AS. Pts were randomized to 3 mos vs. 8 mos of neoadj AS. 5-yr freedom from failure (FFF) did not differ between the Tx arms. In an unplanned subgroup analysis, 5-yr DFS was improved for high-risk pts (71% vs. 42%). (*Crook J et al., IJROBP 2009*) **RTOG 9910** evaluated 2 mos vs. 7 mos of neoadj therapy, and the preliminary report did not show that extending neoadjuvant therapy improved any endpoints. (Pisansky T, ASTRO 2013)

Which studies support the role of long-term AS in localized high-risk prostate cancer pts treated with EBRT?

An OS benefit of long-term AS in high-risk pts after EBRT was 1st shown in **RTOG 8531.** Multiple subsequent RCTs have also shown improved prostate cancer outcomes: **the Casodex Early Prostate Cancer trial, EORTC 22863, RTOG 9202, and EORTC 22961.**

Describe the study design and results of RTOG 8531, which studied the benefit of the long-term AS in locally advanced prostate cancer.

RTOG 8531 enrolled 945 men with cT3 (nonbulky), pT3 after prostatectomy, or N1 prostate cancer. All were treated with EBRT (definitive dose: 65–70 Gy; postop dose: 60–65 Gy) and randomized to adj AS indefinitely or observation with AS at relapse. **Adj AS improved 10-yr OS (49% vs. 39%), 10-yr CSM (16% vs. 22%), 10-yr LF (23% vs. 38%), and 10-yr distant failure (24% vs. 39%)** (WP). On subset analysis, benefits were limited to the subset with Gleason ≥7 and were especially important in the subset with Gleason ≥8. (*Pilepich MV et al., IJROBP 2005*)

Describe the study design and results of the Casodex Early Prostate Cancer trial, which studied the benefit of the long-term adj Casodex in locally advanced prostate cancer.

The Casodex Early Prostate Cancer trial randomized 8113 men with prostate cancer to observation or long-term Casodex after local therapy (RT, prostatectomy, observation). The duration of Casodex was either 2 yrs or until progression. In the subgroup of RT pts (1,730 men), after a median follow-up of 7.2 yrs, adj long-term Casodex did not result in OS or PCSS. However, in the subgroup of locally advanced pts (cT3-T4 or N1), there was an OS and PCSS benefit. These findings, however, were the results of an unplanned subset analysis. (*See WA et al., J Cancer Res Clin Oncol 2006*)

Describe the study design and results of EORTC 22863, which studied the benefit of long-term AS in locally advanced prostate cancer.

EORTC 22863 enrolled 412 men with cT3-T4/any grade or cT1-T2/WHO grade 3 prostate cancer. All were treated with EBRT (70 Gy) and randomized to 3 yrs of adj AS (beginning with EBRT) or observation with AS at relapse. Long-term AS improved **5-yr OS (78% vs. 62%), CSS (94% vs. 79%), LF (1.7% vs. 16.4%), and distant failure (9.8% vs. 29.2%).** (*Bolla M et al., Lancet 2002*)

Describe the study design and results of RTOG 9202, which studied the benefit of the long-term AS in locally advanced prostate cancer.

RTOG 9202 enrolled 1,541 men with cT2c-T4, PSA <150. All were treated with 2 mos of neoadj AS and 2 mos of concurrent AS + EBRT (65–70 Gy). Pts were randomized to an additional 2 yrs of adj AS or observation with AS at relapse. Long-term AS was not associated with OS in the entire cohort, although it did show improved 10-yr CSS (89% vs. 84%), local progression (12% vs. 22%), and DM (15% vs. 23%). In an unplanned subgroup analysis, long-term AS improved 10-yr OS in pts with Gleason ≥8 (45% vs. 32%). (*Horwitz EM et al., JCO 2008*)

Describe the study design and results of the EORTC 22961 RCT, which compared short-course and long-term AS with EBRT in localized prostate cancer.

EORTC 22961 enrolled 1,113 men with cT2c-T4/N0 or cT1c-T2b/pN1-N2 prostate cancer and randomized to EBRT (70 Gy) with 6 mos vs. 3 yrs of neoadj, concurrent, and adj AS. **Men receiving 3 yrs of AS had superior OS (5-yr OS 85% vs. 81%) and CSM (5-yr CSM 3.2% vs. 4.7%).** Long-term overall QOL did not significantly differ between the 2 arms. (*Bolla M et al., NEJM 2009*)

What is the appropriate duration of long-term AS in localized high-risk prostate cancer pts treated with EBRT?

RTOG 9202 and EORTC 22961 suggested that long-term (2–3 yrs) AS is superior to short-course AS in high-risk pts. However, the optimum duration of long-term AS has not been well studied.

What is the role of pelvic nodal RT in localized intermediate- and high-risk prostate cancer?

The major RCTs that established the role of RT in locally advanced prostate cancer generally irradiated pelvic nodes. However, the role of pelvic nodal RT in localized prostate cancer has been specifically studied in 3 RCTs: **RTOG 7706, RTOG 9413, and GETUG-01,** and none showed a cancer control benefit to irradiating pelvic nodes. Yet, all of these trials included men who may have been at low risk for harboring nodal Dz. Pelvic nodal RT may still be warranted in men at very high risk of harboring nodal Dz, although who these pts are is controversial.

What is the appropriate EBRT dose for intermediate- and high-risk prostate cancer?

Men with intermediate- and high-risk prostate cancer who do not rcv AS should be treated to total EBRT doses of ≥74 Gy (in 2 Gy/fx). There have been at least 4 EBRT dose escalation studies including intermediate- and high-risk pts: the **MDACC dose escalation trial, PROG 9505, the Dutch dose escalation trial, and the MRC RT01 trial.** All 4 RCTs have shown at least improved biochemical control with dose-escalated EBRT. The role of high-dose EBRT is less clear in the setting of AS. The Dutch dose escalation trial allowed AS, but only a minority of men rcv it (22%). (*Peeters ST et al., JCO 2006*) The **MRC RT01** trial mandated neoadj and concurrent AS, and 5-yr outcomes favored dose escalation.

Describe the study design and results of the MDACC RCT that studied the benefit of dose escalation in localized prostate cancer.

The MDACC dose escalation trial enrolled 301 pts with cT1b-T3 prostate cancer. None were treated with AS. 21% were low risk, 47% were intermediate risk, and 32% were high risk. Pts were randomized to 70 Gy vs. 78 Gy. **Dose escalation improved 8-yr FFF (78% vs. 59%).** This improvement was seen in the low- and high-risk subsets but not in the intermediate-risk subset. **8-yr CSS was not significantly different (99% vs. 95%) nor was 8-yr OS (78% vs. 79%).** (*Kuban D et al., IJROBP 2008*)

Describe the study design and results of the PROG 9509 RCT, which studied the benefit of dose escalation in localized prostate cancer.

The **PROG 9509** RCT on dose escalation enrolled 393 pts with T1b-T2b, PSA <15 ng/mL prostate cancer. Pts were randomized to 70.2 Gy or 79.2 Gy. CD RT to the prostate only was given by proton RT prior to 50.4 Gy with photon RT to the prostate and seminal vesicle. **Dose escalation improved 5-yr freedom from biochemical failure (80% vs. 61%) and 5-yr LC (48% vs. 55%).** In an unplanned analysis, a significant improvement in freedom from biochemical failure was seen in both low- and intermediate-risk subsets. (*Zietman AL et al., JAMA 2005*)

Describe the study design and results of the MRC RT01 RCT, which studied the benefit of dose escalation in the setting of neoadj and concurrent AS for localized prostate cancer.

The **MRC RT01** trial enrolled 843 men with cT1b-T3a, PSA <50 prostate cancer. All men were treated with 3–6 mos of neoadj and concurrent AS and randomized to EBRT 64 Gy or 74 Gy. The **dose escalation arm improved 5-yr bPFS (71% vs. 60%).** LC, freedom from salvage AS, and DMFS favored the dose escalation arm, although these endpoints were not statistically different. (*Dearnaley DP et al., Lancet Oncol 2007*)

What is the role of primary AS alone for localized high-risk prostate cancer?

AS alone for localized high-risk prostate cancer may be considered for men who cannot tolerate local management or who have a short life expectancy (<5 yrs). However, **SPCG-7** and Warde P et al., showed that the addition of EBRT to long-term AS conferred a survival advantage in high-risk men.

Describe the design and results of the Scandinavian RCT (SPCG-7) that studied the long-term AS +/− EBRT in locally advanced prostate cancer.

SPCG-7 enrolled 875 men with cT1b-T2, N0 WHO grade 2–3 or cT3, any grade, N0 prostate cancer. All men were treated with total AS for 3 mos → an antiandrogen alone (flutamide) indefinitely. Pts were randomized to EBRT (70 Gy) starting after 3 mos of AS or no local therapy. With median follow-up of 7.6 yrs, the addition of **EBRT improved 10-yr OS (70% vs. 61%) and 10-yr CSS (88% vs. 76%).** The 10-yr prostate cancer–specific mortality was reduced by half with EBRT (12% vs. 24%). (*Widmark A et al., Lancet 2009*)

Describe the design and results of the Warde RCT that studied the long-term AS +/− EBRT in locally advanced prostate cancer.

Warde P et al. randomized 1,205 patients with prostate cancer initially who had cT3-4 disease (later broadened to include cT2 w/ PSA >40 or PSA >40 and Gleason >8) to either lifelong AS alone (bilateral orchiectomy or LHRH agonist) +/− EBRT (pelvis to 45 Gy → prostate (65–69 Gy) or prostate alone (65–69 Gy). Addition of RT to AS resulted in improved OS (HR 0.77), 7-yr OS to 74% vs. 66% (*Warde P et al. Lancet 2011*).

What is the role of definitive prostate RT in men with node+ prostate cancer?

There has been no RCT to determine whether men with node+ prostate cancer benefit from local RT. A retrospective review by *Zagars et al.* suggested that **EBRT in addition to long-term AS confers an OS benefit to node+ pts.** (*J Urol 2001*) Subset analyses from **RTOG 8531** suggest that long-term AS + EBRT confers OS benefit compared to EBRT alone in node+ pts. However, long-term biochemical control (PSA <1.5 ng/mL) was still poor (10% at 9 yrs). (*Lawton C et al., JCO 2005*)

▶ TOXICITY

What are the most common acute and late side effects of definitive prostate RT?

Acute side effects: fatigue, urinary urgency/frequency, proctitis/diarrhea

Late side effects: erectile dysfunction (inability to maintain an erection for intercourse), cystitis, proctitis (frequency/bleeding)

Estimate the rate of erectile dysfunction in previously potent men 2+ yrs after Tx with definitive prostate RT.

~50% of men who were previously potent will no longer be able to maintain erections for intercourse 2+ yrs after definitive prostate RT. (*Robinson JW et al., IJROBP 2002*)

Does the use of short-course or long-term AS affect acute or late GU and GI RT toxicity in prostate cancer pts?

No. Multiple studies have evaluated the effect of AS on GU and GI RT toxicity. There appears to be no strong effect.

What are the common short-term and long-term side effects of AS?

Short-term side effects: hot flashes, decreased libido, fatigue

Long-term side effects: gynecomastia, anemia, decreased muscle mass, decreased bone density, obesity, mood changes, dyslipidemia, insulin resistance, possibly diabetes and coronary artery Dz

(*Higano CS, Urology 2003; Keating NL et al., JCO 2006*)

What are common side effects associated with antiandrogen therapy, and how long is the Tx course?

Common side effects of bicalutamide, which is most commonly prescribed due to its favorable toxicity profile, include **breast tenderness and gynecomastia** (50%) as well as **loss of libido, diarrhea, and hepatotoxicity.** It is generally prescribed for the 1st 2–4 wks with a GnRH analog.

55

Adjuvant and Salvage Treatment for Prostate Cancer

Updated by Jing Zeng

What % of newly diagnosed prostate cancers are cT3 Dz or higher?

12%–28% of men with newly diagnosed prostate cancer have cT3 Dz or higher.

In which portion of the prostate is ECE most commonly found?

ECE is most commonly found in the **posterolat portion of the prostate, near the prostatic neurovascular bundle.**

Name the most important factors in predicting Dz recurrence in pts undergoing local therapy for prostate cancer.

Pre-Tx PSA, Gleason score, ECE, and +margins are the most important factors in predicting Dz recurrence in pts undergoing local therapy for prostate cancer.

What is the ASTRO/ American Urological Association (AUA) definition of biochemical recurrence s/p radical prostatectomy?

The AUA definition of biochemical recurrence s/p radical prostatectomy is a serum **PSA ≥0.2,** confirmed by a 2nd determination also ≥0.2. (*Valicenti R et al., IJROBP 2013*)

What is the mean time to PSA nadir after RT for localized prostate cancer?

The mean time to PSA nadir after RT for localized prostate cancer is **~18 mos.** Though there are contradictory reports, it seems that the rate of decline in PSA does not appear to correlate with risk of Dz recurrence.

Is there an absolute PSA nadir that defines Tx failure after RT for localized prostate cancer?

The PSA nadir after RT for localized prostate cancer is a strong prognostic indicator of Tx success, but there is no absolute level below which the PSA must fall in order to define Tx success vs. failure.

What is the original ASTRO criterion (1996 consensus panel) for defining biochemical recurrence after RT for localized prostate cancer?

In order to be sure that the PSA is truly rising, the original ASTRO criteria for defining biochemical recurrence after RT for localized prostate cancer required **3 consecutive PSA rises** following a nadir. The date of biochemical recurrence was defined as halfway between the nadir and date of 1st rise or any rise enough to provoke initiation of therapy.

What is the Phoenix criterion (2005 consensus panel) for defining biochemical recurrence after RT for localized prostate cancer?

Partly to eliminate concerns about the "backdating" associated with the original ASTRO definition, the Phoenix criterion for defining biochemical recurrence after RT for localized prostate cancer is a PSA rise of **≥2 ng/mL above the PSA nadir,** even after the discontinuation of androgen deprivation therapy (ADT). The date of recurrence is the date of the PSA that triggers the definition. This definition is also considered to be useful for pts treated with EBRT and neoadj hormone therapy.

What is the concept of "PSA bounce" in pts who rcvd RT for localized prostate cancer? How should it be managed?

After RT for localized prostate cancer, serum PSA typically falls. However, **it can rise transiently,** called a *PSA bounce,* usually around **12–18 mos after Tx.** This can occur even without Dz recurrence. Using the Phoenix definition of biochemical failure, a PSA bounce can trigger a false failure in **10%–20% of pts.** There is no definitive method to distinguish a PSA bounce from recurrent Dz. The PSA should be rechecked 3–6 mos later and managed accordingly.

▶ WORKUP/STAGING

For men with rising PSA (and no other Sx of Dz) after definitive local Tx for prostate cancer, what is the utility of imaging studies, such as bone scan, CT, MRI, ProstaScint, and PET?

For men with rising PSA (and no other Sx of Dz) after definitive local Tx for prostate cancer, the **likelihood of a positive bone scan is <5% unless the PSA is >40 ng/mL.** CT also has limited utility unless the PSA value is relatively high or there is a short PSA doubling time (PSA-DT). MRI may be more sensitive in detecting mets, but its benefits must be weighed against its costs. ProstaScint remains controversial. PET scans are considered investigational, and FDG-PET is problematic b/c of the low metabolic rate of prostate cancer and the excretion of the PET agent into the bladder.

What is the utility of prostate Bx for men with a rising PSA (and no other Sx of Dz) after definitive prostate RT?

For post-RT pts with prostate cancer, **TRUS prostate Bx is typically not recommended unless local salvage options are being considered,** such as prostatectomy. Bx should be performed at least 18 mos after RT completion, since a positive result <2 yrs after Tx does not correlate well with Dz progression.

What is the utility of prostate bed Bx for men with a rising PSA (and no other Sx of Dz) after radical prostatectomy?

Utility of the prostate bed Bx is controversial, and most recurrences are at the anastomotic site. Palpable prostate bed nodules should probably be biopsied and perhaps given higher doses of RT.

▶ **TREATMENT/PROGNOSIS**

What is the prognostic significance of PSA-DT after local therapy for prostate cancer?

After radical prostatectomy for prostate cancer, PSA-DT can help predict MFS and CSS. PSA-DT <3 mos confers a 20-fold higher risk of prostate cancer death than PSA-DT ≥3 mos. **For pts with PSA-DT <3 mos, 5-yr cause-specific mortality after biochemical failure is 35% and 75% for Gleason ≤7 and ≥8 Dz, respectively.**

Name 5 prognostic factors associated with a favorable outcome after salvage RT post prostatectomy.

Prognostic factors associated with a favorable outcome after salvage RT post prostatectomy:
1. +Margin
2. Low PSA at recurrence
3. Long recurrence-free interval
4. Long PSA-DT
5. Low prostatectomy Gleason score

(*Stephenson AJ et al., JCO 2007*)

What are the indications for adj RT after prostatectomy, and what studies support its role?

The indications for adj RT after prostatectomy have been refined due to reports from 3 RCTs that included men with **pT3N0 prostate cancer or positive surgical margins** and showed improved 10-yr biochemical PFS with adj RT compared to observation: **SWOG 8794, EORTC 22911, and ARO 96-02.** The SWOG 8794 study, which has the longest follow-up, found an OS benefit with adj RT. Exploratory analyses of the EORTC study suggest that the benefit may be limited to men <70 yo or with +margins after surgery.

Describe the study design and results of the SWOG 8794 RCT that compared adj RT and observation in pts with high-risk features after prostatectomy.

SWOG 8794 enrolled 431 men with pT3N0 prostate cancer or +margin after prostatectomy and randomized to adj RT (60–64 Gy). **Adj RT improved MS (15.2 yrs vs. 13.3 yrs).** Global QOL was initially worse in the adj RT arm but was similar after 2 yrs of follow-up and superior thereafter. (*Thompson IM et al., J Urol 2009*)

Is there any evidence that salvage RT post prostatectomy improves survival compared with observation?

Yes. There are no RCTs comparing salvage RT post prostatectomy against other Tx strategies. However, there is a suggestive retrospective series from the Johns Hopkins Hospital (*Trock BJ et al., JAMA 2008*) that evaluated 635 pts s/p prostatectomy with biochemical recurrence. Tx included observation, RT alone, or RT + hormone therapy. Adjusted for prognostic factors, **cancer-specific survival was prolonged in pts who rcvd salvage RT, regardless of hormone therapy (5-yr CSS 96% vs. 88%).**

Are there randomized data comparing adj vs. salvage RT in men with locally advanced prostate cancer or biochemical recurrence s/p prostatectomy?

No. There are no published randomized trials comparing adj vs. salvage RT in men with locally advanced prostate cancer or biochemical recurrence s/p prostatectomy. The 3 randomized trials on adj therapy **(SWOG 8794, EORTC 22,911, and ARO 96-02)** compared adj RT vs. observation, without strict salvage guidelines at the 1st sign of Dz recurrence. **Nonrandomized series on salvage RT appear to produce results somewhat comparable to adj RT.**

What should be the Tx volume in adj and salvage RT post prostatectomy?

The appropriate Tx volume in adj and salvage RT post prostatectomy has not been prospectively determined. Randomized trials in adj RT **(SWOG 8794, EORTC 22,911, and ARO 96-02)** used **small-field RT and did not include regional pelvic nodal irradiation.** **RTOG-0534** is an ongoing trial looking at extent of pelvic RT, but only in men also receiving hormone therapy.

What should be the RT dose in adj and salvage RT post prostatectomy?

There are no randomized studies addressing the issue of dose in adj and salvage RT post prostatectomy. **Retrospective series typically report better outcomes when doses are >65 Gy.** The ASTRO consensus panel recommends >64 Gy. Often, pts with higher levels of pre-RT PSA or with palpable nodules will rcv higher doses of PORT. (*Valicenti R et al., IJROBP 2013*)

Are there randomized data supporting the addition of hormone therapy to salvage RT post prostatectomy?

No. There are no published randomized trials addressing the addition of hormone therapy to salvage RT post prostatectomy. **RTOG-9601,** which randomized pts to salvage RT ± Casodex, has not shown a significant difference in OS at median follow-up of 7.1 yrs, but there was an improvement in freedom from PSA progression and metastasis (*ASTRO 2010*). RTOG-0534 is investigating the addition of 4–6 mos of ADT to salvage radiation, and EORTC 22,043-30,041 is looking at the addition of ADT to adjuvant radiation patients. Based on retrospective series, **it is reasonable to recommend hormone therapy for pts with very unfavorable risk factors, such as high Gleason score or high pre-RT PSA.**

Is there a role for salvage prostatectomy for biochemical recurrence after RT for prostate cancer?

Yes. For biochemical recurrence after RT for prostate cancer, salvage prostatectomy can provide long-term Dz control in a significant portion of pts. However, salvage prostatectomy is associated with a higher risk of urinary incontinence and rectal injury, though pts treated with modern IMRT may have better outcomes. Careful pt selection is key. Outcome is better with pts with lower preop PSA. Based on retrospective series, **5-yr PFS is up to 86% for a PSA <4, 55% for a PSA 4–10, and 28% for a PSA >10.**

Is there a role for cryotherapy for biochemical recurrence after RT for prostate cancer?

This is **uncertain.** There are no prospective studies comparing cryotherapy against prostatectomy in the salvage setting post-RT with biochemical recurrence. Relative efficacy and safety are uncertain between the 2 modalities. Because cryotherapy can destroy tissue beyond the prostate, it may be an option for pts with extraprostatic extension of Dz.

Is there a role for brachytherapy for biochemical recurrence after EBRT for prostate cancer?

This in **uncertain.** There are not sufficient data to support the widespread use of LDR or HDR brachy for biochemical recurrence after EBRT for prostate cancer over the other available modalities, such as prostatectomy and cryotherapy. Small series have shown promise with good Dz control and low levels of toxicity in carefully selected pts, but further study is needed before it is considered a standard approach.

What is the optimal timing of ADT for biochemical recurrence after local therapy for prostate cancer?

Optimal timing of ADT for biochemical recurrence after local therapy for prostate cancer is controversial. In advanced prostate cancer, there is survival benefit to early initiation of ADT. Proponents of early ADT argue that even in the biochemical recurrence setting, early ADT can delay Dz progression and prolong survival. However, there are significant side effects associated with ADT, and there is no clear evidence of survival benefit compared with initiating therapy when there is clinical evidence of mets or Sx. **1 strategy is to choose early ADT in pts with high-grade Dz or short PSA-DT.**

▶ **TOXICITY**

What is the rate of urinary incontinence and anastomotic stricture with salvage prostatectomy for biochemical recurrence after RT for prostate cancer?

The rate of toxicity with salvage prostatectomy for biochemical recurrence after RT for prostate cancer is lower in modern series compared with older series due to decreased fibrosis with modern RT techniques and improved surgical techniques. In modern series, the rate of many acute and late complications are similar to standard prostatectomy. However, there are still significant rates of **urinary incontinence (30%–50%) and anastomotic stricture (17%–32%).**

Name 5 side effects associated with ADT.

Side effects associated with ADT include **hot flashes, loss of libido, decreased muscle mass, mild anemia, and loss of bone density.**

56 Metastatic Prostate Cancer

Updated by Phillip J. Gray

What % of newly diagnosed prostate cancer pts present with advanced Dz?

~10%–20% of pts present with advanced Dz (local and/or metastatic).

Has the incidence of metastatic prostate cancer changed with the introduction of the PSA?

Yes. The introduction of the PSA into general practice in the early 1990s appears to have decreased the incidence of metastatic prostate cancer; a SEER database analysis showed a 52% decrease in the incidence of metastatic prostate cancer Dx from 1990–1994. (*Stephenson RA et al., World J Urol 1997*)

How are most cases of metastatic prostate cancer identified?

The majority of metastatic prostate cancer cases are identified by an **isolated biochemical (PSA-only) recurrence;** a much smaller % of pts are detected by signs/Sx of metastatic Dz.

In what % of pts with advanced prostate cancer are serum PSA values abnl?

~**95%** of pts with metastatic Dz also have an abnl PSA, which is the most sensitive and specific marker for recurrence.

What is the anticipated natural Hx of prostate cancer after biochemical failure following local therapy?

Following local therapy and subsequent biochemical failure, the median time to development of mets is 8 yrs, and the median time to death is 13 yrs. (*Pound CR et al., JAMA 1999*)

What are common predictors of a poorer prognosis after biochemical failure following local therapy?

Poor prognostic factors after biochemical failure following local therapy:
1. **Prostate-specific antigen doubling time (PSA-DT) ≤3 mos**
2. **Gleason score ≥8**
3. **T3b Dz**
4. **LN involvement**

(*D'Amico AV et al., J Urol 2004; Katz MS et al., JCO 2004; Stephenson RA et al., JAMA 2004; Zhou P et al., JCO 2005*)

What are the common sites of mets from prostate cancer?

The most common sites are the **bones of the axial skeleton.** These lesions are usually osteoblastic but can be lytic as well.

▶ WORKUP/STAGING

What imaging modalities are commonly used for a metastatic workup?

Imaging modalities most commonly used for workup of suspected metastatic prostate cancer include whole body bone scan (technetium-99m bone scintigraphy), CT abdomen/pelvis with contrast, and chest imaging with CXR or CT. X-ray radiographs or MRI should be used if bone scan findings are equivocal.

How accurate are bone scans and CT scans at predicting mets following biochemical failure?

Bone scan and CT scan are rarely positive until PSA values of ≥30 ng/mL are reached in the absence of prior androgen suppression (AS). These scans are also more likely to be positive with higher PSA velocities. (*Cher ML et al., J Urol 1998; Kane CJ et al., Urology 2003*)

How sensitive and specific is MRI at detecting metastatic Dz?

The role of MRI in this setting has not been thoroughly evaluated. A prospective study of 66 pts with high-risk prostate cancer found the sensitivity/specificity of axial MRI to be 100%/88% compared to bone scan–X-ray sensitivity/specificity of 63%/64% in detecting mets. (*Lecouvet FE et al., JCO 2007*)

What is ProstaScint?

ProstaScint is indium-111 capromab pendetide, which is a radiolabeled monoclonal antibody used to target prostate-specific membrane antigen. It is FDA approved for detecting localized Dz recurrence after radical prostatectomy but not metastatic Dz. Data are mixed regarding the utility of ProstaScint and it is not commonly included as part of the workup for recurrent prostate cancer.

Is there a role for prostate Bx after biochemical failure in pts initially treated with RT?

Based on an ASTRO consensus statement (1999), re-Bx should be considered if the pt is considering additional local therapy and is >2 yrs s/p completion of RT. (*Cox JD et al., JCO 1999*)

▶ TREATMENT/PROGNOSIS

What is 1st-line systemic therapy for metastatic prostate cancer?

AS by orchiectomy or, more commonly, the use of a GnRH agonist is considered 1st-line therapy for metastatic prostate cancer.

What is the premise behind androgen deprivation in the Tx of prostate cancer?

Seminal studies by *Huggins C et al.* revealed that androgen deprivation through castration or estrogen administration leads to the death of prostate cancer cells. (*Cancer Res 1941*)

Is GnRH agonist therapy superior to orchiectomy for the Tx of metastatic prostate cancer?

Randomized trials and meta-analyses have confirmed equivalent long-term outcomes. Secondary to the irreversibility and psychological morbidity associated with orchiectomy, GnRH agonists are generally considered 1st-line therapy. This therapy has been shown to mainly improve PFS, not OS. (*Kaisary AV et al., Br J Urol 1991; Turkes AO et al., J Steroid Biochem 1987; Vogelzang NJ et al., Urology 1995*)

What are 3 commonly used GnRH agonists?

Most commonly used GnRH agonists:
1. Goserelin (Zoladex)
2. Leuprolide (Lupron)
3. Triptorelin (Trelstar)

All 3 are available as depot formulations.

What other modalities of AS are utilized?

GnRH antagonists, antiandrogens (AAs; nonsteroidal competitive androgen receptor [AR] antagonists), estrogens, and ketoconazole (antifungal agent, blocks cytochrome P450 enzymes involved in steroidogenesis). The recently approved drug **abiraterone** works by inhibiting 17-α hydroxylase, an important enzyme in testosterone synthesis. **Enzalutamide** is a novel AR antagonist that prevents binding of AR to DNA.

Should AS be initiated for biochemical recurrence after definitive RT in the absence of clinically evident mets?

The data are mixed, and the answer is therefore **controversial.** There are ongoing RCTs designed to address this issue (Early vs. Late Androgen Ablation Therapy [ELAAT], Ontario Clinical Oncology Group [OCOG]). Until these data are available, in our practice, the authors initiate AS in pts with high-risk features (such as Gleason score >7 and rapid PSA-DT). (*Faria SL et al., Urology 2006; Walsh PC et al., J Urol 2001*)

Should AS be initiated for radiographically evident but asymptomatic mets?

Yes. Studies have shown improved PFS with upfront AS compared with deferring therapy until signs and Sx of clinical progression. (*MRC Prostate Cancer Group, Br J Urol 1997; Nair B et al., Cochrane Database Syst Rev 2002*)

Is intermittent AS efficacious as continuous AS?

This is **uncertain.** The premise behind the use of intermittent AS is to help reduce side effects, cost, and progression to hormone-refractory Dz. Phase II studies have validated feasibility and improved QOL, and phase III trials are ongoing with preliminary data and a recent meta-analysis suggesting at least similar outcomes. (*Hussain M et al., JCO 2006; Salonen AJ et al., J Urol 2008; Shaw GL et al., BJU Int 2007; Niraula S et al., JCO 2013*)

Can AAs be used as monotherapy for AS?

Randomized trial data are **mixed.** A meta-analysis of several trials showed a trend toward OS benefit with medical/surgical castration compared to nonsteroidal AA therapy. (*Seidenfeld J et al., Ann Int Med 2000*) As a result, **common practice involves both use of GnRH alone or in combination with a nonsteroidal AA.**

Should GnRH analogs be used alone or in combination with AAs (combination androgen blockade [CAB])?

Possibly. Several randomized trials and meta-analyses have shown a small but significant OS benefit with CAB. (*PCTCG, Lancet 2000; Samson DJ et al., Cancer 2002*) GnRH monotherapy may also cause an initial flare of Sx, which can be prevented by preceding therapy with a short course of AAs. (*Kuhn JM et al., NEJM 1989*) CAB should be recommended if the side effects can be tolerated.

Typically, how long after initiating AS does it take before a pt's prostate cancer becomes androgen independent?

Androgen independence usually occurs **within 2–3 yrs of starting AS.** (*Eisenberger MA et al., NEJM 1998; Sharifi N et al., BJU Int 2005*)

What is the anticipated 5-yr OS for metastatic prostate cancer treated with CAB?

A meta-analysis by the Prostate Cancer Trialists Collaborative Group reported a **25.4%** 5-yr OS rate for pts with metastatic prostate cancer treated with CAB. (*PCTCG, Lancet 2000*)

How are pts with castrate-resistant prostate cancer commonly treated?

If CAB is being administered, withdrawal of the AA may result in PSA decline. If a GnRH analog is being given, switching to AA may help. Additionally, megestrol acetate may be used. Multiple new agents are now available, including **abiraterone, enzalutamide,** and **sipuleucel-T.** Palliative focal or systemic radiotherapy may be considered, as appropriate, in conjunction with a bisphosphonate.

What additional therapy should be offered to patients with castrate-resistant prostate cancer and clinically detectable bone metastases?

Denosumab or zoledronic acid, which have been shown in randomized trials to improve bone mineral density and decrease the risk of fracture. (*Michaelson MD et al., JCO 2007; Smith MR et al., NEJM 2009*)

What are the initial therapy options for patients with newly diagnosed castrate-resistant prostate cancer?

For patients with symptomatic metastases, **docetaxel is considered 1st-line therapy.** The utility of this regimen was demonstrated in 2 randomized trials: **TAX 327** and **SWOG 9916.** (*Tannock IF et al., NEJM 2004; Petrylak DP et al., NEJM 2004*) For patients not considered candidates for docetaxel therapy, **mitoxantrone, abiraterone, or enzalutamide** are all considered acceptable regimens. For patients who are asymptomatic or minimally symptomatic **sipuleucel-T (Provenge)** is considered an appropriate therapy. Sipuleucel-T, a form of autologous active cellular immunotherapy, was demonstrated to improve OS in a recent phase III randomized trial. (*IMPACT trial, Kantoff PW et al., NEJM 2010*)

What additional chemotherapy is available to patients who fail initial therapy with docetaxel?

The novel taxane **cabazitaxel** is considered the preferred 2nd-line agent for patients with symptomatic bone mets from castration-resistant prostate cancer. Cabazitaxel/prednisone has been shown to improve OS in patients who have failed docetaxel in a phase III randomized trial. (*de Bono JS et al., Lancet 2010*)

What novel radiopharmaceutical is available for patients with symptomatic bone mets from castration-resistant prostate cancer and what is its mechanism of action?

Radium-223 (Xofigo) has recently been approved for use in patients with symptomatic bone mets and no visceral mets. In the recent randomized phase III ALSYMPCA (ALpharadin in SYMptomatic Prostate CAncer) trial, radium-223 was demonstrated to improve OS and reduced skeletal-related events. (*Parker C et al., NEJM 2013*) Radium-223 is the first α-particle emitter to be approved for routine clinical practice. The short range and high RBE of the α-particles produced by radium-223 theoretically results in more rapid cell killing and less marrow toxicity compared with previously tested β-emitters such as strontium-89 and samarium-153.

What novel therapies are being considered for metastatic prostate cancer?

Novel therapies considered for metastatic prostate cancer:
1. Gene transfer immunotherapies are designed to express immune-stimulating compounds (e.g., GM-CSF [Gvax] and Prostvac). Phase III data are pending.
2. Gene transfer cytoreduction is designed to express lytic viruses (e.g., CV706/E1a) that preferentially target prostate cancer cells.
3. Monoclonal antibody therapies (e.g., cetuximab, trastuzumab) are being explored in phase I–II studies.
4. Novel tyrosine kinase inhibitors such as cabozantinib (XL184) are being tested in phase III trials.

▶ TOXICITY

What are the common short-term and long-term side effects of AS?

<u>Short-term effects</u>: hot flashes, ↓ libido, fatigue
<u>Long-term effects</u>: gynecomastia, anemia, ↓ muscle mass, ↓ bone density, obesity, mood changes, dyslipidemia, insulin resistance, possibly diabetes and coronary artery Dz

(*Higano CS, Urology 2003; Keating NL et al., JCO 2006*)

What are common side effects associated with AA therapy, and how long is the Tx course?

Common side effects of bicalutamide, which is the most commonly prescribed AA due to its favorable toxicity profile, include breast tenderness and gynecomastia (50%) as well as loss of libido, diarrhea, and hepatotoxicity. It is generally prescribed for the 1st 2–4 wks with a GnRH analog.

57 Brachytherapy for Prostate Cancer

Updated by Anand Shah and György Kovács

▶ BACKGROUND

What are the 2 most common types of prostate brachytherapy (brachy)?

Most common types of prostate brachy:
1. LDR using permanently implanted iodine-125 (**I-125**) or palladium-103 (**Pd-103**) radioisotopes.
2. HDR using temporarily implanted iridium-192 (**Ir-192**).

Which prostate cancer pts are good candidates for LDR brachy monotherapy?

According to the American Brachytherapy Society (ABS) guidelines, low-risk pts with the following characteristics are good candidates for LDR brachy monotherapy:
1. cT1–T2a
2. Gleason score ≤6
3. PSA <10

Select intermediate-risk patients may be candidates, absent other risk factors.

(*Davis BJ et al, Brachytherapy 2012*)

Why is the presence of seminal vesicle involvement a contraindication to prostate brachy monotherapy?

Seminal vesicle involvement is a contraindication to brachy monotherapy b/c seminal vesicles are **technically challenging to implant** with acceptable dose coverage and involvement is associated with **higher risk of regional spread** as well as **mets,** rendering LC potentially less effective.

List the relative contraindications to prostate LDR brachy.

Relative contraindications to prostate LDR brachy:
1. Severe pre-existing urinary outlet obstruction Sx (International Prostate Symptom Score [IPSS] >20)
2. Previous pelvic RT
3. Transurethral resection defects
4. Large median lobes
5. Prostate gland >60 cc
6. Inflammatory bowel disease

(*Davis BJ et al, Brachytherapy 2012*)

Why is a prostate size >60 cc a contraindication to prostate brachy?

Large prostate volumes >60 cc are considered a relative contraindication to brachy b/c they have been associated with a **higher rate of postimplant urinary retention and prolonged obstructive urinary Sx.** Implantation is also more technically difficult. (*Davis BJ et al., Brachytherapy 2012*)

Is neoadj hormonal therapy (NHT) effective at shrinking prostate size and decreasing the risk of retention?

Prostate volume may be reduced by 25%–40% after 3 mos of androgen deprivation therapy (ADT). Additionally, after 6 mos, there is no further volume reduction. It is controversial whether this decreases the risk of urinary retention. A large retrospective series demonstrated that in pts with IPSS scores ≥15, urinary retention occurred in 25% of those not taking NHT vs. 5% in those taking NHT ($p = 0.039$). (*Stone RG et al., J Urol 2010*)

Why is the presence of pre-existing urinary Sx a contraindication to brachy?

Obstructive and irritative urinary Sx are common after brachy, and **pre-existing Sx increase the risks and severity** of these side effects.

What are the advantages of prostate brachy over EBRT?

Advantages of prostate brachy over EBRT:
1. Decreased integral dose to the pt, particularly to the rectum and bladder, which allows for dose escalation
2. Simplified targeting of RT (i.e., no issues with setup variation, prostate motion, etc.)
3. Shorter Tx course

What is the purpose of ADT prior to brachy?

The purpose of ADT prior to brachy is to **downsize large glands prior to implant,** thereby potentially:
1. Decreasing urinary Sx postimplant
2. Decreasing operative time and # of seeds required
3. Decreasing rectal dose due to smaller gland size
4. Decreasing chance of pubic arch interference

Note: Several large retrospective studies have failed to show that androgen suppression improves cancer control outcomes in combination with LDR brachy.

▶ **WORKUP/STAGING**

What is the purpose of the preimplant volume study in prostate cancer pts being treated with LDR brachy?

A volume study is done prior to implant to **assess prostate volume and architecture** (presence of median lobe size, assessment for pubic arch interference) and to **develop a preliminary seed distribution plan** for ordering seeds.

What is pubic arch interference, and how can it be avoided?

Pubic arch interference is when the needle paths are obstructed by the pubic arch. It occurs more frequently in pts with large glands and affects the ant and lat needles. To evaluate for interference, TRUS can be used to compare the largest prostate cross-section with the narrowest portion of the pubic arch. Other than hormonal downsizing, the use of an extended lithotomy position (Trendelenburg) may also alleviate some pubic arch interference.

What sources are typically used in permanent seed prostate brachy?

I-125 and Pd-103 are the sources typically used in prostate brachy. Cesium-131 (Cs-131) has also been utilized more recently.

What are the half-lives of the 3 most common sources used in prostate brachy?

Half-lives of the 3 most common sources:
1. I-125 (60 days)
2. Pd-103 (17 days)
3. Cs-131 (10 days)

What doses are typically prescribed when using monotherapy with I-125, Pd-103, and Cs-131?

Doses typically prescribed for brachy monotherapy:
I-125: **140–160 Gy**
Pd-103: **110–125 Gy**
Cs-131: **115 Gy**

How far outside the prostate gland are Rx IDLs able to reach?

Rx IDLs are able to reach **3 mm** outside the prostate gland.

What can be done to place sources into the tissues surrounding the prostate to provide extracapsular coverage?

In order to reliably place sources into tissues surrounding the prostate, a possible technical solution is to place **linked seeds embedded in Vicryl sutures** in the peripheral portions of the prostate.

Prior to the closed transperineal approach, what other method of seed implantation was used?

Prior to the transperineal approach, an **open retropubic laparotomy** method of seed implantation was used.

In prostate LDR brachy, to what do D90 and V100 refer and what are the recommended values for these parameters?

In prostate LDR brachy, the **D90 refers to the min dose that covers 90% of the postimplant prostate volume** (given as a % of the prescribed dose). The goal **D90 is >90%** of the Rx dose. The **V100 refers to the volume of the prostate receiving 100% of the Rx dose.** The goal **V100 is >90%.** Although D90 and V100 are strongly correlated, D90 is used to describe how hot or cold an implant is with respect to the Rx dose and V100 is used to describe how well the implant covers the desired target.

In prostate brachy, why is the D90 parameter used and not the D100?

D90 is used instead of D100 to evaluate postimplant dosimetry b/c **retrospective studies have identified D90 as a better predictor of long-term biochemical control.** D90 may be a better predictor of outcomes b/c it is less sensitive to small differences in the way a prostate is contoured between users on postimplant CTs. (*Potters L et al., IJROBP 2001*)

In prostate brachy, to what do RV100 and Ur150 refer?

RV100 is the volume of the rectum in cubic cm receiving 100% of the Rx dose. Ur150 is the volume of the urethra receiving 150% of the Rx dose.

What are the goals for RV100 and Ur150 in prostate brachy planning?

Reasonable goals are to limit RV100 to <0.5 cc and Ur150 to <30% of the urethra.

What isotope is typically used in HDR brachy for prostate cancer?

Ir-192 is typically used for HDR brachy to treat prostate cancer.

What is the half-life for Ir-192?

The half-life for Ir-192 is **73.8 days.**

What are the dose/ fractionation schedules that have been used with HDR brachy as monotherapy for low-risk prostate cancer?

HDR dose/fractionation schedules for prostate cancer monotherapy (*Demanes DJ et al, IJROBP 2011*):
1. William Beaumont Hospital schedule: 38 Gy in 4 fx (9.5 Gy/fx) bid (1 implant/day required)
2. California Endocurietherapy Center schedule: 42 Gy in 6 fx (7 Gy/fx) in 2 separate implants 1 wk apart

Have there been any studies comparing EBRT + brachy boost to EBRT alone?

Yes. *Hoskin PJ et al.* enrolled 218 pts with T1-T3, localized prostate cancer and PSA <50 and randomized to EBRT alone (55 Gy/20 fx [2.75 Gy/ fx]) or EBRT + HDR brachy (EBRT 35.75 Gy/13 fx [2.75 Gy/fx] and then 8.5 Gy HDR × 2 over 24h). Median PSA RFS; using the RTOG/ASTRO Phoenix definition) was 9.7 yrs (combined) vs. 6.2 yrs (EBRT alone). No difference in OS. The results of this study are difficult to interpret given the nonstandard fractionation in the control arm. (*Radiother Oncol 2012*)

TREATMENT/PROGNOSIS

Estimate the long-term (8–10 yrs) biochemical control in low-risk pts treated with LDR brachy.

Estimates of long-term (8–10 yrs) biochemical control vary from **87%–94%.** (*Koukourakis G et al., Adv Urol 2009*)

Does the addition of NHT confer an RFS advantage over brachy monotherapy?

This is **uncertain.** Retrospective comparisons do not suggest that NHT improves RFS. In a matched pair analysis by *Potters L et al.,* NHT in addition to brachy did not improve 5-yr PSA RFS (87.1% vs. 86.9%, *p* = 0.935). (*JCO 2000*)

What are the data comparing the efficacy of I-125 and Pd-103 implantation for prostate brachy?

I-125 and Pd-103 appear similarly efficacious. The **Seattle Isotope trial** randomized low-risk prostate cancer pts to I-125 vs. Pd-103 and found no difference in 3-yr biochemical freedom from failure (89% vs. 91%, *p* = 0.76) and no differences in morbidity. (*Wallner K et al., IJROBP 2003*)

Describe the PSA bounce and its prognostic significance following brachy as monotherapy for prostate cancer.

The PSA bounce is the abrupt rise and fall in the PSA value following brachy Tx. Bounces of ≥0.2 ng/mL may occur in 40% of pts with a median onset of 15 mos and a magnitude of 0.76 ng/mL. Younger pts appear more likely to have a bounce. Bounces of >2 ng/mL (i.e., biochemical failure by Phoenix definition) may occur in 15% of pts. However, PSA bounce does not appear to predict for clinical failure. (*Crook J et al., IJROBP 2007*)

TOXICITY

What are the most common acute and late side effects from prostate LDR brachy?

Obstructive and irritative urinary Sx and impotence are side effects that are generally experienced due to prostate seed implantation. Rectal toxicity is relatively rare.

Are phosphodiesterase inhibitors effective for prostate brachy–related erectile dysfunction (ED)?

Yes. ~50% of pts who have ED after prostate brachy can achieve erections useful for intercourse with the use of phosphodiesterase inhibitors.

How does the intensity and timing of urinary irritation differ between men treated with I-125 vs. Pd-103?

Irritative Sx are more intense and occur earlier but resolve more quickly in prostate brachy pts treated with Pd-103 compared to I-125. In the Seattle Isotope trial, at 1-mo postimplant, I-125 implanted pts had a mean morbidity American Urological Association (AUA) score of 14.8 compared with 18.6 for the Pd-103 pts (*p* = 0.0009). At 6 mos, mean AUA scores were 12 for I-125 implanted pts and 9.9 for Pd-103 pts. (*Herstein A et al., Cancer 2005*)

Estimate the incidence of late rectal bleeding in prostate cancer pts treated with LDR brachy monotherapy. Is there a difference in the incidence between I-131 vs. Pd-103 brachy?

In the Seattle Isotope trial, the overall incidence of late rectal bleeding was **9%.** There was **no significant difference** between I-125 and Pd-103 pts, though there was a trend toward more radiation proctitis in the I-125 arm. (*Herstein A et al., Cancer 2005*)

What acute toxicities are associated with HDR brachy?

Similar to LDR therapy, prostate HDR brachy pts experience **frequency, urgency, and urinary retention acutely.**

What are the late toxicities that have been associated with prostate HDR brachy?

Potential late toxicities associated with prostate HDR brachy: urethral stricture (most common), prolonged dysuria, urinary retention, hematuria, and urinary incontinence. Rectal pain and rectal bleeding can also occur.

58 Bladder Cancer

Updated by Brian C. Baumann and John P. Christodouleas

▶ BACKGROUND

How prevalent is bladder cancer in the U.S.?

Bladder cancer is the **4th most commonly diagnosed cancer in men** behind prostate, lung, and colorectal malignancies and the **9th most commonly diagnosed cancer in women.**

How many cases are diagnosed and how many deaths occur annually in the U.S.?

There are **~73,000 cases** of bladder cancer and **~15,000 deaths** annually.

What are common risk factors for bladder cancer?	Common risk factors include: 1. **Smoking** 2. Chronic bladder irritation (nephrolithiasis, urinary tract infection, etc.) 3. Chemical exposures (Cytoxan, amino biphenyl, naphthylamine, etc.) 4. Prior pelvic irradiation 5. *Schistosoma haematobium* infection (associated only with squamous cell carcinoma [SCC])
What is the median age at diagnosis?	The median age is **65 yrs.**
Is bladder cancer more common in men or women?	In the U.S., urothelial bladder cancer is diagnosed **3 times more frequently in men** than women. For squamous histology, the incidence between men and women are equal.
What is the most common histologic subtype in developed and developing countries?	In developed countries, **~90% of bladder cancers are urothelial carcinomas, formerly called transitional cell carcinomas.** In developing countries, SCCs often predominate.
What are the different histopathologic types of bladder cancer in order of decreasing frequency?	The most common histology in the U.S. is urothelial carcinoma (94%) > SCC (3%) > adenocarcinoma (2%) > small cell tumors (1%).
What % of newly detected bladder tumors are Ta/Tis/T1 lesions?	~70% of bladder cancers are exophytic papillary tumors, with 70% of these confined to the mucosa (Ta/Tis) and 30% confined to the submucosa (T1).
What % of patients have distant metastases at diagnosis?	**~8%** have metastatic disease at presentation, usually involving bones, lungs, or liver.

▶ WORKUP/STAGING

What is the most common presenting Sx of bladder cancer?	The most common presenting Sx is **painless hematuria.**
What are the initial steps in the workup of suspected bladder cancer? What additional workup is needed after a cancer diagnosis is established?	1. Perform **urine cytology and cystoscopy.** 2. If a lesion is identified that is solid, of high grade, or suspicious for muscle invasion, then **CT/MRI of the abdomen and pelvis** ideally prior to Bx so induced inflammatory changes do not result in overstaging. 3. Perform a **transurethral resection of bladder tumor (TURBT) and EUA.** 4. If a cancer diagnosis is made, **image the upper urinary tract** (CT or MRI urography, intravenous pyelogram, renal US, retrograde pyelogram, or ureteroscopy).

5. For muscle-invasive disease, obtain **chest imaging** (CXR or CT) and consider bone scan if the patient is symptomatic or has an elevated alkaline phosphatase level.
6. Recommended blood work includes **CBC/CMP.**

For adequate clinical staging, what should be present in the initial TURBT pathologic specimen?

The Bx specimen should contain **muscle from the bladder wall** to properly stage the tumor.

What are the indications for re-resection after initial TURBT?

Repeat resection should be performed when there is:
1. Incomplete resection of gross tumor
2. High-grade disease and no muscle in specimen
3. Any T1 lesion

What is the AJCC 7th edition (2011) T-stage criteria for bladder cancer?

Ta: noninvasive papillary carcinoma
Tis: CIS ("flat tumor")
T1: tumor invades subepithelial connective tissue
T2a: tumor invades superficial muscularis propria (inner half)
T2b: tumor invades deep muscularis propria (outer half)
T3a: microscopic invasion of perivesical tissue
T3b: macroscopic invasion of perivesical tissue
T4a: tumor invades prostatic stroma, uterus, vagina
T4b: tumor invades pelvic wall, abdominal wall

Can a TURBT be used to define the pathologic tumor (pT) stage?

No. pT stage is defined by an evaluation of a cystectomy specimen. TURBT findings are included in the clinical T-stage (cT) staging.

What is the probability of pathologic pelvic nodal involvement based on the pT stage of a bladder tumor?

Pelvic node involvement by pT stage (*Stein JP et al., JCO 2001*):
Overall: 24% LN+
pT0-T1: 5%
pT2: 18%
pT3 a: 26%
pT3b: 46%
pT4: 42%

Can the cT stage reliably predict occult pathologic pelvic node involvement?

No. cT stage does not reliably predict occult pathologic node involvement because there is significant discordance between cT stage and pT stage. (*Goldsmith B et al., IJROBP 2014*)

What is the AJCC 7th edition (2011) N- and M-stage criteria for bladder cancer?

N0: no regional LN involvement
N1: single +LN in true pelvis (hypogastric, obturator, external iliac, or presacral)
N2: multiple LNs in true pelvis
N3: mets to common iliac LN
M0: no distant mets
M1: positive distant mets

Define the AJCC 7th edition (2011) bladder cancer stage grouping based on TNM status.	**Stage 0 a:** Ta, N0, M0 **Stage 0is:** Tis, N0, M0 **Stage I:** T1, N0, M0 **Stage II:** T2, N0, M0 **Stage III:** T3 or T4 a, N0, M0 **Stage IV:** T4b or N+ or M1

Define the AJCC 7th edition (2011) bladder cancer stage grouping based on TNM status.

Stage 0 a: Ta, N0, M0
Stage 0is: Tis, N0, M0
Stage I: T1, N0, M0
Stage II: T2, N0, M0
Stage III: T3 or T4 a, N0, M0
Stage IV: T4b or N+ or M1

Estimate the 5-yr OS by stage.

5-yr OS rates for bladder cancer based on SEER data:
Stage 0: 98%
Stage I: 88%
Stage II: 63%
Stage III: 46%
Stage IV: 15%

▶ **TREATMENT/PROGNOSIS**

Which pts with noninvasive bladder cancer can be observed after maximum TURBT?

Observation is indicated for non–muscle invasive bladder cancer pts after max TURBT with all of the following characteristics:
1. Completely resected
2. Ta
3. Grade 1
4. No residual abnormality on urine cytology

What are the indications for adj therapy in pts with non–muscle invasive bladder cancer (NMIBC) treated with TURBT?

Pts with NMIBC should be treated with intravesicular therapies after TURBT if:
1. Grades 2–3
2. T1
3. Tis
4. Multifocal or residual Dz

What agents are commonly used for intravesicular therapy following TURBT for NMIBC?

Intravesicular immunotherapy (bacillus Calmette-Guerin [**BCG**]) was superior to intravesicular chemotherapy (mitomycin) for preventing tumor recurrence following TURBT for NMIBC based on 4 meta-analyses. Intravesicular therapy is usually initiated 3–4 wks after resection.

Is NMIBC likely to recur?

Yes. Pts with resected non–muscle invasive Dz have a >50% chance of recurrence within 5 yrs.

Which subsets of pts with NMIBC are at highest risk of having a muscle invasive bladder cancer (MIBC) recurrence?

Pts with CIS or high grade T1 NMIBC are at highest risk of developing a MIBC recurrence.

How is a recurrence of NMIBC treated?

Ta or low-grade T1 disease that recurs is treated with repeat TURBT + intravesicular BCG. Recurrent high-grade T1 or CIS disease is treated more aggressively, often with cystectomy. TURBT + concurrent chemo/ RT is a noncystectomy option for medically inoperable or selected operable pts with recurrent high-grade T1.

What are the Tx options for pts with node– MIBC (cT2-T4a, N0) who are medically operable?

For **medically operable** pts with node– MIBC, standard Tx options include:
1. Radical cystectomy (RC) + lymph node dissection (LND) +/– neoadj or adj chemo
2. Selective bladder preservation for pts without high-risk features
3. Partial cystectomy + LND +/– neoadj chemo

What is involved in an RC?

RC removes the bladder, distal ureters, pelvic peritoneum, prostate, seminal vesicles, uterus, fallopian tubes, ovaries, and anterior vaginal wall. Urine can be diverted via a conduit to the abdominal wall or to an orthotopic neobladder.

What regions are typically included in the pelvic LND?

LND typically includes the distal common iliac, internal and external iliac, and obturator nodes but many surgeons advocate an "extended" LND that includes the proximal common iliacs and presacral nodes.

What are the 3 most common types of urinary diversions?

The 3 most common urinary diversions are:
1. Noncontinent diversion with a bowel conduit (e.g., ileal conduit)
2. Continent nonorthotopic catheterizable diversion (e.g., Indiana pouch)
3. Continent orthotopic diversion (e.g., Studer pouch)

Estimate the 5-yr OS after RC for MIBC.

5-yr OS after RC is ~60% for stage T2 and ~40% in stages T3-T4a with most patients dying with DM. (*Grossman HB et al., NEJM 2003*)

Is there evidence to support neoadj chemo prior to RC in MIBC?

Yes. Multiple RCTs suggest a **~5% OS benefit** to neoadj chemo + RC compared to RC alone. (*Grossman HB et al., NEJM 2003; Sherif A et al., Eur Urol 2004*)

What is the argument against standard use of neoadj chemo for MIBC?

Neoadj chemo may represent **overtreatment** of subsets of pts who actually have pT0-2, pN0 disease. Some favor adj chemo for subsets of MIBC found to **have pT3-4 and/or N+ Dz.** Small series suggest a benefit of adj chemo after RC, but neoadj and adj chemo paradigms have not been compared.

What % of MIBC pts have pT0 at the time of RC?

~15% of MIBC pts have pT0 at the time of RC. Neoadj chemo improves pT0 rate to ~38%. (*Grossman HB et al., NEJM 2003*)

Name 3 predictors of pelvic failure after RC?

The 3 strongest predictors of pelvic failure (isolated and co-synchronous with DM) are **pT3-4 disease, +margins,** and **<10 benign or malignant lymph nodes identified** in the LND specimen. (*Baumann BC et al., ASTRO 2013*)

Where are pelvic recurrences after RC typically found?

In pT3-4 patients with –margins, failures occur predominantly along the pelvic sidewalls (obturator and iliac regions). In pT3-4 patients with +margins, most pelvic failures are still found along the sidewalls, but recurrences in the cystectomy bed and presacral region increase significantly. (*Baumann BC et al., IJROBP 2013*)

Is there a role for postop RT (PORT) in MIBC pts with +margins?

Yes. PORT is commonly offered to MIBC pts with +margins because 5-yr the pelvic recurrence rate is ~68% and long-term survival after isolated pelvic recurrence is <5%. (*Herr HW et al., JCO 2004*)

Is there a role for PORT in MIBC pts with –margins?

Possibly. There are no RCTs comparing PORT to observation specifically in margin– pts. However, the RCT by *Zaghloul M et al.* randomized pts with locally advanced MIBC with or without +margins to observation, hyper-fx PORT, or standard fx PORT. (*IJROBP 1992*) PORT significantly improved the 5-yr disease-free survival (DFS) in the hyper-fx and standard fx PORT arms (49% and 44%, respectively) compared with the observation arm (25%). Most pts in this trial had SCC. The value of PORT for urothelial MIBC treated with modern surgery and chemotherapy is being studied.

Is there a role for preop RT?

Possibly. Preop RT was commonly used in the past but abandoned when several small RCTs performed in the 1970s and 1980s showed no survival benefit. These trials had limited power and included early-stage pts unlikely to benefit. (*Huncharek M et al., Anticancer Res 1998*) A small RCT of SCC and urothelial cancer pts compared preop RT vs. PORT and found similar efficacy and toxicity. (*El-Monin HA et al., Urol Oncol 2013*)

What factors are used to select MIBC pts for selective bladder preservation?

Ideal candidates for selective bladder preservation have:
1. Good baseline bladder function
2. Unifocal, cT2-3 tumors
3. Limited CIS
4. No hydronephrosis
5. A visibly complete TURBT

Only 6%–19% of medically operable MIBC pts are good candidates for selective bladder preservation. (*Sweeney P et al., Urol Clin N Am 1992*)

What is the difference between continuous-course and split-course selective bladder preservation paradigms?

The **continuous course paradigm** completes the entire course of planned chemo/RT and assesses response with TURBT ~3 mos after. The **split-course paradigm** involves an induction chemo/RT phase, a planned break with response assessment ~3 wks after, and a consolidation chemo/RT phase.

Is there evidence that concurrent chemo-RT is superior to RT alone in MIBC?

Yes. The **BC2001** randomized MIBC to concurrent chemo/RT vs. RT alone. 2-yr local-regional DFS favored chemo/RT (67% vs. 54%). (*James ND et al., NEJM 2012*)

Is there a role for neoadj chemotherapy prior to chemo-RT for bladder preservation?

RTOG 8903 randomized MIBC pts to neoadj methotrexate/cisplatin/vinblastine (MCV) + cisplatin/ RT vs. cisplatin/RT alone. Neoadj MCV did not improve pCR, DM, or OS and was poorly tolerated, with only 67% of patients completing the prescribed therapy. (*Shipley WU et al., JCO 1998*)

Describe the concurrent chemo and RT regimen used in BC2001.

In the concurrent chemo/RT arm of **BC2001,** MIBC pts were treated with **5-FU + mitomycin** and **64 Gy/32 fx qd or 55 Gy/20 fx qd.** The trial included a 2nd randomization to either standard whole bladder RT (PTV: noninvolved bladder + 1.5-cm margin + 2-cm margin around any extravesicular Dz) or to reduced high-dose volume RT, where dose to uninvolved bladder was 80% of max. Pelvic nodes were not intentionally targeted. (*James ND et al., NEJM 2012*)

Describe the chemo and RT used in RTOG 8903.

In the concurrent chemo/RT alone arm of **RTOG 8903,** MIBC pts were treated with induction **cisplatin q3 wks + 39.6 Gy/22 fx qd** targeting the small pelvis (whole bladder, perivesicular, obturator, external iliac and internal iliac nodes). Complete responders were treated with consolidation **cisplatin q3 wks + 5.4 Gy/3 fx** to the small pelvis followed by a boost to the tumor bed of **19.8 Gy/11 fx (total 64.8 Gy).** (*Shipley WU et al., JCO 1998*)

How are locally recurrent NMIBC and MIBC treated after bladder preservation?

Recurrent NMIBC may be treated with TURBT + intravesicular therapy. Recurrent MIBC is treated with prompt RC.

Estimate the CR rate at initial assessment and 5-yr OS after selective bladder preservation.

60%–80% of pts have a CR at initial post-Tx TUBRT after selective bladder preservation. **5-yr OS 40%–60%.** OS after selective bladder preservation appears comparable to OS after RC, but the 2 Txs have not been compared in an RCT.

What are the Tx options for pts with node– MIBC (cT2-T4 a, N0) who are medically inoperable?

For **medically inoperable** pts with node– MIBC, the most well-established option is **definitive chemo/RT.** Pts unfit for definitive chemo/RT should have maximal safe TURBT and can be offered observation, RT alone, or chemo alone.

How does the chemo-RT technique differ for medically operable and inoperable pts?

For medically inoperable pts, only **continuous-course paradigm** is used, since salvage RC is not an option. Similar doses and target volumes are used, though there is a stronger case for pelvic nodal radiation in inoperable pts because they often have more advanced disease and there is no concern about complicating the urinary diversion of a salvage RC.

What are the Tx options for locally advanced bladder tumors (e.g., cT4b or cN+)?

For cT4b or cN+ bladder cancers, Tx options are:
1. Definitive chemo/RT → cystectomy (if possible) or adj chemo
2. Induction chemo → cystectomy (if possible) or definitive chemo/RT or additional chemo

Estimate the 5-yr OS for medically inoperable or locally advanced MIBC treated with definitive chemo-RT.

SWOG 9312 was a single arm trial including 53 pts with cT2-4, any N, who were medically inoperable, unresectable, or refused surgery. Tx included max TURBT → cisplatin/5-FU + 60 Gy → adj cisplatin/5-FU. **5-yr OS ~32%.**

What are the 1st-line chemo regimens for bladder cancer?

Gemcitabine + cisplatin (GC) or **dose-dense MVAC** (methotrexate, vinblastine, doxorubicin, and cisplatin) are considered 1st-line chemo regimens for neoadj, adj, or palliative chemo (per NCCN 2014).

How is metastatic bladder cancer treated?

Cisplatin-based combination chemo is the preferred initial Tx. GC, or dose-dense MVAC are frequently used. GC is often preferred over MVAC because of similar efficacy and reduced toxicity. (*von der Maase H et al., JCO 2000*) For patients with impaired renal function or ECOG performance status ≥2, carboplatin-based chemo is often used. Local therapy (surgery or RT) may be considered depending on the extent of response to palliative chemo.

How is mixed histology or pure nonurothelial bladder cancers treated?

Tumors of mixed histology with urothelial elements generally have a poorer prognosis but should be treated like pure urothelial carcinoma. Tumors with a small cell component are treated with neoadj chemo using small-cell regimens followed by RC or RT. Tx of SCC or adenocarcinoma uses chemo specific to the lesion's histology.

▶ **TOXICITY**

What are the operative mortality rates and perioperative complication rates following radical cystectomy?

Operative mortality rates are 2%–5% with short-term complication rates of 28%–57%. In a randomized trial of open vs. robotic cystectomy, short-term grade ≥3 morbidity was 22%–24% with no difference in morbidity between the 2 techniques. (*Laudone VP et al., AUA 2013 abstract*)

What are the toxicities associated with RT for organ preservation?	<u>Short-term complications</u>: transient urinary frequency/urgency, dysuria, hematuria, bladder spasms, diarrhea, radiation dermatitis, fatigue <u>Relatively common long-term complications:</u> chronic urinary frequency/urgency, erectile dysfunction, diarrhea <u>Uncommon long-term complications:</u> chronic hematuria, dysuria, hematochezia, bowel obstructions or fistulas, 2nd cancers or fractures in the irradiated field
What is the impact of organ preservation approaches on QOL for patients with bladder cancer?	QOL for patients after bladder preservation therapy is good. Urodynamic studies and patient-reported outcomes from the Massachusetts General Hospital found that 78% of patients retained normal bladder function with 85% reporting little-to-no urinary urgency. Bowel symptoms were reported by 22%. 50% reported normal erectile function. (*Zietman ZS et al., J Urol 2003*)
How many patients require cystectomy for palliation of Tx-related toxicities following bladder preservation?	Cystectomies performed for palliation of bladder preservation–related toxicities are very uncommon with rates of **0%–2%.** (*Rodel C et al., JCO 2002; Shipley WU et al., J Urol 2002*)
What is the recommended follow-up for patients with MIBC treated with bladder preservation?	**Urine cytology, cystoscopy + Bx, imaging of the upper urinary tracts, abdomen, pelvis q3–6 mos for the first 2 yrs,** and then at increasing intervals. **LFTs, BMP, and chest imaging performed q6–12 mos.**

59 Seminoma

Updated by Reid F. Thompson

▶ BACKGROUND

Clinically, what are the 2 main subgroups of testicular germ cell tumors (GCTs)?	**Seminomatous and nonseminomatous** germ cell tumors (NSGCTs) are the 2 main subgroups of testicular GCTs. 60% are pure seminoma, 30% are NSGCTs, and 10% are mixed (pts with mixed histology are typically considered to have NSGCTs).

What is the estimated annual incidence and mortality from testicular cancer in the U.S.? Has the incidence been increasing or decreasing?

In the U.S., the annual testicular cancer **incidence is ~8,000 and mortality is ~380.** From 1973–1998, the **incidence in testicular GCTs rose 44%** in the U.S. (mostly seminoma).

What is the most common age group for testicular seminoma?

Testicular seminoma is most common in those **25–40 yrs of age.**

In the U.S., what is the relative incidence of testicular tumors in white men vs. black men?

Testicular cancer is **5.4 times more common in white men** than black men.

What is the best established risk factor for testicular cancer?

A **Hx of cryptorchidism** increases the risk of testicular cancer by ~5 times. The higher the undescended testicle (inguinal canal vs. intra-abdominal), the higher the risk. Orchiopexy prior to puberty lowers this risk. 5%–20% of tumors in pts with a Hx of cryptorchidism develop in the contralat, normally descended testis. The risk is greatest in cases of bilat cryptorchidism.

In a pt with a prior Dx of testicular cancer, what is the cumulative incidence (at 25 yrs) of contralat testicular seminoma?

At 25 yrs following the primary Dx, the cumulative incidence of contralat testicular seminoma is **3.6%.**

What is the most common chromosomal abnormality in testicular GCTs?

A **12p isochromosome** (i.e., a chromosome with 2 copies of the short arm of chromosome 12) is the most common testicular GCT chromosomal abnormality.

Name the layers of tissue surrounding the testes from outer to inner.

Layers of tissue surrounding the testes (outer to inner):
1. Skin
2. Tunica dartos
3. External spermatic fascia
4. Cremaster muscle
5. Internal spermatic fascia
6. Parietal layer of tunica vaginalis
7. Visceral layer of tunica vaginalis
8. Tunica albuginea

Compare and contrast lymphatic drainage of the left vs. right testis.

Lymphatic drainage from testicular tumors goes directly to the para-aortic (P-A) nodes. The left testicular vein drains to the left renal vein, and nodal drainage is primarily to the P-A nodes, directly below the left renal hilum. The right testicular vein drains to the IVC; paracaval and interaortocaval nodes are most commonly involved. Lymphatic drainage from the right testes commonly crosses over to the left, but the reverse is rare.

What is the chance of pelvic/inguinal nodal involvement from testicular cancer? What increases this risk?	Pelvic/inguinal nodes are rarely (<3%) involved by testicular cancer. Risk of involvement increases with: 1. Prior scrotal or inguinal surgery 2. Tumor invasion of the tunica vaginalis or lower onethird of epididymis 3. Cryptorchidism
What is the DDx of a testicular mass?	The DDx of a testicular mass includes tumor, torsion, hydrocele, varicocele, spermatocele, and epididymitis.
What is the classic presentation of testicular cancer?	A **painless testicular mass** is the classic presentation of testicular cancer. However, up to 45% of pts will present with pain.

▶ WORKUP/STAGING

What imaging modality is preferred for primary evaluation of a testicular mass?	**Transscrotal US** is preferred for primary evaluation of a testicular mass. Testicular tumors are typically hypoechoic.
What is the preferred primary surgical Tx for a unilat testicular tumor?	**Transinguinal orchiectomy** is the preferred surgical Tx for unilat testicular tumor.
What are 3 tumor markers that should be drawn before orchiectomy for testicular tumor?	Before orchiectomy for a testicular tumor, levels of β-HCG, AFP, and LDH should be drawn.
What are the half-lives of β-HCG and AFP?	The half-life for β-**HCG is 22 hrs.** The half-life for **AFP is 5 days.**
How commonly are β-HCG and AFP elevated in testicular seminoma vs. NSGCT? What are unrelated etiologies for elevated β-HCG and AFP?	β-HCG is elevated in 15% of seminomas. AFP is never elevated in seminoma. 1 or both markers will be elevated in 85% of NSGCTs. The use of marijuana can elevate β-HCG, and reagent cross-reaction with LH can cause falsely elevated results. Hepatocellular carcinoma, cirrhosis, and hepatitis can elevate AFP.
What imaging studies, labs, and evaluation should be ordered following transinguinal orchiectomy for seminoma?	Following transinguinal orchiectomy for seminoma, chest imaging (CXR), CT abdomen/pelvis, AFP, β-HCG, and LDH should be ordered. If the CT is positive, bone scan should be added. Pts should also have fertility evaluation and consider sperm banking.
Describe the AJCC 7th edition (2011) TNM and S staging for testicular tumors.	**T1:** limited to testis and epididymis with no LVSI or tunica vaginalis involvement **T2:** LVSI or involvement of tunica vaginalis **T3:** involvement of spermatic cord **T4:** scrotal invasion

N1: single or multiple regional nodes, all ≤2 cm in greatest dimension

N2: single or multiple regional nodes, any >2–5 cm in greatest dimension

N3: single or multiple regional nodes, any >5 cm in greatest dimension

M1 a: nonregional nodal or pulmonary Dz

M1b: nonpulmonary visceral mets

S0: normal LDH, β-HCG, and AFP

S1: LDH <1.5 times normal, β-HCG <5,000 mIU/mL, and AFP <1,000 ng/mL

S2: LDH 1.5–10 times normal, β-HCG 5,000–50,000, or AFP 1,000–10,000

S3: LDH >10 times normal, β-HCG >50,000, or AFP >10,000

Summarize the AJCC 7ᵗʰ edition (2011) stage grouping for testicular tumors.

Stage I: no Dz beyond testis/scrotum (i.e., T1-4N0M0S1-3)

Stage II: regional nodal involvement and S0-S1 tumor markers (IIA = N1, IIB = N2, IIC = N3)

Stage III: S2-S3 tumor markers with N1-S3 Dz, or M1 Dz

What is the stage group distribution for testicular seminoma at presentation?

Most testicular seminoma pts present with stage I Dz (70%–80%), 15%–20% have stage II Dz, and 5% have stage III Dz.

In addition to AJCC staging, what is another common staging system for testicular seminoma?

In addition to AJCC staging, **Royal Marsden staging** is also used for testicular seminoma. This staging is largely similar to the AJCC stage grouping:

Stage I: confined to testis

Stage IIA: node <2 cm

Stage IIB: node 2–5 cm

Stage IIC: node 5–10 cm

Stage IID: node >10 cm

Stage III: nodes above/below diaphragm

Stage IV: extralymphatic mets

▶ **TREATMENT/PROGNOSIS**

Following transinguinal orchiectomy, what is the optimal Tx for stage I seminoma, stages IIA–IIB seminoma, and stage IIC or greater seminoma?

Following transinguinal orchiectomy, pts with **stage I seminoma** may rcv **surveillance,** adj RT, or single-agent chemo. Pts with **stages IIA–IIB Dz** should rcv **adj RT.** Pts with **stage IIC or greater Dz** should be treated with **multiagent chemo.**

For pts undergoing surveillance for stage I seminoma, estimate the 10-yr relapse rate and 10-yr CSS rate.

For pts undergoing surveillance for stage I seminoma, the **10-yr relapse rate is 15%–20%** but nearly all relapses can be salvaged. **10-yr CSS is ~99.6%.** (*Mortensen MS et al., ASCO 2013 abstract*)

For pts undergoing surveillance for stage I seminoma, where do most relapses occur?

85% of relapses are in the **P-A nodes.** Observation should therefore include regular CT assessment of the abdomen and pelvis.

What pathologic factors are associated with increased risk of relapse following transinguinal orchiectomy for stage I seminoma?

Pathologic factors associated with risk of relapse following transinguinal orchiectomy include:
1. tumor size >4 cm
2. LVSI
3. β-HCG >200 IU/L
4. Rete testis invasion

(*Warde P et al., JCO 2002; Mortensen MS et al., ASCO 2013 abstract*)

Following P-A relapse in pts observed following transinguinal orchiectomy for stage I seminoma, what are the appropriate Tx options?

Following P-A relapse in pts observed following transinguinal orchiectomy for stage I seminoma, **retroperitoneal RT** (for nodes <5 cm) **or multiagent chemo** are reasonable Tx options.

For pts treated with P-A RT following transinguinal orchiectomy for stage I seminoma, what is the relapse rate? Where do relapses occur?

For pts treated with P-A RT following transinguinal orchiectomy for stage I seminoma, relapse occurs in **0.5%–5%** of pts. Most relapses occur within 2 yrs. In-field relapses are extremely rare; most relapses are mediastinal, lung, left supraclavicular, or (if risk factors are present) inguinal. Surveillance should include regular CXR.

What data support the option of adj chemo for stage I seminoma following transinguinal orchiectomy?

MRC-UK randomized 1,447 stage I seminoma pts between adj RT (2 Gy/fx to 20 or 30 Gy) and 1 cycle of carboplatin. There was no difference in 3-yr relapse rates (3.4% for RT vs. 4.6% for carboplatin). (*Oliver R et al., Lancet 2005*)

In a stage I seminoma pt, what factors would favor active treatment over surveillance?

In a stage I seminoma pt, concern over pt adherence with follow-up may favor active treatment.

Why is P-A RT not part of the definitive management of pts with stage IIC seminoma?

P-A RT is not part of the definitive management of pts with stage IIC seminoma due to **high rates of distant failure** (mediastinal, lung, supraclavicular, or bone). Thus, chemo is needed. In 1 series, 5-yr RFS among IIC pts treated with orchiectomy and RT alone was only 44%. (*Chung PW et al., Eur Urol 2004*)

What is the appropriate Tx for pts with stages I–IIB seminoma following relapse after adj P-A RT?

Pts with stages I–IIB seminoma who relapse following adj P-A RT should be treated with **salvage chemo.**

How should seminoma pts with stage IIC or greater be treated?

4 cycles of cisplatin/etoposide (+/– bleomycin) are appropriate for seminoma pts with stage IIC or greater.

What is the appropriate RT field for stage I seminoma pts?

Stage I seminoma pts (if receiving adj RT) should have the P-A nodes treated. **MRC-UK TE 10** randomized 478 pts to P-A RT +/– pelvic RT and found equivalent RFS (96%). (*Fossa SD et al., JCO 1999*) 4 pelvic failures occurred in the P-A group (vs. none in the P-A + pelvic group).

For adj stage I seminoma, what are the borders for a P-A field?

Borders for a P-A field (for adj stage I seminoma):
Superior: T10-11 has been the historical standard, however, cranial reduction to T11-12 reduces kidney, stomach, and small bowel dose without compromise in RFS. (*Bruns F et al., Acta Oncol 2005*)
Inferior: L4-L5
Lateral: 2 cm on vertebral bodies. If left-sided primary, give 1-cm border on left renal hilum and sacroiliac joint. CT-based planning using vascular and nodal anatomy may help avoid marginal misses. (*Martin JM et al., Radiother Oncol 2005*)

What is the appropriate field for a stages IIA–IIB seminoma pt?

A stages IIA–IIB seminoma pt should have a "dogleg" or "hockey stick" field treated (including P-A and ipsi pelvic nodes). The sup border is at T10-11, and the inf border is at the obturator foramen. Per **MRC-UK TE 10**:
Superior: T10-11
Inferior: mid obturator foramen
Ipsilateral: renal hilum down as far as disc between 5th lumbar and 1st sacral vertebrae (L5-S1), then diagonally to lat edge of acetabulum, then vertically downward to mid obturator level
Contralateral: inclusion of processus transversus in P-A area down to L5-S1, then diagonally in parallel with ipsi border, then vertically to median border of obturator foramen

What is a reasonable dose and fractionation schedule for stage I seminoma?

For stage I seminoma, common prescription doses include:
Stage IA. **25 Gy** in 1.25 Gy/fx
Stage IB. **25.5 Gy** in 1.5 Gy/fx
Stage IC. **20 Gy** in 2 Gy/fx

The **MRC-UK TE 18** trial compared 2 Gy/fx to 20 Gy vs. 30 Gy and found equivalent relapse rates at 5 yrs. (*Jones WG et al., JCO 2005*)

What is a reasonable dose and fractionation schedule for stages IIA–IIB seminoma?

For stage IIA–IIB seminoma, the "dogleg" field may be treated with a similar dose-fractionation as stage I. Gross LAD may be boosted with an additional 5–10 Gy in 2 Gy/fx (~30 Gy for IIA, ~35 Gy for IIB).

What pathologic subtype of seminoma can be uniformly treated with orchiectomy alone?	**Spermatocytic seminoma** can be treated with orchiectomy alone. This tumor is seen in older pts and, while the precursor cell is unknown, is probably not a true seminoma.

▶ **TOXICITY**

What RT dose can induce temporary azoospermia? Doses greater than what may cause permanent aspermia?	RT doses as low as 0.2–0.5 Gy will cause temporary azoospermia. Doses >0.5 Gy can cause extended or permanent aspermia.
What should be done to reduce the testicular RT dose during Tx for testicular seminoma?	During RT for testicular seminoma, a **clamshell should be used** to reduce the dose to the contralat testis.

60 Testicular Nonseminomatous Germ Cell Tumor

Updated by Reid F. Thompson and Thomas J. Guzzo

▶ **BACKGROUND**

Approximately how many cases of germ cell tumor (GCT) are diagnosed annually in the U.S.?	**~8,000 cases/yr** in the U.S.
What % of testicular malignancies are GCTs?	**~95%** of testicular malignancies are GCTs.
What is the most common solid tumor in men age 15–34 yrs?	**GCT** is the most common solid tumor in men age 15–34 yrs.
How has the incidence of GCTs changed in the past 40 yrs?	The incidence of GCTs has **more than doubled** in the past 40 yrs.

Name 5 risk factors for GCTs.

Risk factors for GCTs:
1. Prior personal Hx of GCT
2. Positive family Hx
3. Cryptorchidism
4. Testicular dysgenesis
5. Klinefelter syndrome

How are GCTs classified?

GCTs are classified as **seminomatous or nonseminomatous.**

What % of testicular GCTs are nonseminomatous germ cell tumors (NSGCTs)?

40% of testicular GCTs are NSGCTs.

Name 5 histologic types of NSGCTs.

Histologic types of NSGCTs:
1. Embryonal cell carcinoma
2. Choriocarcinoma
3. Yolk sac tumor
4. Teratoma
5. Mixed

In what 2 ways are teratomas classified?

Teratomas are classified as either **mature or immature** depending on whether they contain adult-type differentiated cell types (mature) or partial somatic differentiation similar to that found in a fetus (immature).

What is a teratoma with malignant transformation?

A teratoma with malignant transformation is a teratoma that **histologically resembles a somatic cancer,** such as an adenocarcinoma or a sarcoma.

How does the presence of a seminoma component influence outcomes in pts with histologically confirmed NSGCTs?

The presence of a seminoma component within a histologically confirmed NSGCT has **no major impact on the clinical outcome.** Such pts are treated based on the NSGCT algorithm.

What is the median age of presentation for pts with NSGCTs, and how does this compare to the median age of presentation for pts with seminomatous germ cell tumors (SGCTs)?

The median age of presentation for NSGCTs is 27 yrs vs. age 36 yrs for SGCTs and 33 yrs for mixed tumors.

How does the presence of pure choriocarcinoma affect the prognosis?

Pure choriocarcinoma typically presents with widespread mets and a very high β-HCG and has a **poor prognosis.** Note that elements of choriocarcinoma are found in 10% of NSGCTs and do not affect the prognosis.

Which histology of NSGCTs is most commonly associated with an elevated AFP?

Yolk sac tumors are composed of cells that produce AFP.

What is the most common GCT histology in childhood?

Yolk sac tumors are the most common histology of GCT in childhood.

▶ **WORKUP/STAGING**

Per NCCN 2014, what 3 blood tests should be performed in the workup of a suspicious testicular mass?

There are 3 blood tests that should be performed in a man with a suspicious testicular mass: **AFP, β-HCG, and a chemistry panel including LDH.**

What is the half-life of AFP?

The half-life of AFP is **5–7 days.**

What is the half-life of β-HCG?

The half-life of β-HCG is **24–36 hrs.**

How should a pt with pure seminoma histology and an elevated AFP be classified?

A pt with pure seminoma histology and an elevated AFP should be **considered and treated as an NSGCT pt. AFP is not considered to be elevated in SGCT.**

Per NCCN 2014, what imaging study should be performed in the workup of a suspicious testicular mass?

CXR and testicular ultrasound should be performed in the workup of a suspicious testicular mass.

How is the AJCC 7th edition (2011) staging for NSGCTs different from staging for SGCTs?

The AJCC staging is the **same for both** NSGCTs and seminomas. See seminoma staging for details.

How should an NSGCT be definitively diagnosed?

Definitive Dx of an NSGCT should be via a radical inguinal orchiectomy. Do not Bx a testicular mass (separate inguinal lymphatic drainage of scrotum).

Per NCCN 2014, what should be discussed preoperatively with a pt who has a testicular mass?

The **pros and cons of sperm banking** should be discussed prior to orchiectomy.

Per NCCN 2014, what imaging study should be ordered postoperatively after Dx of NSGCT?

CT abdomen/pelvis ± chest imaging should be performed postoperatively after the Dx of NSGCTs.

Per the International Germ Cell Cancer Collaborative Group, what 5 factors must be met to be classified as *good*-risk NSGCT?

Per the International Germ Cell Cancer Collaborative Group (*JCO 1997*), good-risk NSGCT must meet all of the following:
1. Testicular or retroperitoneal primary tumor
2. No nonpulmonary visceral mets
3. AFP <1,000 ng/mL
4. β-HCG <5,000 mIU/mL
5. LDH <1.5 times the upper limit of normal

Per the International Germ Cell Cancer Collaborative Group, what 3 factors must be met to be classified as *intermediate*-risk NSGCT?

Per the International Germ Cell Cancer Collaborative Group (*JCO 1997*), intermediate-risk NSGCT must meet both of the following:
1. Testicular or retroperitoneal primary tumor
2. No nonpulmonary visceral mets

and any of the following intermediate risk factors:
3a. AFP 1,000–10,000 ng/mL
3b. β-HCG 5,000–50,000 mIU/mL
3c. LDH 1.5–10 times the upper limit of normal

Per the International Germ Cell Cancer Collaborative Group, the presence of any of which 5 factors leads to classification of *poor*-risk NSGCT?

Per the International Germ Cell Cancer Collaborative Group (*JCO 1997*), poor-risk NSGCT has any of the following:
1. Mediastinal primary tumor
2. Nonpulmonary visceral mets
3. AFP >10,000 ng/mL
4. β-HCG >50,000 mIU/mL
5. LDH >10 times the upper limit of normal

▶ TREATMENT/PROGNOSIS

Per NCCN 2014, what is the Tx of stage I good- or intermediate-risk NSGCT?

The Tx of stage I good- or intermediate-risk NSGCT is **observation** after orchiectomy (preferred for stage IA) if compliant vs. retroperitoneal lymph node dissection (RPLND) vs. bleomycin/etoposide/cisplatin (BEP) chemo × 2 cycles (stage IB only).

What is the risk of relapse after orchiectomy alone for stage I good- or intermediate-risk NSGCT if tumor markers are normal postoperatively?

The risk of relapse after orchiectomy alone for stage I good- or intermediate-risk NSGCT if tumor markers are normal postoperatively is **~30%.**

Per NCCN 2014, how should pts with stage I NSGCT be monitored in an observation protocol?

Observation in pts with stage I NSGCT should consist of visits, tumor markers, and CXR q1–2 mos for yr 1, q2 mos for yr 2, q3 mos for yr 3, q4 mos for yr 4, q6 mos for yr 5, and q12 mos if >6 yrs. CT abdomen/pelvis should be done q3-4 mos for yr 1, q4–6 mos for yr 2, q6-12 mos for yrs 3-4, q12 mos for yr 5, and q12-24 mos if >6 yrs..

What did the MRC trial TE08 show for pts with stage I NSGCT?	**MRC TE08** randomized 414 pts with stage I NSGCT s/p orchiectomy with normal serum markers (10% high risk with LVI) to CT chest/abdomen at 3 and 12 mos vs. CT scans at 3, 6, 9, 12, and 24 mos. At median follow-up of 3.3 yrs, 2-yr RFS was 79% with 2 scans vs. 84% with 5 scans (NSS). The 1st indication of relapse was markers in 39% and CT abdomen in 39%. The conclusion is that CT scans at 3 and 12 mos after orchiectomy might be reasonable in low-risk pts and that chest CT may be unnecessary. (*Rustin GJ et al., JCO 2007*)
What is the chance of positive nodes on RPLND despite a negative CT scan in pts with stage I NSGCT?	The risk of positive nodes on RPLND despite negative CT scan in pts with stage I NSGCT is **30%.**
What is the relapse rate in pts with stage I NSGCT after orchiectomy → RPLND?	The relapse rate in pts with stage I NSGCT after orchiectomy → RPLND is **5%–10%,** most commonly to the lungs.
Per NCCN 2014, how should pts with NSGCT and persistently positive tumor markers after orchiectomy be treated?	Pts with NSGCT and persistently positive tumor markers after orchiectomy should be treated with either BEP × 3 cycles or cisplatin/etoposide (EP) × 4 cycles.
What did the German Testicular Study Group AUO trial AH 01/94 show for pts with stage I NSGCT?	The **AUO AH 01/94** trial randomized 382 pts with clinical stage I NSGCT to RPLND vs. BEP × 1 cycle. At median follow-up of 4.7 yrs, 2-yr RFS was 92% with surgery and 99% with BEP (HR 7.9, SS). The authors concluded that 1 course of BEP is superior to RPLND in clinical stage I Dz. (*Albers P et al., JCO 2008*) Some question the quality of RPLND in this study.
Per NCCN 2014, how should pts with stage II NSGCT with a +node diagnosed only after RPLND be treated?	pN1 (1-5 nodes <2cm) may be observed (preferred) or offered 2 cycles of BEP or EP chemo. pN2 (extranodal extension or any number of nodes <5cm) chemotherapy is preferred over surveillance. pN3 (any number of nodes >5cm) should receive 3 cycles of BEP or 4 cycles of EP. Node should be observed.
Per NCCN 2014, what is the Tx of pts with bulky stage II or III NSGCT?	Pts with bulky stage II or III NSGCT should be treated with either BEP × 3 cycles or EP x 4 cycles (good risk) or BEP × 4 cycles (intermediate risk).
What is the role of RT in the primary Tx of NSGCT?	Although RT may be used for palliation of metastatic Dz, there is no established role for RT in the primary Tx of NSGCT.

Per NCCN 2014, what is the follow-up for pts with NSGCT with CR to chemo and/or RPLND?

Surveillance of pts with NSGCT after CR to chemo and/or RPLND should consist of visits, tumor markers, and CXR q2–3 mos for yrs 1–2, q3-6 mos for yr 3, q6 mos for yr4, q6-12 mos for yr 5, and q12 mos if >6 yrs. CT abdomen/pelvis should be done q6 mos for yr 1, q6–12 mos for yr 2, q12 mos for yrs 3–5, and as clinically indicated if >6 yrs.

▶ TOXICITY

What is the major toxicity associated with RPLND?

The major toxicity associated with RPLND is **retrograde ejaculation resulting in infertility;** however, nerve-sparing techniques can preserve ejaculation in 95% of cases.

What is the pathognomonic complication of bleomycin chemo?

The pathognomic complication of bleomycin chemo is bleomycin-induced pneumonitis.

61 Penile Cancer

Updated by Jing Zeng

▶ BACKGROUND

What is the estimated annual incidence of penile cancer Dx in the U.S.? What % of male cancers does this represent? How is this different in developing countries?

There are ~**1,500 new cases/yr** of penile cancer in the U.S., representing **<1% of male cancers. In developing countries, it can account for up to 10% of all male cancers.**

Name 4 factors associated with the risk of developing penile cancer.

Risk factors for penile cancer:
1. Lack of circumcision
2. Phimosis
3. HPV infection (45%–80% of cases are related)
4. HIV infection

Others factors that may also be associated include chronic inflammation, poor hygiene, trauma, lichen sclerosus, smoking, and PUVA therapy.

What causes condyloma acuminata?

Condyloma acuminata, more commonly known as genital warts, are associated with **HPV infection.** They are usually benign but can undergo malignant transformation.

What is the difference between erythroplasia of Queyrat (EQ) and Bowen Dz?

Both EQ and Bowen Dz are CIS conditions. **EQ** occurs within the penile mucocutaneous epithelium (**glans and prepuce**), whereas **Bowen Dz** occurs within follicle-bearing epithelium (**penile shaft**).

What are the 2 most common anatomic locations for penile cancer?

The **glans and prepuce** are the 2 most common locations for penile cancer. Less common locations include the coronal sulcus and the shaft. Lesions can appear as a mass, ulceration, or inflammation.

To what LNs do penile cancers primarily drain to 1st?

Inguinal LNs are the initial site of nodal involvement in penile cancers → iliac and pelvic nodes.

What is the anatomic position of the penis?

The anatomic position of the penis is **erect;** the descriptors dorsal and ventral refer to the anatomic position.

Approximately what % of men with penile cancer and palpable inguinal LAD have pathologically +nodal mets?

Overall, ~**58%** of palpable inguinal nodes in pts with penile cancer are actually positive for cancer mets on pathology. The rest of the nodes are reactive.

In men with penile cancer and clinically −nodes, what is the likelihood of occult nodal mets?

In men with penile cancer and clinically −nodes, the likelihood of occult nodal mets depends on the tumor stage, grade, and presence of LVI. Roughly, it can be **11%–20% for T1 lesions** and up to **60%–75% for T2-T3 lesions.**

What % of men with penile cancer present with DM lesions?

Hematogenous spread of penile cancer is rare until late in the Dz course and is found in only **1%–10%** of men at initial presentation.

What are the most common sites for DM in penile cancer?

Lung, liver, and bone are the most common sites for DM in penile cancer.

What is the most common histology in penile cancer?

Squamous cell carcinoma accounts for 95% of penile malignancies. Other histologic subtypes such as sarcoma, urethral tumors, lymphoma, and basal cell carcinoma are extremely rare.

► **WORKUP/STAGING**

What is the workup for penile cancer?	Penile cancer workup: H&P, basic labs, biopsy, MRI or US of penis for depth of invasion. **Consider PET/CT and inguinal sentinel LN Bx.**
How should clinically negative LNs in penile cancer be evaluated?	Clinically negative LNs in penile cancer should be evaluated with **CT, MRI, or PET scan,** but the false+ rate and false– rate (FNR) are both high regardless of the imaging modality. Inguinal sentinel LN Bx is promising (FNR 7%).
Should clinically negative nodes in penile cancer undergo inguinal dissection?	The toxicity of inguinal LND should be weighed against the likelihood of occult nodal mets in penile cancer. **LND may be considered for ≥T2 tumors or for high-grade lesions.** (*Solsona E et al., J Urol 2001*) Recent studies suggest that dynamic sentinel LN Bx may be a reasonable alternative. (*Leijte JA et al., JCO 2009*)
How should clinically +LNs in penile cancer be evaluated?	Historically, palpable inguinal LNs in penile cancer can be managed by a 6-wk trial of antibiotics. The current most popular approach is FNA +/– antibiotics.
What is the AJCC 7th edition (2011) T staging for penile cancer?	**Tis:** CIS only **Ta:** noninvasive verrucous carcinoma **T1 a:** invades subepithelial connective tissue without LVI and is not poorly differentiated (i.e., grades 3–4) **T1b:** invades subepithelial connective tissue with LVI or is poorly differentiated **T2:** invades corpora spongiosum or cavernosum **T3:** invades urethra **T4:** invades other adjacent structures
What is the AJCC 7th edition (2011) clinical and pathologic N staging for penile cancer?	**cN1:** palpable mobile unilat inguinal LN **cN2:** palpable mobile multiple or bilat inguinal LN **cN3:** palpable fixed inguinal nodal mass or pelvic LAD **pN1:** single inguinal LN **pN2:** multiple or bilat inguinal LN **pN3:** LN ECE or pelvic LN
What is the AJCC 7th edition (2011) stage grouping for penile cancer?	**Stage I:** T1 a, N0, M0 **Stage II:** T1b-T3, N0, M0 **Stage IIIa:** T1-3, N1, M0 **Stage IIIb:** T1-3, N2, M0 **Stage IV:** T4 or N3 or M1

▶ TREATMENT/PROGNOSIS

How are noninvasive penile cancers treated?	CIS of the penis can be treated with **topical 5-FU or imiquimod** with good LC and excellent cosmetic outcome. Other methods that are acceptable include **laser surgery, cryotherapy, photodynamic therapy, and local excision.** Fulguration alone has a high recurrence rate and is not an acceptable option.
What are the Tx options for pts with early-stage penile cancer (T1-T2, <4 cm)?	Early-stage penile cancer Tx options include **penectomy (partial or total)** or an organ preservation approach using **EBRT, brachytherapy, or CRT** (cisplatin based). Circumcision should always precede RT to minimize complications.
How are locally advanced (T3-T4) penile cancers managed?	For locally advanced penile cancers, consider **CRT, with surgery reserved for salvage or total penectomy.** Induction chemo → penile-preserving Tx is under investigation.
What surgical margin is typically required for total or partial penectomy for Tx of invasive penile cancer?	For penile cancer resection, historically, a **2-cm proximal margin is needed to ensure a 10–15-mm histologic margin,** which appears to give good LC. More recently, studies suggest that margins as small as 5–10 mm may be adequate. (*Minhas S et al., BJU Int 2005*)
What length of corpus cavernosum is required in order for 50% of men to be able to have sexual intercourse?	~45% of men are able to have adequate sexual intercourse with about **4–6 cm** of corpus cavernosum.
What residual penile length is required for men to be able to urinate in the standing position?	**~2.5–3 cm** of residual penile length is required for men to be able to urinate in the standing position.
Name 3 penile-sparing techniques for treating penile cancer.	**Mohs surgery, laser therapy** (mostly for smaller T1-T2 tumors), and **RT** are all penile-sparing techniques for treating penile cancer.
What surgical procedure should accompany any RT for penile cancer?	**Circumcision** should accompany any RT for penile cancer in applicable pts. This allows for better inspection and staging of the lesion as well as helps to alleviate some of the side effects of RT.
In megavoltage EBRT for penile cancer, should bolus be used?	**Yes.** Bolus should be used in megavoltage EBRT for penile cancer for dose buildup at the surface (usually a wax or plastic cast with the penis suspended above the abdomen or secured against the abdomen if also treating nodes).

In EBRT for penile cancer, what is the CTV and what dose is typically prescribed?

In EBRT for penile cancer, the **CTV can be the entire penile length** depending on size and extent of the primary, and typically goes to **45–50 Gy,** with a 10–20 Gy boost to the tumor + a 2-cm margin. Pelvic fields + inguinal nodes are treated to 45 Gy if the pelvic nodes are included in the Tx. Boost to any clinically **gross Dz (60–70 Gy).**

What types of penile cancer lesions are acceptable for brachytherapy?

Penile cancer lesions that can be treated with brachytherapy are typically **<4 cm in diameter** and have **<1 cm of corpora invasion (T1-T2).**

What are 2 ways of delivering brachytherapy in penile cancer, and what is the dose prescribed?

Brachytherapy for penile cancer can be delivered by either (1) using **molds containing sources** such as iridium-192 (less appropriate for pts with short penile length) or (2) using **interstitial implants** by placing catheters 1–1.5 cm apart, perpendicular to the penile axis and afterloading with sources. The **target dose is 55–60 Gy,** with the urethral dose limited to 50 Gy.

How are pts with penile cancers simulated for EBRT?

Simulation for EBRT for penile cancer Tx: supine position and frog-legged, Foley catheter, and penis surrounded with bolus material. If treating pelvic and inguinal nodes, the penis is secured cranially into the pelvic field.

What data support the use of concurrent CRT in treating penile cancer?

There are **no data** directly supporting the use of concurrent CRT in treating penile cancer, but extrapolation from cervical cancer and anal cancer data have led to the increasing use of concurrent cisplatin-based CRT.

What are the common chemotherapy agents given for penile cancer, for either localized or metastatic disease?

Cisplatin-based chemotherapy is the standard for penile cancer patients. If given neoadj, TIP (paclitaxel, ifosfamide, and cisplatin) is a reasonable 1st-line regimen. With radiation, cisplatin, 5-FU, or mitomycin-C can be used. For metastatic disease, TIP or 5-FU/cisplatin are reasonable regimens. Although metastatic penile cancer is chemosensitive, responses are brief and incomplete, and eventual progression is inevitable.

What is the most important prognostic factor in predicting survival in penile cancer pts without DMs?

Inguinal LN mets is the most important prognostic factor in predicting survival in penile cancer pts without DMs.

What is the overall cure rate for surgically treated penile cancer pts +/− node– Dz?

The **5-yr survival** for penile cancer pts **without nodal Dz is 80%–100%,** while the 5-yr survival for pts **with nodal mets is 32%–50%.**

What are the expected LC rates for pts managed with EBRT or brachytherapy for penile cancers?	LC estimates vary widely, likely depending on pt selection. In a well-selected pt with T1-T3 penile cancer treated with EBRT or brachytherapy, LC (i.e., penile preservation rate) is **80%–90%** (5–10 yrs follow-up). (*Crook JM et al., IJROBP 2005*)
How does surgery compare to RT as the initial modality in the management of penile cancers?	Retrospective comparisons between surgery and RT suggest that surgery is associated with superior initial LC as a primary modality, though these studies suffer from significant selection bias. **Overall LC does not appear to differ when allowing for surgical salvage.** The benefit of RT is penile preservation. Long-term OS appears similar between the 2 modalities.

Estimate the MS in men with localized, regional (node+), or metastatic penile carcinoma.	MS in men with penile carcinoma:
	    Localized: 4 yrs
	    Regional: 2.5 yrs
	    Metastatic: 7 mos
	
	(*Rippentrop M et al., Cancer 2004*)

► **TOXICITY**

How should pts with penile cancer who rcv definitive therapy be followed?	Penile cancer pts treated with penectomy with nodal dissection can be followed q4 mos for 2 yrs, then q6 mos for an additional 3 yrs. **Pts treated with penile-sparing therapy or those who did not undergo LND should be followed q2 mos for yrs 1–2, then q6 mos for an additional 3 yrs.**
Name 3 acute side effects that may occur during RT for penile cancer.	**Urethral mucositis, edema, and secondary infection** are experienced by nearly all pts during RT for penile cancer.
Name 5 long-term complications from RT for penile cancer.	**Telangiectasia, superficial necrosis, urethral stricture, fistula formation, meatal stenosis, and dyschromia** are all common long-term toxicities from RT for penile cancer.
What doses increase the risk of urethral strictures from fibrosis or stenosis?	Doses **>60 Gy** increase the risk of urethral stenosis and fibrosis.
What are the side effects from inguinal LND in pts with clinically –nodes in penile cancer?	Side effects from inguinal LND include **lower extremity edema, wound complications, and DVT.**
What are the doses that cause sterilization?	**2–3 Gy** is sufficient for sterilization.

62 Urethral Cancer

Updated by Reid F. Thompson

▶ BACKGROUND

What is the estimated annual incidence of urethral cancer in the U.S.?

~500 cases/yr of urethral cancer in the U.S.

Is there a racial or sex predilection for urethral cancer?

Yes. The incidence of urethral cancer is greater in **women** at a 4:1 ratio. It is **higher in white women and black men.**

At what age does urethral cancer incidence peak?

The peak incidence of urethral cancer occurs in **women age 40–50 yrs** and in **men age 75–84 yrs.** It is very rare in men <55 yrs.

What are the conditions or exposures associated with urethral cancer?

Exposures associated with urethral cancer include possibly HPV in women. Many men have long-standing urethral infections, Hx of STDs, stricture, trauma, or urethritis.

Is there an association between urethral cancer and other malignancies?

Yes. There is an association between bladder cancer and urethral cancer. The risk of urethral cancer in men with bladder cancer has been reported as 4%–18%. A recent series of women with bladder cancer reports a 2% incidence of concurrent urethral cancer. (*Stenzl A et al., J Urol 1995*)

What are the avg length and anatomic divisions of the female urethra?

The avg length of the adult female urethra is **4 cm.** It is anatomically divided into the **distal one-third (ant urethra) and proximal two-thirds (post urethra).**

In a female, what type of epithelium does the proximal and distal urethra have?

The distal two-thirds of the female urethra has stratified squamous epithelium. The proximal one-third has transitional epithelium.

What are the avg length and anatomic divisions of the male urethra?

The avg length of the adult male urethra is **21 cm.** It is divided into **ant (distal) and post (proximal) portions,** which are further subdivided from most distal to proximal as follows:

Anterior urethra: glandular, penile, bulbar
Posterior urethra: membranous, prostatic

In a male, what type of epithelium does the proximal and distal urethra have?	In the male urethra: 1. Squamous epithelium is present in the glandular and penile regions. 2. Pseudostratified or stratified columnar epithelium is present in the post proximal portion of the penile and bulbomembranous portions. 3. Transitional cell epithelium is present in the prostatic portion.
What is the histologic prevalence of urethral cancers?	Squamous cell carcinomas (SCCs) are the most common urethral cancers in both men and women → transitional cell carcinomas (TCCs) and adenocarcinoma.
What is the most common site of origin of urethral cancer in men?	In men, urethral cancer occurs most frequently in the **bulbomembranous urethra** (~60%). It occurs mainly as squamous metaplasia. The next most common sites are the penile urethra and prostatic urethra.
What is the main pattern of spread in urethral cancer?	The main pattern of spread is **direct extension.**
What is the lymphatic drainage for the urethra?	Traditionally, the distal urethra in women and glandular and penile urethra in men are drained by inguinal nodes, and the more proximal regions (bulbar and prostatic in men) are drained by pelvic nodes. However, crossover can occur, particularly with direct extension of Dz.
What portion of urethral cancer pts will be LN+ at Dx?	**14%–30%** of pts will be LN+ at Dx.
Are most clinically apparent nodes pathologically positive in urethral cancer?	**Yes.** ~75% of clinically apparent LNs are pathologically positive for cancer. This is in contrast to penile cancer, where ~50% of enlarged LNs are involved.
What % of urethral cancer pts have DM at Dx? What are the most common sites of mets?	**10%** of pts have metastatic Dz at Dx. The most common sites of mets are the **lung, liver, and bone.**
What are the most common presenting Sx of urethral cancer?	In women, hematuria and obstructive Sx are the most common. In men, a palpable mass and obstructive Sx are more common.

▶ WORKUP/STAGING

What is the workup of urethral cancer?	Urethral cancer workup: H&P, including palpation of length of urethra in men, inguinal nodal examination, and bimanual examination. The pt should have a cystourethroscopy with Bx, retrograde urethrography, CT/MRI pelvis, and basic labs. Consider PET or bone scan if mets are suspected.

What is the AJCC 7th edition (2011) T and N staging for primary tumors of the urethra?	**Tis:** CIS

What is the AJCC 7th edition (2011) T and N staging for primary tumors of the urethra?

Tis: CIS
Ta: noninvasive verrucous/papillary/polypoid carcinoma
T1: invasion of subepithelial connective tissue
T2: invasion of corpus spongiosum, prostate, or periurethral muscle
T3: invasion of corpus cavernosum, prostatic capsule, ant vagina, or bladder neck
T4: invasion of other adjacent organs
N1: mets to single LN <2 cm
N2: mets to single LN >2 cm or multiple +nodes

What is the AJCC 7th edition (2011) T staging for urothelial carcinoma (TCC) of the prostate?

Tis pu: CIS with involvement of prostatic urethra
Tis pd: CIS with involvement of prostatic ducts
T1: invasion of urethral subepithelial connective tissue
T2: invasion of prostatic stroma, corpus spongiosum, or periurethral muscle
T3: invasion of corpus cavernosum, beyond prostatic capsule, bladder neck
T4: invasion of adjacent organs

▶ TREATMENT/PROGNOSIS

What factors affect the Tx strategy of urethral cancer?

Location (ant vs. post), size, DOI, and presence of nodal mets or DMs are the major factors affecting prognosis and Tx strategy.

Does location correlate to the stage/prognosis of urethral cancer?

Yes. Proximal lesions more often present at a higher stage and thus carry a worse prognosis.

What types of surgical resections have been used for male urethral cancer pts?

Multiple forms of conservative resections have been used for very early Dz (Tis-T1), including transurethral resection, laser ablation, and microsurgical resection. Radical resections, which have been the historical standard, include partial and total penectomy and penectomy with cystoprostatectomy.

What are the desired margins for a partial penectomy in urethral cancer?

A **2-cm margin** is desired for a partial penectomy.

What is the expected outcome for early-stage (Tis-T1) male pts treated with surgery alone?

Based on the MSKCC experience, among 10 male pts (Tis-T1) treated with various surgical strategies, **DFS at 5 yrs was 83%.** (*Dalbagni G et al., Urology 1999*)

What is the expected outcome for advanced-stage (≥T2) male pts treated with surgery alone?

Based on the MSKCC experience, among 36 male pts (T2-T4) treated with various surgical strategies, **DFS at 5 yrs was 45%.** (*Dalbagni G et al., Urology 1999*) Of note, 6 pts were treated with surgical salvage after initial Tx with RT.

What are the outcomes for early-stage (Tis-T1) male pts treated with RT alone?

There are very few data for RT alone in treating male pts with urethral cancer. Only very small series are available. A series of 5 men with early-stage urethral cancer described LC in 4 of those men. (*Heysek R et al., J Urol 1985*)

What types of surgical resections have been used for female urethral cancer pts?

Early-stage Dz (Tis-T1) has been treated with local excision, laser excision, transurethral resection, and partial urethrectomy. Radical resection for locally advanced Dz (≥T2) includes ant exenteration, which involves removal of pelvic nodes, the uterus, and appendages, and en bloc resection of pubic symphysis and inf rami.

In locally advanced female urethral cancer (≥pT2), what is the 5-yr OS and LF after ant exenteration alone?

The **5-yr OS is <20%, with a >66% LF rate** in female pts with locally advanced urethral cancer treated with exenteration alone. (*Narayan P, Urol Clin N Am 1992*)

What are the outcomes for early-stage (variable definition of early stage includes ant, node– pts without T stage) urethral cancer in female pts treated with RT alone?

A meta-analysis of RT alone in female pts with urethral cancer showed a **5-yr OS of 75% with early-stage Dz and 34% with advanced-stage Dz.** (*Kreig R, Oncology 1999*)

What is the OS for female pts with advanced Dz (variable in definition but in general refers to >T1 Dz, post Dz, or node+ Dz) treated with combined surgery and RT?

Meta-analysis of 34 pts treated in this manner revealed **5-yr OS of 29%.** (*Kreig R et al., Oncology 1999*) The single-largest series revealed a 25% OS at 5 yrs among the 20 pts treated. (*Grabstald H et al., JAMA 1966*)

What is the typical single-modality RT Tx for female urethral cancer?

RT is often given as brachytherapy alone or brachytherapy + EB. Typical Tx includes brachytherapy alone to 50–60 Gy and EBRT to 40–45 Gy → brachytherapy to 20–25 Gy. Inguinal nodes should be included.

What are the outcomes for advanced-stage pts treated with CRT?

A number of case reports have shown good results with combined RT and 5-FU/mitomycin-C in both men and women with advanced Dz. A retrospective study of 18 pts from the University of Texas–San Antonio, including male and female pts, demonstrated that among the 8 advanced-stage pts (T3-4N1M1), DFS was 45.2 mos for those treated with CRT compared with 23.3 mos for those treated with surgery alone. Chemo from this study was based on histology and included 5-FU/cisplatin for SCC and carboplatin/taxol for TCC. There were 8 total high-stage pts in this study. (*Eng T et al., Am J Clin Oncol 2003*)

TOXICITY

What are the expected acute and late RT toxicities associated with Tx of urethral cancer?	<u>Acute toxicities</u>: dermatitis, urinary Sx, diarrhea <u>Late toxicities</u>: urethral stricture/stenosis, urethrovaginal fistulas, incontinence

63 Renal Cell Carcinoma

Updated by Phillip J. Gray and Thomas J. Guzzo

 BACKGROUND

Order the following 5 tissues from outermost to innermost: renal cortex, Gerota's fascia, adrenal gland, perirenal fat, and renal capsule.	From outermost to innermost: 1. Gerota's fascia 2. Perirenal fat 3. Adrenal gland (which is embedded in the perirenal fat sup to the kidney) 4. Renal capsule 5. Renal cortex
Name 3 environmental risk factors for renal cell carcinoma (RCC).	Environmental risk factors for RCC: 1. Cigarette smoking 2. Phenacetin exposure (found in analgesics) 3. Heavy metal exposure
Name the most important nonenvironmental risk factor for RCC.	Obesity. The risk of RCC increases by 7% per unit increase in BMI. (*Bergstrom A et al., Br J Cancer 2001*)

Familial RCC makes up what % of RCC cases? Name 5 familial syndromes.	Familial RCC makes up ~4% of RCC cases. Familial syndromes:
	1. Von Hippel-Lindau
	2. Birt-Hogg-Dube syndrome
	3. Tuberous sclerosis
	4. Hereditary papillary RCC
	   a. HRCC (met proto-oncogene)
	   b. Familial leiomyomatosis
	   c. RCC (fumarate hydratase)
	5. Familial clear cell RCC

What is the estimated annual incidence of new RCC cases in the U.S.?	**~58,000 cases/yr** of new RCC in the U.S.
Has the incidence of RCC been increasing or decreasing over the past 30 yrs? Is there a sex predilection?	The incidence of RCC has been **increasing** by 2%/yr over the past 30 yrs according to NCI SEER data. **Men** appear to be more commonly diagnosed with RCC than women.
In which decade of life is RCC typically diagnosed?	RCC is typically diagnosed in the **7th decade of life.**
RCC represents what % of all urinary tract tumors?	RCC represents ~6% of all urinary tract tumors.
What benign tumors can exist in the kidney?	Benign tumors of the kidney: 1. Angiomyolipomas 2. Fibromas 3. Lipomas 4. Lymphangiomas 5. Oncocytomas 6. Hemangiomas
What % of RCC pts will present with a palpable mass on physical exam?	~10% of RCC pts will have a palpable mass at the time at presentation.
RCC pts are at increased risk of having what other type of synchronous urinary cancer?	RCC pts have an RR of 1.5 of having a synchronous bladder cancer, though the authors do not screen for bladder cancer in RCC pts. This increased risk may be related to smoking.
What is the classic triad of RCC? With what other clinical Sx can pts with RCC present?	Pts with RCC present with classic triad Sx of hematuria, flank pain, and a palpable mass. Sx of fever, night sweats, and weight loss suggest the presence of metastatic Dz.
What are some paraneoplastic syndromes associated with RCC? In what % of pts would these syndromes be found?	Paraneoplastic syndromes associated with RCC: 1. Hypercalcemia 2. Elevated LFTs 3. Hypertension These paraneoplastic syndromes arise in **20%** of pts.
What % of RCC pts present with bilat kidney involvement?	**3%** of RCC pts will have bilat involvement at Dx.
What are 4 pathologic subtypes of RCC?	Pathologic subtypes of RCC: 1. Clear cell 2. Chromophilic (or papillary) 3. Chromophobic 4. Collecting duct
What is the most common pathologic subtype of RCC?	**Clear cell** is the most common subtype of RCC (~70%), demonstrating large clear cells with abundant cytoplasm.

What is the most common histologic grading system for RCC?

The most common histologic grading system for RCC is the **Fuhrman grading system** from I–IV based on nuclear roundness, size, nucleoli presence, and the presence of clumped chromatin.

Sporadic RCC is characterized by what genetic mutation?

Sporadic RCC is characterized by a **mutation in the VHL tumor suppressor gene on chromosome 3p25,** which is silenced in >50% of sporadic RCC.

▶ **WORKUP/STAGING**

How is RCC diagnosed?

RCC requires a tissue Dx. Often, nephrectomy is both diagnostic and therapeutic. Percutaneous Bx can also be employed for surgically unfit pts, those considering active surveillance, or at the time of ablative therapy.

What % of biopsied pts have benign Dz?

~33% of small renal masses may be characterized as benign according to the specimen obtained. The risk of benign pathology is inversely proportional to the size of the renal mass.

What imaging is important in the initial workup of RCC?

Imaging workup typically includes contrast-enhanced CT or MRI scan of the abdomen and chest imaging. Consider bone scan and MRI brain if clinically indicated.

Summarize the AJCC 7th edition (2011) T staging for RCC.

T1: limited to kidney and ≤7 cm
T1 a: ≤4 cm
T1b: 4–7 cm
T2: limited to kidney and >7 cm
T2 a: >7 cm but ≤10 cm
T2b: >10 cm
T3: invades into major veins or perinephric tissues but not into ipsilateral adrenal gland and not beyond Gerota's fascia
T3 a: grossly extends into renal vein or its segmental branches, or extends into perirenal and/or renal sinus fat but not beyond Gerota's fascia
T3b: extends into vena cava below diaphragm
T3 c: extends into vena cava above diaphragm or invades wall of vena cava
T4: invades beyond Gerota fascia, including contiguous extension into ipsilateral adrenal gland

Summarize the AJCC 7th edition (2011) stage grouping for RCC.

Stage I: T1N0M0
Stage II: T2N0M0
Stage III: T1-2N1M0 or T3N0-1M0
Stage IV: T4 or M1

What other staging systems are widely used for RCC?

The Flocks and Kadesky system (with or without Robson modification) and Jewett-Strong classification system have been used to stage RCC.

| Name 3 prognostic factors for RCC. | Prognostic factors for RCC:
1. TNM stage
2. Performance status
3. Fuhrman grade |

▶ TREATMENT/PROGNOSIS

Describe 5 invasive Tx for locally confined RCC.	Invasive Tx for locally confined RCC: 1. Open nephrectomy 2. Laparoscopic nephrectomy 3. Percutaneous CT-guided cryosurgery 4. Percutaneous radiofrequency ablation 5. Partial nephrectomy
Are there any studies comparing laparoscopic resection with that of open resection in pts with RCC?	**Yes.** There are retrospective data that compared laparoscopic resection vs. open resection of RCC. There was no difference in DFS. (*Luo JH et al., World J Urol 2009; Marszalek M et al., Eur Urol 2009*)
Are there surgical options for pts with bilat RCC or unilat RCC with a diseased contralat kidney?	**Yes.** Pts with bilat RCC or a diseased contralat kidney can be treated with a partial nephrectomy provided the lesion is amenable to a nephron-sparing approach.
When is recurrence most likely to occur following surgery for RCC?	The median time for recurrence after surgery for RCC is ~2 yrs. Most recurrences occur within 5 yrs.
Name 4 predictors of RCC recurrence after nephrectomy.	Predictors of RCC recurrence after nephrectomy: 1. Nuclear grade (Fuhrman grade) 2. TNM stage 3. DNA ploidy 4. Genetic RCC syndromes
What are the most common sites of RCC recurrence after nephrectomy?	Most common sites of RCC recurrence after nephrectomy: 1. Lung 2. Bone 3. Regional LNs
What follow-up imaging is recommended for RCC pts after nephrectomy?	RCC pts after nephrectomy should be followed with **CXR/CT chest and CT/MRI abdomen.**
For how long should pts with RCC treated with nephrectomy be followed?	Pts with RCC treated with nephrectomy should be followed **for life** (sporadic RCC recurrences have been documented ≥40 yrs later).
Are there any prospective randomized studies examining the role for adj therapy in pts with RCC treated with initial nephrectomy?	**Yes.** IFN α-2b within 1 mo after surgery vs. Tx only after postsurgical relapse demonstrated no EFS or OS benefit. (*Messing EM et al., JCO 2003*) A phase III randomized comparison of adjuvant sunitinib, sorafenib, or placebo is ongoing.

What is the 1ˢᵗ-line Tx for pts with metastatic RCC?

1ˢᵗ-line Tx for pts with metastatic RCC:
1. Cytoreductive nephrectomy
2. Metastasectomy for oligometastases
3. Sunitinib
4. Temsirolimus
5. Bevacizumab and IFN
6. High-dose recombinant interleukin-2
7. Sorafenib

Cytotoxic chemo for non–clear cell histologies may be considered.

What is the mechanism of action of sorafenib? Of sunitinib?

Sorafenib inhibits multiple kinase pathways, including Raf kinase, PDGF, VEGF receptor 2 and 3, and c-Kit. Sunitinib also inhibits multiple kinase pathways, including PDGF, VEGF, c-Kit, RET, CSF-1R, and flt3.

Is there a role for palliative nephrectomy in pts with RCC?

Yes. Palliative nephrectomy is still encouraged to relieve local Sx of pain or intractable hematuria; as well as systemic Sx related to the primary tumor.

What are the data for using cytoreductive surgery in combination with immunotherapy?

Cytoreductive surgery utilized before immunotherapy **may delay time to progression and improve survival of pts with metastatic Dz** (median duration of survival 17 mos vs. 7 mos, SS). (*Mickisch GH et al., Lancet 2001*)

Is there a role for resection of metastatic lesions in pts with RCC?

Yes. A retrospective study by *Kavolius JP et al.* suggests that curative resection of metastatic lesions in pts with RCC improves survival compared with the subtotal resection of pts or those with noncurative salvage attempts (44%, 14%, and 11%, respectively). (*JCO 1998*)

Is there a role for RT in patients with RCC?

Yes. RCC is widely regarded as a radioresistant tumor. When clinically and technically appropriate, consider SRS for pts with RCC brain mets. (*Jagannathan J et al., Neurosurgery 2010; Te BS et al., Clin Genitourin Cancer 2007*) Several recent studies have identified good outcomes using stereotactic body radiotherapy to treat primary RCC in patients who are not operative candidates. Postoperative radiotherapy can improve local control but does not appear to affect OS or DFS. (*Tunio MA et al., Ann Oncol 2010*)

▶ **TOXICITY**

What toxicities are associated with sorafenib and sunitinib?

Sorafenib and sunitinib are associated with fatigue, diarrhea, HTN, rash, hand-foot syndrome (sorafenib), and mucositis (sunitinib).

Part IX Gynecology

64 Cervical Cancer

Updated by Jing Zeng

▶ BACKGROUND

What is the annual incidence of cervical cancer in the U.S.?

~12,000 cases/yr of cervical cancer in the U.S.

What is the mean age of presentation for cervical cancer?

The mean age of presentation for cervical cancer is **in the 40s** in the U.S.

List the 7 lifestyle factors associated with an increased risk of cervical cancer.

Lifestyle factors associated with increased risk of cervical cancer:
1. Early onset of sexual activity
2. Larger number of sexual partners
3. Exposure to high-risk partners
4. Hx of STD
5. Smoking
6. High parity
7. Prolonged use of oral contraceptives

HPV is detectable in what % of cervical cancer?

HPV is detectable in **>99%** of cervical cancer.

Roughly what % reduction in mortality has been achieved with PAP screening for cervical cancer?

There has been an **~70% reduction** in cervical cancer mortality with PAP screening.

What does ASCUS stand for (on a PAP result), and how should it be managed?

ASCUS stands for **A**typical **S**quamous **C**ells of Unknown **S**ignificance. About two-thirds can resolve spontaneously. Pts can undergo **repeat PAP in 6 mos and then colposcopy if abnl.**

How should LGSIL seen on PAP be managed?

LGSIL resolves spontaneously ~40% of the time; therefore, like with ASCUS, pts can undergo **repeat PAP in 6 mos with colposcopy if abnl.**

How should a HGSIL result from a PAP be managed?	All pts with HGSIL should undergo **colposcopy with Bx.** One-third of these pts can still resolve spontaneously, but waiting without further investigation is not recommended due to concern for progression.
What % of HGSIL progresses to invasive cancers?	**~22%** of HGSIL progress to invasive cancer. This is in contrast to ASCUS (<1%) and LGSIL (~5%).
What % of cervical cancers are caused by HPV-16 and -18?	**>70%** of cervical cancers are caused by HPV-16 and -18.
What HPV subtypes cause the most cases of benign warts?	HPV subtypes **6 and 11** cause most cases of benign warts.
In the U.S., what % of cervical cancers are squamous cell carcinomas vs. adenocarcinomas?	With regard to cervical cancers in the U.S., **80% are squamous cell carcinomas,** while **~20% are adenocarcinomas.**
List 5 histologic subtypes of adenocarcinoma of the cervix.	Subtypes of adenocarcinoma of the cervix: 1. Mucinous 2. Adenosquamous 3. Endometrioid 4. Clear cell 5. Glassy cell
Name 3 common presenting Sx of cervical cancer.	Common presenting Sx of cervical cancer: 1. Abnl vaginal bleeding 2. Postcoital bleeding 3. Abnl vaginal discharge
What specific area of the cervix is the most common point of origin for cervical cancer?	The **transformation zone** is the most common point of origin for cervical cancer. It is a dynamic area between the original and present squamocolumnar junction.

 WORKUP/STAGING

What should be included in the workup for a cervical mass?	Pelvic mass workup: H&P, including a careful pelvic exam in the office, basic labs, and EUA with Bx, with cystoscopy and proctoscopy (if concern for invasion) for any visible lesions. Imaging studies such as CT, PET, and MRI can be obtained for treatment decision making and planning purposes (but do not enter FIGO staging of the pt).
What are the areas at risk for local extension of cervical cancer?	Cervical cancer can spread locally to the **corpus, parametria, and vagina.** These should be carefully assessed during a physical exam. Tumor size and parametrial involvement are best assessed by rectovaginal exam. Cervical tumors can also spread to bladder anteriorly or rectum posteriorly, but this is rare in North America.

Name 3 routes of lymphatic drainage from the cervix.

Routes of lymphatic drainage from the cervix:
1. Lat to the external iliac nodes
2. Post into common iliac and lat sacral nodes
3. Post-lat into internal iliac nodes

What imaging studies are included in FIGO staging of cervical cancer? What common imaging modalities are not allowed?

CXR, barium enema, and intravenous pyelogram data are included in FIGO staging of cervical cancer, as are procedures such as cystoscopy, proctoscopy, and hysteroscopy. **CT, PET, MRI, bone scan, lymphangiography, and laparotomy/laparoscopy data are not allowed** to be used for staging but can be used for decisions regarding management.

What is the utility of PET scans in cervical cancer?

PET is generally fairly sensitive (85%–90%) and specific (95%–100%) for detection of para-aortic (P-A) nodes in pts with locally advanced cervical cancer.

In what group of cervical cancer pts is evaluation of the urinary tract required?

Cervical cancer **pts with more than stage IB1 disease** require imaging of the urinary tract. This can be performed with CT, MRI, or intravenous pyelogram.

What is the FIGO (2010) staging for cervical cancer?

Stage IA: microscopic Dz, with ≤5 mm DOI and ≤7 mm horizontal spread. It is further delineated into IA1 (tumors ≤3 mm depth and ≤7 mm wide) and IA2 (tumors >3 mm but ≤5 mm deep and ≤7 mm wide)

Stage IB: clinically visible tumor or >IA2, with IB1 ≤4 cm, and IB2 being bulky tumors >4 cm

Stage IIA: invades beyond uterus/cervix; involves the upper two-thirds of the vagina without parametrial invasion with IIA1 lesions ≤4 cm and IIA2 lesions >4 cm

Stage IIB: invades beyond uterus/cervix and into parametria but not into pelvic wall or lower 3rd of vagina

Stage IIIA: invades lower 3rd of vagina but no extension into pelvic wall

Stage IIIB: invades pelvic sidewall and/or causes hydronephrosis or nonfunctioning kidney

Stage IVA: invades beyond true pelvis or mucosa of bladder or rectum (must be Bx proven); bullous edema of bladder or rectum does not count

Stage IVB: DMs

How does the AJCC (TNM) staging system for cervical cancer compare with the FIGO system?

In AJCC cervical cancer staging, the **T stage corresponds to the FIGO stage, except for FIGO stage IVB.** Node+ patients are AJCC stage IIIB. Stage 0 exists in the AJCC but not in the FIGO system.

What factors are predictive of pelvic nodal involvement in cervical cancer?

Factors that predict for nodal involvement in cervical cancer include **DOI, FIGO stage, tumor size, and LVSI** (10% without vs. 25% with). It is controversial whether histologic subtype is an independent predictor for nodal involvement, although some studies show adenocarcinomas having higher rates of distant metastasis.

Estimate the risk of pelvic LN involvement based on the following DOIs of a cervical cancer: <3 mm, 3–5 mm, 6–10 mm, and 10–20 mm.

Risk of pelvic nodal involvement by DOI:
 ≤3 mm: <1%
 3–5 mm: 1%–8%
 6–10 mm: 15%
 10–20 mm: 25%

Estimate the risk of pelvic LN involvement based on the FIGO stage of cervical cancer.

Pelvic LN+ rates for cervical cancer based on the FIGO stage:
 Stage IA1: 1%
 Stage IA2: 5%
 Stage IB: 15%
 Stage II: 30%
 Stage III: 50%
 Stage IVA: 60%

Estimate the risk of P-A nodal involvement based on the FIGO stage of cervical cancer.

P-A LN+ rates for cervical cancer based on the FIGO stage:
 Stage IA: 0%
 Stage IB: 5%–8%
 Stage IIA: ~10%
 Stage IIB: ~15%
 Stage III: 30%
 Stage IVA: 40%

What are the 5-yr OS rates based on the FIGO stage?

5-yr OS based on FIGO stage:
 Stage IA: 93%
 Stage IB: 75%–80%
 Stage IIA: 80%
 Stage IIB: 65%–70%
 Stage IIIA: 35%
 Stage IIIB: 35%–40%
 Stage IVA: 10%
 Stage IVB: 0%
 (AJCC 7th edition, 2011)

▶ TREATMENT/PROGNOSIS

What is the most important prognostic factor in cervical cancer?

Tumor stage is the most important prognostic factor in cervical cancer since FIGO staging is based on prognostic factors. Per stage, extent of nodal involvement is the next most important factor.

What is removed in a radical trachelectomy as Tx for cervical cancer?

In a radical trachelectomy, **all cervical cancer is removed with a margin,** but the internal os is left behind and stitched closed, with a small meatus for menses to escape. This procedure allows future pregnancy, delivered via a C-section. This procedure should be reserved for women desiring fertility preservation and with stage IA1 as well as select cases of IA2 and small IB1 and tumors <2.0 cm in size.

How should pts with preinvasive cervical cancer (HGSIL or CIN III) be managed?

Pts with preinvasive cervical cancer should be managed with **colposcopy → conization, LEEP, laser, cryotherapy, or simple hysterectomy.**

In which subset of cervical cancer pts is simple hysterectomy adequate as definitive management?

Pts with IA1 Dz can be treated with simple abdominal hysterectomy. A cone should be done 1st to ensure that there are no foci of invasion beyond 3 mm identified. Sometimes, conization is also adequate for IA1, but there must be DOI <3 mm and no LVSI or dysplasia at the margin. (*Van Nagell J et al., Am J Obstet Gynecol 1983*) All other pts (≥IA2) should get radical hysterectomy with pelvic LND.

What is the difference between a class II and class III radical hysterectomy (Piver-Rutledge-Smith classification)?

In a class II modified radical hysterectomy (Piver-Rutledge-Smith classification), there is removal of the uterus, ureters are unroofed to remove parametrial and paracervical tissue medial to the ureters and 1–2 cm of vaginal cuff, and the uterine artery is ligated at the ureter. In a class III surgery, there is removal of parametrial and paravaginal tissue to the pelvic sidewall, ligation of the uterine artery at the ureter, and removal of the upper half to two-thirds of the vagina.

What stage of cervical cancer can be treated with brachytherapy alone?

Stage IA cervical cancer can be treated with brachytherapy alone with LDR 65–75 Gy or HDR 7 Gy × 5–6 fx, with LC of 97%. (*Grisby P et al., IJROBP 1992*)

When treating cervical cancer pts with brachytherapy, is there a Dz control or toxicity difference between LDR and HDR?

This is **uncertain.** In *Teshima T et al.,* pts with stages I–III cervical cancer were randomized to HDR cobalt-60 or LDR cesium-137 therapy. There was no SS difference in 5-yr CSS between the 2 groups (stage I, 85%–93%; stage II, 73%–78%; stage III, 47%–53%). Moderate to severe complications were higher in HDR (10% vs. 4%). (*Cancer 1993*)

Where is point A, and what should it correspond to anatomically?

Point A is **2 cm above the external cervical os and 2 cm lat to the central canal/tandem.** This should correspond to the paracervical triangle, where the uterine vessels cross the ureter.

Where is point B, and what should it correspond to anatomically? How does the dose to point B typically relate to the dose to point A?

Point B is **5 cm lat from the midline at the same level as point A** (2 cm above the external cervical os). It is supposed to represent the obturator nodes. The **dose to point B is usually <20% of the dose to point A using current ring and tandem systems.**

Before CT-based planning, how were the bladder, rectum, and vaginal points defined for cervical cancer brachytherapy?

Before CT-based planning, the bladder point was 5 mm behind the post surface of the Foley balloon on a lat x-ray filled with 7 cc radiopaque fluid and pulled down against the urethra. The rectum point was 5 mm behind the post vaginal wall between the ovoids at the inf point of the last intrauterine tandem source or mid vaginal source. The vaginal point was the lat edge of the ovoids on AP film and mid ovoid on lat film. In the present age of CT planning, an alternative is to contour the organs and calculate the max dose to the organ using 3D planning.

What are the dose limits to the bladder, rectum, and vaginal points in cervical cancer brachytherapy?

In cervical cancer brachytherapy, typically the **max allowed dose to the rectal point is 75 Gy, the max bladder point dose is 80 Gy, and the max vaginal dose is 120 Gy. With 3D planning, dose limit to 2cc of bladder is ≤90 Gy equivalent 2Gy dose (EQD2) (normalized therapy dose), rectum dose to 2cc (D2cc) ≤75 Gy EQD2.** (*Viswanathan A et al., Brachy 2012*)

What RT dose can cause ovarian failure? What about sterility?

Ovarian failure can occur with **5–10 Gy** of RT. Sterility can occur **after 2–3 Gy.**

What are the typical LDR and HDR in cervical cancer Tx?

In cervical cancer brachytherapy, **LDR is usually 0.4–0.8 Gy/hr, while HDR is much higher, at least 12 Gy/hr. Typically, 1 treatment of 5.5–6.0 Gy takes approximately 5–10 min to deliver.**

What should be the dose to point A in RT for cervical cancer (sum of EBRT + brachytherapy)? Does it depend on the stage of Dz?

In cervical cancer radiotherapy, the cumulative dose to point A should be **at least 75 Gy for stage IA Dz, 80–85 Gy for stages IB–IIB Dz, and 85–90 Gy for stages III–IVA Dz,** so **staging is a factor** in determining the dose.

What is the role for definitive surgery vs. definitive RT for the management of early stage (IB–IIA) cervical cancers? What study tested these 2 modalities?

In *Landoni F et al.,* pts with stages IB and IIA cervical carcinoma were randomized to surgery (class III) vs. RT for definitive therapy. Adj RT was allowed for the surgery group based on preset criteria. 5-yr OS and DFS were equal (83% and 74%, respectively, for both groups). 64% of surgery pts rcvd adj RT. Grades 2–3 morbidity was higher in the surgery arm (28% vs. 12%). (*Lancet 1997*)

What are the benefits of surgery over RT for the Tx of early-stage cervical cancers?

Benefits of surgery over RT include **shorter Tx time, preservation of ovarian function, possibly better sexual functioning after Tx, no 2nd malignancy risk, avoidance of long-term RT sequelae, and psychologically easier for many patients to understand. Surgery can also better identify the accurate anatomic extent of disease.**

For pts with early-stage cervical cancer treated with radical or modified radical hysterectomy, what are 3 major indications for adj therapy?

For pts with early-stage cervical cancer treated with radical or modified radical hysterectomy, major indications for adj therapy include **+/close margin, LN mets, and microscopic parametrial invasion.** Other indications include tumor >4 cm, deep stromal invasion, or LVI.

What adverse features after surgery are indications for adj RT alone without chemo?

Cervical cancer pts after radical hysterectomy to –margins and –nodal status but have ≥2 risk features (+LVSI, >4-cm tumors, more than one-third stromal invasion) may benefit from PORT.

The Gynecologic Oncology Group's study **GOG 92** enrolled 277 stage IB cervical cancer pts who underwent surgery and had –nodes but >1 adverse feature: more than one-third stromal invasion, LVI, or tumor >4 cm. Compared to observation, there was a pelvic RT (46–50.4 Gy) RR of recurrence by 46% (21% vs. 14%, $p = 0.007$) and trend to OS benefit by ~10% (71% vs. 80%, $p = 0.074$). (*Rotman M et al., IJROBP 2006*)

When is adding chemo to adj RT after radical hysterectomy beneficial compared with RT alone for the surgical management of early-stage cervical cancer (IA2–IIA)?

In **GOG 109,** high-risk pts (with at least 1 of the following features: +margin, +nodes, or microscopic parametrial invasion) with stage IA2, IB, and IIA cervical cancer treated with radical hysterectomy and pelvic lymphadenectomy were randomized to standard pelvic field RT (49.3 Gy) vs. RT + cisplatin/5-FU for 4 cycles. CRT was superior in both 4-yr OS (81% vs. 71%) and 4-yr PFS (80% vs. 63%). (*Peters W et al., JCO 2000*)

What subset of pts from GOG 109 did not benefit from adding chemo to adj RT?

The subset analysis of **GOG 109** demonstrated that **pts with tumors ≤2 cm and only 1 +node** did not benefit from CRT compared with RT alone. (*Monk B et al., Gyn Oncol 2005*)

For pts with bulky (>4 cm) early-stage cervical cancer, is there an advantage to adding adj hysterectomy to definitive RT?

In **GOG 71,** pts with tumors >4 cm were randomized to RT alone vs. RT + adj hysterectomy. RT consisted of EBRT + brachytherapy (80 Gy to point A for the RT-alone group, and 75 Gy to point A for the surgery group). At median 9.6-yr follow-up, there was no difference in OS or severe toxicity. There was a trend to improved LR (26% vs. 14%, $p = 0.08$). (*Keys HM et al., Gyn Oncol 2003*)

An option is to give upfront CRT and assess for response at 2 mos. If residual Dz is evident, then salvage surgery can be considered. A downside to adjuvant hysterectomy is the potential for complications due to the high-dose radiation delivered to the area, including a relatively high dose to the posterior bladder wall.

For stage IB2 cervical cancer pts, what is the advantage of preop CRT compared with preop RT alone?

In **GOG 123,** stage IB2 cervical cancer pts were randomized to preop RT vs. CRT → adj simple hysterectomy. RT was whole pelvis (WP) + brachytherapy to a point A dose of 75 Gy. CRT added weekly cisplatin 40 mg/m^2. CRT was superior in 3-yr pCR (52% vs. 41%), OS (83% vs. 74%), and pCR (52% vs. 41%). *Note:* Adj and immediate hysterectomy was included in this trial prior to the results of GOG 71 being available. (*Keys HM, NEJM 1999*)

In stage IB cervical cancer, is there a role for neoadj chemo prior to surgery?

Controversial. GOG 141 looked at stage IB2 pts randomized to radical hysterectomy with nodal dissection +/– neoadj vincristine/cisplatin × 3 cycles. The study closed early, but there was comparable LC and OS in both groups, and PORT was needed in 45%–52% of pts. (*Eddy GL et al., Gyn Oncol 2007*)
A phase III trial from Italy looked at neoadj chemo + surgery vs. radiation alone for stages IB2 to III patients and found superior OS and PFS in the chemo + surgery arm. Benefit was significant only for stages IB2 to IIB group (*Benedetti-Panici P et al., JCO 2002*)
EORTC 55994 is currently testing the question whether preop CRT is better than preop chemo alone.

In locally advanced cervical cancer, what is the OS advantage of definitive CRT over RT alone?

The benefit of CRT over RT alone in locally advanced cervical cancer was evaluated in **RTOG 90-01.** (*Eifel P et al., JCO 2004*) This study randomized stages IIB–IVA, large stages IB–IIA (>5 cm), or LN+ pts and randomized to RT to the pelvis and P-A nodes vs. pelvis RT + 3 cycles of cisplatin/5-FU. Both arms had brachytherapy with a point A dose of 85 Gy. 8-yr OS was 67% vs. 41%, benefiting the CRT.

Which chemo agents are most effective in CRT for cervical cancer?

Weekly cisplatin at 40 mg/m^2 is the current standard to be given with definitive RT. **GOG 120** randomized cervical cancer pts stages IIB–IVA to RT + 3 different chemo arms. RT was WP + brachytherapy (to 81 Gy at point A). Chemo was weekly cisplatin 40 mg/m^2, or hydroxyurea, or cisplatin/5-FU/hydroxyurea. Cisplatin arms had better 4-yr OS (65% vs. 47%) and reduced recurrence (34%–35% vs. 54%). Toxicity was less with cisplatin alone or hydroxyurea alone. The benefit of adding 5-FU is unknown b/c of the confounding effect of hydroxyurea. (*Rose P et al., NEJM 1999*)

To what subset of pts is adding P-A fields to the pelvic field beneficial in the definitive Tx of cervical cancer?

There are 2 indications where the P-A field should be added to the definitive management of cervical cancer pts: (1) pts with +P-A Dz and (2) pts with +pelvic nodal Dz and not receiving CRT. 2 studies have addressed this:

RTOG 79-20 randomized 337 pts with stage IIB Dz without clinical or radiographic evidence of P-A Dz to the WP (45 Gy) alone vs. WP + P-A field (extended-field radiation therapy [EFRT]) (45 Gy). No chemo was given. Adding the P-A field improved 10-yr OS (55% vs. 44%) without improvement in LC or DM. However, there was slightly increased toxicity with the P-A field (8% vs. 4%). (*Rotman M et al., JAMA 1995*)

RTOG 90-01 randomized 386 pts with locally advanced cervical cancers (stages IIB–IVA or IB–IIA with ≥5 cm) or with a +pelvic LN (no P-A nodal Dz) to WP RT + chemo vs. WP + P-A field alone (EFRT). All pts were treated with post-EBRT brachytherapy of 85 Gy to point A. Chemo was cisplatin 75 mg/m^2 + 5-FU 1,000 mg/day × 4 days per 21-day cycle for 3 cycles. Pelvic CRT was superior to EFRT in 8-yr OS (67% vs. 41%), DFS (61% vs. 46%), LRF (18% vs. 35%), and DM (20% vs. 35%). There was a slight increase in P-A nodal failure in the CRT arm (8% vs. 4%, p = N SS). (*Morris M et al., NEJM 1999; Eifel P et al., JCO 2004*)

Describe the borders of typical AP and lat fields in cervical cancer Tx.

In cervical cancer therapy, the typical borders of an AP field are sup to L4-5 or L5/S1, inf to 3 cm below the most inf vaginal involvement or inf obturator foramen, and lat 2 cm from the pelvic rim. Lat beams would have the same sup and inf extent, with the ant edge to 1 cm ant of the pubic symphysis and post edge to include the entire sacrum. For common iliac nodal involvement, extend the field to cover up to L2. For P-A nodal involvement, extend the field to the top of T12. The borders can be tailored for early-stage vs. more advanced Dz. In the CT planning era, the alternative is to contour the organs and nodes of interest to ensure adequate coverage.

What is a typical EBRT prescription for cervical cancer?

Typically, cervical cancer pts treated with EBRT rcv RT to the WP to 45 Gy in 1.8 Gy/fx. Sidewall boosts usually go to 50–54 Gy. Persistent or bulky parametrial tumors usually rcv 60 Gy. P-A nodes go to 45 Gy if treated. Bulky nodes go to 60 Gy with 3D-CRT or IMRT.

What should be the total dose to point A and point B in patients with stage IB2 or higher disease? When should Tx of inguinal nodes be considered in cervical cancer?	For most patients with stage IB2 or higher disease, point A dose should be at least 80 Gy and point B dose should be at least 55 Gy. In cervical cancer, Tx of inguinal nodes should be considered **if Dz involves the lower 3rd of the vagina.**
Does overall Tx time in cervical cancer impact outcome? Ideally, how long should the RT Tx take?	**Yes.** Prolonged overall RT Tx time in cervical cancer is associated with poorer outcomes. Ideally, **EBRT and brachytherapy should be completed within 7 wks.** The effect is more notable in more advanced-stage pts (stages III–IV).

▶ **TOXICITY**

List 3 procedure-related complications seen in cervical cancer intracavitary brachytherapy.	Procedure-related complications seen in cervical cancer intracavitary brachytherapy: 1. Uterine perforation (<3%) 2. Vaginal laceration (<1%) 3. DVT (<1%)
Name the most common acute side effects associated with RT for cervical cancer.	**Skin irritation, fatigue, hemorrhoids, colitis-diarrhea, cystitis-frequency/dysuria, and nausea** are all possible acute side effects from cervical cancer RT.
Name the common long-term side effects associated with cervical cancer RT.	Common long-term side effects of cervical cancer radiation include permanent alteration in bowel habit, menopause in the premenopausal age group, chronic cystitis with frequency, and vaginal stenosis with dyspareunia and postcoital bleeding. The major severe long-term toxicities are most commonly bowel related: rectosigmoid stenosis, requiring possible colostomy, and major rectal bleeding. Hematuria, ureteral stricture, fistula, SBO, and hip fracture or sacral insufficiency fracture can also occur.
What should pts do regularly to prevent vaginal stenosis after receiving RT for cervical cancer?	**Routine use of a vaginal dilator** is essential to preventing vaginal stenosis in pts who have undergone RT for cervical cancer.

65 Ovarian Cancer

Updated by Surbhi Grover

▶ BACKGROUND

In the U.S., where does ovarian cancer rank as a cause of cancer death in women?

In the U.S., epithelial ovarian cancer (EOC) is the **5th leading cause of cancer mortality** in women. It is the 2nd most common gyn malignancy and the leading cause of death in this group.

What is the annual incidence and mortality of ovarian cancer in the U.S.?

Annually, there are **~22,000 new Dx and ~14,600 deaths** from ovarian cancer in the U.S. (*ACS, Facts and Figures 2009*)

What is the median age at Dx of ovarian cancer?

The median age at Dx of ovarian cancer is **63 yrs.** The incidence increases with age and is most prevalent during the 8th decade of life.

Is routine screening for ovarian cancer recommended?

No. Routine screening is not recommended for ovarian cancer. A prospective randomized trial failed to show that screening with transvaginal US and CA125 led to the detection of more early-stage cancers. (*Partridge E et al., Obstet Gynecol 2009*) However, preliminary data from the ongoing UKCTOCS (United Kingdom Collaborative Trial of Ovarian Cancer Screening) trial, which compares US and CA125 vs. US vs. no screening, suggests that more early-stage cancers are being detected with multimodal screening. (*Menon U et al., Lancet Oncol 2009*)

What are the histopathologic subtypes of ovarian cancer in order of decreasing frequency?

Ovarian cancer subtypes: EOC (80%) > ovarian stromal tumors > germ cell neoplasms > carcinosarcomas/malignant mixed müllerian tumors (MMMTs)

What risk factors are associated with the development of ovarian cancer?

Risk factors associated with the development of ovarian cancer:
1. Nulliparity
2. Advanced age at time of 1st birth (>35 yrs)
3. HRT
4. High fat/lactose diet
5. Hx of ≥2 1st-degree relatives with ovarian cancer
6. Family Hx of *BRCA1/2* or *HNPCC*
7. Older age

(*Finch A et al., JAMA 2006*)

445

What is the role of prophylactic oophorectomy in BRCA1/2-positive women?

Prophylactic oophorectomy has been shown to reduce the risk of ovarian and fallopian tube malignancies in *BRCA1/2* women; however, the risk of primary peritoneal cancer persists. (*Finch A et al., JAMA 2006; Rebbeck TR et al., J Natl Cancer Inst 2009*)

What factors portend a ↓ risk for the development of ovarian cancer?

Factors associated with ↓ lifetime risk of ovarian cancer:
1. Younger maternal age at 1st birth (≤25 yrs)
2. Use of oral contraception
3. Breastfeeding

What are the regional LN drainage routes from the ovaries?

Regional LNs of the ovaries include **internal iliac, obturator, sacral, external iliac, common iliac, para-aortic, and inguinal LNs.**

What are the most common sites of DMs for ovarian cancer?

Common sites of DMs from ovarian cancer include the **liver parenchyma, lung, bone, and axillary and supraclavicular LNs.** Whereas intra-abdominal spread to the peritoneum and diaphragmatic and liver surfaces is common, these are formally FIGO III Dz.

What are the common presenting signs and Sx of ovarian cancer?

The NCCN (2014) has released the following consensus guidelines for ovarian cancer Sx: **bloating, abdominal/pelvic pain, difficulty eating, early satiety, new urinary Sx (frequency/urgency >12 days/mo), palpable abdominal/pelvic mass, and ascites.** Identification of such Sx should prompt a workup for ovarian cancer.

▶ WORKUP/STAGING

What is CA125, and what is its utility in ovarian cancer?

CA125 is a **mucinous protein encoded by the *MUC16* gene and is used to assess response to Tx and predict prognosis after Tx for ovarian cancer.** Due to its low sensitivity and specificity as a diagnostic test, it is not used as a screening tool.

What are the initial steps in the workup of pts with an undiagnosed pelvic mass?

Pts with signs/Sx suspicious for ovarian cancer should undergo a full H&P, including a thorough family Hx and pelvic examination, CBC, CMP, CA125, US, CT abdomen/pelvis, and CXR. Final staging is determined through surgical/pathologic evaluation of the abdomen and pelvis. (NCCN 2014)

What is the FIGO staging system for ovarian cancer?

Stage IA: limited to 1 ovary with capsule intact; no tumor on ovarian surface; no malignant cells in ascites or peritoneal washings

Stage IB: limited to both ovaries with capsules intact; no tumor on ovarian surface; no malignant cells in ascites or peritoneal washings

Stage IC: limited to 1 or both ovaries with any of the following: ruptured capsule, tumor on ovarian surface, malignant cells in ascites, or peritoneal washings

Stage IIA: extension and/or implants on uterus and/or tube(s); no malignant cells in ascites or peritoneal washings

Stage IIB: extension to and/or implants on other pelvic tissues; no malignant cells in ascites or peritoneal washings

Stage IIC: pelvic extension and/or implants (T2 a or T2b) with malignant cells in ascites or peritoneal washings

Stage IIIA: microscopic peritoneal mets beyond pelvis (no macroscopic tumor)

Stage IIIB: macroscopic peritoneal mets beyond pelvis ≤2 cm in greatest dimension

Stage IIIC: peritoneal mets beyond pelvis >2 cm in greatest dimension and/or regional LN mets

Stage IV: DM (excludes peritoneal mets)

If a pt with ovarian cancer is found to have a liver met, what stage is she?	In ovarian cancer, the stage implications of a liver met depend on whether the met was on the liver capsule or in the parenchyma. **Liver capsule mets are T3/stage III,** and **liver parenchymal mets are M1/stage IV.**
What is the difference between the FIGO and AJCC TNM staging for ovarian cancer?	As of 2010, the **FIGO and AJCC staging systems do not differ for ovarian cancer.**
What % of pts with newly diagnosed ovarian cancer present with advanced-stage Dz?	~70% of all newly diagnosed ovarian cancer pts present with advanced-stage Dz (stage I, 20%; stage II, 12%; stage III, 45%; stage IV, 23%). Dx at earlier stages is difficult due to the location of the ovaries.

▶ TREATMENT/PROGNOSIS

What is the general Tx paradigm for ovarian cancer?	Ovarian cancer Tx paradigm: pts with suspected ovarian cancer should undergo a comprehensive diagnostic and therapeutic laparotomy for surgical staging and cytoreduction, respectively. This should include **peritoneal lavage; total abdominal hysterectomy with bilat salpingo-oophorectomy; and resection of suspicious LNs, including bilat pelvic/periaortic nodes in stage IIIB pts with a goal to cytoreduce to <1 cm of gross residual Dz.**

Are there situations where unilat salpingo-oophorectomy may be considered in pts with ovarian cancer?

For a young woman with **early-stage Dz or a low malignant potential tumor wishing to preserve fertility,** a unilat salpingo-oophorectomy may be considered.

How should early-stage ovarian cancer be treated?

The gold standard for Tx of all stages of ovarian cancer is **surgery.** For stages IA-B, grade 1, non–clear cell tumors treated with complete cytoreductive staging laparotomy, 5-yr OS rates approach 95% and no adj therapy is indicated. For pts with suspected stages IA-B, grade 1, non–clear cell tumors who have had incomplete surgical staging, consider completion staging or adj chemo. For all other stages, consider adj chemo. (*Young RC et al., NEJM 1990; Trimbos JB et al., J Natl Cancer Inst 2003*)

What trials support the use of chemo in the postsurgical setting for pts with ovarian cancer?

The ICON1/ACTION trials randomized mostly stages I–II ovarian cancer pts (some advanced-stage pts in ICON1) to postsurgical platinum-based chemo (4–6 cycles) vs. observation. Adj chemo significantly increased 5-yr OS (82% vs. 74%) and RFS (76% vs. 65%). Subset analysis of the ACTION Adjuvant Chemo Therapy In Ovarian Neoplasm) trial suggested that some early stage pts who have been optimally staged may not benefit from adj chemo. (*Trimbos JB et al., J Natl Cancer Inst 2003*)

What is the ideal duration of adj chemo for early-stage ovarian cancer?

The Gynecologic Oncology Group's study **GOG 157** randomized 427 stages IA-B (grade 2–3), IC, and II ovarian cancer pts to 3 vs. 6 cycles of adj carboplatin and paclitaxel. The estimated 5-yr probability of recurrence (25.4% vs. 20.1%) and OS were not significantly different. Neurotoxicity, anemia, and granulocytopenia were significantly higher in the longer-therapy arm. Thorough surgical staging was incomplete or inadequately documented in 29% of included pts. (*Bell J et al., Gynecol Oncol 2006*) **GOG 175** is exploring the role of consolidative paclitaxel after 3 cycles of adj carboplatin/paclitaxel.

How should advanced-stage ovarian cancer be treated?

GOG 158 randomized 792 advanced-stage ovarian cancer pts with residual Dz ≤1 cm to adj paclitaxel/cisplatin vs. paclitaxel/carboplatin. There was no significant difference in outcome, yet there were more GI, renal, and hematologic toxicities with cisplatin. (*Ozols R et al., JCO 2003*) **GOG 47** and **GOG 111** had previously established the benefits of platinum- and taxane-based chemo in the postop setting, respectively. (*Omura G et al., Cancer 1986; McGuire WP et al., NEJM 1996*)

What is the role of neoadj chemo in the Tx of ovarian cancer?

Generally, neoadj chemo may be considered for pts with inoperable, bulky, advanced-stage, Bx-proven ovarian cancer. (*Hou JY et al., Gynecol Oncol 2007; Steed H et al., Int J Gynecol Cancer 2006*) The EORTC Gynaecological Cancer Group/NCIC Clinical Trials Group randomized primary debulking surgery +/− neoadj chemo in stages IIIC and IV ovarian, fallopian tube, and peritoneal cancer. Neoadj chemo was **not inferior** to primary surgery. Median OS was 29 mos vs. 30 mos for initial surgery and neoadj chemo arms, respectively. (*Vergote I et al., NEJM 2010*)

What is the ~5-yr stage-adjusted survival of pts with ovarian cancer treated with standard of care therapy?

Survival by stage for treated ovarian cancer pts:
Stage I: 80%
Stage II: 60%
Stage III: 30%
Stage IV: 10%

What is the role of RT in the Tx of ovarian cancer?

In the postsurgical setting, whole abdomen irradiation (WAI) has resulted in similar outcomes when compared with chemo (with melphalan) in the Tx of ovarian cancer pts, yet it has led to more toxicity. (*Smith JP et al., Natl Cancer Inst Monogr 1975; Chiara S et al., Am J Clin Oncol 1994*) As a result, the use of RT in the adj setting has fallen out of favor. There are no known recent phase III randomized trials comparing WAI to current standard of care chemo in the adj setting.

Is there a role for consolidative RT after cytoreductive surgery and adj chemo for ovarian cancer?

Consolidative RT may improve cancer control in subgroups of pts, but very few institutions recommend it because of concern for toxicity. A prospective randomized trial compared consolidative RT vs. chemo vs. observation in 172 pts with stage III EOC initially treated with cytoreductive surgery and adj chemo. In the subgroup with complete surgical and pathologic remission, pts receiving RT had significantly improved 5-yr PFS (56% vs. 36% vs. 35%). However, Tx-related side effects were also more frequent in pts receiving RT, including severe, late GI toxicity in 10%. (*Sorbe B et al., Int J Gynecol Cancer 2003*) Small institutional studies have also reported on the feasibility and apparent benefit of WAI as a consolidative Tx after standard of care therapy (laparotomy and platinum/taxane chemo) in advanced-stage ovarian cancer. (*Rochet N et al., BMC Cancer 2007*)

Has the utility of IMRT been investigated for WAI?

Yes. The feasibility of applying IMRT to WAI has been reported both in concept and practice and is shown to allow excellent PTV coverage with better sparing of organs at risk. (*Hong L et al., IJROBP 2002; Rochet N et al., Strahlenther Onkol 2008*)

Is there a role for WAI in persistent, chemo-refractory ovarian cancer?

This is **uncertain.** There are no prospective, randomized data available. *Cmelak AJ et al.* retrospectively analyzed 41 women with persistent or recurrent ovarian carcinoma after initial Tx with surgical debulking and chemo who were treated with WAI (median dose: abdomen, 28 Gy; pelvis, 48 Gy). 5-yr DSS for pts with residual Dz <1.5 cm before WAI was 53% vs. 0% if >1.5 cm. 29% failed to complete WAI secondary to acute toxicity. Late toxicity requiring surgery occurred in 3 pts. The authors recommend WAI in pts who have failed initial chemo with small-sized residual tumor burden. (*Gynecol Oncol 1997*)

Can RT be used to effectively palliate recurrent, cisplatin-refractory, focal ovarian cancer lesions?

This is **uncertain.** There are no prospective, randomized data available. *Corn BW et al.* retrospectively analyzed the efficacy of RT in palliating focally recurrent, symptomatic ovarian cancer lesions. Complete palliative response was 51%, overall palliative response was 79%, and median duration of palliation was 4 mos. The likelihood of obtaining a complete symptomatic response was related to a Karnofsky performance status ≥70% and a biologic effective dose 10 >44 Gy. (*Cancer 1994*)

Describe the WAI fields used to treat ovarian cancer pts.

Pts being planned to rcv WAI should undergo CT simulation. An AP/PA open-field technique is historically used with borders as follows:
Superior: top of diaphragm
Inferior: obturator foramen
Lateral: peritoneal reflection

What dose is prescribed when treating ovarian cancer pts with WAI?

Pts being treated with WAI should rcv **30 Gy** in 1.5 Gy/fx with a para-aortic boost to 45 Gy and pelvic boost to 50 Gy. Kidney and liver blocks should be applied at 15 Gy and 25 Gy, respectively.

How should pts with a rising CA125 be managed following CR to initial therapy in the absence of clinical or radiographic evidence of Dz recurrence?

Pts who are chemo naive should be treated the same as newly diagnosed pts (**complete surgical staging +/− chemo, if appropriate**). Tx options for pts who have previously rcvd chemo include observation until clinical relapse, hormonal therapy (e.g., tamoxifen), systemic therapy, or clinical trial enrollment.

What is the median time to clinically or radiographically detectable Dz after an isolated CA125 relapse?	The median time to clinical relapse in the setting of a rising CA125 is **3–6 mos.**
Are most relapses of ovarian cancer local or distant?	~80% of relapsed ovarian cancers are **local.**
How should ovarian cancer relapses be managed?	Pts with platinum-sensitive relapsed ovarian cancer (relapse ≥6 mos after initial chemo) should be treated with platinum-based combination chemo. (*Fung-Kee-Fung M et al., Curr Oncol 2007*) In cases of platinum-resistant Dz, single agents such as docetaxel, gemcitabine, etoposide, pemetrexed, and others can be used. (*Mutch DG et al., JCO 2007*) Response rates in the latter are 20%–30%.

▶ **TOXICITY**

What is the most common severe toxicity experienced by ovarian cancer pts treated with WAI?	**Grades 3–4 diarrhea** occurs in ~30% of ovarian cancer pts treated with WAI. (*Chiara S et al., Am J Clin Oncol 1994*)

66 Endometrial Cancer

Updated by Surbhi Grover

▶ **BACKGROUND**

What is the incidence of endometrial cancer in the U.S.?	Endometrial cancer is the most common gyn malignancy in the U.S., with an incidence of **~44,000 cases/yr** annually. It is the 2nd most common cause of gyn cancer deaths.
What are the 2 forms of endometrial cancer?	Forms of endometrial cancer: 1. Type I: endometrioid, 70%–80% of cases, estrogen related 2. Type II: nonendometrioid, typically papillary serous or clear cell, high grade, not estrogen related, aggressive clinical course

What are the risk factors for endometrial cancer?

Risk factors for endometrial cancer:
1. Exogenous unopposed estrogen
2. Endogenous estrogen (obesity, functional ovarian tumors, late menopause, nulliparity, chronic anovulation/polycystic ovarian syndrome)
3. Tamoxifen
4. Advancing age (75% postmenopausal)
5. Hereditary (HNPCC)
6. Family Hx
7. HTN

What are protective factors for endometrial cancer?

Protective factors for endometrial cancer include **combination oral contraceptives and physical activity.**

What is the most common clinical presentation of endometrial cancer?

Endometrial cancer presents with **abnl vaginal bleeding** in 90% cases.

What % of postmenopausal women with abnl vaginal bleeding have endometrial cancer?

Only **5%–20%** of postmenopausal women with abnl vaginal bleeding have endometrial cancer.

What are the 3 layers of the uterine wall?

The 3 layers of the uterine wall are the **endometrium, myometrium, and serosa.**

What is the primary lymphatic drainage of the uterus?

The primary lymphatic drainage of the cervix and lower uterine segment is to the **pelvic LNs** (parametrial, internal and external iliacs, obturator, common iliac, presacral). The fundus has direct drainage to the para-aortic (P-A) nodes. The round ligament can drain directly to the inguinal nodes.

What % of endometrial cancer pts with positive pelvic LNs will also harbor Dz in the P-A LNs? What is the chance of P-A nodal involvement if pelvic nodes are negative?

33%–50% of pts with pelvic LN involvement also have involvement of the P-A nodes. Isolated P-A nodal involvement with negative pelvic LNs is detected in ~1% of surgically staged cases, though the rate may be higher when dissection is extended above the IMA to the perirenal nodes, especially on the left where direct route of spread might occur.

What determines the grade of endometrial tumors?

The grade of endometrial tumors depends on the **glandular component:**

Grade I: ≤5% nonsquamous solid growth pattern

Grade II: 6%–50% nonsquamous solid growth pattern

Grade III: >50% nonsquamous solid growth pattern

What is the risk of LN involvement by DOI and grade per Gynecologic Oncology Group's GOG 33?

According to **GOG 33,** the risk of LN involvement is <5% for tumors limited to the endometrium (all grades) and 5%–10% for tumors invading the inner and middle 3rd of the myometrium (all grades). For tumors invading the outer 3rd of the myometrium, the risk is ~10% for grade 1, ~20% for grade 2, and ~35% for grade 3. (*Creasman WT et al., Cancer 1987*)

What are the most aggressive histologies of endometrial cancer?

The most aggressive histologies of endometrial cancer are **papillary serous, clear cell, and pure squamous cell.**

What % of endometrial cancers are adenocarcinoma?

75%–80% of endometrial cancers are adenocarcinomas.

According to the American College of Obstetricians and Gynecologists (ACOG), how should women be screened for endometrial cancer?

According to the ACOG, there is **no appropriate cost-effective screening test** for endometrial cancer.

▶ WORKUP/STAGING

Per the NCCN (2014), what is the workup for endometrial cancer?

NCCN endometrial cancer workup: CBC, PAP smear, endometrial Bx, and CXR. If extrauterine Dz is suspected, consider CA125, MRI/CT, cystoscopy, and sigmoidoscopy.

What are the sensitivity and specificity of an endometrial Bx?

Endometrial Bx has **90%–98% sensitivity and 85% specificity.**

When is D&C recommended?

D&C is recommended **if endometrial Bx is nondiagnostic.**

What is involved in the surgical staging of pts with endometrial carcinoma?

Surgical staging for endometrial cancer:
1. Vertical incision/or laparoscopy
2. Peritoneal washing/cytology (controversial)
3. Exploration of all peritoneal surfaces with Bx of any lesions
4. Total abdominal hysterectomy (TAH)/bilateral salpingo-oophorectomy (BSO)
5. Uterus bivalved in operating room
6. Omental Bx (omentectomy for uterine papillary serous carcinoma [UPSC]/clear cell carcinoma [CCC])
7. Pelvic/P-A LN sampling vs. dissection

During the surgical staging procedure for endometrial cancer, what features are an indication for P-A nodal sampling? Approximately what % of pts have these features?

P-A sampling should take place in endometrial cancer pts with the following:
1. Gross P-A Dz
2. Positive pelvic LN
3. Gross adnexal mass or peritoneal disease
4. More than one-third myometrial involvement

~25% of pts have these features, but they account for 98% of all positive P-A LNs.

Per the NCCN (2014), when is cystoscopy or sigmoidoscopy indicated?

Per the NCCN, cystoscopy or sigmoidoscopy is indicated **only for Sx or advanced lesions.**

What is the AJCC 7ᵗʰ edition (2011)/FIGO (2008) pathologic staging for endometrial cancer?

Stage T1a/IA: limited to endometrium or less than one-half of myometrium
Stage T1b/IB: invades half or more of myometrium
Note: Endocervical glandular involvement only is considered AJCC T1 and FIGO stage I.
Stage T2/II: invades connective tissue of cervix but does not extend beyond uterus
Stage T3a/IIIA: tumor involves serosa and/or adnexa by direct extension of mets
Stage T3b/IIIB: vaginal involvement or parametrial involvement
Stage T4/IVA: tumor invades bladder mucosa (bullous edema is not sufficient) and/or bowel mucosa
Stage N0: no regional LN mets
Stage N1/IIIC1: regional LN mets to pelvic nodes
Stage N2/IIIC2: regional LN mets to P-A nodes
Stage M1/IVB: DMs

Note: Per the AJCC 7ᵗʰ edition (2011) and FIGO (2008), positive cytology no longer alters stage.

▶ TREATMENT/PROGNOSIS

What is the primary Tx modality for endometrial cancer?

Surgery is the primary Tx modality for endometrial cancer.

What is resected in a TAH?

TAH removes **the uterus and a small rim of vaginal cuff.**

What is resected in a modified radical hysterectomy?

Modified radical hysterectomy:
1. Removal of uterus and 1–2 cm of vaginal cuff
2. Wide excision of parametrial and paravaginal tissues (including median one half of cardinal and uterosacral ligaments)
3. Ligation of uterine artery at ureter

What is resected in a radical hysterectomy?

Radical hysterectomy:
1. Resection of uterus and upper vagina
2. Dissection of paravaginal and parametrial tissues to pelvic sidewalls
3. Ligation of uterine artery at its origin at internal iliac artery

Pelvic and P-A lymphadenectomy is recommended in which pts with endometrial cancer?

Although controversial, LNs are commonly assessed at the time of initial surgery for endometrial cancer. Pelvic lymphadenectomy may not be indicated in women with Dz clinically confined to the uterus. The ASTEC (A Study in the Treatment of Endometrial Carcinoma) trial randomized 1,408 pts with endometrial cancer that was clinically confined to the uterus to standard surgery (TAH + BSO, peritoneal washing, palpation of P-A nodes) vs. standard surgery + pelvic lymphadenectomy. Those at intermediate or high risk for recurrence (independent of nodal status) were further randomized to rcv pelvic RT or not. There was no benefit to pelvic lymphadenectomy in terms of OS or RFS. (*ASTEC Study Group et al., Lancet 2009*)

What is the risk of lymphedema following surgery for uterine malignancies?

According to an MSKCC retrospective review of 1,289 pts, the rate of lymphedema at a median follow-up of 3 yrs was 1.2%. When ≥10 LNs were removed, the rate of symptomatic lymphedema was 3.4%. (*Abu-Rustum NR et al., Gyn Oncol 2006*)

What are considered negative prognostic factors for endometrial cancer?

Negative prognostic indicators for endometrial cancer:
1. LVSI
2. Age >60 yrs
3. Grade 3/nonendometrioid histology
4. Deep myometrial invasion
5. Tumor size
6. Lower uterine segment involvement
7. Anemia
8. Poor Karnofsky performance status

What adj therapy is indicated for completely surgically staged endometrial cancers limited to the endometrium?

No adj therapy is indicated for endometrial cancers limited to the endometrium, except for grade 3, where vaginal cuff brachytherapy is considered. In grade 3 tumors with adverse risk factors and incomplete surgical staging, pelvic RT is considered.

What adj therapy is indicated for completely surgically staged endometrial cancers that invade less than half of the myometrium?

Endometrial cancers that invade less than half of the myometrium could be **observed or treated with adj vaginal cuff brachytherapy.**
Note:
1. If the tumor is grade 3 with adverse risk factors, pelvic RT should be considered.

2. If the tumor is incompletely surgically staged and grade 1–2, consider observation or vaginal brachytherapy +/– RT.

3. Endocervical glandular involvement favors the use of vaginal brachytherapy.

What adj therapy is indicated for completely surgically staged endometrial cancers that invade half or more of the myometrium?

Endometrial cancers that invade half or more of the myometrium can be **observed or treated with adj vaginal cuff brachytherapy.**
Note:

1. If grade 3 or any grade with adverse prognostic factors, whole pelvic RT +/– brachytherapy should be considered.

2. If the tumor is incompletely surgically staged, consider pelvic RT + vaginal brachytherapy. For incompletely staged grade 3 tumors, consider chemo as well.

3. Endocervical glandular involvement favors the use of vaginal brachytherapy.

What adj therapy is indicated for completely surgically staged, stage II endometrial cancer?

Adj pelvic RT and vaginal brachytherapy is indicated for endometrial cancers that invade the cervical stroma. If grade 3, consider chemo.

What adj therapy is indicated for completely surgically staged, stage III endometrial cancer?

Adj chemo +/– **RT** should be given for stage III endometrial cancer. RT in addition to chemo is needed if there is gross residual Dz or unresectable Dz.

Describe the whole pelvic RT field for endometrial cancer. What total doses are typically prescribed?

Borders of the whole pelvis (WP) RT field for endometrial cancer:
  Superior: L4-5 or L5/S1
  Inferior: bottom of obturator foramen
  Lateral: 1.5–2.0 cm lateral to pelvic brim
  Anterior: front of pubic symphysis
  Posterior: split sacrum to S3

Treat to 45–50 Gy.

What is the border of an extended RT field for endometrial cancer, and when should extended fields be used?

The sup border of an extended RT field for endometrial cancer is **T10-11 or T11-12.** It should be used if there are **positive P-A LNs.**

According to the American Brachytherapy Society (ABS), what are the Tx site and depth for vaginal cuff brachytherapy for endometrial cancer?

According to the ABS, for endometrioid carcinoma of the endometrium, the proximal 3–5 cm of the vagina (approximately one-half) should be treated. For CCC, UPSC, or stage IIIB, the target is the entire vaginal canal. Prescribe to 0.5 cm beyond the vaginal mucosa. (*Nag S, IJROBP 2000*)

What LDR and HDR are typically used for adj intracavitary RT alone for endometrial cancer?

For adj intracavitary RT therapy alone, the LDR is 50–60 Gy over 72 hrs (0.7–0.8 Gy/hr). The HDR is 21 Gy (7 Gy × 3) at 0.5 cm depth.

What LDR and HDR are commonly used for adj intracavitary RT given with WP RT for endometrial cancer?

When given in combination with WP RT, LDR doses of 30–40 Gy and HDR doses of 10–15 Gy (5 Gy × 2 or 3) at 0.5 cm depth are commonly used.

How are nonbulky vaginal cuff recurrences treated in endometrial cancer pts with no prior RT?

For nonbulky vaginal cuff recurrences in pts with no prior RT, a **combination of pelvic RT and brachytherapy** is typically used. Treat to 45 Gy pelvic RT and assess the response. If the residual is <0.5 cm, add HDR vaginal brachytherapy at 7 Gy × 3 to 0.5 cm depth of the vaginal mucosa. (*Nag S et al., IJROBP 2000*)

How are vaginal cuff recurrences that are bulky or within a previously irradiated field treated in endometrial cancer pts?

For endometrial cancer pts with vaginal cuff recurrences that are bulky (>0.5 cm thickness) or in a previously irradiated field, **consider interstitial brachytherapy or IMRT.**

When do inguinal nodes need to be included in the RT fields for endometrial cancer?

In cases with **distal vaginal involvement,** the entire vagina and inguinal nodes need to be included in EBRT fields.

How should inoperable endometrial cancer be treated with RT?

Consider pelvic RT to 45 Gy → intracavitary RT boost using 2 tandem intrauterine applicators to 6.3 Gy × 3 prescribed to 2-cm depth (serosal surface). If pelvic RT is contraindicated, consider definitive intracavitary RT alone (7.3 Gy × 5 prescribed to 2-cm depth). (*Nag S et al., IJROBP 2000*)

Describe the design and of PORTEC-1 (Post Operative Radiation Therapy in Endometrial Carcinoma).

In **PORTEC-1,** 714 pts with more than one-half myometrial invasion and grades 2–3 or one-half or more myometrial invasion and grades 1–2 underwent TAH/BSO with washings *with no lymphadenectomy* and were randomized to adj EBRT (46 Gy) vs. observation. EBRT reduced LRR from 14% to 5% at 10 yrs. 75% of LRs were in the vaginal vault. There was no difference in 10-yr OS. Note that with central pathology review, there was a significant shift from grade 2 to grade 1. (*Creutzberg CL et al., Lancet 2000; Scholten AN et al., IJROBP 2005*)

Describe the design and results of GOG 99.

In **GOG 99,** 392 endometrial cancer pts with myometrial and/or occult cervical invasion underwent TAH/BSO, pelvic and P-A LN sampling, and peritoneal cytology and then were randomized to observation vs. WP RT (50.4 Gy). Inclusion criteria were revised during the trial to include only high-intermediate–risk pts defined as: (1) age >70 yrs with 1 risk factor (grade 2 or 3, LVI, outer one-third myometrial invasion), (2) age >50 yrs with 2 risk factors, and (3) any age with 3 risk factors. RT improved LR from 12% to 3%. The greatest benefit in LR was in high-intermediate–risk pts from 26% to 6% vs. low-intermediate–risk pts from 6% to 2%. There was no change in OS, but the study was not powered to detect this. *Conclusion:* Limit pelvic RT to high-intermediate–risk pts. The major flaw of this study is that grade 2 was grouped with grade 3 even though grade 2 Dz tends to behave more similarly to grade 1. (*Keys HM et al., Gyn Oncol 2004*)

Describe the design and results of the Aalders Norwegian study.

The Aalders Norwegian study enrolled 540 pts with surgical stage I endometrial cancer s/p TAH/BSO (with no lymphadenectomy). **All pts rcvd vaginal cuff brachytherapy (~40 Gy LDR at 0.5 cm or ~24 Gy HDR at 0.5 cm).** They were then randomized to no further therapy vs. pelvic RT (40 Gy with central shielding after 20 Gy). Overall, the pelvic RT arm had decreased 9-yr LR (7% to 2%) but more DM (5% vs. 10%). There was no difference in 9-yr OS. On subset analysis of pts with invasion of one half or more of the myometrium and grade 3 Dz, pelvic RT improved 9-yr OS (72% to 82%) and improved 9-yr LR (20% to 5%). There was no change in DM. There was no difference in OS, LR, or DM for pts with invasion of one half or more of the myometrium and grade 1–2 Dz. (*Aalders J et al., Ob Gyn 1980*)

Describe the design and results of GOG 122.

In **GOG 122,** 388 pts with endometrial tumors invading beyond the uterus (all histologies) underwent TAH/BSO and surgical staging with <2-cm residual tumor. P-A LNs were allowed, but mets to the chest or supraclavicular nodes were not allowed. Pts were randomized to whole abdomen irradiation (30 Gy AP/PA +15 Gy boost to pelvic +/– P-A LNs) vs. chemo (doxorubicin/cisplatin q3wks × 8 cycles). At 5 yrs, chemo had improved stage-adjusted OS (55% vs. 42%) and PFS (38% vs. 50%). Chemo had increased grades 3–4 heme toxicity (88% vs. 14%) and increased GI, cardiac, and neurologic toxicity. Note: Results were questioned b/c although this was a randomized trial, the analysis was based on stage-adjusted results that may not be justified. (*Randall ME et al., JCO 2006*)

Describe the design and results of PORTEC-2.

PORTEC-2 randomized 427 pts with intermediate-high–risk endometrial cancer defined as:

1. Age >60 yrs and less than one-half myometrial invasion and grade 3
2. Age >60 yrs and one-half or more myometrial invasion and grades 1–2
3. Invasion of cervical glandular epithelium and grades 1–2
4. Invasion of cervical glandular epithelium and grade 3 with less than one-half myometrial invasion

All pts were s/p TAH/BSO without pelvic LND and were randomized to EBRT (46 Gy) vs. vaginal brachytherapy alone (HDR 21 Gy in 3 fx or LDR 30 Gy). At median follow-up at 3.8 yrs, vaginal brachytherapy was similar to EBRT with respect to 5-yr outcomes: vaginal relapse (1.8% vs. 1.6%), isolated pelvic relapse (1.5% vs. 0.5%), LRR (5.1% vs. 2.1%), or OS (85% vs. 80%). However, there were significantly higher rates of acute grades 1–2 GI toxicity in the EBRT group. The authors concluded that vaginal brachytherapy should be standard in intermediate-high–risk endometrial cancer. (*Nout RA et al., Lancet 2010*)

Describe the design and results of the Finnish randomized trial comparing adj EBRT vs. interdigitated CRT in endometrial cancer.

The Finland trial included 156 endometrial cancer pts with (1) less than one-half myometrial invasion and grade 3 or (2) one-half or more myometrial invasion or extrauterine extension up to stage IIIA and any grade.

All were s/p TAH/BSO (with pelvic LAD in 80%) and randomized to split-course pelvic EBRT (28 Gy × 2 with a 3-wk break) vs. interdigitated CRT (28 Gy → chemo → 28 Gy → chemo, where chemo used was cisplatin/epirubicin/cyclophosphamide). There was no difference in 5-yr DFS, LR, or DM. Note the atypical Tx paradigms including split-course therapy. (*Kuoppala T et al., Gyn Oncol 2008*)

Describe the design and results of the Japanese GOG (JGOG) 2033.

JGOG 2033 enrolled 385 pts with more than one-half myometrial invasion, including pts with stages II–III Dz. All were s/p TAH/BSO and surgical staging and were randomized to 40–50 Gy EBRT AP/PA vs. ≥3 cycles of chemo (cyclophosphamide/doxorubicin/cisplatin). At 5 yrs, there was no difference in PFS, OS, or toxicity. An unplanned subset analysis defined high-intermediate risk:

1. Stage I and age >70 yrs or grade 3 Dz
2. Stage II or +cytology

In this subset, chemo improved PFS (83.8% vs. 66.2%). The authors concluded that adj chemo is a reasonable alternative to RT in intermediate-risk endometrial cancer. (*Susumu N et al., Gyn Oncol 2007*)

Describe the design and results of the Nordic Society of Gynaecological Oncology (NSGO)-EORTC trial that evaluated adj RT ± chemo in high-risk endometrial cancer.

The NSGO-EORTC trial enrolled 367 endometrial cancer pts with surgical stages I–II, positive peritoneal fluid cytology or positive pelvic LNs. Most had ≥2 risk factors: grade 3, deep myometrial invasion, or DNA nondiploidy. Pts with serous, clear cell, or anaplastic carcinomas were eligible regardless of risk factors. Pts were randomized to RT vs. RT + chemo (various regimens allowed). RT was pelvic EBRT (44 Gy) +/– vaginal brachytherapy. 5-yr PFS favored the RT + chemo arm (82% vs. 75%). (*Hogberg T et al., ASCO 2007 abstract*)

Describe the design and results of GOG 94—the study of UPSC and CCC.

GOG 94 was a phase I–II trial enrolling 21 pts with UPSC or CCC of the uterus s/p TAH/BSO, pelvic/P-A nodal sampling, and peritoneal washing. Pts were treated with whole abdomen irradiation (30 Gy/20 fx) and pelvic boost (19.8 Gy/11 fx). At 5 yrs, >50% failures were within the RT field, and 5-yr PFS was 38% for UPSC and 54% for CCC. The authors concluded that chemo likely is necessary for these radioresistant histologies. (*Sutton G et al., Gyn Oncol 2006*)

▶ TOXICITY

What is the RT tolerances of proximal and distal vagina?

The RT tolerance of the mucosa of the proximal vagina is 120 Gy and distal vagina is 98 Gy. (*Hintz BL et al., IJROBP 1980*)

At what RT dose does ovarian failure occur?

Ovarian failure occurs after **5–10 Gy.**

At what RT dose does sterilization occur in women?

Sterilization in women occurs after **2–3 Gy.**

What are the expected acute and late RT toxicities associated with RT Tx for endometrial cancer?

Acute toxicities: diarrhea, proctitis, abdominal cramps, fatigue, bladder irritation, drop in blood counts, n/v

Late toxicities: vaginal dryness and atrophy, pubic hair loss, vaginal stenosis and fibrosis (recommend vaginal dilators), urethral stricture, fistula formation, SBO, chronic urinary and bowel frequency

67 Uterine Sarcoma

Updated by Surbhi Grover

▶ BACKGROUND

What % of uterine malignancies are sarcomas?

Sarcomas account for ~4% of uterine malignancies.

What are the 3 most common histologic subtypes of uterine sarcoma?

Most common uterine sarcomas (in order of frequency):
1. Carcinosarcoma, also referred to as malignant mixed müllerian tumor (MMMT)
2. Leiomyosarcoma (LMS)
3. Endometrial stromal sarcoma (ESS)

How does uterine sarcoma typically present?

Typical presentation by histologic subtype:
MMMT: vaginal bleeding
LMS and ESS: similar Sx and signs as uterine fibroids

What is the incidence of nodal mets?

MMMT: 30% (20%–38%), even in clinically early-stage Dz (similar to endometrial adenocarcinoma)
LMS: 8% (6.6%–9.1%), usually associated with extrauterine Dz
ESS: traditionally thought to be low. (A recent study of 831 pts with ESS showed a 10% incidence.) (*Chan JK et al. Br J Cancer 2008*)

How does the risk of DM compare between endometrial cancer and uterine sarcoma?

In general, **uterine sarcoma has a higher rate of metastatic Dz** than endometrial cancer.

What is the most common site of mets in uterine sarcoma?

In uterine sarcoma, the most common site of mets is the **lung.**

For which histologic subtype of uterine sarcoma is grade most important?

Grade is most important for **ESS.** Low-grade ESS is a hormone-sensitive low-grade malignancy with an indolent course, whereas high-grade ESS is characterized by an aggressive clinical course that cannot be differentiated from other high-grade uterine sarcomas such as LMS and MMMT. Some consider ESS low grade by definition and categorize high-grade tumors as high-grade undifferentiated sarcoma.

In MMMT, which component (epithelial or sarcomatous) dictates prognosis and treatment?

In MMMT, it is the **epithelial component** that dictates prognosis and treatment, not the sarcomatous component. Most have serous or high-grade endometrioid histology as the epithelial component and behave as their pure uterine cancer counterpart with respect to recurrence, routes of spread, and indications for adjuvant treatment.

▶ WORKUP/STAGING

What is the FIGO (2008) staging for uterine sarcoma?

MMMT is still staged according to the FIGO system for endometrial adenocarcinoma.
LMS and ESS staging:
  Stage I: limited to uterus
  Stage IA: <5 cm
  Stage IB: >5 cm
  Stage II: extends to pelvis
  Stage IIA: adnexal involvement
  Stage IIB: extends to extrauterine pelvic tissue
  Stage III: invades abdominal tissues (not just protruding into abdomen)
  Stage IIIA: 1 abdominal site
  Stage IIIB: >1 abdominal site
  Stage IIIC: mets to pelvic LNs, para-aortic (P-A) LNs, or both
  Stage IVA: invades bladder or rectum
  Stage IVB: DM

How should the initial workup for uterine sarcoma differ from the workup for endometrial cancer?

The initial workup for uterine sarcoma is identical to the workup for endometrial cancer, but it should include a CT chest b/c of the increased risk of pulmonary mets. There is also anecdotal evidence that PET/CT may be useful.

▶ TREATMENT/PROGNOSIS

What is the primary Tx modality for uterine sarcoma?

Uterine sarcoma primary Tx modality: simple hysterectomy and bilateral salpingo-oophorectomy (BSO) is the mainstay. Ovarian preservation may be considered in young pts with early-stage LMS and ESS. The role of RT, chemo, and HRT is still controversial.

What is the role of LND in the Tx of uterine sarcoma?

Pelvic LND, P-A LND, or both for uterine sarcoma is considered controversial. They usually are recommended in MMMT and undifferentiated sarcoma. They usually are not recommended in LMS and ESS without extrauterine Dz.

Is there a benefit to postop pelvic RT for the management of uterine sarcomas?

The role of adj RT remains **controversial.** The issue has been addressed in at least 1 randomized trial and 2 important retrospective studies. In general, the data suggest an LC benefit for MMMT but limited, if any, OS benefit with adj RT. The LC and OS benefits of adj RT in LMS, which has a high DM rate, are unclear but likely limited.

EORTC 55874 randomized 224 pts with stages I–II high-grade uterine sarcoma (46% LMS, 41% carcinosarcoma, 13% endometrial stromal tumor) s/p total abdominal hysterectomy/BSO, washings (75%), and optional nodal sampling (25%) to either (1) observation or (2) pelvic RT to 50.4 Gy. The results suggest that pelvic RT improves LC but not OS or PFS for MMMT; however, there is no benefit for LMS. (*Reed NS, Eur J Cancer 2008*)

A SEER-based study found that adj RT offered survival benefits in pts with early MMMT but not in LMS. (*Wright JD et al., Am J Obstet Gynecol 2008*)

A retrospective series from Mayo Clinic included 208 pts with uterine LMS. Pelvic RT had no impact on DSS ($p = 0.06$), but it was associated with a significant improvement in LR. (*Giuntoli R et al., Gyn Oncol 2003*)

What is the role of whole abdomen irradiation (WAI) in MMMT?

GOG 150 is a randomized trial of WAI vs. 3 cycles of cisplatin/ifosfamide/mesna (CIM) as postsurgical therapy in stages I–IV carcinosarcoma of the uterus. Neither Tx was particularly effective. Vaginal recurrence increased and abdominal recurrence fell in the chemo group. Serious late adverse events increased significantly in the group receiving WAI. (*Wolfson AH et al., Gynecol Oncol 2007*)

For which pts with MMMT is pelvic irradiation typically indicated?

Similar to epithelial cancers, pelvic irradiation is typically recommended for MMMT with **age >60 yrs, deep myometrial involvement, cervical involvement, nodal involvement, or residual Dz (micro- or macroscopic).**

For which pts with LMS is pelvic irradiation typically indicated?

Although controversial, pelvic irradiation may be considered in **pts with uterine LMS with micro- or macroscopic residual Dz,** particularly in the context of a clinical trial.

How do the RT fields for uterine sarcoma differ from those used for endometrial carcinoma?

The **RT fields are the same** for uterine sarcoma and endometrial carcinoma.

| Does the prognostic index developed for soft tissue sarcomas apply to uterine sarcomas? | **No.** The prognostic index for soft tissue sarcomas does not apply to uterine sarcomas. |

 TOXICITY

| What are the expected acute and late toxicities associated with RT Tx for uterine sarcoma? | <u>Acute toxicities</u>: n/v, diarrhea, mucositis, fatigue, bladder irritation
<u>Late toxicities</u>: vaginal dryness and atrophy, pubic hair loss, vaginal stenosis and fibrosis (recommend vaginal dilators), urethral stricture, fistula formation, SBO |

68 Vulvar Cancer

Updated by Surbhi Grover

 BACKGROUND

Approximately how many pts are affected by vulvar cancer per yr in the U.S.? What is the incidence of vulvar cancer in the U.S.?	**~3,500** pts are affected by vulvar cancer per yr in the U.S. The incidence is **1/100,000 people.**
Vulvar cancer accounts for what % of gyn malignancies? What % of all malignancies in women are vulvar malignancies?	Vulvar cancer represents **3%–5% of all gyn malignancies.** This comprises **1%–2% of all cancers in women.**
What are the risk factors for vulvar cancer?	Risk factors for vulvar cancer: 1. Increasing age 2. HPV 3. Vulvar intraepithelial neoplasia (VIN) 4. Bowen Dz (squamous cell CIS) 5. Paget Dz (lesions arising from Bartholin, urethra, or rectum) 6. Smoking 7. Immune deficiency 8. Lichen sclerosis

What HPV subtypes are associated with vulvar cancer?

HPV subtypes associated with vulvar cancer include **6, 16, 18, and 33.**

What is the function of HPV-associated oncoproteins?

It is thought that HPV-associated oncoproteins **bind and inactivate tumor suppressor proteins** such as Rb, p53, and p21.

What are the 7 subsites of the vulva?

Subsites of the vulva:
1. Labia majora
2. Labia minora
3. Mons pubis
4. Clitoris
5. Vaginal vestibule
6. Perineal body
7. Posterior fourchette

What are the most common presenting Sx of pts with vulvar cancer?

Common presenting Sx of vulvar cancer: pruritus, vulvar discomfort or pain, dysuria, oozing, or bleeding.

In which subsites does vulvar cancer most commonly arise?

70% of vulvar cancers arise from the **labia majora/minora.**

How is "locally advanced" vulvar cancer defined?

Locally advanced vulvar cancer is defined as **a vulvar tumor burden that cannot be resected without exenterative surgery.**

What % of vulvar cancers are locally advanced at Dx?

30% of vulvar cancers are locally advanced at Dx.

What are the 1st-, 2nd-, and 3rd-echelon LN regions in vulvar cancer, and which subsite is associated with skip nodal mets?

LN regions in vulvar cancer:
1st echelon: superficial inguinofemoral
2nd echelon: deep inguinofemoral and femoral
3rd echelon: external iliac nodes

The **clitoris** can drain directly to the deep inguinofemoral or pelvic nodes.

What are the 2 strongest predictors of LN involvement in vulvar cancer?

The 2 strongest predictors of LN involvement in vulvar cancer are **tumor grade and DOI.**

Estimate the risk of inguinal LN involvement based on the DOI of a cervical tumor: <1 mm, 1–3 mm, 3–5 mm, and >5 mm.

LN involvement by cervical tumor DOI:
$\leq$1 mm: <5%
1–3 mm: 8%
3–5 mm: 27%
5 mm: 34%

(*Hacker NF et al., Cancer 1993*)

Estimate the risk of inguinal LN involvement based on the vulvar cancer FIGO stage.

LN involvement by the vulvar cancer FIGO stage:
Stage I: 17%
Stage II: 40%
Stage III: 30%–80%
Stage IV: 80%–100%

What histology constitutes the vast majority of vulvar cancers? Name 3 other histologies of tumors found on the vulva.	The most common vulvar histology is **squamous cell carcinoma** (80%–90%). Other histologies include **melanoma, basal cell, Merkel cell, sarcoma, and adenocarcinomas of the Bartholin glands.**
What % of vulvar cancers are multifocal?	**~5%** of vulvar cancers are multifocal.

▶ WORKUP/STAGING

What is the Bx approach for small (<1 cm) vulvar lesions?	For small (<1 cm) vulvar lesions, **excisional Bx with a 1-cm margin, including the skin, dermis, and connective tissue.**
What is the Bx approach for large (>1 cm) vulvar lesions?	For large (>1 cm) vulvar lesions, **wedge Bx including surrounding skin.** These should be taken from the edge of the lesion to include the interface between normal skin and the tumor to determine whether there is invasion of adjacent epithelium. (*Baldwin P et al., Curr Obst Gyn 2005*)
What is the basic workup of vulvar cancer?	Vulvar cancer workup: 1. H&P 2. Labs: CBC (to check for anemia); UA (to r/o infection), HIV testing (to r/o immunodeficiency) 3. EUA if adequate assessment cannot be done due to pain while awake, routine PAP smear of cervix, and colposcopy of the vagina and rest of vulva. Other investigations such as cysto or sigmoid only if clinically indicated 4. DRE to r/o multifocal Dz; rectal exam is part of pelvic assessment 5. Imaging: CT abdomen/pelvis (if clinical inguinal adenopathy present) and CXR, but consider PET and MRI (in advanced disease only) 6. Stage-specific inguinal nodal evaluation
Which pts with vulvar cancer do not require inguinal LND?	In vulvar cancer, **all pts with clinically suspicious nodes** require bilat inguinal LND unless there are bulky unresectable nodes. For pts with no clinically suspicious nodes, the need for nodal evaluation depends primarily on DOI. **If the DOI is <1 mm, a nodal evaluation may not be needed unless there is lymphovascular invasion or a high grade.**

Which patients can have sentinel lymph node dissection (SLD) for nodal evaluation?

Patient with low-risk disease: clinically node–, unifocal T1/T2 disease (<4 cm). The **GROINSS-V** (Groningen International Study on Sentinel Nodes in Vulvar Cancer) study evaluated safety of SLD in early stage vulvar cancer. 403 patients with T1/T2 (<4 cm) SCC with DOI >1 mm and clinically node– underwent SLD. Inguinal LND was omitted in SLD patients. Of the 276 SLD negative patients, only 8 had a groin recurrence at median follow-up of 35 months. In 259 patients with unifocal disease and – SLD, 6 groin recurrences were noted. Significantly lower short-term and long-term morbidity was found in the SLD only group. (*Van der Zee et al., JCO 2008*)

The Gynecologic Oncology Group's **GOG 173** study assessed sensitivity of SLD. 452 women with SCC limited to vulvar 2–6 cm and DOI ≥1 mm underwent lymph node mapping, SLD, and LND. Only 11 patients with a +LN on dissection were negative on SLD. Sensitivity of SLD was 91.7%. In tumors <4 cm, the false– rate was 2%. (*Levenback CF et al., JCO 2012*)

In which pts with vulvar cancer is a unilat (instead of bilat) LND sufficient for workup?

Pts with a well-lateralized primary may undergo a unilat LND only.

Is the staging system for vulvar cancer surgical or clinical?

FIGO **surgical** staging is used for vulvar cancer.

Do imaging results affect the FIGO stage in vulvar cancer?

No. Imaging results are not included in FIGO staging.

Summarize the FIGO (2008) staging for vulvar cancer.

Stage IA: lesion ≤2 cm, confined to vulva or perineum with stromal invasion <1 mm, no nodal mets

Stage IB: lesion >2 cm or with stromal invasion >1 mm, confined to vulva or perineum, no nodal mets

Stage II: lesion of any size with extension to adjacent structures (lower 3rd of urethra, lower 3rd of vagina or anus), no nodal mets

Stage III: lesion of any size with or without extension to adjacent structures (lower 3rd of urethra, lower 3rd of vagina or anus) and positive inguinofemoral LN

Stage IIIA: 1 LN ≥5 mm or 1–2 LNs <5 mm

Stage IIIB: ≥2 LN ≥5 mm or ≥3 LNs each <5 mm

Stage IIIC: node(s) with extracapsular spread

Stage IVA1: lesion invades upper urethra and/or vaginal mucosa, bladder mucosa, rectal mucosa, or fixed to pelvic bone
Stage IVA2: fixed or ulcerated inguinofemoral LN
Stage IVB: DMs, including pelvic LNs

► TREATMENT/PROGNOSIS

What is the Tx for vulvar CIS or VIN?

Pts with vulvar CIS or VIN can be treated with **superficial local excision.** If the labia minora or clitoris is involved, consider laser ablation.

How should the primary of a pt with FIGO stage I or II vulvar cancer be treated?

In a pt with stage I or II vulvar cancer, the primary can be resected via a **WLE,** which includes resection of the tumor + a gross 1.0-cm margin of normal tissue around it.

In a pt with a stage I or II vulvar cancer, does radical vulvectomy improve the LR rate over WLE?

No. In a pt with stage I or II vulvar cancer, radical vulvectomy and WLE have similar recurrence rates (~7%). (*Hacker NF et al., Cancer 1993*)

What is the next step if margins are positive following surgical resection of vulvar cancer?

Re-excise if possible; otherwise, give adj RT. Retrospective data suggests that adj RT improves LC and possibly survival. (*Faul CM et al., IJROBP 1997*)

How are the inguinal nodes treated in vulvar cancer stage IA? Stage IB? Stage II?

Stage IA: lymph node evaluation is not necessary (consider for high-grade lesions).
Stage IB: if the lesion is well lateralized, consider unilat dissection. If there is a midline lesion, then bilat groin nodal dissection is required. SLD for patients with tumor size <4 cm. GROINSS-V II is evaluating the role for adjuvant RT in patients with SLD+ groin.
Stage II: Bilat LND is recommended.

In which vulvar cancer pts is adj RT to the bilat groin and pelvis indicated? What RCT explored this question?

Adj RT to the bilat groin and pelvis is commonly recommended **in pts with ≥2 micromets in inguinal nodes, a single node >5 mm, or a single node with ECE.** In GOG 37, 114 pts s/p radical vulvectomy + bilat inguinal LND were randomized to RT to the pelvis and bilat groin vs. pelvic node dissection if node+. The dose was 45–50 Gy. The 2-yr groin recurrence rate decreased with RT (5% vs. 24%), and there was an OS advantage for RT (68% vs. 54%). All the benefits of RT were for >1 +node. The survival benefit appeared to be due to improved control in the groin. In pts with only 1 +node on the dissection, surgery and RT outcomes were similar. (*Homesley HD et al., Obstet Gynecol 1986*)

In pts with N0 vulvar cancer, does groin RT eliminate the need for inguinal LND? What RCT explored this question?

The need for inguinal node dissection in N0 vulvar cancer prior to groin RT is **controversial.** In **GOG 88,** 58 pts with cN0 vulvar cancer s/p radical vulvectomy were randomized to bilat inguinal femoral and pelvic LND (+nodes rcvd RT) vs. bilat groin-only EBRT (50 Gy). LR, PFS, and OS favored the LND arm. (*Stehman FB et al., Cancer 1992*)

What are the major criticisms of GOG 88?

Major criticisms of **GOG 88:**
1. CT was not used for staging. 50 Gy may not be adequate for pts with gross nodes evident by CT.
2. CT was not required for RT planning. Pts were treated with electron fields prescribed to a depth of 3 cm, which may not adequately cover the inguinal/femoral nodal regions. Retrospective data suggest that adequate RT to groins can result in good LC (~90%). (*Katz A et al., IJROBP 2003*)

What are the relative indications for adj RT to the primary site after WLE?

The relative indications for adj RT to the primary site:
1. +Margins or close margins (<8 mm fixed specimen or <1 cm by frozen section)
2. LVSI
3. DOI >5 mm

(*Heaps JM et al., Gynecol Oncol 1990*)

The most important risk for local recurrence is +margin. Because morbidity of vulvar RT is high, it is not to be done lightly especially if local salvage possible with further excision should relapse occur.

What is the Tx approach for pts with stages III–IV vulvar cancer?

Tx options for stages III–IV vulvar cancer:
1. Surgery (if –margins can be achieved) + PORT
2. Neoadj CRT (phase II) → surgery for those initially unresectable
3. Definitive CRT

What studies support neoadj CRT in initially unresectable vulvar cancer?

GOG 101 was a phase II study of 73 pts with unresectable vulvar cancer given concurrent cisplatin/5-FU + RT. RT was bid to 47.6 Gy. 97% of pts were converted to resectable Dz. (*Moore DH et al., IJROBP 1998*)

Estimate the CR rate for unresectable vulvar cancer pts treated with definitive cisplatin/5-FU + RT.

In small prospective trials, CR rates after definitive cisplatin/5-FU + RT **vary from 47%–80%. GOG 205** is an ongoing trial examining outcomes of T3 or T4 unresectable tumors that rcvd cisplatin and RT → surgery to gross residual Dz.

Estimate the 5-yr OS by FIGO stage.

5-yr estimated OS by FIGO stage:
Stage I: 90%
Stage II: 81%
Stage III: 68%
Stage IV: 20%

(*Gonzalez-Bosquet J et al., Gyn Oncol 2005*)

What are the commonly used adj and definitive RT doses for vulvar cancer?	Commonly used adj and definitive RT doses in vulvar cancer:

1. –Margin, +LVSI: **45–50.4 Gy**
2. Early ECE, close, or focally positive margins: **59.4 Gy**
3. +Margin, gross residual, extensive ECE, +LN: **63–66 Gy**
4. Unresectable Dz: **66–70 Gy** with concurrent weekly cisplatin or cisplatin/5-FU

 ## TOXICITY

What are the acute RT toxicities of the vulva, pelvis, and inguinal nodes?	Acute RT toxicities of the vulva, pelvis, and inguinal nodes include **severe RT dermatitis of the vulva and groins (which results in need for treatment interruption in the majority), n/v, diarrhea, urethritis, cystitis, and decreased blood counts.**
What are the late RT toxicities associated with the vulva and inguinal nodes?	Late RT toxicities of the vulva, pelvis, and inguinal nodes include **vaginal atrophy, itching and discharge, SBO, and femoral neck fracture.**
Estimate the risk of femoral neck fracture after 50 Gy.	50 Gy to the femoral neck is associated with an **11% risk of fracture at 5 yrs.** (*Grisby JS et al., Med Dos 2004*)

69 Vaginal Cancer
Updated by Surbhi Grover

BACKGROUND

Vaginal cancer typically presents in what age group?	70% of primary vaginal malignancies are detected in women **≥60 yo.**
What 3 lifestyle risk factors are associated with increased incidence of vaginal cancer?	Increased risk of vaginal cancer is associated with the # **of lifetime sexual partners, early onset of intercourse, and current smoking.**

What % of cancers involving the vagina are not primary vaginal cancers?	~75% of malignancies involving the vagina originate at other sites.
What is the most common histology for vaginal cancer? What are 5 other rare vaginal cancer histologies?	**Squamous cell carcinoma** is the most common primary vaginal histology. **Melanoma, sarcoma, lymphoma, adenocarcinoma, and clear cell adenocarcinoma** are much more rare.
Increased risk for clear cell adenocarcinoma is linked with what exposure?	In utero exposure to the synthetic estrogen **diethylstilbestrol (DES)** is linked with an increased risk for clear cell adenocarcinoma.
What type of vaginal sarcoma is most common in adults? In children?	<u>Adults</u>: leiomyosarcoma <u>Children (≤6 yo)</u>: embryonal rhabdomyosarcoma (i.e., sarcoma botryoides)
If an elderly woman has had a hysterectomy due to early-stage cervical cancer, is it reasonable to continue PAP smear screening of the vaginal vault?	**Yes.** Though the value of continued screening is not proven, PAP smears of the vaginal vault in elderly women who have had hysterectomy for invasive/preinvasive cervical cancer seems reasonable given the increased risk for vaginal cancer.
What is the nodal drainage of the upper two-thirds of the vagina? Of the lower one-third of the vagina?	The upper two-thirds of the vagina drains to the obturator, internal, external, and common iliac nodes. The lower one-third of the vagina may drain to the inguinofemoral nodes.
What are 4 common presenting Sx of vaginal cancer? What 2 additional Sx may suggest locally advanced Dz?	Vaginal cancer may present with **bleeding, discharge, pruritus, and dyspareunia. Pain or change in bowel/bladder habits may suggest locally advanced Dz.**
Where in the vagina is vaginal cancer most often located?	Vaginal cancer is most often found in the **post wall, sup one-third** of the vagina (the speculum must be rotated to ensure exam of this region).

▶ WORKUP/STAGING

What staging exams/studies contribute to the FIGO stage?	Exams/studies that contribute to the FIGO stage include clinical exam of the pelvis and vagina (possibly under anesthesia), cystoscopy, and proctosigmoidoscopy in women with locally advanced Dz, CXR, LFTs, and alk phos.
What imaging studies do not contribute to the FIGO stage?	Advanced imaging such as **CT, MRI, and PET** do not contribute to the FIGO stage (but still should be used to assess the Dz extent and plan therapy).

What is the FIGO (2008) staging for vaginal cancer?

Stage 0: CIS
Stage I: tumor limited to vaginal wall
Stage II: tumor invades paravaginal tissue but not pelvic sidewall
Stage III: tumor extends to pelvic sidewall
Stage IVA: tumor invades mucosa of bladder/ rectum (bullous edema alone is not sufficient) and/or directly extends outside pelvis
Stage IVB: DMs

A vaginal cancer is never considered a vaginal primary if it involves either of what 2 structures?

Cancer involving the **vulva or cervix** is never considered to be a vaginal primary (even if the bulk of Dz lies in the vagina).

When working up a presumed vaginal cancer primary, what other 3 sites should be evaluated for cosynchronous in situ or invasive Dz?

When working up a presumed vaginal cancer primary, always evaluate for cosynchronous **cervical, vulvar, and/or anal Dz.**

▶ **TREATMENT/PROGNOSIS**

What are 3 appropriate Tx for vaginal intraepithelial neoplasia (VAIN)?

Surgical excision, laser vaporization, and topical 5-FU are all appropriate Tx for VAIN.

VAIN is multifocal in what % of pts?

Up to 60% of pts with VAIN have multifocal Dz. Close follow-up is essential.

In general, what is the preferred definitive Tx modality for vaginal cancer?

Although surgery may be appropriate for early, stage I lesions, **definitive RT** is generally the preferred Tx modality (as morbidity is less compared with radical surgery).

What are the estimates of 5-yr pelvic Dz control and DSS for stages I, II, and III–IVA vaginal cancer managed with definitive RT?

For vaginal cancer managed with definitive RT, 5-yr pelvic Dz control is 86%, 84%, and 71% for FIGO stages I, II, and III–IVA, respectively. 5-yr DSS is 85%, 78%, and 58%, respectively. (*Frank SJ et al., IJROBP 2005*)

Is concurrent CRT) a reasonable consideration in advanced-stage vaginal cancer?

Yes. Extrapolating from the cervical, vulvar, and anal cancer literature, concurrent CRT (typically, cisplatin based) is reasonable to consider for advanced-stage vaginal cancer (i.e., stages III–IVA).

Is vaginal cylinder brachytherapy alone (without EBRT) appropriate in any vaginal cancer pts?

Possibly. Although whole pelvis EBRT combined with brachytherapy is generally preferred, vaginal cylinder brachytherapy alone may be acceptable for pts with VAIN or very early stage I vaginal cancer <5-mm thick.

What brachytherapy technique is commonly required for stages II–III vaginal cancer (in addition to EBRT Tx)?

Interstitial brachytherapy needle implants are commonly required to achieve adequate brachytherapy dose coverage for stages II–III vaginal cancers (the depth-dose characteristics of intracavitary applicators are not favorable enough to treat deep lesions).

Describe the regions that are targeted in whole pelvis RT for vaginal cancer

A whole pelvis field for vaginal cancer typically targets the common, internal, and external iliac nodes, obturator nodes, and the entire vagina (or 3 cm below the Dz extent). If the lower 3rd of the vagina is involved, then the inguinal nodes may be targeted as well (as per vulvar or anal cancer).

What are the appropriate EB and cumulative (EB + brachytherapy) RT doses for vaginal cancer?

Whole pelvis (+/– inguinal nodes) EB doses are typically **45–50 Gy** → brachytherapy boost to a total dose of **70–80 Gy.**

Among pts who fail following definitive RT, what% have LR as a component of their relapse?

~**75%** of pts with relapse following definitive RT for vaginal cancer will experience LF. (*Frank SJ et al., IJROBP 2005*)

▶ **TOXICITY**

What are the 5- and 10-yr grades 3–4 toxicity rates following definitive RT for vaginal cancer?

Grades 3–4 toxicity rates are **10% and 17% at 5 and 10 yrs, respectively,** following RT for vaginal cancer. (*Frank SJ et al., IJROBP 2005*)

What are the 4 most common grades 3–4 late effects following definitive RT for vaginal cancer?

Following definitive RT for vaginal cancer, **proctitis (requiring transfusion), rectal fistula, SBO, and hemorrhagic cystitis** are the most common grades 3–4 toxicities.

What common late effect may limit sexual function as well as follow-up for vaginal cancer?

Vaginal stenosis is very common following RT for vaginal cancer. All pts should use a vaginal dilator.

70 Hodgkin Lymphoma

Updated by Annemarie Fernandes

▶ **BACKGROUND**

At what age does Hodgkin disease (HD) most commonly occur?	HD has a bimodal peak with peaks at **age 15–30 yrs and age ≥55 yrs.**
What are 2 broad histologic categories of HD? Which is more common?	Broad histologic categories of HD: 1. Classic (more common: 95%) 2. Nodular lymphocyte predominant Hodgkin lymphoma (NLPHL: 5%)
What are the subtypes of classic HD, and which is most common in the U.S.?	Subtypes of classic HD: 1. Nodular sclerosing (most common in the U.S.) 2. Mixed cellularity 3. Lymphocyte depleted 4. Lymphocyte rich
What are the 2 most commonly involved LN regions at the initial Dx of HD?	Most commonly involved LN regions at initial Dx of HD: 1. Cervical chains (70% of pts) 2. Mediastinum (50% of pts) 90% of patients have contiguous nodes
Pts who present with mediastinal LAD are most likely to have which subtype of HD?	Pts who present with mediastinal LAD are most likely to have **nodular sclerosing** HD.
In classic HD, what is the most common pathologic feature and CD15, -30, -45, and –20 staining pattern?	Classic HD is characterized by Reed-Sternberg cells in an inflammatory background. In classic HD, tumors are typically **CD15+ and -30+ but CD45– and -20–.**
In NLPHL, what is the common pathologic feature and CD15, -30, -45, and –20 staining pattern?	NLPHL is characterized by lymphocyte-predominant cells, called "popcorn" cells. In NLPHL, tumors are typically **CD15– and -30– but CD45+ and -20+** (i.e., the reverse of classic HD).

Which HD subtype has the best prognosis?	**Lymphocyte-rich** HD has the best prognosis.
Which HD subtype has the worst prognosis?	**Lymphocyte-depleted** HD has the worst prognosis.
Which HD subtype is associated with older age or HIV+ pts?	**Lymphocyte-depleted** HD is associated with older age and HIV+ pts.
Pts with which subtype of HD are at greatest risk of developing a subsequent non-Hodgkin lymphoma?	Pts with **NLPHL** are at greatest risk of developing a subsequent non-Hodgkin lymphoma.
What are the "B Sx" of lymphoma?	B Sx include: 1. Fevers >38°C (100.4 °F) 2. >10% body weight loss in 6 mos 3. Drenching night sweats
How is bulky mediastinal Dz commonly defined?	Bulky mediastinal Dz is commonly defined as a **mass greater than one third of the intrathoracic diameter at T5-6 on an upright PA film.**
How is bulky Dz defined outside of the mediastinum?	Outside of the mediastinum, bulky Dz is variably defined in clinical trials, but **most often is any mass >10 cm.**

▶ WORKUP/STAGING

What kind of Bx is preferred for Dx of HD and why?	**Excisional Bx** is preferred for the Dx of lymphomas b/c **it shows LN architecture.**
What imaging studies are typically ordered as part of the workup of HD?	An **integrated PET/CT** is commonly used in the workup imaging for HD.
What lab work is required as part of the workup of HD?	The following labs have prognostic implications: ESR, CBC, albumin, and LDH. Labs necessary for Tx planning are BUN, Cr, and a pregnancy test in women of childbearing age.
What are common indications for a BM Bx in the workup of HD?	Common indications for a staging BM Bx: 1. B Sx 2. Stages III–IV 3. Bulky Dz 4. >2 sites 5. Recurrent Dz
How is HD staged?	HD is staged using the **Ann Arbor system:** **Stage I:** involvement of 1 LN region or localized involvement of a single extralymphatic organ or site (IE)

Stage II: involvement of ≥2 LN regions on same side of diaphragm or localized involvement of a single associated extralymphatic organ or site and its regional LN with or without involvement of other LN regions on same side of diaphragm (IIE)

Stage III: involvement of LN regions on both sides of diaphragm that may also be accompanied by localized involvement of an associated extralymphatic organ or site (IIIE)

Stage IV: multifocal involvement of ≥1 extralymphatic organ, with or without associated LN involvement, or isolated extralymphatic organ involvement with distant nodal involvement.

Note: Pts with B Sx are designated with a B, otherwise with an A. Pts with splenic involvement are designated with an S. Patients with bulky disease are designated with an X

Involvement of which sites is considered stage IV Dz?

Per the AJCC (7th edition, 2011), pts with involvement of the **BM, liver, pleura, and CSF** have stage IV Dz.

Name the 14 distinct LN regions as per the Rye classification.

LN regions per the Rye classification:
1. Waldeyer ring
2. Occipital, cervical, preauricular, and supraclavicular
3. Infraclavicular
4. Axillary
5. Epitrochlear
6. Mediastinum
7. Right hilum
8. Left hilum
9. Para-aortic
10. Spleen
11. Mesenteric
12. Iliac
13. Inguinofemoral
14. Popliteal

Is involvement of the Waldeyer ring, thymus, or spleen considered extranodal?

No. Per the AJCC (7th edition, 2011), the Waldeyer ring, thymus, and spleen are not classified as extranodal sites.

What does the Waldeyer ring include?

The Waldeyer ring includes:
1. Pharyngeal tonsil (adenoids)
2. Palatine tonsil
3. Lingual tonsil (base of tongue)

What are unfavorable factors for early HD?	Risk factors used to stratify early-stage HD in clinical trials vary.

Unfavorable factors for early HD:
1. Age ≥50 yrs
2. Bulky Dz (at least one-third maximum thorax diameter by the German Hodgkin Study Group [GHSG] or >10 cm by Stanford or NCCN guidelines)
3. ≥4 sites (≥3 sites by GHSG)
4. ESR >50 if no B Sx or >30 if B Sx
5. Presence of extranodal sites
6. Mixed-cellularity or lymphocyte-depleted histology

What are unfavorable factors for advanced HD used in the International Prognostic Score (IPS)?

Unfavorable factors for advanced HD used in the IPS:
WBC ≥15 × 10^9 cells/L
Albumin <4 g/dL
Lymphocytes (ANC) <600 or < 8%
Stage IV
Hgb <10.5 g/dL
Age ≥45 yrs
Male

(Mnemonic: **WALSH AM**)

What % of pts with favorable early-stage HD have occult splenic involvement?

~**30%** of pts with favorable early-stage HD have occult splenic involvement. (*Carde P et al., JCO 1993*)

How many times are HD pts staged with PET/CT?

HD pts are typically staged with PET/CT **at least twice,** once as part of the workup and then again after initial chemo to assess response.

▶ **TREATMENT/PROGNOSIS**

What are the 3 most common multiagent chemo regimens used for HD?

Most common chemo regimens used for HD:
1. **ABVD**
2. **Stanford V**
3. **Dose-escalated BEACOPP**

What agents are included in ABVD chemo for HD?

ABVD includes:
1. Adriamycin
2. Bleomycin
3. Vinblastine
4. Dacarbazine

What agents are included in the Stanford V regimen for HD?

There are 7 drugs in the Stanford V (MOPE-ABV):
1. Mechlorethamine
2. Oncovin (vincristine)
3. Prednisone
4. Etoposide
5. Adriamycin

6. Bleomycin
7. Vinblastine

The Stanford V regimen has reduced doses of mechlorethamine, Adr, and bleomycin compared with ABVD. Although ABVD is sometimes used without consolidation RT, the Stanford V regimen requires consolidation RT.

What agents are included in BEACOPP?

BEACOPP includes:
1. Bleomycin
2. Etoposide
3. Adriamycin
4. Cyclophosphamide
5. Oncovin (vincristine)
6. Procarbazine
7. Prednisone

Escalated-dose BEACOPP is typically used for advanced-stage HD with poor prognostic factors. It is more commonly used in Europe than in the U.S.

What is the common Tx strategy for stages I–II classic HD?

Chemotherapy followed by consolidation RT. Patients with favorable risk disease are generally treated with ABVD × 2 cycles followed by 20 Gy IFRT according to the HD10 study. Patients with unfavorable risk disease are generally treated with ABVD × 4 cycles followed by 30 Gy involved-field radiation therapy (IFRT) according to the HD11 study. Areas of residual disease are boosted to 30–36 Gy.

What are common Tx strategies for stages III–IV classic HD?

Common Tx strategies for stages III–IV classic HD:
1. ABVD × 6–8 cycles +/– IFRT to initial bulky Dz and/or residual PET+ sites at restaging
2. Stanford V + IFRT to initial bulky Dz and residual PET+ sites
3. Escalated-dose BEACOPP + IFRT to initial bulky Dz and residual PET+ sites

What is the Tx paradigm for stages I–II NLPHL?

Stages I–II NLPHL Tx paradigm: Tx is similar to Tx for a low-grade non-Hodgkin lymphoma. Stages I–II NLPHL can be treated with **RT alone (regional-involved node radiotherapy is not appropriate if treated with RT alone)** or chemo + IFRT (if B Sx are present).

What is the Tx paradigm for stages III–IV NLPHL?

Stages III–IV NLPHL Tx paradigm: **observation, palliation (with chemo or RT), or definitive Tx with chemo +/– RT.** If CD 20+, R-CHOP can be used as the chemotherapy regimen.

What are the commonly used RT doses in HD after initial chemo?

Sites without bulky Dz are typically treated to 30 Gy after chemo. Sites of initial bulky Dz are typically treated to 36 Gy after chemo.

Describe the evidence that suggests improved outcomes with CRT compared with RT alone in early-stage favorable HD.

In the 1990s, CRT vs. RT alone was evaluated in at least 4 major randomized trials:

1. **EORTC H7 F** (*Noordijk EM et al., JCO 2006*)
2. **EORTC H8 F** (*Ferme C et al., NEJM 2007*)
3. **German HD7** (*Engert A et al., JCO 2007*)
4. **SWOG S9133** (*Press OW et al., JCO 2001*)

Although the chemo and RT techniques varied in these studies, long-term relapse rates consistently favored the CRT arms. In **EORTC H8 F**, 10-yr OS was significantly improved with CRT (97% vs. 92%), but long-term OS was not significantly different in the other studies.

Summarize the evidence for and against the elimination of consolidative RT in pts who achieve a CR after chemo in HD.

The outcomes after chemo alone in early and advanced HD have been evaluated in at least 4 major RCTs:

1. **EORTC GELA H9 F** randomized favorable stages I–II HD pts with a CR after epirubicin/bleomycin/vinblastine/prednisone (EBVP) × 6 cycles to 36 Gy IFRT vs. 20 Gy IFRT vs. no RT. 4-yr EFS was similar between the 36 Gy and 20 Gy arms (87% vs. 84%, respectively) but was significantly lower in the no-IFRT arm (70%). (*Noordijk EM et al., ASCO 2005 abstract*)
2. **EORTC H10** compared ABVD alone in pts who have a PET CR after 2 cycles vs. ABVD + INRT. Risk of early relapse in nonirradiated patients with stages I–II HD was significantly higher than in standard combined modality treated patients, even in this selected group of patients with an early negative PET. (*Raemakers JM, JCO, 2014*)
3. ***Laskar S et al.*** randomized a diverse cohort of pts in India (stages I–IV, +/– bulky Dz and/or B Sx, adults and children, all of whom had a CR after ABVD × 6 cycles) to IFRT or observation. A majority of pts had mixed cellularity histology (most common in India). IFRT improved 8-yr EFS (88% vs. 76%) and 8-yr OS (100% vs. 89%), especially in pts <15 yo, with B Sx, bulky Dz, and advanced stages. (*JCO 2004*)
4. **NCI-Canada/ECOG** randomized stages I–II nonbulky pts to ABVD × 4–6 cycles (4 if CR after 2nd cycle) vs. **Sub-total nodal irradiation (STNI) to 35 Gy** (+ ABVD × 2 cycles if unfavorable risk). STNI decreased 12-yr OS (87% vs. 94%) due to toxicity, but improved rates of freedom from disease progression (92% vs. 87%). (*Meyer RM et al., NEJM 2012*)

Summarize the evidence to support the use of IFRT instead of more extensive RT in HD pts receiving CRT.

At least 4 RCTs have compared IFRT to more extensive RT in HD pts receiving CRT:
1. **Groupe Pierre-et-Marie-Curie (GPMC)** (*Zittoun R et al., JCO 1985*)
2. **German HD8** (*Klimm B et al., Ann Oncol 2007*)
3. **Milan study** (*Bonadonna G et al., JCO 2004*)
4. **EORTC H8-U** (*Ferme C et al., NEJM 2007*)

The 5–12-yr OS outcomes were similar in all of these studies, suggesting that more extensive RT than IFRT is not necessary.

Summarize the evidence to support the use of IFRT at 20 Gy after induction chemo in favorable stages I–II HD pts.

The use of <30 Gy in favorable stages I–II HD pts after initial chemo has been studied in at least 2 RCTs:
1. **HD10** from the German Hodgkin Study Group randomized pts to 2 vs. 4 cycles of chemo followed by 20 Gy vs. 30 Gy IFRT (2×2 factorial design). 5-yr PFS, freedom from Tx failure, and OS were similar between the chemo comparison and the RT dose comparison. (*Engert A et al., NEJM 2010*)
2. **EORTC GELA H9 F** (see above)

Summarize the evidence to support consolidative RT after partial response or bulky disease in advanced stage disease.

1. *Aleman et al.* randomized those with stages III–IV HD who achieved a CR after 4 or 6 cycles of MOPP-ABV to IFRT or observation. Patients with PR after 6 cycles received IFRT to 30 Gy with a 4–10 Gy boost. Rates of EFS and OS in patient with PR + IFRT were similar to those of patients in CR. In patients with CR, there was no difference in 8-yr EFS (observation, 77% vs. IFRT, 73%) or 8-yr OS (observation, 85% vs. IFRT, 78%). (*IJROBP 2007*)
2. *HD12* randomized patients to 2 BEACOPP regimens and patients with initial bulky disease or partial response to chemotherapy to consolidative RT to 30 Gy vs. no consolidative RT. RT improved FFTF in patients with residual disease after chemotherapy but not in patients with initially bulky disease with a complete response. (*Borchmann P, JCO 2011*)

What are the historic fields used to treat HD?

The **mantle field** is a classic comprehensive field including major nodal regions above the diaphragm. **Total lymphoid irradiation (TLI)** treats a mantle field and "inverted Y" to include the para-aortic lymph nodes, pelvic lymph nodes, and spleen. **Subtotal lymphoid irradiation (STLI)** excludes the pelvic lymph nodes.

What is the difference between IFRT vs. regional-field radiation therapy (RFRT) vs. involved nodal radiation therapy (INRT) vs. involved site radiation therapy (ISRT)?

IFRT covers the involved lymphoid region (defined by Rye classification and delineated by *Yahalom et al.* [*Ann Oncol 2002*]). RFRT covers the involved regions + the immediately adjacent LN regions. INRT and ISRT cover only the prechemo tumor volume and are currently under investigation. INRT relies on ideal prechemotherapy imaging with PET/CT in the treatment planning position, while ISRT is used when ideal prechemotherapy imaging is not available. For this reason, the CTV cannot be reduced to the same extent as with INRT; therefore, clinical judgment is used along with imaging to create a larger CTV in order to accommodate these uncertainties. (*Specht L et al., IJROBP, 2013*)

Describe the IFRT borders for the cervical/supraclavicular region

Upper: 1–2 cm above mastoid
Lower: 2 cm below clavicle
Lateral: Include medial two-thirds of clavicle
Medial: Ipsilateral transverse process (if (+) supraclavicular fossa (SCV), extend to contralateral transverse process and block larynx)

Describe the IFRT borders for the mediastinal region

Upper: C5-C6
Lower: 5 cm below carina or 2 cm below prechemo border
Lateral: postchemo volume with 1.5-cm margin. Hilum to be included with 1 cm margin (1.5-cm margin if involved)

Describe the IFRT borders for the axillary region.

Upper: C5-C6
Lower: tip of scapula or 2 cm below the lowest axillary node
Medial: Ipsilateral cervical transverse process
Lateral: Flash axilla

Describe the IFRT borders for the abdominal region

Upper: Top of T11 and at least 2 cm above prechemo volume
Lower: Bottom of L4 and at least 2 cm below prechemo volume
Lateral: transverse process or at least 2 cm from postchemo volume

Describe the IFRT borders for the pelvic region

Upper: Middle of sacroiliac joint
Lower: 5 cm below the lesser trochanter
Lateral: Greater trochanter and 2 cm lateral to prechemo volume
Medial: Obturator foramen and at least 2 cm medial to prechemo volume

Describe INRT.

INRT relies on ideal prechemotherapy imaging. The prechemotherapy PET/CT is fused with the postchemotherapy radiation planning CT. The prechemotherapy GTV (based on prechemotherapy CT and PET imaging) is drawn. The CTV is then created by modifying the prechemotherapy GTV based on the postchemotherapy CT scan to respect normal structures that were never involved by lymphoma. For details regarding INRT as well as ISRT, see *Specht L et al.* (*IJROBP 2013*)

▶ **TOXICITY**

In pts treated for HD, what is the RR for a 2ⁿᵈ solid malignancy after 30 yrs?

In pts who survive >5 yrs, the **overall RR is 2–3** for a solid malignancy after 30 yrs compared to the general population. (*Hodgson DC et al., JCO 2007*)

Which type of secondary cancer occurs sooner after HD Tx: leukemias or solid malignancies?

Leukemias tend to occur <5 yrs after Tx, whereas solid malignancies typically occur >7 yrs after Tx.

71 Non-Hodgkin Lymphoma
Updated by Annemarie Fernandes

▶ **BACKGROUND**

What is the pathologic definition of non-Hodgkin lymphoma (NHL)?

NHL is a **monoclonal expansion of malignant B or T cells that lacks the pathologic characteristics of Hodgkin disease** (HD) (no Reed-Sternberg cells) and is typically characterized by nodal/focal involvement vs. the more disseminated presentation of leukemias.

How does the clinical presentation of NHL differ from that of HD?

NHL typically involves more nodes at presentation, is more likely to be extranodal, is more likely to spread in a noncontiguous fashion, and has a prognosis that is more strongly affected by histologic subtype than HD.

What are the most common presenting signs or Sx of NHL?

Painless adenopathy (axillary, inguinal, femoral) is the most common presenting sign of NHL. ~30% of pts have B Sx. Waxing and waning adenopathy suggests an indolent form of NHL. Tumor bulk may cause intestinal obstruction, urinary tract obstruction, or nerve compression.

What are the B Sx?

The B Sx include fever >38°C (100.4 °F), >10% body weight loss in 6 mos, or drenching night sweats.

What is the NCI working formulation for NHL?

The NCI's working formulation groups NHL by clinical aggressiveness or grade with subgroups based on cell type or presentation.

> Low-grade NHL: follicular (grades 1–2), chronic lymphocytic leukemia (CLL), MALT, mycosis fungoides
>
> Intermediate-grade NHL: follicular (grade 3), mantle cell, diffuse large B-cell lymphoma (DLBCL), T/natural killer (NK) cell, peripheral T cell, anaplastic large cell
>
> High-grade NHL: Burkitt, lymphoblastic

What is the WHO classification of NHL?

The WHO classification divides NHL into B- and T-cell/NK cell neoplasms. The **indolent, aggressive, and highly aggressive** subgroups roughly correlate to the aforementioned working formulation groups.

Is there a relationship between clinical aggressiveness and curability of NHL?

Advanced-stage indolent NHL is rarely curable. Intermediate-grade NHL may be curable even in advanced stages.

Without Tx, what is the life expectancy for pts with NHL of varying aggressiveness?

Pts with indolent NHL have survival measured in yrs. Pts with aggressive NHL have survival measured in mos, and those pts with highly aggressive Dz have an expected survival of wks.

What % of NHL is indolent, and what are the most prevalent subtypes?

~**35%** of NHL is indolent by the WHO classification. 95% of indolent NHL are **follicular lymphoma** (FL) (grades 1–2; 65%), **small lymphocytic lymphoma** (SLL) (18%), and **marginal zone B-cell lymphoma or MALT lymphoma** (12%).

What are the common cytogenetic abnormalities associated with indolent NHL?

t(14;18) is seen in 90% of FLs. This results in overexpression of antiapoptotic Bcl-2. **Chromosome 13 deletion, t(14;19),** and **trisomy 12** are associated with SLL and CLL. **Trisomy 3** (60%) and **t(11:18)** (25%–40%) are associated with MALT lymphoma. **c-myc overexpression t(8:14)** is associated with Burkitt lymphoma.

How is FL graded?

FL demonstrates a mix of centrocytes (small, cleaved cells) and centroblasts (large, noncleaved cells). **Grade correlates to the density of centroblasts** (e.g., 0–5 centroblasts/high-power field (hpf), grade 1; >15 centroblasts/hpf, grade 3a).

What is SLL?	SLL is the same Dz entity as CLL but with a **predominant manifestation in the spleen, liver, or nodes** as opposed to peripheral blood or BM.
What is Richter syndrome? What is its rate of occurrence?	Richter syndrome is the **transformation of SLL or CLL into DLBCL.** It occurs in **~5% of cases.**
How is bulky mediastinal Dz commonly defined?	Bulky mediastinal Dz is commonly defined as a **mass greater than one-third of the intrathoracic diameter at T5-6 on upright PA film.**
How is bulky Dz defined outside of the mediastinum?	Outside of the mediastinum, bulky Dz is variably defined in clinical trials, but most often is **any mass >10 cm.**

▶ WORKUP/STAGING

What are the pertinent focused aspects of the physical exam in a person with suspected NHL?	The physical exam should include complete nodal assessment including epitrochlear and popliteal groups. Cervical adenopathy palpable above the hyoid bone should prompt an ENT exam. (The Waldeyer ring is more frequently involved in NHL than in HD.) Exam of extranodal at-risk sites including the liver, spleen, testicles, bones, abdomen, and flanks is appropriate.
What lab studies should be performed?	Laboratory studies should include CBC with differential, CMP, LDH, β_2-microglobulin, serum protein electrophoresis, HIV, hepatitis B virus (essential as it may reactivate with rituximab Tx), and hepatitis C virus. BM Bx should be performed for all lymphomas. LP should be performed for CNS Sx, testicular or paranasal sinus involvement, or immunodeficiency.
What imaging studies should be performed?	The imaging workup should include CT C/A/P. PET is appropriate in most cases. MRI brain should be performed for CNS Sx, testicular or paranasal sinus involvement, or immunodeficiency.
How is NHL staged?	NHL is staged similar to HD using the **Ann Arbor (AA) system:** **Stage 1:** involvement of 1 LN region or localized involvement of 1 extralymphatic organ or site (IE) **Stage 2:** involvement of ≥2 LN regions on the same side of diaphragm or localized involvement of 1 associated extralymphatic organ or site and its regional LN, with or without involvement of other LN regions on same side of diaphragm (IIE)

Stage 3: involvement of LN regions on both sides of diaphragm, which may also be accompanied by localized involvement of an associated extralymphatic organ or site (IIIE)

Stage 4: multifocal involvement of ≥1 extralymphatic organ, with or without associated LN involvement, or isolated extralymphatic organ involvement with distant nodal involvement

Note: Pts with B Sx are designated with a B, otherwise with an A. Pts with splenic involvement are designated with an S. Patients with bulky disease are designated with an X.

What is a major limitation to the AA staging of NHL (as opposed to HD)?

NHL **typically spreads in a less contiguous fashion** compared to HD and thus stage I NHL is very rare (10%).

How is NHL practically staged?

NHL is practically divided into **limited stage and advanced stage.** Limited stage consists of AA stages I–II pts with ≤3 adjacent LN regions, no B Sx, and no bulky (≥10 cm) lesions. Advanced stage includes all other pts. For FL, practical division is between AA stages I–II, nonbulky, nonabdominal Dz, and all others.

▶ TREATMENT/PROGNOSIS

What are prognostic factors for NHL?

Although grade remains the most important factor, several attempts have been made to combine multiple prognostic factors into a single numerical prognostic index to determine prognosis within a grade stratification of NHL. The most well known is the **International Prognostic Index (IPI)** based on aggressive NHL. Derivatives of the IPI include **age adjusted, stage adjusted,** and **the follicular lymphoma International Prognostic Index (FLIPI).**

What factors are included in the IPI?

IPI factors: **A**ge >60 yrs, ECOG **P**erformance status ≥2, **L**DH > normal, >1 **E**xtranodal group, AA **S**tages III–IV (Mnemonic: **APLES**)

Estimate the 5-yr OS based on the number of IPI factors.

Number of IPI factors as associated with 5-yr OS:
    <u>Low</u>: 0–1 factors → 73%
    <u>Low-intermediate</u>: 2 factors → 51%
    <u>High-intermediate</u>: 3 factors → 43%
    <u>High</u>: 4–5 factors → 26%

What were the Dz characteristics and the Tx strategies employed for the British Columbia pts whose outcome data were used to generate the IPI formulation?

The data used to generate the IPI come from 308 pts with stage I–IIA nonbulky DLBCL treated at the British Columbia Cancer Agency from 1980–1998. All pts rcvd 3 cycles of doxorubicin-containing chemo and involved-field radiation therapy (IFRT) (30 Gy for small-volume Dz, 35 Gy for larger-volume Dz). (*Shenkier TN et al., JCO 2002*)

What is the revised IPI (R-IPI) for intermediate-risk NHL incorporating the use of rituximab (Rituxan)?

The R-IPI incorporates the same 5 factors as the standard IPI but with substantial changes in the prognosis of these pts:

Estimate the 5-yr OS based on the number of R-IPI factors.

Number of **R-IPI factors** as associated with 5-yr OS:
0 factors: 94%
1–2 factors: 79%
3–5 factors: 55%

(*Sehn LH et al., Blood 2007*)

What factors are included in the FLIPI?

FLIPI factors: **H**gb <12 g/dL, **A**ge >60 yrs, **S**tages III–IV, ≥**5** extranodal **S**ites, **L**DH > normal (Mnemonic: FLIPI is a **HASSL**). *Note:* These are FLIPI-specific nodal sites, not AA nodal groups.

Estimate the 5-yr OS based on the number of FLIPI factors.

Number of **FLIPI factors** as associated with 5-yr OS:
0–1 factors: 90%
2 factors: 80%
3–5 factors: 55%

(*Solal-Celigny P et al., Blood 2004*)

What was demonstrated by the Stanford retrospective series supporting RT alone in the management of stages I–II, low-grade FL?

The Stanford series of 177 pts treated from 1961–1994 (*MacManus MP et al., JCO 1996*) demonstrated an MS of 13.8 yrs, 5-, 10-, and 15-yr RFS of 55%, 44%, and 40%, respectively, and 5-, 10-, and 15-yr OS of 82%, 64%, and 44%, respectively. RT included IFRT, EFRT, and total lymphoid irradiation. Doses ranged from 35–50 Gy. Age <60 yrs was associated with better OS and freedom from recurrence (FFR). Only 5 of 47 pts who had FFR at 10 yrs relapsed subsequently. RT to both sides of the diaphragm was associated with better 10-yr FFR (67% vs. 36%).

What was demonstrated in the retrospective Stanford series of stages I–IIA, low-grade FL not treated immediately?

In this series of highly selected patients, 43 pts (11 pts stage I) with a median age of 58 yrs rcvd no initial Tx for various reasons. At a median follow-up of 86 mos, 63% had not been treated. Estimated OS at 5, 10, and 20 yrs were 97%, 85%, and 22%, respectively. (*Advani R et al., JCO 2004*)

Has adj chemo demonstrated a benefit in randomized trials of early-stage, low-grade FL?

No. 5 randomized trials have failed to demonstrate significant benefit from RT → adj chemo (cyclophosphamide/vincristine/prednisone [CVP], chlorambucil, or cyclophosphamide HCl/doxorubicin/Oncovin/prednisone [CHOP]) in early-stage FL:

1. *Nissen NI et al., Cancer 1983*
2. *Monfardini S et al., IJROBP 1980*
3. *Carde P et al., Radiother Oncol 1984*
4. *Yahalom J et al., Cancer 1993*
5. *Kelsey SM et al., Med Oncol 1994*

What is the clinical evidence for combined modality Tx in the management of early-stage, low-grade FL?

A prospective series from MDACC followed 102 pts (83% FL) with low-grade NHL treated with 10 cycles of chemo and IFRT to 30–40 Gy after 3 cycles. 10-yr FFP and OS for pts with FL were 72% and 80%, respectively. (*Seymour JF et al., JCO 2003*) Other retrospective series have also demonstrated good outcomes.

What is the evidence for reduced doses of RT to control FL?

A U.K. phase III trial randomized patients with indolent lymphomas (both follicular and marginal zone) to 40–45 Gy in 20–23 fx vs. 24 Gy in 12 fx. With a median follow-up of 5.6 yrs, there was no difference in in-field failure, OS, or PFS. (*Lowry et al., R&O, 2011*)

The Follicular Radiotherapy Trial (FoRT) phase III trial presented at ASTRO 2012 (*Hoskin PJ et al., Lancet Oncol, 2014*) randomized patients (follicular or marginal zone) to either 24 Gy or 4 Gy and found better CR with 24 Gy (68 % vs. 49%) and better local PFS, which was the primary endpoint. HR for time to local progression of 3.42 (95% CI 2.10–5.57, $p <0.0001$).

What remains the Tx standard for localized, low-grade FL?

Locoregional RT to 24–30 Gy remains standard. However, observation and combined modality Tx are considered viable options depending on the pt and Dz characteristics.

What are the basic Tx principles for stages III–IV, low-grade FL?

No Tx is considered curative. Several randomized trials have indicated that therapy can be deferred without reducing survival. Tx is reserved for the following:

1. Symptomatic Dz
2. Threatened end organ dysfunction
3. Cytopenias
4. Bulky Dz
5. Steady Dz progression
6. Clinical trial
7. Pt preference

What is the evidence for radioimmunotherapy in advanced state FL?

SWOG S0016 randomized pts with advanced stage FL to R-CHOP × 6 vs. CHOP-RIT with Bexxar (I-131-tositumomab, a CD-20 radiotherapeutic antibody). There was no difference in 2-yr PFS (80% vs. 76%) or 2-yr OS (93% vs. 97%). (*Press OW et al., JCO 2013*)

What is the role of RT for stages III–IV, low-grade FL?

In advanced-stage indolent lymphomas, RT is reserved for **palliation of Sx.**

What is a typical RT Tx for symptomatic stages III–IV FL?

Traditionally, **>20 Gy.** A phase II study of RT for symptomatic local masses with indolent NHL demonstrated a 65% CR and 22% PR with a median duration of response of 22 mos with 2 Gy × 2. (*Johannsson J et al., IJROBP 2002*)

What is the role of RT in the Tx of SLL?

RT is used for **palliation of symptomatic lesions** in SLL. Consider 2 Gy × 2 regimens.

What is the role of RT in treating nodal marginal zone lymphomas?

RT is used for **palliation of symptomatic lesions** in advanced-stage nodal marginal zone lymphomas.

What is the most common initial multiagent chemo used in the management of intermediate- or high-grade NHL?

The most common initial multiagent chemo used in NHL is **R-CHOP,** which uses the following drugs:
1. Rituximab
2. Cyclophosphamide
3. Hydroxydaunomycin (Adriamycin)
4. Oncovin (vincristine)
5. Prednisone

What are the current indications for RT in early-stage, intermediate- or high-grade NHL?

The inclusion of RT in early-stage, intermediate- or high-grade NHL is very **institution dependent.** It may be included as consolidation after 3–4 cycles of R-CHOP in favorable Dz, in pts with a PR to chemo, or in pts with bulky Dz. The inclusion of rituximab to CHOP in advanced Dz has resulted in significant OS benefit, and the results of trials including rituximab in the management of localized Dz may obviate the inclusion of RT for most localized NHL. Alternatively, improved systemic control may further increase the importance of LC and thus RT in early-stage Dz.

What is the present Tx paradigm for advanced stage, intermediate- or high-grade NHL?

Advanced-stage, intermediate- or high-grade NHL Tx paradigm: R-CHOP × 6–8 cycles. IFRT may be considered for initially bulky sites.

Estimate the prognosis of limited-stage aggressive B-cell lymphoma treated with R-CHOP and IFRT.

Long-term outcomes with R-CHOP and IFRT are limited. **SWOG 0014 (phase II)** enrolled 60 pts with limited-stage aggressive NHL and at least 1 adverse risk factor and treated with R-CHOP × 3 + IFRT: 4-yr PFS was 88%, and OS was 92%. (*Persky DO et al., JCO 2008*)

What is the long-term DFS for pts with localized DLBCL treated with RT alone? What were the typical Tx doses used in clinical trials?

Using **45–50 Gy** to maximize LC, **only 40% of pts with localized DLBCL had long-term DFS** based on historical RT-alone data. (*Chen MG et al., Cancer 1979; Sweet DL et al., Blood 1981; Kaminski MS et al., Ann Intern Med 1986*)

What was demonstrated in the initial publication of the SWOG 8736 study comparing chemo alone to abbreviated CRT in localized intermediate-grade NHL?

In **SWOG 8736,** 401 pts with stage I or IE (including bulky Dz) and stage II or IIE (nonbulky) intermediate-grade NHL were randomized to CHOP × 8 cycles vs. CHOP × 3 + IFRT. RT doses of 40–55 Gy were employed. At 5-yr follow-up, PFS and OS favored the combined therapy group (OS: 82% vs. 72%). (*Miller TP et al., NEJM 1998*) However, 8-yr data (in abstract form) suggest no difference in OS or PFS between the 2 groups and increased late relapses in the RT arm. (*Miller TP et al., ASH 2001 abstract 3024*)

What was demonstrated in the ECOG E1484 study randomizing postchemo complete responders to observation vs. IFRT?

In **ECOG E1484,** 352 pts with intermediate-grade, bulky stages I–IE or nonbulky stages II–IIE Dz were administered CHOP × 8 cycles. Complete responders (215 pts) were randomized to IFRT vs. observation. At 6 yrs, DFS favored IFRT (73% vs. 56%), but OS was equivalent. FFS was equivalent in partial responders administered IFRT (40 Gy) and in CR pts (30 Gy). Failure at initial sites was greater in pts not given IFRT. (*Horning SJ et al., JCO 2004*)

What was demonstrated in the GELA LNH-93-1 study comparing aggressive chemo vs. standard chemo and RT in pts ≤60 yo?

In **GELA LNH-93-1,** 647 pts ≤60 yo with low-risk (IPI 0), stages I or II, intermediate-risk NHL (extranodal or bulky Dz allowed) were randomized to doxorubicin/cyclophosphamide/vindesine/bleomycin/prednisone (ACVBP) × 3, then methotrexate/etoposide/ifosfamide/cytarabine vs. CHOP × 3, then IFRT to 30–40 Gy. ACVBP without RT improved 5-yr EFS (82% vs. 74%) and OS (90% vs. 81%) regardless of the presence of bulky Dz. However, ACVBP is considered to be a toxic regimen (dose intensity 150% of CHOP; requires hospitalization to administer; associated with high rates of secondary acute myeloid leukemia and lung cancer). (*Reyes F et al., NEJM 2005*)

What was demonstrated in the GELA LNH-93-4 study evaluating pts age >60 yrs with low-risk, localized, intermediate-grade NHL?

In **GELA LNH-93-4,** 576 pts age >60 yrs with low-risk (age-adjusted IPI 0), stage I or II NHL (bulky [8%] or extranodal [56%] Dz allowed) were randomized to CHOP × 4 vs. CHOP × 4 + IFRT to 40 Gy. The 5-yr EFS (~62%) and OS (~70%) were equivalent in both Tx arms. (*Bonnet C et al., JCO 2007*)

What is the present Tx paradigm for relapsed intermediate- or high-grade NHL?

Relapsed intermediate- or high-grade NHL Tx paradigm: high-dose chemo + stem cell transplant

▶ **TOXICITY**

What are the expected RT toxicities associated with Tx of NHL?	The RT toxicities depend on the site of Tx. B/c of high rates of long-term survival in these pts, particularly important late effects are **coronary artery Dz, hypothyroidism, and 2ⁿᵈ malignancies.** The later age at presentation, when compared to HL, should be considered when considering risk of 2ⁿᵈ malignancies.

72 MALT Lymphoma (Gastric and Ocular Adnexa and Other Sites)

Updated by Annemarie Fernandes

▶ **BACKGROUND**

What does MALT stand for? Where is MALT generally located?	MALT stands for **mucosa-associated lymphoid tissue.** It is located in the **Peyer patches of the bowel and lymphoid tissues of the H&N** (nasopharynx [adenoids] or oropharynx [tonsils]).
What is the etiology of MALT lymphomas?	The etiology of MALT lymphomas is **chronic inflammation** from infection or autoimmune disorder.
What are the most common locations of MALT lymphoma in the body?	The most common locations of MALT lymphoma are the GI tract (stomach > small intestine > colon), lung, thyroid, salivary gland, tonsil, breast, and orbit.
What types of infectious or autoimmune conditions are associated with MALT lymphoma in the stomach? Ocular adnexa? Salivary gland? Skin? Thyroid?	Infections or autoimmune conditions associated with MALT: Stomach: *Helicobacter pylori* Ocular adnexa: *Chlamydia psittaci* Salivary gland: Sjögren Skin: *Borrelia burgdorferi* Thyroid: Hashimoto thyroiditis

What is the natural Hx of MALT lymphomas?

The natural Hx includes an **indolent clinical course,** as in low-grade lymphoma.

From where do MALT lymphomas typically arise in the lymphoid follicle?

MALT lymphomas typically arise from the **marginal zone** of the lymphoid follicle (and therefore are also termed as *extranodal marginal zone lymphoma*).

What are some important cytogenetic abnormalities in MALT lymphomas?

Important cytogenetic abnormalities include **t(11;18) (q21:q21) and trisomy 3.**

What is the immunophenotype of MALT lymphoma?

MALT lymphoma is a **low-grade B-cell lymphoma that is CD20+, CD35+, CD5–, and CD10–.**

▶ WORKUP/STAGING

What is the typical stage of MALT lymphomas?

Ann Arbor staging for IAE (80%) is typical for MALT lymphomas.

What is the typical presentation of a pt with gastric MALT?

The typical presentation of gastric MALT is **dyspepsia (#1), epigastric pain or discomfort, n/v, GI bleed, and B Sx (rare).**

What workup should be included in a pt with suspected MALT lymphoma of the stomach?

Suspected MALT lymphoma of the stomach workup: Complete H&P (with emphasis on B Sx and evaluation of all LNs, including the Waldeyer ring [15% association; check hepatosplenomegaly]), CBC/CMP, LDH, CXR, CT abdomen/pelvis, esophagogastroduodenoscopy (EGD) with Bx, and EUS (to assess depth of invasion [DOI]). Test for *H. pylori* infection with a rapid urease test (RUT) on the Bx specimen and test for t(11;18) with FISH or PCR. Consider BM Bx in pts with suspected systemic Dz.

What is the sensitivity and specificity of the RUT for *H. pylori*? What are other alternatives if the RUT is negative?

The sensitivity and specificity of RUT are >90%. However, if the test on the tissue sample is negative and the clinical suspicion is high, preferred noninvasive tests are (1) *H. pylori* serum serology (antibody), (2) urea breath test, or (3) stool antigen test.

How is the Ann Arbor system used for staging MALT lymphoma of the GI tract?

Ann Arbor staging for MALT lymphoma of the GI tract if no B Sx:
  Stage IAE: confined to GI tract
  Stage IIAE: GI confined + nodal involvement below diaphragm
  Stage IIIAE: GI focus + nodes above diaphragm
  Stage IVAE: GI + both sides of diaphragm + other extranodal involvement (BM, liver, etc.)

▶ **TREATMENT/PROGNOSIS**

What is the 1ˢᵗ-line therapy used for the Tx of gastric MALT lymphoma?

If there is documented *H. pylori* infection, use **antibiotics against *H. pylori*** (triple therapy of clarithromycin/Flagyl/proton-pump inhibitor [PPI] or clarithromycin/amoxicillin/PPI).
If there is lymphoma but the pt is *H. pylori*–, consider RT as a primary therapeutic approach, especially if there are chromosomal abnormalities.

How is the eradication of *H. pylori* determined?

To determine the eradication of *H. pylori,* a **urea breath test should be done 1 mo after antibiotic use.** If there is persistence of tumor and *H. pylori* infection, switch to a different antibiotic regimen.

What response rate is expected from 1ˢᵗ-line Tx of gastric MALT lymphoma?

75%–80% of pts have a CR. (*Wündisch T et al., JCO 2005*)

What is the typical response period to antibiotics in MALT lymphoma?

In MALT lymphoma, regression is slow and can take a **median of 15 mos (range: 5 mos–3 yrs).**

How should response be assessed when using antibiotics for gastric MALT lymphoma?

Response to antibiotics in MALT lymphoma is assessed by **EGD with visual inspection and Bx q3mos.** Dz should at least be stable or responding. If Dz if progressing, consider RT. If Dz is stable or regressing and the pt is asymptomatic, repeat the EGD in 3 mos. After CR is attained, monitor for relapse with EGD every 6 mos for 2 yrs and then as clinically indicated.

What are 3 tumor characteristics that portend a poor response to the use of antibiotics for the Tx of gastric MALT lymphoma?

Tumor characteristics that portend a poor response with antibiotics for MALT lymphoma include **t(11;18), trisomy 3, and DOI beyond the submucosa** (muscularis/serosa/adjacent organs). (*Sackmann M et al., Gastroenterology 1997*) There is an 86% CR with DOI < submucosa and 0% if invasion is beyond the submucosa.

What are the options for antibiotic-resistant MALT lymphomas?

Given the indolent nature of the Dz, there are many options. Involved-field radiation therapy (IFRT) should be considered upfront for early stage disease with excellent CR (98%), 5-yr DFS (77%), and 5-yr OS (98%) rates. Single-agent immunotherapy with rituximab (Rituxan) or chemo with chlorambucil can be considered after RT failure or in advanced disease.

When should RT be considered for the Tx of gastric MALT lymphoma?	RT for MALT lymphoma should be considered in the following situations: 1. *H. pylori*– with stage IAE lymphoma, with or without initial use of antibiotics, and pt has no documented response to Tx 2. t(11;18) 3. Invasion beyond submucosa (muscularis/serosa/adjacent organs) 4. Documented progression after initial use of antibiotics 5. Documented failure of 2nd course of antibiotics 6. Rapid symptomatic progression of Dz
What are some important prognostic factors for MALT lymphomas?	Important prognostic factors for MALT lymphomas: 1. Age 2. Histology 3. DOI 4. LN involvement 5. Tumor size, cytogenetics
What are the factors in the follicular lymphoma International Prognostic Index (FLIPI) used for predicting the prognosis in MALT?	FLIPI for predicting the prognosis in MALT: **H**gb <12 g/dL **A**ge >60 yrs **S**tage III–IV Dz **S**ites >3 nodal **L**DH abnl (Mnemonic: FLIPI is a **HASSL**)
Is there a benefit of adding chemo in low-risk (<1 FLIPI) MALT?	**No.** Trials have demonstrated no additional survival benefit. Thus, IFRT remains the standard 1st-line modality. Considerations are made with rituximab + IFRT or radioantibody therapy in the future.
What are some factors that would predict for poor response to RT alone?	Factors that predict for poor response to RT alone: 1. Stage II Dz 2. FLIPI >1 factor 3. B Sx 4. Tumor bulk 5. Age >60 yrs
How should pts with poor-risk MALT lymphoma be managed?	Pts with poor-risk MALT lymphoma should be managed with a combined modality, using **chemo + IFRT.**
What is the 3rd-line therapy for Tx of gastric MALT lymphoma?	The 3rd-line therapy for MALT lymphoma is **chemo (rituximab, single-agent Cytoxan) or total gastrectomy + chemo.**
What is the Tx paradigm for DLBCL of the stomach?	DLBCL of the stomach Tx paradigm: rituximab/cyclophosphamide/hydroxydaunomycin (Adriamycin)/Oncovin (vincristine)/prednisone (R-CHOP) + IFRT

What are the simulation procedures for RT planning for Tx of MALT lymphoma of the stomach?

CT patient in a fasting state, supine and with oral contrast. Use methods to determine respiratory excursion. The field should encompass the entire stomach + perigastric LNs +/– celiac nodes at T12-L1 + a 2-cm margin.

Princess Margaret has reported on AP/PA or 4-field 3D-CRT technique. (*Goda JS, Cancer 2010*) In selected patients, 4-field 3D-CRT may significantly reduce kidney dose, and IMRT may provide incremental improvements in left kidney and liver dose (MSKCC: *Della Biancia C et al., IJROBP 2005*) **Rx dose: 30 Gy** in 1.5 Gy/fx for 20 fx. Consider boosting to the area of residual Dz to 36 Gy.

What are the long-term outcomes with the use of IFRT for Tx of gastric MALT lymphoma?

92% recurrence-free rate at 10 yrs. (*Goda JS, Cancer 2010*)

What is the most common nongastric MALT?

Orbital MALT is the most common nongastric MALT and is generally found in the **elderly** with a median age of 60 yrs.

With which areas of the eye is orbital MALT usually associated?

The **conjunctiva, eyelids, lacrimal gland, and retrobulbar areas** are usually associated with orbital MALT.

What organism is often associated with orbital MALT?

C. psittaci is often associated with orbital MALT, with studies showing eradication of the organism with antibiotics (doxycycline) to result in a CR (65% lymphoma regression rate).

How should RT be performed for the Tx of orbital MALT?

The whole orbit should be treated. Orthovoltage, electrons, or 3D conformal photons have been used, but volumetric arc therapy (VMAT) may give better conformality. Proton beam therapy is being investigated.

Dose: **25–30 Gy** in 10–20 fx has been used, with >95% LC but with high incidence of late toxicity, arguing for using the lower end of range, 25 Gy. (*Goda JS, IJROBP 2011*)

What is the typical natural Hx of orbital MALT?

The typical natural Hx of orbital MALT includes a **high distant relapse rate** (PMH: 10-yr recurrence-free survival rate was only 67%: *Goda JS, Cancer 2010*), generally in the contralateral eye or other MALT sites (20%–50%) but high survival in the long term.

What is typically associated with MALT of the salivary gland?

Typical associations of MALT of the salivary gland include **Sjögren syndrome, a median age of 50 yrs, and bilateral parotids.**

What are the fields, volumes, and doses used for MALT of salivary gland?	Treat the whole parotid (superficial and deep lobe) with IMRT or 3D-CRT to 30 Gy in 20 fx. For pts with stage IIE Dz (cervical nodal involvement), encompass the ipsilateral cervical LN stations. Treat the bilateral parotid if there is bilateral involvement. A dental evaluation should be performed.
What are the long-term outcomes for MALT of the salivary gland treated with radiation?	A 10-yr recurrence-free rate of 68% has been reported with the contralateral parotid gland as the predominant site of failure. (*Goda JS, Cancer 2010*)
What is typically offered for MALT of the lung?	**Surgical resection** is typically offered for MALT of the lung; however, RT should also be considered given the high response rate. Use observation for clear margins and no mediastinal nodal involvement. If the tumor is unresectable or there are + margins, consider IFRT. RT-induced 2nd malignancies must be considered for a young person getting RT.
How is MALT of the skin managed?	MALT of the skin is managed by **surgical excision for smaller lesions. If large, use electrons with bolus.**
What is the regimen used for management of advanced low-grade lymphoma?	For advanced low-grade lymphoma, use **systemic agents;** however, no agents are curative. **Palliative RT** is very effective, especially for extensive symptomatic Dz. A high response rate (80%–90%) is seen with the use of 4 Gy (2 Gy × 2).

▶ TOXICITY

To what RT doses should the kidneys and liver be limited in MALT of the stomach?	Keep the mean dose to both kidneys to <20 Gy (or 20% of left kidney to <20 Gy). The dose to the liver should be V25 <50%.
What are some toxicities for using IFRT for Tx of MALT lymphoma of the stomach?	**Anorexia and n/v** are toxicities associated with IFRT for MALT lymphoma of the stomach and can be lessened with prophylactic daily antiemetics prior to treatment. Very rarely is ulceration or outlet obstruction seen.

73 Plasmacytoma/Multiple Myeloma

Updated by Robert Prosnitz

▶ BACKGROUND

What is the cell of origin in multiple myeloma (MM), and what does this cell usually secrete?

Mature B cells are the cell of origin in MM, and they usually secrete **immunoglobulins** that are also known as M proteins.

Approximately how many cases of MM are diagnosed annually in the U.S.?

~15,000 cases/yr of MM are diagnosed in the U.S.

What % of plasma cell tumors are MM? Solitary plasmacytoma (SP)?

MM constitutes 90% of plasma cell tumors, while **SP constitutes 10%** of plasma cell tumors.

Is there a racial or sex predilection for MM?

Yes, with regard to race. The incidence of MM is **greater in blacks** than whites (2:1). However, the incidence is **similar among men and women.**

What is the avg decade of life in which pts present with MM?

On avg, pts present with MM in the **5th–6th decades of life.**

What environmental exposure is most strongly associated with MM?

Ionizing RT is strongly linked to MM, as seen in A-bomb survivors in Hiroshima.

What are the 2 forms of SP?

The 2 forms of SP are **solitary bone plasmacytoma (SBP)** and **solitary extramedullary plasmacytoma (SEP).**

What environmental or genetic alterations are consistently associated with MM?

There are **no strong genetic or environmental patterns associated with MM.** There may be a modest but increased risk of MM with exposure to RT (latency 20+ yrs) or the chemical alachlor, a commonly used pesticide.

What % of pts with SBP will progress to MM at 10 yrs?

SBP will progress to MM in **50%–80%** of pts at 10 yrs. (*Hu K et al., Oncology 2000*)

What % of pts with SEP will progress to MM at 10 yrs?

SEP will progress to MM in **10%–40%** of pts at 10 yrs. (*Hu K et al., Oncology 2000*)

What is the most common site of SEP?

The most common site of SEP is the **H&N** region (80% of SEP); the nasal cavity and paranasal sinuses are the most common subsites for SEP.

What is the relationship between secretory patterns in SBP vs. SEP?

Most pts with SBP have a secretory tumor, whereas most pts with SEP have a nonsecretory tumor.

What is the relationship between LN involvement in SBP vs. SEP?

SBP rarely involves LNs, but SEP will have LN involvement 30%–40% of the time.

What 3 lab abnormalities may prompt a clinician to evaluate for a plasma cell neoplasm?

Laboratory abnormalities that may prompt evaluation for a plasma cell neoplasm:
1. Unexplained normochromic/normocytic anemia
2. Unexplained renal insufficiency
3. Hypercalcemia

What lab tests are used for screening of a plasma cell abnormality?

Serum protein electrophoresis (SPEP) and **urine protein electrophoresis** (UPEP) are lab tests used to screen for a plasma cell abnormality. A positive screen on these tests results when a monoclonal population (or spike) is detected.

What is the common pattern of bone Dz in MM?

Lytic bone lesions are the most common bone abnormality seen on imaging of pts with MM.

What is monoclonal gammopathy of undetermined significance (MGUS), and how often will it transform to MM?

MGUS is a **condition with clonal proliferation of an immunoglobulin in the absence of clinical, radiographic, or lab evidence of MM.** The risk of transformation from MGUS to MM is 1% per yr.

What is 1 factor that predicts the risk of transformation from MGUS to MM?

The risk of transformation from MGUS to MM is predicted by the **initial size of the M-protein peak.**

What is the most common clinical Sx seen at Dx of MM or SP?

Bone pain is the most common clinical Sx seen at Dx of MM or SP. A subset of these pts will present with a pathologic fracture.

What is POEMS syndrome?

POEMS syndrome (polyneuropathy, organomegaly, endocrinopathy, M protein, and skin changes) is a **variant of MM with solitary or limited sclerotic bone lesions** that often responds to radiotherapy with a spontaneous improvement in neuropathy.

What 3 diagnostic criteria are required for MM?

Criteria requisite for Dx of MM (all are required):
1. Clonal plasma cells of ≥10% (on either BM Bx or a Bx from other tissue)
2. Monoclonal protein in serum or urine
3. Evidence of end organ damage

(*No author, Br J Haematol 2003*)

Name 7 factors that can be used as evidence of end organ damage in MM.

Factors that can be used as evidence of end organ damage in MM:
1. Hypercalcemia
2. Renal insufficiency
3. Anemia
4. Bone lesions
5. Frequent severe infections
6. Amyloidosis
7. Hyperviscosity syndrome

(*No author, Br J Haematol 2003*)

What is the difference between symptomatic MM and asymptomatic (smoldering) MM?

Smoldering (or asymptomatic) MM requires the presence of serum monoclonal protein ≥3 g/dL and/or bone marrow plasma cells ≥10% but no evidence of end organ damage attributable to plasma cell dyscrasia. (*No author, Br J Haematol 2003*)

What 3 criteria are necessary for the Dx of MGUS?

Criteria necessary for the Dx of MGUS:
1. Serum monoclonal protein <3 g/dL
2. BM plasma cell <10%
3. No end organ damage attributable to plasma cell dyscrasia

(*No author, Br J Haematol 2003*)

What 4 criteria are necessary for the Dx of SP?

Criteria necessary for the Dx of SP:
1. Solitary bone lesion on skeletal survey
2. Histologic evidence of plasmacytoma by Bx
3. <5% plasma cells on marrow aspirate
4. No other end organ damage attributable to plasma cell dyscrasia

(*No author, Br J Haematol 2003*)

▶ WORKUP/STAGING

What is β_2-microglobulin (β_2M)?

β_2M is a component of major histocompatibility complex class 1 molecules. Increasing levels of β_2M are associated with a worse prognosis in MM.

What are the 2 most commonly used staging systems for MM?

The 2 most commonly used staging systems for MM are the **Durie-Salmon Staging and the International Staging System** (ISS).

What 2 factors are used to stage pts in the ISS system, and how are they grouped?

The 2 factors used in the ISS system are **β_2M and albumin.** They are used to stage pts as follows:
Stage I: β_2M <3.5 mg/L, albumin ≥3.5 g/dL
Stage II: β_2M <3.5 mg/L, albumin <3.5 g/dL, or β_2M ≥3.5 and <5.5
Stage III: β_2M ≥5.5

What is the MS of MM by ISS stage?

MS of MM by ISS stage:
  Stage I: 62 mos
  Stage II: 44 mos
  Stage III: 29 mos

(*Greipp PR et al., JCO 2005*)

What is the Durie-Salmon staging scheme for MM?

The Durie-Salmon staging scheme for MM:
  Stage I: all of the following are required:
    a. Hgb >10 g/dL
    b. normal calcium
    c. skeletal survey with no lytic bone lesions
    d. serum paraprotein level <5 if IgG (<3 if IgA)
    e. urinary light chain excretion <4 g/24 hrs

  Stage II: not fitting stage I or III
  Stage III: 1 or more of the following:
    a. Hgb <8.5 g/dL
    b. calcium >12
    c. skeletal survey with ≥3 lytic lesions
    d. serum paraprotein level >7 if IgG (>5 if IgA)
    e. urinary light chain excretion >12 g/24 hrs

The Durie-Salmon staging system gives a subclassification of A or B based on what factor?

The Durie-Salmon staging subclassification distinguishes pts based on **serum Cr:** A, Cr <2 mg/dL; B, Cr ≥2 mg/dL.

Besides a careful H&P, what lab and radiographic studies are necessary to evaluate a pt with newly diagnosed or suspected MM?

The lab and radiographic workup of MM includes CBC with differential, LDH, calcium, and albumin levels, β_2M, 24-hr total protein, SPEP/UPEP, skeletal survey, and unilat BM aspirate and Bx (with BM flow cytometry or immunohistochemistry). Other studies that may be helpful in select cases include MRI for suspected vertebral compression or tissue BM to Dx an SP.

What is the role of a bone scan in the workup and staging for plasma cell neoplasms?

There is **no role for routine staging** with a bone scan in pts with plasma cell neoplasms b/c the lesions are primarily lytic with little evidence of bone repair and consequent low isotope uptake.

▶ **TREATMENT/PROGNOSIS**

What is the recommended management of smoldering (asymptomatic) MM?

The recommended management of smoldering MM is **close observation** (expectant management).

What is the recommended management of SBP?

The recommended management of SBP is **involved-field RT to ≥45 Gy.**

What is the recommended management of SEP?	The recommended management of SEP is either **involved-field RT to ≥45 Gy, surgery, or surgery + RT.**
In what subgroup of pts with SEP may combined modality therapy (surgery → RT) be preferred?	In 1 study of **pts with SEP in the upper aerodigestive tract,** surgery → RT yielded improved OS in retrospective comparison of surgery or RT alone. (*Alexiou C et al., Cancer 1999*)
What is the role of RT in the Tx of MM, and what dose should be given?	The role of RT in the management of MM is for the **palliation of symptomatic bone mets, prevention of pathologic fractures, and the relief of cord compression.** The dose of RT given in MM is generally **20–36 Gy in 1.5–2 Gy/fx.**
Why is the dose of RT for the management of SP higher than the dose used in MM?	RT used in MM is for palliation of Sx, and doses of 20–30 Gy are generally sufficient to palliate this radio-responsive tumor. By definition, SP is a localized neoplasm, and a curative paradigm is employed. Dose escalation is used under the assumption that **complete eradication of tumor can occur at higher doses.**
What is the role of bisphosphonates in the management of MM?	Bisphosphonates are given with 1st-line antimyeloma therapy b/c they have been shown to **decrease the risk of skeletal events** (41% vs. 24%) and **decrease bone pain.** (*Berenson JR et al., NEJM 1996*)
What is the initial management of transplant candidate pts with MM?	The recommended management of potential transplant candidates with MM is **induction bisphosphonate/bortezomib/dexamethasone +/– thalidomide.**
What is the initial management of nontransplant candidate pts with MM?	The recommended management of nontransplant candidates with MM is **induction bisphosphonate/melphalan/prednisone + either bortezomib or thalidomide.**
What type of BM transplant (BMT) is preferred in the management of MM?	In 1 study, an autologous transplant followed by a nonmyeloablative allograft was superior in terms of OS in comparison to tandem autologous graft in the management of MM. (*Bruno B et al., NEJM 2007*)
What is the preferred conditioning regimen for pts receiving a myeloablative BMT in MM?	**High-dose melphalan** is the preferred conditioning regimen in pts with MM undergoing BMT. A randomized study of high-dose melphalan vs. total body irradiation (8 Gy in 4 fx) + low-dose melphalan showed worse hematologic toxicity and worse OS in pts treated with RT. (*Moreau P et al., Blood 2002*)
What RT Tx portal should be used in the management of SBP?	If toxicity allows, **treat the entire involved bone with a 2–3-cm margin** in RT Tx of SBP. In the spine, include 1 vertebral body above and 2 vertebral bodies below the lesion.

What RT Tx portal should be used in the management of SEP?

The Tx portal recommended in the primary management of SEP is the **extraosseous SP + primary draining LNs.**

What is the recommended follow-up for pts with SP?

Recommended SP follow-up: clinical evaluation + quantitative immunoglobulins, M protein, CBC, CMP, LDH, and β_2M q3 mos for 1 yr. A bone survey should take place q6–12 mos for the 1st 2 yrs. After 2 yrs, continued clinical evaluation and annual bone survey is appropriate.

74 Mycosis Fungoides
Updated by Lauren M. Hertan

▶ BACKGROUND

What subtypes of disorders are encompassed in the general term *cutaneous T-cell lymphoma (CTCL)*?

Subtypes of CTCL:
1. Mycosis fungoides (MF)
2. Sézary syndrome
3. Adult T-cell leukemia/lymphoma
4. Primary cutaneous CD30 anaplastic lymphoma
   The following are sometimes considered under the umbrella term of CTCL:
5. Lymphomatoid papulosis
6. Pagetoid reticulosis
7. Follicular mucinosis

What is MF?

A low-grade non-Hodgkin's lymphoma caused by skin-homing CD4+ T cells that form cutaneous lesions.

MF comprises what % of all lymphomas? What % of all CTCL?

MF comprises ~2% of all lymphomas but is the most common type of primary cutaneous lymphoma. MF comprises 50% of all CTCLs.

What is the median age at presentation in MF?

The median age at presentation of MF is **55–60 yrs.**

Is there a race and sex predilection for MF?

Yes. Black race (2:1) and male gender (2.2:1) are known risk factors for having MF.

What do MF pts have an increased susceptibility to?

MF pts have an increased susceptibility to **infections and other malignancies,** possibly due to an impaired immune system.

What is the histopathologic hallmark of MF?

The histopathologic hallmark of MF is the **Pautrier abscess** (sometimes called microabscess), which refers to the clustering of CD4 T cells around an antigen-presenting dendritic cell in the epidermis. Although this is a classic MF finding, it is present in only 20% of early-stage Dz.

What molecular study can be done to Dx early MF?

PCR for the T-cell receptor has been effective at identifying a malignant T-cell clone population in those who go on to develop MF.

What is the most common presentation of early MF?

The most common presentation of early MF is the **presence of erythematous, scaly, and pruritic macules** on an area of skin not commonly exposed to the sun.

What are the clinical presentations/phases of MF?

Clinical presentations/phases of MF:
1. Premycotic (erythematous macule) phase
2. Patch phase
3. Plaque phase
4. Tumor phase
5. Erythroderma (>80% surface area involvement)

When MF progresses from patch to plaque, what is seen under the microscope?

When MF progresses from patch to plaque, it is apparent that the **lymphoid clones begin to invade deeper into the dermis** and the **Pautrier abscesses are seen.**

What % of MF pts present with LN involvement?

~**15%** of MF pts have LN involvement at the time of diagnosis, but this varies based on T stage.

What is a Sézary cell?

Sézary cells are defined as any **atypical lymphocyte with moderately to highly infolded or grooved nucleus.**

What is Sézary syndrome?

Sézary syndrome is an aggressive T-cell lymphoma defined as erythroderma + evidence of circulating T cells that satisfy any of the below criteria:
1. A Sézary cell count ≥1,000 cells/μL
2. CD4/CD8 ratio ≥10
3. Chromosomal abnl T-cell clone
4. Increased lymphocyte count with T-cell clone detected in the blood
5. Abnl expression of pan T-cell markers (CD2, CD3, CD4, CD5).

▶ **WORKUP/STAGING**

What is the workup of MF?

Hx: focus on B Sx and skin lesions with attention to duration, distribution, changes, and associated pain or pruritus.

Physical exam: focus on entire skin (including soles, perineum, nails, and auditory canals) and LNs. Delineate skin involvement with photographs. Perform a minimum of 2 Bx of involved skin, with pathologic evaluation including T-cell receptor gene analysis.

Blood work: obtain a Sézary cell count and a T-cell receptor gene analysis, CBC, CMP, and LFTs.

Imaging: CXR for early stage, CT C/A/P or PET/CT for suspected stages IIA–IV to assess for extracutaneous manifestations. If concerning LN, excisional biopsy. Consider BM Bx in pts with blood or visceral involvement.

Describe the difference between a patch and a plaque.

A patch does not have elevation or induration. A plaque has elevation or induration.

Describe the T classification system for MF.

T1: limited patch/plaque (<10% total skin surface):
(a) patch only
(b) plaque +/– patch
T2: generalized patch/plaque (≥10% total skin surface):
(a) patch only
(b) plaque +/– patch
T3: tumor(s) ≥1 cm in diameter
T4: generalized erythroderma covering ≥80% of body surface area

Describe the N and M classification system for MF.

N0: uninvolved
N1: clinically abnl peripheral LN, histopathologically Dutch grade 1 or NCI LN 0-2:
(a) T-cell clone negative
(b) T-cell clone positive

N2: clinically abnl peripheral LNs, histopathologically Dutch grade 2 or NCI LN 3:
(a) T-cell clone negative
(b) T-cell clone positive

N3: clinically abnl peripheral LN, histopathologically Dutch grades 3–4 or NCI LN 4, clone positive or negative
M0: no visceral involvement
M1: visceral involvement

Describe the B classification of MF.	**B0:** absence of significant blood involvement: ≤5% of peripheral blood lymphocytes are Sézary cells: (a) clone negative (b) clone positive **B1:** low blood tumor burden: >5% of peripheral blood lymphocytes are Sézary cells, but pt not B2: (a) clone negative (b) clone positive **B2:** high blood tumor burden: ≥1,000/µL Sézary cells with a positive T-cell clone
Describing the stage grouping of MF.	**Stage IA:** T1, N0, M0, B0-1 **Stage IB:** T2, N0, M0, B0-1 **Stage IIA:** T1-2, N1-2, M0, B0-1 **Stage IIB:** T3, N0-2. M0, B0-1 **Stage IIIA:** T4, N0-2, M0, B0 **Stage IIIB:** T4, N0-2, M0, B1 **Stage IVA1:** any T, N0-2, M0, B2 **Stage IVA2:** any T, N3, M0, any B **Stage IVB:** any T, any N, M1, any B
If MF involves <10% of the body surface area, what T stage is this?	A **T1** MF lesion involves <10% of the body surface area.
How would erythroderma be staged for MF?	Erythroderma constitutes a **T4 lesion** for MF.
What constitutes stage I Dz in MF?	A pt with **T1 or T2, N0, M0, B0-1** would be stage I in MF.
What constitutes stage III Dz in MF?	A pt with **T4, N0-2, M0, B0-1** would be stage III in MF.

▶ **TREATMENT/PROGNOSIS**

What are the Tx options for MF that are limited to the skin?	Tx options for MF limited to skin: 1. Topical nitrogen mustard 2. Topical carmustine (BCNU) 3. Topical steroids 4. Topical imiquimod (immunomodulator that acts on Toll-like receptor 7) 5. PUVA (psoralen + UVA) 6. UVB therapy 7. Local or total skin electron beam therapy (TSEBT)
What is the long-term DFS of pts with a single localized MF lesion treated with topical therapy?	**Long-term DFS is excess of 85%.**

How is PUVA different from UVB therapy?

PUVA stands for psoralen + long-wave ultraviolet radiation (UVA). UVB is less penetrating and its use is limited to thin patches, whereas UVA is more penetrating and can effectively treat some plaques. UVA activates 8-methoxypsoralen, which results in DNA cross-linking and apoptosis.

How are PUVA and UVB administered?

PUVA and UVB are initially administered **q2–3days and then this time interval is gradually increased to q1mo once a CR is achieved.** Pts can be continued on this therapy for several yrs.

What are the response rates of patch or plaque phase MF treated with PUVA or UVB?

Response rates are high (70%–90% CR rate), but long-term DFS remains poor.

What are systemic Tx options for MF?

Systemic Tx options for MF:
1. Interferon-alfa-2a
2. Retinoids
3. Extracorporeal photochemotherapy (photophoresis)
4. Cytotoxic chemo (methotrexate, etoposide, chlorambucil)

Describe photophoresis used in MF pts.

Photophoresis is **often used to treat pts with erythrodermic MF.** It involves the use of leukapheresis to collect a pt's WBCs, which are then treated with PUVA and transfused back to the pt.

How effective is photophoresis in MF?

Overall response rates in erythrodermic MF are around 40%, with ~20% CR rate.

What RT total dose and fractionation should be used in pts with MF?

Several studies have shown an RT dose-response relationship in MF and noted high CR rates (95%–100%) with doses **>30 Gy in 1.5–2 Gy/fx.** (*Hoppe RT et al., IJROBP 1978; Cotter GW et al., IJROBP 1983*) A commonly used RT Rx for TSEBT is 36 Gy in 1.5–2 Gy/fx. For small localized fields or palliation, consider hypofractionation (5 Gy × 3 or 3 Gy × 5).

Describe the Stanford TSEBT setup for MF.

For TSEBT, pts are treated in the standing position, 3.5 m from the electron source with a three-eighths-inch Lucite plate degrader in the beam path. Beams are angled upward and downward 18 degrees to improve homogeneity and decrease photon contamination. Pts are treated using 6 different pt positions (all standing) that result in AP, PA, RAO, LAO, RPO, and LPO fields. (*Hoppe RT et al., Derm Thera 2003*)

In the Stanford TSEBT technique, are all 6 fields treated daily?

No. In the Stanford TSEBT Tx, only 3 fields are treated per day. For each field, both upward and downward (18-degree) angles are treated. (*Hoppe RT et al., Derm Thera 2003*)

In the Stanford TSEBT technique for MF, what 5 areas of skin may be underdosed and would require boosting? How are these areas boosted?

Areas that may be underdosed using the Stanford TSEBT technique:
1. Top of scalp
2. Perineum
3. Soles of feet
4. Inframammary folds in women
5. Under panniculus in obese pts

Boost fields are with conventional electrons or low voltage x-rays at conventional SSDs

In TSEBT for MF, what areas may require shielding?

In TSEBT, shield the **eyes** with internal or external eye shields. Consider shielding the **scalp** (to avoid permanent alopecia) and **hands/feet** (to avoid intense acute reaction) for a portion of the Tx.

How effective is TSEBT for patients with T2 or T3 MF?

The overall response rate is 100%, with a ~60% CR rate (T2 Dz: 75%; T3 Dz: 47%). (*Navi D et al., Arch Dermatol 2011*)

Describe the EORTC criteria for TSEBT.

80% isodose should be ≥4-mm deep to the skin surface and receive a minimum of 26 Gy. The 20% isodose line should be <20 mm from the skin surface. Total dose to bone marrow should be <0.7 Gy.

Is there evidence to support early aggressive Tx with TSEBT and systemic chemo over less aggressive Tx with sequential topical Tx?

No. *Kay et al.* randomized 103 MF pts (all stages) to TSEBT + systemic chemo vs. sequential topical Tx. Although the aggressive arm had a superior CR rate, there was no difference in long-term DFS or OS. The authors concluded that early aggressive Tx is not warranted. (*NEJM 1989*)

What are the Tx options for MF pts that fail 1st-line topical therapies?

Pts that recur after 1st-line therapy for MF can be re-treated with topical therapies before switching to alternative therapies (RT, UV therapy, steroids, or systemic Tx), as many will have a continued response to the same Tx.

Estimate the 5-yr OS of MF pts with stage IA and stage IV Dz.

MF pts with stage IA Dz have a 5-yr OS that is no different from matched normal controls (97%). 5-yr OS for stage IV MF is 27%. (*Kim YH et al., Arch Dermatol 2003*)

► **TOXICITY**

Describe the acute (during and within 6 mos of Tx) toxicities of TSEBT.

During TSEBT, MF pts commonly experience erythema/desquamation (76%), blisters (52%), hyperpigmentation (50%), skin pain (48%), and skin infections (32%). (*Lloyd S et al., J Am Acad Dermatol 2013*) In the 2–6 mos after TSEBT, pts may experience alopecia, loss of fingernails and/or toenails, and hypohidrosis (inability to sweat properly).

Describe the late toxicities of TSEBT.

Late toxicities of TSEBT include chronic dry skin, atrophy, telangiectasias, and premature aging. Additionally, secondary squamous and basal cell carcinomas as well as melanomas have been described.

75 Transplant/Total Body Irradiation

Updated by Delnora L. Erickson and Deborah E. Citrin

Define hematopoietic stem cell transplantation (HSCT).

HSCT is a **procedure to infuse hematopoietic cells** in order to restore normal hematopoiesis and/or to treat cancer.

What is the difference between allogeneic and autologous?

<u>Allogeneic</u>: stem cells from another person
<u>Autologous</u>: stem cells from the affected pt

What is a syngeneic transplant?

A syngeneic transplant uses an **identical twin as the donor.**

Name 3 sources of stem cells.

Umbilical cord blood, BM, and peripheral blood are 3 sources of stem cells.

What source of stem cells is most often used for transplant?

Most stem cells for transplant are obtained from **peripheral blood.**

What is a minitransplant?

A minitransplant, also known as nonmyeloablative or reduced-intensity transplant, **employs less toxic preparatory regimens, targeted to host T cells to facilitate engraftment.**

Name 4 malignancies routinely treated with autologous transplant.

Malignancies routinely treated with autologous transplant:
1. Recurrent Hodgkin Dz
2. Multiple myeloma
3. Chemosensitive aggressive non-Hodgkin lymphoma
4. Refractory testicular cancer

Which type of transplant is associated with a graft vs. tumor effect?

Allogeneic transplants may have graft vs. tumor effect.

Why is there decreased mortality with an autologous transplant in comparison to an allogeneic transplant?

The mortality rate with autologous transplant is lower due to the **absence of graft-vs.-host disease** (GVHD).

What limits the use of allogeneic transplant?

The use of allogeneic transplant is limited by **availability of donors.**

What is the most important risk associated with autologous transplant?

The major risk of autologous transplant is **relapse.**

Allogeneic transplant is used most commonly in what type of malignancy?

Allogeneic transplant is most commonly used to treat **acute leukemias.**

What is a conditioning regimen?

A conditioning regimen is a **Tx used to prepare pts for infusion of hematopoietic cells,** which may be chemo alone or CRT.

What are the 2 main goals of total body irradiation (TBI) as part of an allogeneic ablative HSCT?

1. **Cytotoxicity:** to eradicate residual cancer
2. **Immunosuppression:** to decrease the likelihood of host rejection of donor stem cells

 WORKUP/STAGING

What evaluations should be done prior to TBI?

TBI evaluation: complete H&P, PFTs, LFTs, serum Cr, and fertility counseling to include potential cryopreservation. A dental evaluation should also be done.

TREATMENT/PROGNOSIS

What randomized data support the use of fractionated rather than single-Tx TBI?

A **French (Institut Gustave Roussy) study** of single vs. hyperfractionated TBI randomized 160 pts with various hematologic malignancies to 10 Gy single dose or 14.85 Gy/11 fx. OS at 8 yrs was nonsignificantly higher in the hyperfractionated arm (45% vs. 38%) as well as CSS (77% vs. 63.5%). The rate of interstitial pneumonitis was similar between the 2 arms (14% and 19%); however, the rate of liver veno-occlusive Dz was significantly higher with a single fx (4% vs. 14%). (*Girinsky T et al., JCO 2000*)

What is the main site of recurrence after transplant for lymphoma?

Following transplant for lymphoma, **local tumor** recurrence is the main cause of failure.

In pts receiving BM transplant for refractory lymphoma, is it safe to give local RT prior to transplant?	**Yes.** In the Johns Hopkins Hospital dose-escalation study of locoregional RT prior to Cytoxan/TBI for pts with refractory lymphoma, 21 pts with chemorefractory Dz rcvd RT to current or previous sites of Dz to total doses from 10–20 Gy (all in 5 fx at an LDR of 0.1–0.2 Gy/min) → TBI to 12 Gy in 4 daily fx. 3 of 6 pts at the 20-Gy level had acute grade 3 toxicity. It was concluded that LDR locoregional RT has acceptable toxicity up to 15 Gy/5 fx → Cytoxan/TBI. (*Song D et al., IJROBP 2003*)
Which chemotherapeutics are commonly used in conjunction with TBI as part of HSCT?	**1. Cyclophosphamide** (most commonly used) **2. Etoposide** **3. Ara-C** **4. Fludarabine** (nonmyeloablative)
What pt positions are used for TBI?	TBI pt Tx positions include **supine, lateral recumbent, or standing.**
Why are beam spoilers used for TBI?	Beam spoilers are used to **ensure adequate dose buildup in the skin;** a screen of tissue-equivalent material is positioned between the pt and the beam.
What variation in homogeneity is considered acceptable for TBI?	Homogeneity +/– **10%** is considered ideal for TBI.
Why is the dose rate lowered in TBI?	A LDR is used in TBI to **decrease the incidence of interstitial pneumonitis,** normally 0.05–0.1 Gy/min.
What compensators are often used in TBI?	**H&N compensators** are often used in TBI to improve homogeneity.
What organs are most frequently blocked in TBI?	The **lungs** are most frequently blocked in TBI.
What areas may be boosted in TBI?	When using TBI for lymphomas, the **site of residual Dz** may be boosted to decrease the chance of LR.

▶ **TOXICITY**

What is the major complication of allogeneic transplants?	The major complication of allogeneic transplants is **GVHD.**
What is acute GVHD?	Acute GVHD is the syndrome of **hepatitis, enteritis, and dermatitis occurring secondary to allogeneic transplant.**

What predicts the risk of GVHD and graft rejection?

GVHD and graft rejection risk increase with **human leukocyte antigen disparity.**

What is chronic GVHD?

The chronic form of GVHD **occurs >3 mos after transplant** and can affect many organs such as the GI tract, skin, liver, lungs, and eyes.

Name the acute toxicities from TBI.

Most common acute toxicities from TBI:
1. N/v
2. Diarrhea
3. Xerostomia
4. Parotitis
5. Mucositis
6. Fatigue
7. Alopecia

What is the most common acute side effect?

The most common acute side effect of TBI is **n/v.**

Name 9 chronic toxicities from TBI.

Chronic toxicities from TBI:
1. Cataracts
2. Change in cognitive function
3. Endocrinopathies
4. Interstitial pneumonitis
5. Hepatic dysfunction
6. Renal dysfunction
7. Growth retardation
8. Infertility
9. 2nd malignancies

Part XI Bone

76 Osteosarcoma

*Updated by David V. Eastham
and Deborah A. Frassica*

▶ BACKGROUND

Name the 2 most common types of malignant bone tumors in the pediatric population.

The 2 most common types of malignant bone tumors in the pediatric population are **osteosarcoma (56% of total) and Ewing sarcoma (36% of total)**. (*SEER 2009*) **Both cancers are relatively rare.**

Osteosarcoma is associated with what other pediatric tumor?

Pts with **retinoblastoma** (Rb) have an increased risk of osteosarcoma, both within and outside the irradiated tissue (i.e., the osteosarcoma can occur as a secondary malignancy within bone that rcvd radiation or in distant long bone sites, putatively due to the germline mutation, which increases risk of both Rb and osteosarcoma).

Describe the distribution of osteosarcoma cases as a function of population age.

Osteosarcoma has a **bimodal distribution** as a function of age, with most cases arising during the teenage years with a second spike in an older (age >65 yrs) population, which are often associated with other conditions (Paget Dz, fibrous dysplasia)

What is the incidence of osteosarcoma in the U.S. population?

800 cases/yr of osteosarcoma are diagnosed in the U.S. population, with nearly half occurring in pts >20 y/o. Osteosarcoma is ~2 times more common than Ewing sarcoma.

What are the most common risk factors associated with the development of osteosarcoma?

A high rate of bone production and turnover (as in puberty or Paget Dz) is associated with the development of osteosarcoma. Osteosarcoma is also the most common secondary cancer in adults who received radiation or chemotherapy for a childhood solid tumor.

Describe the sex and ethnicity factors associated with osteosarcoma.

Osteosarcoma is more common in **boys** (> girls) and in **blacks** (> whites).

What is another name for the shaft of a long bone? End of the bone? Flared region between the shaft and end?

The **diaphysis is the shaft** of the bone. The **epiphysis is the end** of the bone, and the growth plate is located in this region. The conical area of bone between the diaphysis and epiphysis is the metaphysis.

Osteosarcoma is most likely to develop in what part of the bone?

Osteosarcoma arises most frequently in the **appendicular skeleton** (80% of cases) at the **metaphyseal** portions of the femur, tibia, and humerus.

Osteosarcoma most commonly arises in which bone?

The distal **femur** is the location in which osteosarcoma most commonly arises. The proximal tibia is 2nd most common. Thus, the most common site is above and below the knee.

Describe the histologic defining feature of osteosarcoma.

Production of immature "osteoid" bone is the defining feature of osteosarcoma. Most are high-grade "intramedullary" tumors.

Describe 2 genetic syndromes associated with osteosarcoma.

Osteosarcoma is associated with **Li-Fraumeni syndrome** as well as **retinoblastoma. Inactivation of tumor suppression pathways is very common in osteosarcoma.**

What is the difference between conventional osteosarcoma and juxtacortical osteosarcoma?

Conventional or "classic" osteosarcoma refers to the most common (75% of all cases) variant of osteosarcoma, which typically presents within areas of rapidly proliferating intramedullary bone. Juxtacortical osteosarcoma refers to a set of more rare osteosarcoma variants that arise adjacent to the outer surface of cortical bone.

Describe juxtacortical osteosarcoma in terms of pathologic grade and prognosis.

Juxtacortical osteosarcoma is usually **low grade (parosteal) or intermediate grade (periosteal).** Parosteal osteosarcoma rarely metastasizes and is **highly curable** with surgery alone. Periosteal osteosarcoma has approximately a 20% risk of metastasis and the role of chemotherapy is controversial. (*Grimer RJ et al., Eur J Cancer 2005*)

What % of osteosarcoma pts have localized Dz at Dx?

90% of pts with osteosarcoma have localized Dz at Dx.

What % of osteosarcoma pts with localized Dz will develop DMs without chemo?

90% of pts with localized Dz will develop mets without chemo. (*Link M et al., Clin Pediatr Oncol 1991*). Chemotherapy is now a standard part of treatment for localized osteosarcoma.

What are the 2 most common presenting Sx of osteosarcoma?

Pts with osteosarcoma typically present with **localized bone pain** (often associated with an injury) of several mos duration and a **soft tissue mass. Diagnosis may be delayed as the symptoms may be attributed to "growing pains."**

▶ WORKUP/STAGING

Define the lab and radiographic studies used in the workup and staging of osteosarcoma.

Osteosarcoma workup: basic labs (CBC, CMP) as well as alk phos, LDH, and ESR. After plain films of the affected bone are obtained, MRI of the primary site and chest imaging are needed. PET or bone scan may be used for systemic staging.

Define 3 principles used in the Bx of a suspected bone tumor.

Principles used in the Bx of a suspected bone tumor:
1. Bx should be performed at the same institution where the definitive resection will take place, preferably by the same surgeon who will undertake the definitive resection.
2. Bx should be placed carefully to avoid contamination of other areas, as may happen with a hematoma formation.
3. The Bx should not increase the extent of subsequent surgery.

What radiographic features distinguish osteosarcoma from Ewing sarcoma?

Osteosarcoma is usually sclerotic, involves the metaphysis, and has periosteal new bone formation (sunburst pattern), whereas Ewing sarcoma is usually lytic, located in the diaphysis, and displays an onion skin effect. (*Lee B et al., Handbook of Radiation Oncology 2007*)

What is the most common site of mets from osteosarcoma?

The **lung** is the most common site of osteosarcoma mets. Hence, chest imaging is important part of osteosarcoma staging.

What are the AJCC 7th edition (2011) TNM stage categories for bone tumors? (Note: Lymphoma and multiple myeloma have separate staging systems)

T1: ≤8 cm
T2: >8 cm
T3: discontinuous tumors in primary bone site
N0: no regional LN mets
N1: regional LN mets
M0: no DMs
M1a: DMs to lung
M1b: DMs to nonpulmonary sites

What is the AJCC stage grouping for bone tumors?

Stage IA: T1N0, low grade
Stage IB: T2–3N0, low grade
Stage IIA: T1N0, high grade
Stage IIB: T2N0, high grade
Stage III: T3N0, high grade
Stage IVA: M1a
Stage IVB: N1 or M1b

▶ TREATMENT/PROGNOSIS

What is the standard Tx paradigm for conventional or high-grade osteosarcoma?

Osteosarcoma standard Tx paradigm: preop chemo → surgical resection → adj chemo.

What data support the use of multiagent chemo in the management of osteosarcoma?

Multiple randomized studies have established the role of adj and neoadj chemo in osteosarcoma management. ***Link et al.*** was 1 of the 1st studies that compared multiagent chemo to no adj management in 36 pts who underwent definitive surgery. At 2 yrs, the RFS was 17% in the control group and 66% in the Tx group. (*NEJM 1986*) More recent studies show doublet chemo using doxorubicin and cisplatin to be better tolerated with no difference in survival for localized, operable osteosarcoma. (*Souhami RL et al., Lancet 1997*)

Define 3 roles for RT in the management of osteosarcoma.

RT is useful in the management of osteosarcoma for pts with close or positive surgical margins that cannot be improved, for surgically inoperable lesions, or for palliation of painful primary tumors in pts with metastatic Dz.

What is the preferred dose of RT for management of an unresectable osteosarcoma or following an R2 resection (definitive paradigm)?

For unresectable Dz, a dose of at least 60–70 Gy is recommended. The preferred dose following an R2 resection is **>55 Gy with boost to 64–68 Gy to the area of highest risk.** In 1 retrospective review, pts receiving doses of >55 Gy had improved LC. (*DeLaney TF et al., IJROBP 2005*)

What radioisotope is currently being investigated for use in the management of osteosarcoma?

Samarium-153 is a bone-seeking radioisotope that has been investigated and found to be safe and effective in a dose-finding study in poor prognosis pts who had been heavily pretreated with chemo. Because of the osteoid production, metastatic Dz outside bone will also take up samarium.

What is the 5-yr survival rate for nonmetastatic and metastatic osteosarcoma treated with chemo and surgery?

The 5-yr survival for nonmetastatic osteosarcoma treated with chemo and surgery is 60%–70%; for metastatic osteosarcoma, survival is ~20%.

77 Chondrosarcoma

Updated by Vincent J. Lee and Deborah A. Frassica

 BACKGROUND

Chondrosarcoma accounts for what % of primary bone tumors?

Chondrosarcoma accounts for **~30%** of primary bone tumors (behind osteosarcoma and multiple myeloma).

What is the most common subtype of chondrosarcoma?

Conventional chondrosarcoma constitutes 85% of chondrosarcomas. The WHO 2013 classification system has reclassified grade 1 conventional chondrosarcoma as an atypical cartilaginous tumor/chondrosarcoma grade I (**ACT/CS1**). Grades 2 and 3 conventional chondrosarcomas are classified as malignant due to metastatic potential.

What are some other subtypes of chondrosarcoma?

Dedifferentiated (10%), mesenchymal (<2%), and clear cell (<2%) are other chondrosarcoma subtypes, classified under the category of malignant by WHO.

How are conventional chondrosarcomas further subdivided?

Conventional chondrosarcomas are further classified by their location in bone. Most are **primary central chondrosarcomas,** based on their location in the medullary cavity. **Secondary peripheral chondrosarcomas** develop from the bone surface.

Which chondrosarcoma subtypes are typically high grade?

Conventional secondary peripheral chondrosarcoma and dedifferentiated chondrosarcoma are typically high grade. Conventional primary central chondrosarcoma can vary in grade from low to high.

What 2 precursor lesions may give rise to conventional chondrosarcoma?

Osteochondroma is a precursor lesion for conventional secondary peripheral chondrosarcoma, and **enchondroma** is a precursor lesion in up to 40% of conventional primary central chondrosarcoma.

Which subtypes occur in older adults? Which subtypes present in younger pts?

Dedifferentiated, conventional primary central, and conventional secondary peripheral chondrosarcoma typically present in older pts. Clear cell and mesenchymal chondrosarcoma can present in any age, but peak incidence occurs in younger adults.

What are the most common locations for conventional primary chondrosarcomas?

Most chondrosarcomas (~75%) arise in the **proximal femur, pelvis, or proximal humerus.**

What are the common presenting symptoms associated with chondrosarcoma?

Conventional chondrosarcoma often presents with **pain of insidious onset** and progressive chronology and **localized swelling.**

Chondrosarcomas of the skull base typically arise from what structures?

Although chondrosarcomas of the skull base may arise from the clivus, most originate **laterally from the spheno-occipital junction** or less commonly from the sphenoethmoid complex.

What is the typical pattern of spread for chondrosarcoma of the skull base?

Chondrosarcomas of the skull base are **locally aggressive and may expand,** destroying bone and compressing adjacent tissues.

What other tumor may often be mistaken for chondrosarcoma at the skull base? How can they be distinguished histologically?

Chordoma (particularly the chondroid variant) may appear similar to chondrosarcoma. Unlike chordomas, chondrosarcomas do not express cytokeratin or epithelial membrane antigen.

▶ **WORKUP/STAGING**

What are the 3 imaging tests commonly ordered for the workup of a possible chondrosarcoma?

Plain radiographs, MRI, and CT are commonly ordered for the workup of a possible chondrosarcoma. CT is best for examining tumor matrix mineralization, while MRI is best for assessing marrow and soft tissue involvement. In addition, CT C/A/P may be indicated to evaluate for metastatic Dz, particularly for high-grade histologies.

What is the characteristic plain film appearance of chondrosarcoma?

Although chondrosarcoma has a variable plain radiograph appearance, mineralization of chondroid matrix may produce a **punctate or ring-and-arc pattern of calcification.**

What 2 subspecialty referrals/workups should be performed prior to Tx of skull base chondrosarcoma?

Baseline neuro-ophthalmology and endocrinology workup is indicated for skull base chondrosarcoma.

What are the AJCC 7th edition (2011) TNM stage categories for bone tumors?

T1: ≤8 cm
T2: >8 cm
T3: discontinuous tumors in primary bone site
N0: no regional LN mets
N1: regional LN mets
M0: no distant mets
M1a: lung metastasis
M1b: distant mets to nonpulmonary sites

What is the AJCC stage grouping for bone tumors?

Stage IA: T1N0, low grade
Stage IB: T2-3N0, low grade
Stage IIA: T1N0, high grade
Stage IIB: T2N0, high grade
Stage III: T3N0, high grade
Stage IVA: M1a
Stage IVB: N1 or M1b

What are the preferred techniques to confirm primary bone cancer?

Core needle or **open biopsy** is recommended to confirm diagnosis. Fine needle aspiration is not suitable due to lower diagnostic accuracy.

▶ TREATMENT/PROGNOSIS

What type of surgical resection is typically recommended for chondrosarcoma?

Wide local excision (i.e., removal of tumor and a cuff of normal tissue) is typically recommended for definitive surgical Tx of chondrosarcoma. For ACT/CS1 intracompartmental chondrosarcomas, **intralesional curettage** followed by **adj cryosurgery** can be used as an alternative to WLE with acceptable outcome.

When is RT recommended for chondrosarcoma? What are the typical doses?

RT is typically recommended following incomplete resection or as palliative treatment for **unresectable chondrosarcoma.** Doses **>60 Gy** are recommended to achieve local control.

What is the recommended definitive Tx for skull base chondrosarcoma?

Maximal surgical resection is recommended for skull base chondrosarcoma. Because complete resection is generally not feasible due to anatomic constraints, adj RT is frequently recommended due to residual Dz.

What adj RT doses are necessary for control of skull base chondrosarcoma?

Adj RT doses **>65 Gy** are needed for control of skull base chondrosarcoma. **IMRT, stereotactic RT, or charged particle therapy** are modalities to consider in the effort to minimize dose to normal critical structures.

When treated with surgical resection and adj RT, what control rates can be expected for skull base chondrosarcoma?

When treated with surgical resection and adj RT (to doses >65 Gy), control rates **>90%** can be expected for skull base chondrosarcoma; these rates are superior to those of chordoma. (*Rosenberg AE et al., Am J Surg Pathol 1999*)

What role does systemic therapy play for chondrosarcoma?

Chemotherapy is not recommended for ACT/CS1 nor for clear cell chondrosarcoma. Its role is undefined for higher-grade chondrosarcomas, although there have been some reports that have advocated a role for chemo for the **mesenchymal subtype.**

What is a reasonable follow-up schedule for low- and high-grade chondrosarcoma?

For follow-up, consider clinical exam, local imaging, and chest imaging q6–12mos for 2 yrs, then annually for a minimum of 10 years, as relapses beyond 5 yrs are more common for chondrosarcomas than for other sarcomas.

78 Chordoma

*Updated by Vincent J. Lee
and Michelle Alonso-Basanta*

▶ BACKGROUND

What are chordomas?

Chordomas are **rare, slow-growing, locally aggressive neoplasms of bone** arising from embryonic remnants of the notochord.

Where do chordomas most commonly arise?

Chordomas most commonly arise in 3 locations in the axial skeleton:
1. Sacrococcygeal region (50%)
2. Spheno-occipital region of the skull base (35%)
3. Vertebral column (15%)

In craniocervical chordomas, the most common sites are the dorsum sellae, clivus, and nasopharynx.

What is the DDx of a tumor involving sacral bone?

Metastatic lesions and **multiple myeloma** make up the overwhelming majority of sacral and spinal neoplasms. **Chordomas** are the most frequently occurring primary malignant bone tumor in both the sacrum and the mobile spine. Other primary sacral tumors include chondrosarcoma, Ewing sarcoma, osteosarcoma, PNET, Paget sarcoma, and benign tumors including giant cell tumor and hemangioma.

What are the most common histologic subtypes seen for chordomas?

Most common histologic subtypes of chordoma:
1. Conventional: most common, no cartilaginous or mesenchymal components
2. Chondroid: 5%–15%, contains cartilaginous components but is distinct from chondrosarcoma
3. Dedifferentiated or sarcomatous transformation: 2%–8%, aneuploid tumors interspersed in areas of conventional chordomas, worse survival

What features characterize conventional chordomas?

Gelatinous, pink or gray masses with solid or cystic areas. Microscopically, characteristic physaliphorous cells are present.

What histologic types of chordomas are most commonly found in the skull base?

Conventional is still the most common, although the **chondroid** type has a predilection for the cranial region (one-third of cranial chordomas are chondroid).

What are the immunohistochemical findings that can help distinguish chordomas from other histologically similar lesions?	**S-100** immunoreactivity distinguishes chordoma from metastatic adenocarcinoma and meningioma, and **epithelial membrane antigen** immunoreactivity distinguishes it from chondroma, chondrosarcoma, and melanoma.
What is the rate of distant metastases for chordoma, and what distant sites can be involved?	Distant metastases have been found in up to 5% of pts at the time of diagnosis. Site of metastasis include lungs, soft tissues, bone, and skin.

▶ WORKUP/STAGING

How do pts with chordomas present clinically?	**Depends on the site of origin,** but pain of a gradual and insidious onset is reported to be the most common presenting symptom regardless of location. Chordomas encroaching on the spinal canal may cause compression of the spinal cord or nerve roots, resulting in neurologic symptoms. Chordomas involving the cervical region may cause dysphagia, dysphonia, or Horner syndrome. Chordomas in the sacral region can create nerve root dysfunction as well as obstipation, constipation, and tenesmus. Pts with base of skull chordomas present with intermittent diplopia, HA, neck pain, or other lower CN findings. Invasion of the cavernous sinus produces diplopia and facial numbness.
Is transrectal biopsy a recommended method to obtain tissue diagnosis for chordoma?	**No.** Due to a propensity to seed along biopsy tracts, transrectal biopsies should be avoided so as to prevent spread of chordoma into the rectum. All biopsy tracts should be marked and removed in subsequent surgery.
What comprises oncologic staging for chordoma?	A complete workup, advanced imaging (MRI/CT), lab studies, and biopsy.
What are the T1-T2 MRI features of chordomas?	T1-T2 MRI features of chordomas: **T1:** intermediate to low signal intensity, with marked but heterogeneous enhancement with gadolinium **T2:** very high signal intensity
What staging system is used for chordomas?	Per the AJCC (2011), chordoma is staged as a **primary bone tumor.**

▶ TREATMENT/PROGNOSIS

What is the mainstay of Tx for chordomas?	**Surgery** is the mainstay of Tx of chordomas, with studies demonstrating a direct correlation between the extent of surgical resection and the length of RFS.

Why is intralesional excision for a vertebral body chordoma a suboptimal surgical treatment?

Intralesional excision has been shown to have a high rate of local recurrence and to negatively affect overall survival. **En bloc spondylectomy** is preferred.

How are sacral amputations classified?

Based on the location of the highest level of nerve root sacrificed: low (sacrifice of at least 1 S4 nerve root or below), middle (sacrifice of at least 1 S3 nerve root), or high (at least 1 S2 nerve root). Total sacrectomy is performed when both S1 nerve roots are sacrificed.

What Tx is most commonly employed after surgical resection?

Because most chordomas are not fully resectable, postop **radiotherapy** is often employed.

Is aggressive management of chordomas at initial presentation (surgery + adj RT) important to improve outcomes compared to the same Tx at the time of recurrence (salvage RT)?

Yes. Adj RT may improve outcomes compared to a strategy of observation, reserving RT for salvage. A retrospective series from France (*Carpentier A et al., J Neurosurg 2002*) found that pts managed aggressively at initial presentation (surgery + RT) compared to those treated aggressively at the time of recurrence (after initial surgery) had improved outcomes (5- and 10-yr survival: 80% and 65% for aggressive vs. 50% and 0% for salvage). A prospective phase II trial incorporating high dose RT given pre- and/or post-operatively reported an 11% local recurrence rate for primary chordomas; findings favored a dose of ~77.4 Gy RBE for primary tumors, and ~70 Gy in the adjuvant setting. (*Delaney TF et al., J Surg Oncol 2014*).

Is conventional fractionated RT an effective Tx for chordomas?

Yes. Conventional fractionated RT is effective for palliating chordomas. Retrospective series of skull base chordomas demonstrated that with 50 Gy (photons only), 85% of pts achieved useful and prolonged pain palliation. However, LC was ~27%, 5-yr PFS was ~23%, and MS was ~62 mos (*Catton C et al., Radiother Oncol 1996*).

What is the role of SRS in the management of chordomas?

There is growing evidence supporting the role of SRS for chordoma. A MSKCC series that included unresectable pts reported a 95% LC rate at a median follow-up of 24 mos with single fraction SRS with a median dose of 24 Gy. (*Yamada Y et al., Neurosurg 2013*)

What other RT modalities can be utilized for skull base chordomas?

Multiple series have reported 5-yr PFS of 59%–73% and 5-yr OS of 79%–80.5% for proton beam therapy, with comparable rates for charged ion therapy. Stereotactic radiosurgery has also been reported to provide improvement in presenting cranial neuropathy; tumor control rates have not yet been defined. (*Muro S et al., Exp Rev Neurother 2007*)

What factor determines the risk for recurrence after Tx with proton beam therapy?

The **volume of residual Dz after surgical resection** determines the risk of recurrence after Tx with proton beam therapy.

In a series from Loma Linda, for residual tumors abutting the brainstem or >25 cc, the control rate was about 50% in the follow-up period (mean, 33 mos); those not abutting the brainstem or <25 cc residual Dz did not have recurrence. (*Hug EB et al., J Neurosurg 1999*)

What is the pattern of recurrence of chordomas after Tx?

LR is most common (95%), while up to 40% of pts will have both LR and distant metastases. The most common sites of distant Dz are lung and bone. (*Fagundes MA et al., IJROBP 1995; McPherson CM et al., J Neurosurg Spine 2006*)

What is the typical LC and OS for chordomas compared to chondrosarcomas after 70 CGE of proton beam therapy?

In the Loma Linda series of 58 pts (33 chordomas and 25 chondrosarcomas), with a mean follow-up of 33 mos, LC was 76% for chordoma and 92% for chondrosarcoma. The 5-yr OS rates were 79% for chordoma and 100% for chondrosarcoma. (*Hug EB et al., J Neurosurg 1999*)

What is the role of chemo or molecularly targeted agents in the management of chordomas?

In chordomas, cytotoxic chemo has not shown clinically significant activity. However, chordomas have been found to overexpress PDGFR-β, and clinical series have reported imatinib to provide symptomatic improvement and stabilization of Dz in some pts.

What is the survival of pts with recurrent Dz who received salvage Tx compared to supportive care?

The outcomes after recurrence are **generally poor,** but salvage Tx (surgery + RT) can be used after recurrence, with 2-yr survival of 63% vs. 21% with supportive care. However, most pts die even with therapy, with 5-yr survival only 6% after recurrence. (*Fagundes MA et al., IJROBP 1995*).

Salvage RT alone is associated with a 2-yr actuarial LC rate of 33%. (*Berson AM et al., IJROBP 1988*)

What are 5 poor prognostic factors for chordomas?

Poor prognostic factors for chordoma:
1. Recurrent Dz
2. Base of skull tumors
3. Female sex
4. Presence of tumor necrosis in pre-Tx Bx
5. Large tumors (>70 cc)

 TOXICITY

What are some common late toxicities that manifest after the Tx of skull base chordomas?

~26% of skull base chordoma pts develop endocrine abnormalities, while 5%–10% of pts develop vision loss, brainstem injury, or temporal lobe injury in 2–5 yrs. (*Berson AM et al., IJROBP 1988; Santoni R et al., IJROBP 1998*). The risk for sacral neuropathy increases with doses >77 Gy (*Delaney TF et al., J Surg Oncol 2014*).

Part XII Soft Tissue Sarcoma

79 General and Extremity Soft Tissue Sarcoma

Updated by Abigail T. Berman and Deborah A. Frassica

▶ BACKGROUND

What is the most common type of sarcoma?

The most common type of sarcoma is **soft tissue sarcoma** (STS).

Approximately how many cases of STS are diagnosed annually in the U.S.? How many deaths occur?

~11,000 cases/yr of STS are diagnosed in the U.S., with **~4,400 deaths/yr.**

What is the median age at Dx of STS?

The median age at Dx of STS is **45–55 yrs.**

What are the 3 most common sites of STS?

The 3 most common sites of STS are the **extremity** (60%), retroperitoneal (15%), and **trunk/H&N** (10% each).

What % of extremity STS involves the lower extremity?

67% of extremity STS involves the lower extremity.

What % of lower extremity STS is at or above the knee?

75% of lower extremity STS is at or above the knee.

What is the most common presentation of STS?

The most common presentation of STS is a **painless mass.**

What is the DDx of a painless mass of the extremity?

Painless mass of the extremity DDx: STS, primary or metastatic carcinoma, lymphoma, desmoid tumor, and benign lesions (lipoma, lymphangioma, leiomyoma, neuroma, Schwannoma, etc.)

What are the 5 most common types of STS?

Most common types of STS:
1. High-grade undifferentiated pleomorphic sarcoma (previously called *malignant fibrous histiocytoma*) (20%–30%)
2. Liposarcoma (10%–20%)
3. Leiomyosarcoma (5%–10%)
4. Synovial sarcoma (5%–10%)
5. Malignant peripheral nerve sheath tumors (5%–10%)

How many different histologic subtypes of STS have been identified?

>50 histologic subtypes of STS have been identified.

What are the chromosomal translocations seen for (1) synovial sarcoma, (2) clear cell sarcoma, (3) Ewing sarcoma/PNET, and (4) alveolar rhabdomyosarcoma?

Chromosomal translocations:
1. Synovial sarcoma: t(X, 18) SYT-SSX
2. Clear cell sarcoma: t(12,22) EWSR1-ATF1
3. Ewing sarcoma/PNET: t(11,22) EWSR1-FLI1
4. Alveolar rhabdomyosarcoma: t(2,13), t(1,13) PAX-FOXO1A

Name 4 genetic syndromes associated with sarcoma and the type of sarcoma associated with each of these syndromes.

Genetic syndromes associated with sarcoma and their type:
1. Gardner (desmoid tumors)
2. Retinoblastoma (bone and STS)
3. NF-1 (benign neurofibromas and malignant peripheral nerve sheath tumors)
4. Li-Fraumeni (bone and STS)

Name 6 environmental risk factors for STS.

Environmental risk factors for STS:
1. Ionizing radiation
2. Thorotrast
3. Chlorophenols
4. Vinyl chloride
5. Arsenic
6. Herbicides

What virus is associated with Kaposi sarcoma (KS)?

Human herpes virus 8 (HHV-8), also known as Kaposi sarcoma–associated herpes virus (KSHV). AIDS-associated (or epidemic KS) KS is 1 of 4 subtypes of KS.

What dose of RT can be used for KS?

Doses of **15 Gy** for oral lesions, **20 Gy** for lesions involving eyelids, conjunctiva, and genitals, and **30 Gy** for cutaneous lesions have been shown to be sufficient to produce an objective response of 92%. (*Kirova YM, Radiother Oncol 1998*)

What is the RR of secondary sarcoma in children who received RT?

According to the Childhood Cancer Survivorship Study, RT is associated with a RR of 3.1 for developing a secondary sarcoma. (*Henderson TO et al., JNCI 2007*)

What is Stewart-Treves syndrome?

Stewart-Treves syndrome is an **angiosarcoma that arises from chronic lymphedema,** most often as a complication of Tx for breast cancer.

Where does STS originate?

STS originates from the **primitive mesenchyme of the mesoderm,** which gives rise to muscle, fat, fibrous tissues, blood vessels, and supporting cells of the peripheral nervous system.

What % of STS have +LNs at Dx?

5% of STS have +LNs at Dx.

Which 5 types of STS have an increased risk of LN mets?

STS types that have an increased risk of LN mets:
1. **S**ynovial sarcoma (14%)
2. **C**lear cell sarcoma (28%)
3. **A**ngiosarcoma (14%)
4. **R**habdomyosarcoma (19%)
5. **E**pithelioid sarcoma (20%)

(Mnemonic: **SCARE**)

What is the most common site of DM from STS?

The most common site of DM from STS is to the **lung** (70%–80%). Retroperitoneal and intra-abdominal visceral sarcomas also tend to metastasize to the liver.

Name 5 factors associated with an increased risk of LR in pts with STS.

Factors associated with an increased risk of LR in pts with STS:
1. Age >50 yrs
2. Recurrent Dz
3. Positive surgical margins
4. Fibrosarcoma (including desmoid)
5. Malignant peripheral nerve sheath tumor

Name 5 factors associated with an increased risk of DM in pts with STS.

Factors associated with an increased risk of DM in pts with STS:
1. High grade
2. Size >5 cm
3. Deep location
4. Recurrent Dz
5. Leiomyosarcoma

▶ WORKUP/STAGING

What is an appropriate workup for a painless mass?

Painless mass workup: H&P, careful exam of the primary site and draining LN regions, basic labs (CBC/BMP/LFTs), CXR, CT/MRI primary site, and a schedule for core Bx or incisional Bx

What is the AJCC 7th edition (2011) TNM classification for STS?	**T1:** tumor ≤5 cm **T1a:** superficial to superficial fascia **T1b:** deep to superficial fascia **T2:** tumor >5 cm **T2a:** superficial to superficial fascia **T2b:** deep to superficial fascia **N1:** regional LN mets **M1:** DMs *Note:* The retroperitoneal location is always considered deep.
What grading system is used by the AJCC for STS, and how many grades are there in this system?	Historically, the AJCC used a 4-grade system but switched to the **French 3-grade system** in their 7th edition (2011).
What are the AJCC 7th edition (2011) stage groupings with TNM and grade for STS?	**Stage IA:** T1a-bN0M0, grade 1 **Stage IB:** T2a-bN0M0, grade 1 **Stage IIA:** T1a-bN0M0, grades 2–3 **Stage IIB:** T2a-bN0M0, grade 2 **Stage III:** T2a-bN0M0, grade 3, or any TN1M0, any grade **Stage IV:** M1
What 2 imaging studies are recommended to evaluate a potential STS?	MRI (+/− **CT scan of the primary site) and chest imaging** are recommended for pts with potential STS.
What type of Bx are recommended to evaluate a concerning soft tissue mass?	Soft tissue masses should be diagnosed using either a **core needle Bx** (preferred) or an **incisional Bx** oriented so that it may be excised during the definitive surgery. Preferably, the Bx should be done by or in coordination with the surgeon who will be performing the definitive surgery.
Under what circumstances are PET, CT, or MRI potentially useful in the workup of STS?	<u>FDG-PET</u>: may be useful for prognostication and grading as well as to determine response to chemo <u>CT abdomen/pelvis</u>: myxoid/round cell liposarcoma, epithelioid sarcoma, angiosarcoma, and leiomyosarcoma <u>MRI spine</u>: myxoid/round cell liposarcoma <u>MRI brain</u>: **alveolar soft part sarcoma (ASPS) or angiosarcoma**

▶ TREATMENT/PROGNOSIS

What is the primary Tx modality for STS?	**Surgery** is the primary Tx modality for STS.

What is the LR rate after surgery alone for STS?

LR after surgery alone **depends on the extent of resection.** LR is 90% after simple excision, 40% after wide excision, 25% after soft part excision, and 7%–18% after amputation.

What prospective trial examined surgery alone?

MDACC treated 88 pts with T1 (<5 cm), any grade STS with limb-sparing surgery (LSS) alone if R0 resection. They found that LR at 10 yrs was 10.6% and that the vast majority of recurrences occurred in high-grade tumors. (*Pisters PW et al., Ann Surg 2007*)

What is the LR rate and DFS after primary RT alone for STS?

2-yr LR is 66% and 2-yr DFS is 17% after primary RT alone for STS. (*Lindberg RD et al., Proc Natl Cancer Conf 1972*)

Surgery alone is adequate for which pts with STS of the extremity?

According to the NCCN, pts with low-grade extremity STS **(stage I)** s/p surgical resection with **>1-cm margins** do not require adj therapy. Consider RT if the margin is ≤1 cm.

What are the management options for a pt with stage II or III resectable STS?

Stage II or III resectable STS management options:
1. Surgery → RT +/– chemo
2. Preop RT → consideration of postop chemo
3. Preop chemo or CRT

What studies support the use of adj RT following LSS in high- and low-grade STS?

There have been 2 RCTs that have evaluated the impact of adj RT after limb-sparing surgery in STS: *Yang et al.,* from the NCI, randomized pts with high- and low-grade STS of the extremity treated with LSS to adj EBRT (63 Gy) or no RT. (*JCO 1998*) Pts with high-grade STS received adj Adr/cyclophosphamide with or without concurrent EBRT. For high-grade pts, 10-yr LC significantly favored RT (100% vs. 80%), but there was no difference in 10-yr DMFS or OS. For low-grade pts, LC favored the RT arm (95 vs. 67%), but there was also no difference in DMFS or OS. Radiation significantly decreased joint motion and worsened edema.

Pisters et al. randomized (in the operating room) pts with high- and low-grade STS who had a complete resection to iridium-192 brachytherapy implant (42–45 Gy) over 4–6 days or no RT. (*JCO 1996*) For high-grade pts, 5-yr LC favored the RT arm (89% vs. 66%), but there was no OS difference. For low-grade pts, LC and OS were not significantly impacted by RT.

What RCT compared preop RT vs. PORT for extremity STS, and what did it show?

The **NCI Canada trial** randomized pts with extremity STS to preop RT (50 Gy in 25 fx + a 16–20 Gy boost for +surgical margins) vs. PORT (50 Gy in 25 fx + a 16–20 Gy boost). The initial field was a 5-cm proximal and distal margin, and boost was a 2-cm proximal and distal margin. The primary endpoint was major wound complications. The trial closed after accruing 190 of the planned 266 pts b/c of significantly greater wound complications with preop RT (35%) vs. PORT (17%), with the highest rates of complications in the ant thigh (45% vs. 38%). 6-wk function was better with PORT. (*O'Sullivan B et al., Lancet 2002*) At median follow-up of 6.9 yrs, there was no difference in LC (93% preop RT vs. 92% PORT), RFS (58% vs. 59%), or OS (73% vs. 67%). Predictors for outcome included surgical margin status for LC and size and grade for RFS and OS. (*O'Sullivan B et al., Proc ASCO 2004*) The decision regarding preop vs. postop therapy was driven by toxicity profiles. In the long term, **PORT was associated with worse fibrosis and joint stiffness** (grade 2 fibrosis was 31% vs. 48%, $p = 0.07$). (*Davis AM et al., Radiother Oncol 2005*)

What are the advantages of preop RT compared to PORT for the management of extremity STS?

Advantages of preop RT for Tx of extremity STS:
1. Lower RT dose
2. Smaller Tx volume
3. Improved resectability
4. Margin-negative resections
5. Better oxygenation of tumor cells
6. Fewer long-term toxicities

What is the evidence that a limb-sparing approach of local excision with PORT yields equivalent outcomes compared to amputation alone in the management of high-grade extremity STS?

The **NCI trial** randomized 43 pts with high-grade extremity STS to amputation at the joint proximal to the tumor vs. limb-sparing resection + RT. Randomization favored limb sparing (2:1). RT was 45–50 Gy → a boost to 60–70 Gy with concurrent adr/Cytoxan → high-dose methotrexate. 4 of 27 pts in the RT group had +margins. There was no difference in 5-yr DFS (78% amputation vs. 71% RT) or OS (88% vs. 83%). There was increased LR with limb sparing (0% vs. 20%). (*Rosenberg SA et al., Ann Surg 1982*)

What is the benefit of adding adj chemo for high-grade extremity STS after surgery?

The SMAC meta-analysis included 1,953 pts with STS s/p WLE +/– adj doxorubicin-based chemo. **Chemo improved LC (HR 0.73), DMFS (HR 0.6710), and OS (HR 0.77).** Number needed to treat: 17 to prevent 1 death. Doxorubicin + ifosfamide better than doxorubicin alone. (*Pervaiz N et al., Cancer 2008*)

Should adj chemo be used in all high-grade STS pts?

This is **controversial.** Adj chemo should not be adopted as standard practice, regardless of histology or tumor size. It is typically reserved for pts with large, high-grade tumors; +margins or gross residual Dz; synovial sarcoma, or round-cell liposarcoma.

Which pts with extremity STS should be treated with neoadj therapy?

Neoadj RT, chemo, or CRT are reasonable options for all pts with **stage II or III extremity STS,** though surgery → adj therapy is also an option for these pts. Neoadj therapy is the preferred option in pts with stage II or III extremity STS when Dz is only potentially resectable or the risk of adverse functional outcomes is high (e.g., in pts who require extensive resection such as disarticulation, amputation, or hemipelvectomy).

Cite 2 studies that demonstrate the efficacy of neoadj CRT for large extremity STS.

The **Harvard retrospective study and RTOG 9514** are 2 studies that demonstrate the efficacy of neoadj CRT for large extremity STS.

What were the results of the Harvard retrospective study for STS?

The Harvard retrospective study of neoadj CRT for large STS reviewed 48 pts with >8-cm extremity STS. Pts were treated with interdigitated sequential CRT as follows: mesna/doxorubicin/ifosfamide/dacarbazine (MAID) → RT (22 Gy in 11 fx) → MAID → RT (22 Gy in 11 fx) → MAID → surgery → MAID × 3. If surgical margins were positive, pts rcvd an additional 16 Gy boost postop. **5-yr LC was 92%, DFS was 70%, and OS was 87%.** Compared with historical controls, there was a significant decrease in DM and a significant increase in DFS and OS. There were 29% wound complications and 2% Tx-related deaths. (*DeLaney TF et al., IJROBP 2003*)

What were the results of RTOG 9514 for STS?

RTOG 9514 was a phase II trial enrolling 64 pts with ≥8-cm grade 2 or 3 STS of the extremity or torso with expected R0 resection. 44% had malignant fibrous histiocytoma, 13% had leiomyosarcoma, and 88% had STS of the extremity. Pts were treated with MAID → RT (22 Gy in 11 fx) → MAID → RT (22 Gy in 11 fx) → MAID → surgery → MAID × 3 → a 14 Gy postop boost if necessary. 91% were R0 resections, and 59% rcvd the full chemo course. 3-yr LRF was 18% (if amputation was considered a failure and 10% if not). **5-yr DFS was 56%, distant DFS was 64%, OS was 71%, and there was a 92% amputation-free rate.** There were 5% Tx-related deaths (mostly secondary AML), and 84% of pts had grade 4 toxicity (mostly hematologic). The authors concluded that the regimen is effective, but substantial toxicity makes this approach controversial. (*Kraybill WG et al., Cancer 2010*) Note that RTOG 9514 used a more intense version of MAID than was used in the Harvard study, which probably worsened toxicity.

What were the results of the EORTC STBSG 62871 trial regarding neoadj chemo for STS?

EORTC STBSG 62871 was a randomized phase II trial enrolling 134 pts with STS ≥8 cm or grade 2 or 3. Pts were randomized to surgery alone vs. neoadj doxorubicin/ifosfamide. PORT was given for marginal surgery, +surgical margins, or LR. There was no difference in 5-yr DFS (52% vs. 56%) or OS (64 vs. 65%), but the study was not sufficiently powered to detect a difference. (*Gortzak E et al., Eur J Cancer 2001*)

What were the results of EORTC 62961 regarding hyperthermia + neoadj chemo for STS?

EORTC 62961 randomized 341 pts with ≥5-cm, grade 2 or 3, deep and extracompartmental STS to neoadj etoposide/ifosfamide/Adriamycin (EIA) vs. neoadj EIA + deep wave regional hyperthermia. Hyperthermia resulted in improved median LRC (3.8 yrs vs. 2 yrs) and median DFS (2.6 yrs vs. 1.4 yrs). (*Issels RD et al., Proc ASCO 2007*)

What were the results of the MSKCC retrospective review regarding IMRT for extremity STS?

The MSKCC reported a retrospective review of 41 pts with extremity STS treated with LSS and IMRT. 51% had close or +surgical margins. IMRT was used preop in 7 pts (mean dose, 50 Gy) and postop in 21 pts (mean dose, 63 Gy). At median follow-up at 2.9 yrs, 5-yr LC was 94% regardless of margin status, DMFS was 61%, and OS was 64%. (*Alektiar KM et al., JCO 2008*)

How long after surgery should adj RT for STS begin?

PORT for STS preferably begins **after healing is completed, by 3–8 wks postsurgery.**

What dose is recommended for adj RT for STS?

A commonly used prescription for adj RT for STS is 50 Gy in 2 Gy/fx → a 10–16 Gy boost for –margins, a 16–20 Gy boost for microscopically +margins, and a 20–26 Gy boost for grossly +margins.

Surgery should take place approximately how long after completion of neoadj RT for STS?

Surgery preferably takes place **3–6 wks after completion of neoadj RT** in order to decrease the risk of wound complications.

What dose is recommended for neoadj RT for extremity STS?

A commonly used Rx for neoadj RT for extremity STS is **50 Gy in 2 Gy/fx.** If postop margins are close or positive, consider a boost using IORT (single 10–16 Gy), brachytherapy (12–20 Gy), or EBRT (10–14 Gy for close margins, 16–20 Gy for microscopically +margins, and 20–26 Gy for grossly +margins).

What are the initial and boost RT Tx volumes for STS in the preop setting?

According to RTOG 0630 (IGRT preop study) revision in 2009, GTV = MRI T1 plus contrast images. CTV = GTV and suspicious edema (on MRI T2) + 3-cm margin longitudinally for intermediate to high-grade tumors ≥8 cm (2 for others) and a 1.5-cm margin radially from the GTV to the CTV. CTV is limited at bone and by the compartment in which tumor arises. A 0.5-cm expansion from CTV to PTV is generally utilized.

What are the initial and boost RT Tx volumes for STS in the postop setting?

In the postop setting, the scar and drainage sites should be included in the GTV. Longitudinal margins should be 5–7 cm. The **boost** volume is the surgical bed + a 2-cm margin to the block/field edge. Try to spare a 1.5- to 2-cm strip of skin.

What are important dose constraints in the extremity?

Per RTOG 0630, no more than 50% of a longitudinal strip of skin/tissue should receive >20 Gy and <50% of a weight-bearing bone should receive 50 Gy.

How is postop brachytherapy performed for the Tx of high-grade STS of the extremity?

Catheters are placed in the operating room after tumor resection, 1 cm apart, with a 2-cm longitudinal and 1–1.5-cm circumferential margin on the tumor bed. Tx begins on or after the 6th postop day to allow for wound healing.

Low-dose rate: 45–50 Gy to tumor bed over 4–6 days

High-dose rate: 3.4 Gy bid × 10 fx (34 Gy in 5 days)

How should pts with unresectable STS be managed?

Consider preop RT, chemo, or CRT. If still deemed unresectable, consider definitive RT, chemo, palliative surgery, observation, or the best supportive care.

What dose of RT is recommended for unresectable STS?

If possible, the dose should be ≥**70–80 Gy** using sophisticated Tx planning (IMRT or proton beam).

▶ TOXICITY

What are the short- and long-term toxicities associated with RT for STS of the extremity?

Toxicities associated with RT for extremity STS:

Short term: wound complications (5%–15% with PORT, 25%–35% with preop RT), dermatitis, recall reactions with doxorubicin and dactinomycin, epilation

Long term: abnl bone and soft tissue growth and development, leg length discrepancy, permanent weakening of bone with the greatest risk of fracture within 18 mos of completion of therapy, fibrosis leading to decreased range of motion, lymphedema, skin discoloration, telangiectasias, 2nd malignancy (≤5%)

What is the recommended follow-up after Tx of STS?

Consider evaluation by occupational/physical therapy for functional restoration, H&P and chest imaging (CXR or CT chest) q3–6mos × 2–3 yrs, then q6mos for the next 2 yrs, then annually. Consider periodic imaging of the primary site (MRI, CT, or US) to assess LR.

80 Hemangiopericytoma and Solitary Fibrous Tumors

Updated by Boris Hristov

▶ BACKGROUND

Are hemangiopericytomas benign or malignant lesions?

Hemangiopericytomas are considered **malignant** lesions (sarcomatous lesions associated with blood vessels).

What is the cell of origin of hemangiopericytomas?

Hemangiopericytomas were originally thought to originate from pericytes of the smooth muscle cells of vessels but are now felt to be of **fibroblastic** origin.

From which other tumor is a hemangiopericytoma difficult to distinguish pathologically?

Solitary fibrous tumor (SFT). The consensus view is that solitary fibrous tumors and hemangiopericytomas belong to the same spectrum of tumors of fibroblastic origin; most hemangiopericytomas are now classified as solitary fibrous tumors (either pleural or extrapleural).

What is the most common location of solitary fibrous tumors?

The most common location is the **lower extremity.** Other sites include the H&N, retroperitoneum, and brain (least common). If in the brain (hemangiopericytomas), they are often meninges based.

What does the prognosis of hemangiopericytomas and solitary fibrous tumors primarily depend on?

The prognosis depends primarily on **tumor location and ability to achieve gross-total resection** (GTR); for example, for CNS tumors, supratentorial tumors have a better prognosis than posterior fossa and base of skull tumors.

What is the rate of local recurrence for resected CNS hemangiopericytomas?

Very high, even after gross-total resection (GTR); as high as 91% in some studies. (*Guthrie BL et al., Neurosurgery 1989*)

▶ WORKUP/STAGING

What are the typical presenting Sx of a pt with SFT or hemangiopericytoma?

Pts with SFTs present with a **firm, painless, localized mass,** typically in the extremities. HA or neurologic symptoms are typical in pts with CNS tumors (hemangiopericytomas).

How do hemangiopericytomas appear on imaging (CT, MRI)?

Hemangiopericytomas typically appear to be **hypervascular lesions with diffuse contrast enhancement** on CT or MRI.

 TREATMENT/PROGNOSIS

What is the Tx paradigm for managing hemangiopericytoma?

Hemangiopericytoma Tx paradigm: **Complete surgical resection** is the mainstay of therapy **+ adj or neoadj RT, chemo, or CRT.** Unresectable cases can be treated with either RT alone or CRT (inferior outcome).

Is there a role for chemo in the management of hemangiopericytoma?

Yes. Chemo may be used either preoperatively or adj. Antiangiogenic therapy is currently being explored, b/c these are highly vascularized tumors.

What is the typical PORT dose used for treating hemangiopericytoma after GTR?

The typical PORT dose is **50–60 Gy** to the surgical bed with the margin varying by site; some studies (*Ghia AJ et al., Neurosurgery 2013*) suggest better LC with doses >60 Gy (HR 0.12, *p* = 0.045)

What is the 5-yr OS for hemangiopericytoma of the meninges?

5-yr OS is **~80%** (*Sonabend AM et al., J Neurosurg 2013*)

What should be strongly considered adj for completely resected CNS hemangiopericytomas?

RT; in a recent SEER analysis of 227 pts (*Sonabend AM et al., J Neurosurg 2013*), GTR plus upfront adj RT was the only treatment that provided a significant survival advantage on multivariate analysis.

▶ **TOXICITY**

What is an important consideration in following pts with a Dx of hemangiopericytoma?

High metastatic propensity despite aggressive initial treatment; as high as 68% at 15 yrs in some studies (*Vuorinen VSP et al., Acta Neurochir 1996*). Therefore, these pts require long-term follow-up care.

81 Desmoid Tumors

*Updated by William K. J. Skinner
and Deborah A. Frassica*

BACKGROUND

What are desmoid tumors (DT)?	DTs are rare, **benign, slow-growing fibroblastic neoplasms** that arise from musculoaponeurotic stromal elements with high recurrence even after complete resection.
What is another commonly used name for DT?	DT is also known as **aggressive fibromatosis (previously called fibrosarcoma grade I of desmoids type).**
Do DTs have metastatic potential?	**No.** DTs do not have metastatic potential but are locally aggressive with a predilection for LR.
Approximately how many cases of DT are diagnosed annually in the U.S.?	**~900 cases/yr** of DT in the U.S.
Is there a sex or racial/ethnic predilection for DT?	**Yes,** with regard to gender. **Women** are slightly more commonly affected than men. There is **no significant racial or ethnic predilection** in DT.
What is the avg decade of life in which pts present with DT?	On avg, DT pts present in the **3rd–4th decades of life.**
What genetic abnormality is associated with DT?	2% of DTs are associated with **mutations to the *APC* gene,** resulting in familial adenomatous polyposis (FAP). Wnt/beta-catenin pathway may play a key role in both FAP and sporadic DT.
What is the clinical syndrome associated with DT?	**Gardner syndrome** is associated with DT, and 10%–20% of pts with this syndrome will develop DT. **S**ebaceous cysts **O**steomas **D**esmoid tumors (Mnemonic: Gardner **SOD**)
What % of DTs are intra-abdominal, and with what clinical syndrome are intra-abdominal DTs associated?	**10%–30%** of DTs are intra-abdominal, and they are associated with **Gardner syndrome. Intra-abdominal DTs are often a source of significant morbidity and mortality.**

What 2 environmental conditions are associated with DT?	Retrospective and anecdotal data suggest an association between DT and (1) antecedent **trauma** and (2) **high estrogen** states (such as pregnancy).
DT appears histologically similar to what tumor?	DT appears histologically similar to **well-differentiated (grade 1) fibrosarcoma.**
Name 3 general anatomic sites in which DT develops.	DT develops in the (1) **trunk/extremity,** (2) **abdominal wall,** and (3) **intra-abdominal compartment.**
What is the typical presentation of an extremity DT?	Most DTs of the extremity present as a **deep-seated painless mass** with a Hx of slow growth.
What is the typical presentation of an intra-abdominal DT?	An intra-abdominal DT can present with **bowel ischemia, obstruction, or complications with ileoanal anastomosis after colectomy for FAP.**
What is the natural Hx of untreated DTs?	Although DTs can regress spontaneously, they usually continue with slow growth and local Sx associated with tumor invasion into surrounding structures.

▶ WORKUP/STAGING

After a careful H&P, what imaging should be done to evaluate for a DT?	An **MRI of the extremity** is recommended to evaluate the extent of a DT preoperatively. A **CT or MRI of the abdomen** may be helpful to evaluate an intra-abdominal or abdominal wall mass.
Full systemic staging of DTs includes what type of imaging?	DTs are benign and do not have metastatic potential. Consequently, **no systemic imaging** is needed outside of the primary tumor.
Can DT be distinguished from malignant soft tissue tumors on the basis of imaging?	**No.** DT cannot be distinguished from malignant soft tissue tumors on the basis of imaging.
Define the staging system for DT.	There is **no defined staging system** for DT. Important features to guide management include location, size, and the ability to resect with a wide margin.
What type of Bx should be done to evaluate a mass suspected of being a DT?	A core needle or open **incisional Bx** is the preferred method for any tumor that may be a malignant soft tissue sarcoma.

▶ TREATMENT/PROGNOSIS

What is considered the primary modality for Tx of DT?	**Surgical resection** is considered the primary modality for Tx of DT. Resection does not appear to affect survival.

What type of primary surgery is recommended for pts with DT?

In pts with DT, **function-preserving surgery** with a goal of wide (2-cm) margin negative resection is preferred.

For what type of pts is nonoperative initial management of DT recommended?

For pts with intra-abdominal DTs that are large, slow growing, involve the mesentery, or encase vessels and/or organs, initial treatment with a nonsurgical approach is recommended.

What is the recurrence rate after margin– surgery vs. margin+ surgery for DT in pts who do not get adj therapy?

In DT Tx with surgery alone, **LR is 13% for –margin resection,** and **LR is 52% for +margin resection.** (*Ballo MT et al., IJROBP 1998*)

Estimate the LR rate by margin status for DT pts who are treated with surgery and then adj RT.

The LR rate for DT treated with surgery and then adj RT is **7% in margin– pts and 26% in margin+ pts.** (*Ballo MT et al., IJROBP 1998*)

What factors should be considered when determining whether or not to offer adj RT for DT?

Factors to be considered when considering adj RT for DT:
1. **Margin status.** Margin– pts are unlikely to benefit
2. **Tumor size.** Large tumors may be considered for PORT even if margin–
3. **Location.** Adj RT for resected **retroperitoneal/intra-abdominal DTs** is associated with significant treatment risks
4. **Salvage options.** Lesions that may undergo repeat resections may be appropriately observed
5. **Pt age.** There should be a high threshold for using adj RT in children

What is the LR rate for DT treated with RT alone?

The LR rate for DT treated with RT alone is **22%.** (*Nuyttens JJ et al., Cancer 2000*)

What dose of RT is needed to control DT with RT alone?

A dose **>50 Gy** is needed to treat DT with RT alone. The recommended dose for gross Dz is 50–56 Gy. The LR for pts treated with RT alone is 60% with doses <50 Gy and ~15% with doses >50 Gy. (*Nuyttens JJ et al., Cancer 2000*)

What dose of RT is recommended after an R1 resection of DT in a pt who cannot be salvaged with repeat resection?

A pt treated with adj RT after an R1 resection should be treated to a dose of **50 Gy in 1.8–2 Gy/fx.**

Define the clinical target volume for RT in the management of DT.

The clinical target volume to include when treating DT with RT includes the tumor bed (and/or gross tumor), a portion of the muscle compartment to cover fascial planes, or neurovascular structures along which tumor may track with a 3–5-cm margin longitudinally and 2 cm in all other directions.

Define 4 nonsurgical, non-RT approaches to DT Tx.

Nonsurgical, non-RT approaches to DT Tx:
1. Hormone ablation (tamoxifen)
2. NSAIDs (sulindac)
3. Low-dose cytotoxic chemo (methotrexate or doxorubicin based)
4. Targeted therapy (imatinib)

Name 1 prognostic classification system for FAP-associated DT.

The **Cleveland Clinic** devised a prognostic stratification system for FAP-associated DT:
Stage I: asymptomatic, ≤10 cm in max diameter, not growing
Stage II: mildly symptomatic, ≤10 cm, not growing
Stage III: moderately symptomatic or bowel/ureteric obstruction of 10–20 cm in max diameter, slowly growing
Stage IV: severely symptomatic or >20 cm, rapidly growing
In a series by *Church et al.,* there were no deaths for stages I–II, but there was a death rate of 15% for stage III and 44% for stage IV. (*Dis Colon Rectum 2008*)

▶ TOXICITY

Define 6 late complications associated with RT Tx to the extremity.

Late complications associated with RT to the extremities:
1. Fibrosis
2. Edema
3. Fracture
4. 2nd malignancy
5. Joint stiffness
6. Neuropathy

Define the dose of RT associated with premature closure of the epiphysis.

The dose of RT associated with premature closure of the epiphysis is **>20 Gy.**

What dose of RT is associated with an increased risk of late complications in Tx of DT of the extremity?

The risk of late complications for pts with DT of the extremity treated with RT is **30% with doses >56 Gy vs. 5% with doses <56 Gy.** (*Ballo MT et al., IJROBP 1998*)

82 Retroperitoneal Soft Tissue Sarcoma

Updated by David V. Eastham and Deborah A. Frassica

Describe the demographics of retroperitoneal soft tissue sarcoma (STS)?

There are **a wide range of ages at presentation, but most pts are in their 50s with about equal numbers of men and women.**

What % of STS are retroperitoneal?

10%–15% of STS are retroperitoneal.

What is the typical presentation of pts with retroperitoneal STS?

Pts with retroperitoneal STS typically present with **vague abdominal complaints.**

What is the median diameter of retroperitoneal STS at presentation?

The median diameter of retroperitoneal STS is **15 cm.**

What are the boundaries of the retroperitoneal space?

Boundaries of the retroperitoneal space:
  Superior: diaphragm
  Inferior: pelvic diaphragm
  Lateral: lat edge of quadratus lumborum, but lat edge of 12th rib is also considered because it corresponds to origin of transversus abdominis aponeurosis
  Anterior: parietal peritoneum where anchors to colon and small bowel
  Posterior: muscular wall composed of psoas and quadratus lumborum in abdomen; iliacus, obturator internus, and pyriformis in pelvis

Which organs are retroperitoneal?

Retroperitoneal organs include the **pancreas, kidneys, adrenal glands, and ureters.**

What is the DDx of a retroperitoneal soft tissue mass? What % are malignant and what are the malignant and benign etiologies?

The DDx of a retroperitoneal mass includes **either malignant or benign tumors. 80% of retroperitoneal neoplasms are malignant.**
Malignant etiology includes:
1. Sarcoma
2. GI stromal tumor (GIST)
3. Lymphoma
4. Germ cell tumor

Benign etiology includes:
1. Desmoid tumor
2. Lipoma
3. Benign peripheral nerve sheath tumor (schwannoma, neurofibroma)

What are the 2 most common histologies of retroperitoneal sarcoma in adults?

The 2 most common histologies for retroperitoneal sarcoma in adults include **liposarcoma and leiomyosarcoma.**

What is the most common histology of retroperitoneal sarcoma in children?

The most common histology of retroperitoneal sarcoma in children is **rhabdomyosarcoma.**

 WORKUP/STAGING

How does staging for retroperitoneal sarcoma differ from the general STS AJCC (7th edition, 2011) staging?

Staging for retroperitoneal STS is according to the AJCC staging for STS except the retroperitoneal location is always considered deep and therefore the T stage will be designated with the letter "b."

Do all pts with suspected retroperitoneal sarcoma require a preop Bx?

No. Preop Bx is not required if the suspicion for retroperitoneal sarcoma is high. However, CT-guided core Bx is necessary in pts undergoing neoadj chemo or RT.

What imaging studies should be performed to stage retroperitoneal sarcoma?

Recommended staging studies for retroperitoneal sarcoma include **CT abdomen/pelvis with contrast, chest imaging, and optional MRI.**

TREATMENT/PROGNOSIS

What is the primary Tx modality for retroperitoneal sarcoma?

Surgery (en bloc resection of the tumor with the goal of attaining –margins) is the primary Tx modality for retroperitoneal sarcoma.

What is the most important treatment factor which predicts survival for retroperitoneal sarcoma?

Postop margin status is the most important factor in predicting survival. MSKCC analysis of >500 pts showed MS= 103 mos if GTR vs. only 18 mos for less than GTR. (*Lewis JJ et al., Ann Surg 1998*)

What are the Tx paradigms for retroperitoneal STS?

Retroperitoneal STS Tx paradigms:
1. Surgery alone
2. Surgery (+/– IORT) → adj RT and/or chemo
3. Neoadj RT and/or chemo → surgery (+/– IORT)

Note: If RT will be included in the Tx, the authors' strong institutional preference is for neoadj RT given the substantial morbidity of adj RT and the limited data supporting this approach.

What % of retroperitoneal sarcomas are amenable to a GTR?

<70% of retroperitoneal sarcomas are amenable to a GTR.

Is recurrence after surgery for retroperitoneal sarcoma more likely to be local or distant?

Most recurrences after surgery for retroperitoneal sarcoma are **local.**

What is the LR rate after GTR (R0 or R1) for retroperitoneal sarcoma?

LR ranges from **50%–95%** in pts who have undergone GTR for retroperitoneal sarcoma.

Summarize the argument in favor of preop RT over PORT.

Preop RT may be superior to PORT for retroperitoneal sarcoma b/c it allows for better tumor volume definition, displacement of normal viscera by tumor (therefore, less normal tissue in Tx volume), smaller Tx fields, and the potential radiobiologic advantage of having normal vasculature/oxygenation in place. Although there has been no RCT comparing preop RT vs. PORT, *Bolla et al.* found significantly worse 5-yr RT-related complication rate with PORT (23% vs. 0%). (*IJROBP 2007*)

Is there a benefit of adding IORT with postop EBRT after the surgical management of retroperitoneal sarcoma?

Possibly. There are at least 2 studies that suggest IORT improves LC when added to EBRT, but it is unclear if this improves OS. An **NCI trial** (*Sindelar WF et al., Arch Surg 1993*) compared IORT + PORT to PORT alone for retroperitoneal STS. 35 pts were randomized to IORT (20 Gy) + postop EBRT (35–40 Gy) vs. PORT (50–55 Gy). Both groups rcvd chemo (doxorubicin/cyclophosphamide/methotrexate). At a min follow-up of 5 yrs, there was no difference in OS between the groups (MS was 3.7 yrs with IORT vs. 4.3 yrs with PORT). There was a significant improvement in "in-field" LR with IORT (40% IORT vs. 80% PORT). RT enteritis occurred in 13% of pts with IORT and 50% of pts with PORT. Peripheral neuropathy was found in 60% of pts with IORT vs. 80% of pts with PORT.

A **Massachusetts General Hospital retrospective review** included 29 pts: 16 treated with IORT (10–20 Gy with intraop electrons) and 13 treated without IORT. All pts rcvs 45 Gy EBRT. LC improved with the addition of IORT (83% vs. 61%). (*Gieschen HL et al., IJROBP 2001*)

What did ACOSOG Z9031 try to address?

ACOSOG Z9031 randomized pts to **surgery alone vs. preop RT + surgery** for primary retroperitoneal sarcoma. The target accrual was 370 pts in 4.5 yrs. The primary endpoint was PFS. This study closed due to poor accrual.

Summarize the outcomes of the Toronto Sarcoma Group and the MDACC prospective trials of preop EBRT for localized intermediate- or high-grade retroperitoneal sarcoma.

The Toronto Sarcoma Group and the MDACC prospective trials enrolled 72 pts with intermediate or high-grade retroperitoneal sarcoma. 75% were primary, and 25% were recurrent. Pts were treated preop to a median dose of 45 Gy with concurrent low-dose doxorubicin. 89% underwent laparotomy with curative intent 4–8 wks after RT. 60% had an intraop or postop boost. At median follow-up of 3.4 yrs, the RR was 52% after GTR. 5-yr LRFS was 60%, DFS was 46%, and OS was 61%. (*Pawlik TM et al., Ann Surg Oncol 2006*) Results compared favorably to historical controls.

What EBRT dose is typically used for preop RT for retroperitoneal sarcoma? What phase I study tested tolerability of this preop RT dose with concurrent doxorubicin?

Retroperitoneal STS is typically treated to **50.4 Gy** preop. Based on the **MDACC phase I trial** enrolling 35 pts with potentially resectable intermediate- or high-grade retroperitoneal sarcoma, preop RT can be safely administered to 50.4 Gy with concurrent weekly doxorubicin. At this dose, there was 18% grade 3–4 nausea. (*Pisters PW et al., JCO 2003*)

Summarize the outcomes of the retrospective study by the French Federation Cancer Sarcoma Group regarding adj RT for retroperitoneal sarcoma.

The French Federation Cancer Sarcoma Group retrospectively reviewed 145 pts with localized nonmetastatic retroperitoneal sarcoma. 65% underwent GTR, and 41% had adj RT. 5-yr OS was 46%. 5-yr LRC was 55% with adj RT vs. 23% with surgery alone. (*Stoeckle E et al., Cancer 2001*). These results should be interpreted cautiously, as selection bias may have favored the RT arm in this study and adj RT is associated with significant RT-related morbidity.

In the preop radiotherapy management of retroperitoneal sarcoma, does the whole tumor volume need to be treated? What prospective study studied this question?

This is **uncertain.** *Bossi A et al.* was a prospective trial enrolling 18 pts with retroperitoneal sarcoma. (*IJROBP 2007*) Pts were treated with neoadj IMRT limited to the postabdominal wall, and planning was compared to standard RT fields. All pts successfully completed RT and surgery. There were 2 LRs, 1 within the high-dose region and 1 marginal recurrence that would not have been covered by the standard CTV. The authors concluded that limiting the CTV to the postabdominal wall is feasible.

Is there a benefit of IMRT over 3D-CRT for the preop management of retroperitoneal sarcoma?

Yes. The Emory retrospective review compared 3D-CRT with IMRT for 10 pts with retroperitoneal sarcoma and showed improved tumor coverage with better sparing of organs at risk with IMRT. (*Koshy M et al., Sarcoma 2003*)

 TOXICITY

What are acute and late toxicities associated with RT for retroperitoneal sarcoma?

Acute and subacute toxicities: n/v, diarrhea, fatigue, wound complications, duodenitis

Late toxicities: SBO (as well as stenosis and perforation), peripheral neuropathy, 2nd malignancy

Part XIII Skin

83 Melanoma

Updated by Anna O. Likhacheva

▶ BACKGROUND

What is the incidence of melanoma in the U.S.?

~**75,000 cases/yr** of melanoma in the U.S. (and **rising**)

What are some risk factors for developing melanoma?

UV RT, fair complexion, light hair/eyes, numerous benign nevi or larger atypical nevi (>5 mm, variable pigmentation, asymmetric, indistinct borders), personal Hx of melanoma (900 times), family Hx of melanoma, and polyvinyl chloride exposure

In terms of UV exposure, what is the most important risk factor associated with development of melanoma?

Intermittent intense exposure to UVA and UVB, such as Hx of blistering burns in childhood, is the most important risk factor for developing melanoma.

What are the sex differences in terms of body distribution of melanoma lesions?

<u>Males</u>: lesions predominantly on trunk (e.g., upper back)
<u>Females</u>: lesions predominantly on extremities

What % of melanomas derive from melanocytic nevi?

~**15%** of melanomas derive from melanocytic nevi.

What % of melanomas are derived from noncutaneous sites?

<**10%** of melanomas are from noncutaneous sites.

What are the common noncutaneous melanoma sites?

The **GI, ocular, and gyn areas** are the most common noncutaneous sites.

What % of melanoma pts have LN involvement at Dx, and how does this differ by T stage?

15% of pts have LN involvement at Dx, **with 5% being T1 and 25% being ≥T2.**

What % of melanoma pts present with DM at Dx?	**5%** of pts present with DM at Dx.
What proportion of DM pts present with DM from an unknown melanoma primary?	**One-third** of DM pts or 1%–2% of all pts present with mets from an unknown primary.
What are the 5 subtypes of melanoma?	Superficial spreading, nodular, lentigo maligna, acral lentiginous, and desmoplastic variant
Which of the 5 melanoma subtypes is the most common?	**Superficial spreading** (70%) is the most common subtype → nodular (25%).
What are typical features of desmoplastic melanoma?	Features of the desmoplastic subtype include older pts (60–70 yo), more infiltrative, higher rate of perineural invasion, **higher LF rates,** and **lower nodal met/DM rates.**
Which melanoma subtype has the best prognosis?	**Lentigo maligna** melanoma has the best prognosis.
What is the LN+ rate and 5-yr OS for lentigo maligna melanoma?	For lentigo maligna melanoma, the **LN+ rate is only 10%,** with **5-yr OS at 85%** after WLE alone.
What subtype commonly presents in dark-skinned populations, and what body locations does it commonly affect?	**Acral lentiginous,** which **commonly affects the palms/soles and subungual areas,** is the most common melanoma subtype in dark-skinned populations.
Which subtype of melanoma is most common and has the worst prognosis?	**Superficial spreading** is the most common subtype. This subtype also has the worst prognosis.
What is the name for lentigo maligna involving only the epidermis (Clark level I)?	**Hutchinson freckle** is lentigo maligna of the epidermis.
What are 3 commonly used immunohistochemical stains for melanoma?	**S100, HNB-45, and Melan-A** stains are commonly used for melanoma.

▶ WORKUP/STAGING

A pt presents with a pigmented lesion. What in the Hx can help to determine if this is a suspicious lesion?	Changes in **A**symmetry, **B**orders, **C**olor, **D**iameter (>6 mm), and **E**nlargement (Mnemonic: **ABCDE**)

Per the latest NCCN guidelines, for what melanoma pts should imaging be performed?

Per the NCCN, imaging should be performed for **specific signs/Sx or stage ≥III** (not recommended for stages IA–II).

What are some common DM sites for melanoma?

The **skin, SQ tissues, distant LNs, lung, liver, viscera, and brain** are common melanoma DM sites.

What is the preferred method of tissue Dx for a suspected melanoma?

For suspected melanoma, **full-thickness or excisional Bx** (elliptical/punch) with a 1–3-mm margin is preferred for tissue Dx.

Why should wider margins on excisional Dx be avoided?

Avoid wide margins **to permit accurate subsequent lymphatic mapping.**

For what locations is full-thickness incisional or punch Bx adequate?

Full-thickness incisional and punch Bx are adequate for the **palms/soles, digits, face, and ears or for very large lesions.**

When is a shave Bx sufficient?

Shave Bx is sufficient **when the index of suspicion for melanoma is low.**

How do the Breslow thickness levels correspond to the latest AJCC (7th edition, 2011) T staging for melanoma?

The Breslow thickness levels are identical to and define the AJCC T staging of malignant melanoma:

T1: ≤1 mm
T1a: no ulceration and mitosis $<1/mm^2$
T1b: ulceration or mitosis $\geq 1/mm^2$
T2: 1.01–2 mm
T3: 2.01–4 mm
T4: >4 mm
    a: no ulceration
    b: with ulceration

Into what further categories are T2–T4 broken down?

What is considered N1, N2, and N3 in melanoma staging?

All regional LN mets:
N1: 1
N2: 2–3
N3: ≥4, or matted, or in-transit mets with mets to regional node(s)

For melanoma nodal groups, into what further categories are N1–N2 stages broken?

N1a: micromets
N1b: macromets
N2a: micromets
N2b: macromets
N2c: satellite or in-transit mets without nodal mets

How do M1a, M1b, and M1c differ in a pt with metastatic melanoma?

M1a: skin, SQ, distant LNs
M1b: lung only
M1c: viscera or other sites with ↑ LDH

Describe the overall stage groupings per the latest AJCC classification.

Stage 0: Tis
Stage IA: T1aN0
Stage IB: T2aN0 or T1bN0
Stage IIA: T3aN0 or T2bN0
Stage IIB: T4aN0 or T3bN0
Stage IIC: T4bN0
Stage III: any N+
Stage IV: any M1

With regard to the pathologic staging of melanoma, how does regional nodal involvement figure into stages IIIA, IIIB, and IIIC Dz?

Stage IIIA: nonulcerative primary with LN micromets
Stage IIIB: ulcerative primary + LN micromets or nonulcerative primary + LN macromets/ in-transit mets
Stage IIIC: ulcerative primary + LN macromets/ in-transit mets or N3 Dz

What are the Clark levels? Under what circumstance does the Clark level need to be known on the pathology report for a pt with melanoma?

Clark levels:
Level I: epidermis only
Level II: invasion of papillary dermis
Level III: filling papillary dermis, compressing reticular dermis
Level IV: invading reticular dermis
Level V: SQ tissue
The Clark level should be provided on the pathology report for lesions ≤1 mm.

What are the similarities and differences between clinical and pathologic staging for melanomatous lesions?

Both require microstaging of the primary after resection:
Clinical staging: clinical exam + radiology allowed (after complete resection)
Pathologic staging: pathology assessment of LN after dissection

What should the pathology report reveal about the primary tumor in a pt with a newly diagnosed melanoma after surgical resection?

The pathology report should list the **Breslow thickness, ulceration status, mitotic rate, deep/ peripheral margins, evidence of satellitosis, and Clark level** (only for lesions ≤1 mm).

What are some adverse features on pathology after surgical resection for a melanoma?

Adverse pathology features after surgical resection include **+margins (+ deep margin), LVSI, and a mitotic rate >1/mm^2.**

For clinical staging purposes, what stage designates regional nodal involvement?

Stage III designates nodal involvement in melanoma staging.

What is the most powerful prognostic factor for recurrence and survival for pts with melanoma?	**Sentinel LN status** is the most powerful prognostic factor.
What are 3 favorable clinical factors at presentation for pts with a newly diagnosed melanoma?	**Female sex, young age, and extremity location** are all favorable prognostic factors.
What are 5 poor prognostic factors on pathology in melanoma?	**Increasing thickness, # of nodes involved, ulceration, Clark level (if <1 mm), and satellitosis** are 5 poor prognostic factors in melanoma.
What are microsatellites as seen with melanoma?	With melanoma, microsatellites are **discrete nest of cells >0.05 mm that are separated from the body of the primary lesion by collagen or fat.**
What are satellite metastases as seen with melanoma?	**Gross cutaneous or subcutaneous intralymphatic mets,** observed **≤2 cm from primary** Dz.
What are the in-transit mets seen with melanoma?	**Gross cutaneous or subcutaneous intralymphatic mets,** observed **>2 cm from primary** Dz, but **before reaching the 1st echelon nodes.**
In order of frequency, which melanoma sites have the highest LR rates after surgery?	Melanoma sites with the highest LR rates after surgery (in descending order of frequency): **H&N (9.4%)** > distal extremities (5%) > trunk (3%) > proximal extremities (1%) (*Balch CM et al., Ann Surg Oncol 2001*)
What are the comparative OS rates of melanoma pts by stage at presentation?	OS rates of melanoma pts by stage: Stage I: 80%–90% Stage II: 40%–60% Stage III: 30% Stage IV: <10%

▶ TREATMENT/PROGNOSIS

What is the general paradigm for the management of melanoma lesions?	Melanoma lesion management paradigm: 1. WLE → sentinel LN Bx (if >0.6 mm thick or >0 mitotic rate). 2. If sentinel LN Bx is positive, then full LND is required.
When is WLE alone adequate as Tx of melanoma?	WLE alone is adequate for **in situ or stage IA lesions** without adverse features on Bx.

When should sentinel LN Bx be considered or recommended with WLE for melanoma?

Sentinel LN Bx with WLE for melanoma should be considered/recommended for **stage IA with adverse features, stage ≥IB, or Clark level IV–V.**

What evidence demonstrates improved survival outcomes for prophylactic LND in the management of melanoma?

For lesions >1.6-mm thick, retrospective data by **Milton et al.** (*Br J Surg 1982*) and **Urist et al.** (*Ann Surg 1984*) have demonstrated improved survival. A randomized study by **Balch et al.** (*Ann Surg Oncol 2000*) has shown improved survival for pts with nonulcerated lesions, lesions 1–2-mm thick, and limb lesions.

What is the LN recurrence rate for pN+ melanoma pts after LND?

After LND, the LN recurrence rate for pN+ pts is **30% at 10 yrs.** (*Lee RJ et al., IJROBP 2000:* no adj RT; 45% rcvd chemo)

What min surgical margins are required by T stage for the optimal surgical management of melanoma?

Min surgical margins for optical surgical management:
  Tis: 5 mm
  T1: 1 cm
  T2: 1–2 cm
  T3–T4: 2 cm

Which randomized trials support the surgical margins currently used in the management of melanoma?

Balch et al. (*Ann Surg Oncol 2001*): 2 cm vs. 4 cm for >T2; no difference in outcome

Thomas et al. (*NEJM 2004*): 1 cm vs. 3 cm; 3 cm resulted in better LC for >T2 lesions, but no OS benefit

When is elective iliac or obturator LND necessary after resection of a lower extremity melanoma?

Elective iliac or obturator LND is necessary if there are **clinically positive superficial nodes, ≥3 superficial +LNs, or if pelvic CT shows LAD.**

When is primary RT ever indicated for Tx of melanoma?

Primary RT is indicated for **medically inoperable pts or lentigo maligna of the face** (cosmetic outcome better); this is given as 50 Gy/20 fx or 7–9 Gy × 6 biweekly (*Farshad A et al., Br J Dermatol 2002*), 1.5-cm margin, 100–250 kV photons.

If primary RT is used for medically inoperable pts, what modality can be added to improve the efficacy of RT?

Hyperthermia (*Overgaard J et al., Lancet 1995*) improves LC (46% vs. 28%) without added toxicity.

How were RT and hyperthermia administered to pts with melanoma in the Overgaard study?

In the *Overgaard J et al.* study, pts were given 24 or 27 Gy in 3 fx over 8 days ± hyperthermia (43°C × 60 min), which improved LC. (*Lancet 1995*)

When is adj RT indicated for resected melanoma?

Adj RT indications for resected melanoma:
>   <u>Primary site</u>: +/close margins, desmoplastic histology
>   <u>Nodal site</u>: >3 +LNs or matted LNs, >3 cm, +ECE, or incomplete nodal assessment
>   *Note:* Per the latest NCCN guidelines, consider RT for stage III pts (category 2b)

What RCT showed that adj RT improves lymph node field control?

ANZMTG 01.02/TROG 02.01. (*Burmeister et al., Lancet Oncol 2013*) 217 pts at high risk for further LN relapse randomized to adj RT (**48 Gy/20 fx**) or observation, 40-mo median follow-up. LN field relapse was significantly lower in adj RT arm (HR = 0.56; $p = 0.041$), but no difference in RFS and OS.

Define what is considered high risk for further lymph node field relapse per TROG 02.01?

≥1 parotid LN, ≥2 cervical or axillary LN, ≥3 inguinal LN; ECE; ≥3 cm cervical LN, or ≥4 cm axillary or inguinal LN.

Which studies suggest that RT can make up for a lack of formal neck dissection in H&N pts?

MDACC data by **Ballo et al.** (*Head Neck 2005*): cN+ in neck s/p local excision only with adj RT; 5-yr LC 93%
Ang et al. (*IJROBP 1994*): high-risk pts ± LND; 5-yr LC 88%

What is the only proven adj systemic therapy that improves DFS and OS in pts with resected high-risk stage III melanoma?

High-dose IFN-alfa, using the Kirkwood schedule (20 mU/m^2/day intravenously, 5–7 days/wk for 4 wks → 10 mU/m^2/day SQ, 3 × wk for 48 wks). However, **NCCTG 83–7052** did not demonstrate benefit of IFN (costly Tx at $50–$60K/pt).

What RT fractionation scheme is commonly used in the adj setting for melanoma of the H&N?

Biweekly 6 Gy/fx × 5 (30 Gy) based on the *Ang et al.* study (MDACC data): 5-yr LRC was 88%, OS was 47%, and there was min acute/late toxicity. (*IJROBP 1994*)

Is there a benefit to hypofractionating RT for melanoma in the adj setting?

No. RTOG 8305 showed no difference between 8 Gy × 4 fx and 2.5 Gy × 20 fx. (*Sause WT et al., IJROBP 1991*)

What did the University of Florida experience/ study (*Chang DT et al., IJROBP 2006*) demonstrate regarding adj nodal RT in pts with melanoma lesions of the H&N?

The University of Florida study showed excellent 5-yr LC (87%) and no difference between hypofractionation (6 Gy × 5 fx) and standard (60 Gy in 30 fx) dosing. The major cause of mortality was DM.

What is generally recommended for a pt with nodal recurrence after primary management for melanoma?	Recommendations for a pt with nodal recurrence after primary management include restaging, FNA or LN Bx → LND if no previous dissection → consideration for adj RT and/or INF, a clinical trial, or observation.
How is salvage RT delivered in melanoma pts with isolated axillary nodal recurrences?	After axillary LND, RT to the axilla alone is sufficient (the supraclavicular region may be omitted), using 6 Gy × 5 fx (30 Gy) per MDACC data. (*Beadle BM et al., IJROBP 2009*) The 5-yr LC rate was 88%.
What systemic agents are currently being used or explored for use for met melanoma?	**Ipilimumab,** a monoclonal antibody to the immune checkpoint receptor CTLA-4. (*Hodi FS et al, NEJM 2010; Robert C et al., NEJM 2011; Margolin K et al., Lancet Oncol 2012*) Other immune checkpoint inhibitors such as anti-PD1 or PDL1 are being tested in earlier phase clinical trials. In a phase I trial, combining anti-CTLA4 and anti-PD1 monoclonal antibody showed a response rate of 53%, much higher than single agents alone. (*Wolchok JD et al., NEJM 2013*) **Vemurafenib,** a specific inhibitor of V600E mutated BRAF (~50% of all melanomas). (*Chapman PB et al., NEJM 2011; Sosman JA et al., NEJM 2012*) In the phase III randomized trial (*Chapman et al.*) that compared vemurafenib to dacarbazine, vemurafenib had a response rate of 48% (vs. 5%) and an improved OS.

▶ TOXICITY

What is the rate of lymphedema when treating different LN regions with hypofractionated RT?	The rates for lymphedema are **39% for the groin, 30% for the axilla, and 11% for H&N sites.** (MDACC data: *Ballo MT et al., Head Neck 2005*)
What is the α/β ratio of melanoma?	For melanoma, the α/β ratio is **2.5.** (*Overgaard J et al., Lancet 1995*)
When using a hypofractionated regimen (e.g., 6 Gy × 5 [30 Gy]), at what dose does the practitioner come off the spinal cord and small bowel?	**24 Gy** is the dose tolerance of the spinal cord/small bowel when hypofractionating with 6 Gy/fx.

What are the main toxicities of concurrent IFN and RT in the adj Tx of stage III melanoma?

In stage III melanoma, the use of concurrent IFN and RT in adj Tx can cause **acute skin toxicity as well as increased grade 3–4 subacute and late toxicities** (fibrosis, SQ necrosis, myelitis, mucositis, pneumonitis, lymphedema). Up to 50% of pts can develop grade 3 toxicities.

What are the latest NCCN follow-up recommendations for melanoma by stage?

NCCN melanoma follow-up recommendations:
1. Annual skin exam for life (all stages)
2. For stages IA–IIA: H&P q3–12mos for 5 yrs, then annually; routine labs/imaging not recommended
3. For stages IIB–IV: H&P q3–6mos for 2 yrs, then q3–12mos for 3 yrs, then annually; routine labs for 1st 5 yrs; consider imaging (CXR, PET/CT, annual MRI brain)

84 Squamous Cell and Basal Cell Carcinomas (Nonmelanoma Skin Cancers)

Updated by Anna O. Likhacheva

▶ BACKGROUND

What is the incidence of nonmelanoma skin cancer (NMSC) in the U.S.?

>2 million cases/yr in the U.S. and **rising** (exceeds incidence of all other cancers combined)

Which is more common: basal cell carcinoma (BCC) or squamous cell carcinoma (SCC)?

BCC (80%) is more common than SCC (20%).

What is the sex predilection for skin cancers?

Males are more commonly affected than females **(4:1).**

What is the most common genetic mutation in NMSC?	**p53** mutations
What signaling pathway is involved in BCC pathogenesis?	Sonic hedgehog signaling pathway
What are the areas represented by the letters H, M, and L?	<u>H</u>: "mask areas" (central face, eyelids, eyebrows, periorbital nose, lips, chin, mandible, preauricular, postauricular, temple, ear), genitalia, hands, feet <u>M</u>: cheek, forehead, scalp, neck, pretibial <u>L</u>: trunk and extremities (except pretibial, hands, feet, nails, ankles) (*Connolly et al., Dermatol Surg 2012*)
What does the "mask area" correspond to?	**Midface, where the embryologic fusion lines lie** (high risk for deep invasion and high risk for LR).
What are the high-risk factors for BCC?	Area L ≥20 mm, area M ≥10 mm, area H ≥6 mm, ill-defined borders, recurrent, poorly differentiated, immunosuppressed, prior RT, PNI, aggressive histology (morpheaform, sclerosing, mixed infiltrative, micronodular)
What are the high-risk factors for SCC?	Those listed above for BCC **and** rapidly growing, neurologic symptoms, moderately or poorly differentiated, unfavorable histology (adenoid, adenosquamous, desmoplastic), ≥2-mm thick or Clark level IV or V.
What genetic/inherited disorders are associated with skin cancer?	**Phenylketonuria, Gorlin syndrome (PTCH), xeroderma pigmentosa, and albinism** have a genetic/inherited association with skin cancer.
What is the incidence of PNI and mets with BCC?	<u>PNI</u>: 1% <u>Mets</u>: <0.1% (nodes > distant sites)
What is the incidence of PNI and mets with SCC?	<u>PNI</u>: 2%–15% <u>Mets</u>: nodes: 1%–30% (1% grade 1, 10% grade 3, 30% from burns); distant: 2% (lung > liver > bones)
What are the major determinants of LN spread for SCC?	Poor differentiation, size/depth (>3 cm/>4 mm), PNI/LVI, location (lips, scars/burns, ear), and recurrent lesions
What LN regions are most commonly involved in SCC?	The **upper cervical and deep parotid regions** (with the H&N as the most frequent site) are most commonly involved in SCC.
Sun exposure at what stage of life correlates with BCC vs. SCC?	<u>BCC</u>: early in life/childhood <u>SCC</u>: decade preceding Dx

What is Bowen Dz?	Bowen Dz is **SCC in situ.**
What is erythroplasia de Queyrat?	Erythroplasia de Queyrat is **Bowen Dz of the penis.**
What is a Marjolin ulcer?	Marjolin ulcer is **SCC arising in a burn scar.**
Which is more common when the ear is the primary site: BCC or SCC?	External ear: BCC more common Internal/canal: SCC more common
What is the most common site for sebaceous carcinomas?	Ocular adnexa
What is the most common primary in a pt with SCC of intraparotid LN?	SCC of the skin

► WORKUP/STAGING

On what is the latest AJCC (7th edition, 2011) T staging based for SCC/ BCC?	**T1:** ≤2 cm (<2 high-risk features) **T2:** >2 cm (≥2 high-risk features) **T3:** invasion of maxilla, mandible, orbit, or temporal bone **T4:** skeletal invasion, PNI of skull base
Per the latest AJCC classification, to what other site is N staging for skin cancer similar?	Skin cancer N staging is similar to that of the **H&N:** **N1:** single, ipsi ≤3 cm **N2a:** single, ipsi 3–6 cm **N2b:** multiple, ipsi ≤ 6 cm **N2c:** bilat or contralat LNs ≤6 cm **N3:** LNs >6 cm
What defines stage groupings I, II, III, and IV?	**Stage I:** T1N0 **Stage II:** T2N0 **Stage III:** T3N0 or T1–3N1 **Stage IV:** N2–3, or T4, or M1
What are considered high-risk features for staging per the 7th edition of AJCC?	High-risk features include **>2-mm DOI/thickness, Clark level ≥IV, +PNI, poor differentiation, an ear or hair-bearing lip site.**
For what is a "pearly papule" lesion pathognomonic?	**BCC lesions**
How does SCC appear on the skin?	SCC is **flesh toned and variably keratotic.**
On H&P, what aspects should be the focus of the exam?	Palpate extent of tumor, CN exam for H&N lesions, regional LN evaluation, audiometry/otoscopy for cancers of the ear, and CT/MRI to verify extent

▶ **TREATMENT/PROGNOSIS**

Name 4 Tx options for NMSC

SCC/BCC of the skin Tx options:
1. Surgery (WLE, Mohs surgery, surgical excision with complete circumferential peripheral and deep margin assessment)
2. Curettage and electrodesiccation (C&E)
3. Superficial therapies
4. Primary RT

Describe Mohs surgery.

In Mohs surgery, a superficial slice of skin is taken and then sectioned into quadrants. Additional layers are taken in the quadrants that show persistent Dz.

When are C&E and superficial therapies appropriate for skin cancer?

Low-risk NMSC. (Cannot evaluate histologic margins with these techniques.)

List the superficial therapies.

Topical 5-FU, imiquimod, photodynamic therapy, cryotherapy

What % of BCC recurs if margin+ at the time of resection?

BCC recurs in **30% for a +lat margin and >50% for a +deep margin.**

What % of SCC recurs if margin+ at the time of resection?

Nearly 100% of SCCs recur if margin+.

When is RT preferred as the primary Tx modality for skin cancer?

RT is preferred for pts >60 yo and who are not candidates for primary surgery. RT should be offered for lesions of the central face, lip, eyelid, and ears if surgery will lead to inferior cosmetic or functional outcomes.

What is the best predictor of LC after definitive RT?

T stage is the best predictor for LC

What is the LC after definitive RT for BCC vs. SCC?

LC is similar for BCC and SCC with T1 lesions (95%) and lower for SCC than BCC if T2 (75%–85%) or T3 (50%).

What should be done with +margin resection?

Re-excise if possible, otherwise adj RT.

What are 3 indications for adj RT to the primary site with skin cancer?

Indications for adj RT to the primary in skin cancer:
1. +Margin (per NCCN)
2. PNI of named nerve (per NCCN)
3. Invasion of bone, cartilage, or skeletal muscle

What are relative contraindications to RT in the Tx of skin cancers?

Relative contraindications to RT for skin cancer include areas prone to trauma (hand dorsum or beltline) or with poor blood supply (below knees/elbows), age <50 yrs, post-RT recurrence, Gorlin syndrome, CD4 count <200, high occupational sun exposure, and exposed area of bone/cartilage.

When should adj nodal RT be considered after surgical resection for skin cancers?

Consider adj nodal RT after surgical resection for **multiple (>1) +LNs, large (>3 cm) LNs, ECE.**

What fields and dose schemes are typically employed with photons/orthovoltage in the Tx of skin cancers?

Treat the tumor/tumor bed + 1–2 cm to **60–66 Gy (2 Gy/fx),** especially for involvement of cartilage, or to **50–55 Gy (2.5–3 Gy/fx).** For the elderly/poor performance status, 3.5–4 Gy × 10 fx or 10 Gy × 2 fx can be used.

What is the margin/dose modification if electrons are used? Why?

If electrons are used, add an additional 0.5-cm margin on the skin surface and use 10%–15% higher daily/total dose b/c of bowing out of isodose curves and a lower RBE (0.85–0.9) of electrons.

What is the Rx point if orthovoltage (100–200 kV) RT is employed?

Dmax (90% of the IDL has to encompass the tumor). Do not use this if the lesion is >1-cm deep.

When treating with electrons, how deep should the 90% IDL extend in relation to the lesion?

The IDL should extend at least **5–10 mm deeper than the deepest aspect of the lesion.**

When treating skin lesions with electrons, what rule is typically employed to choose the correct beam energy?

Electron energy (in MeV) should be **>3 times the lesion depth** (i.e., a 9-MeV beam is needed for a 2-cm lesion depth).

What is the RT volume if a named nerve is involved by SCC?

The RT volume should include nerve retrograde to the skull base. Consider IMRT/elective nodal RT.

Where do basosquamous skin cancers occur? What is the Tx paradigm?

Basosquamous skin cancers occur on the **face.** These are treated like SCC, as they have similar rates of nodal mets.

What kind of shields are used, and where should they be placed? Why?

Wax-covered lead shields are used b/c of backscattered electrons with low E beams. They are typically placed behind/downstream of tumor, as hotspots occur upstream of the shield.

How is SCC of the pinna approached?

For SCC of the pinna, use RT with **2.5–4 Gy/fx to 45–65 Gy in 2–3 fx/wk** to the lesion + a 1–2-cm margin (using bolus and shielding as necessary).

When should surgery be recommended for pinna lesions?

Recommend surgery **when cartilage is involved or with tumor extension to the canal.**

When is adj RT generally recommended for ear lesions?

Pinna: if +margin, ≥T3
Middle ear/mastoid: if ≥T2

Can definitive RT be done for canal/middle ear lesions?	**Yes.** Good outcomes have been reported with RT alone for T1 lesions. (*Ogawa K et al., IJROBP 2007*)
What RT fields/margins are used for middle ear/canal lesions?	For middle ear/canal lesions, include the **entire canal/temporal bone + a 2–3-cm margin and ipsi regional nodes** (preauricular, postauricular, level II).
How should fx size be tailored for skin cancer depending on the RT field size used?	The larger the field size, the smaller the fx size should be.
If simple excision is performed for BCC, what are the min margins required?	Low risk: 4 mm High risk: 10 mm
What is the 1st step to take when the pt has a +margin after excision?	Send the pt back to the surgeon to be evaluated for re-excision if there is a +margin.
What is the preferred RT modality for bone-invasive skin cancer? For cartilage invasion?	Megavoltage photons are the preferred Tx modality for bone invasion b/c of a more homogenous distribution compared to orthovoltage due to the f-factor; however, this is not so with cartilage invasion, as orthovoltage beams have little difference in distribution in cartilage regardless of energy.
If treating recurrent BCC or morpheaform BCC, what type of margins should be used?	Because these tumors infiltrate more extensively, an **extra 0.5–1-cm margin** should be added on the surface.
How long should be the wait for a skin graft to heal before starting RT?	**6–8 wks** of healing time is required after skin grafting before RT can be initiated.
How should an SCC of the mastoid be treated?	Treat SCC of the mastoid with **mastoidectomy or temporal bone resection → PORT.**
How should the RT doses be modified based on tumor size/extent for ear primaries?	Conventional fx of 1.8–2 Gy: Small thin lesions <1.5 cm: 50 Gy Larger tumors: 55 Gy Min cartilage/bone involvement: 60 Gy Cartilage/bone involvement: 65 Gy

 TOXICITY

What are some toxicities expected after RT for skin cancer?	Telangiectasia, skin atrophy, hyperpigmentation, skin necrosis, fibrosis, osteonecrosis, chondritis; xerostomia/hearing loss for the ear

If cartilage is in the RT field, what should the dose/fx be kept below?	The dose should be kept at **<3 Gy/fx** to reduce chondritis.
What is the incidence of skin necrosis after RT?	Skin necrosis occurs in **3%** of pts (in 13% if fx size is >4–6 Gy).
To what dose should middle ear/canal lesions be limited? Why?	Limit middle ear/canal lesions to **65–70 Gy** b/c of higher rates (>10%) of **osteoradionecrosis** with doses >70 Gy.
What must be done to reduce the toxicities to normal tissues from skin irradiation in the H&N region?	To reduce toxicities to normal tissues, use **lead shielding** to block the lens, cornea, nasal septum, teeth, and gums. Use **dental wax** on the side from which the beam enters to absorb backscatter.
Per the latest NCCN guidelines, what should be the follow-up intervals for pts with nonmelanoma skin cancers?	NCCN nonmelanoma skin cancer follow-up intervals: 1. Complete skin exam for life at least once/yr 2. For local Dz: H&P q3–6 mos for yrs 1–2, q6–12 mos for yrs 3–5, then annually 3. For regional Dz: H&P q1–3 mos for yr 1, q2–4 mos for yr 2, q4–6 mos for yrs 3–5, then q6–12 mos for life

85 Merkel Cell Carcinoma

Updated by Anna O. Likhacheva

▶ BACKGROUND

What is the annual incidence of Merkel cell carcinoma (MCC) in the U.S.?	**~500 cases/yr** of MCC in the U.S.
What is the median age of Dx for MCC?	The median age of Dx is **75 yrs** (90% >50 yrs). MCC presents earlier in immunosuppressed pts.
What is the cell type of origin for MCC?	**Neuroendocrine** (dermal sensory cells)—aka primary **small cell cancer,** trabecular cell, or anaplastic cancer of the skin.
What virus is associated with MCC?	Merkel cell polyomavirus (detected in 43%–100%)

What is the prognosis of MCC as compared to other skin cancers?	Of skin cancers, MCC has the **worst prognosis** (even worse than melanoma).
What % of pts have LN involvement at Dx?	**20%** have LN involvement at Dx.
DMs develop in what % of pts with MCC?	**50%–60%** of MCC pts develop DMs.
Is MCC a radiosensitive or radioresistant tumor?	MCC is considered **radiosensitive.**
What demographic group does MCC affect predominantly?	**Elderly whites males** are primarily affected by MCC (male:female ratio, 2:1).
Where do most MCCs arise anatomically?	**H&N region (50%)** > extremities (33%)
MCC tumors at which sites have a particularly poor prognosis?	**Vulva and/or perineum** MCC is associated with a particularly poor prognosis.
To what tumor type is the histologic appearance of MCC similar?	The histologic appearance of MCC is similar to **small cell carcinoma of the lung.**
What are the histologic subtypes of MCC?	Histologic subtypes of MCC: 1. Small cell 2. Intermediate cell 3. Trabecular
What histologic subtype of MCC has the best prognosis?	**Trabecular** MCC has the best prognosis.
What are 2 important prognostic factors in MCC?	Prognostic factors in MCC: 1. Thickness/DOI 2. LN status

▶ WORKUP/STAGING

What is the workup for MCC?	MCC workup: H&P, CBC, CMP, CT C/A/P, and MRI or **PET for H&N primaries** to assess nodal status
What imaging is required at a min for MCC staging?	**CT chest/abdomen** is required for staging.
What markers should be included in the immuno panel?	CK-20 (specific for MCC) and TTF-1 (specific for lung and thyroid)

Why obtain chest imaging at staging?

To **r/o the possibility of small cell lung cancer with mets to the skin** as an etiology, especially when CK-20–.

Outline the informal staging system commonly utilized by various institutions for MCC.

Informal staging system for MCC:
Stage I: localized
Stage II: LN+
Stage III: DMs

Outline the 7th edition (2011) AJCC TNM staging.

T1: ≤2 cm
T2: >2 cm and ≤5 cm
T3: >5 cm
T4: invades bone, muscle, fascia, or cartilage
N1a: micromets
N1b: macromets (clinically detectable, path confirmed)
N2: in-transit mets (between primary and nodal basin or distal to primary)
M1a: mets to skin, SQ tissue, or distant LN
M1b: mets to lung
M1c: mets to all other visceral sites

What is the definition of in-transit mets or N2 Dz per the latest AJCC classification?

N2 Dz is defined as tumor distinct from the primary tumor and either between the primary and the nodal basin or distal to the primary.

Outline the latest AJCC stage groupings for MCC.

Stage IA: T1pN0
Stage IB: T1cN0
Stage IIA: T2–3pN0
Stage IIB: T2–3cN0
Stage IIC: T4N0
Stage IIIA: any TN1a
Stage IIIB: any TN1b–2
Stage IV: M1

▶ TREATMENT/PROGNOSIS

What is the Tx paradigm for MCC?

MCC Tx paradigm: surgery (WLE or Mohs) with sentinel LN Bx +/– LND +/– adj RT +/– adj chemo

What are some commonly used chemo agents for MCC?

Agents used in MCC: cisplatin/carboplatin +/– etoposide

What surgical margins are recommended for WLE?

1–2 cm (NCCN 2014)

When is adj RT indicated for MCC?	Historically, adj RT has been included in the Tx course for the majority of MCC pts. A study by *Allen PJ et al.* (*JCO 2005*) suggested that adj RT was of no benefit in margin– pts with surgically staged low-risk nodal Dz. A SEER analysis of 1665 cases showed adj RT to be associated with better OS. (*Mojica P et al., JCO 2007*) Strong indications for RT include: 1. **Tumor >2 cm** 2. **+/Close margins** 3. **Angiolymphatic invasion** 4. **LN+ or no LN evaluation** 5. **Immunocompromised pts**
Per the NCCN, what RT doses are commonly used for MCC?	Commonly used total doses for MCC: <u>Negative margins</u>: **50–56 Gy** <u>Positive margins</u>: **56–60 Gy** <u>Gross residual or unresectable</u>: **60–66 Gy** <u>Clinically negative LN</u>: **46–50 Gy** <u>Clinically positive LN</u>: **60–66 Gy**
What RT margins are typically used for MCC?	For MCC, the typical RT margin is **5 cm around the primary tumor** (i.e., not the scar).
When are regional LNs covered in the RT volume for MCC?	**Regional LNs are typically covered for all MCC pts.** Retrospective data suggest that the inclusion of regional LNs in the RT field is associated with superior outcomes. (*Eich HT et al., Am J Clin Oncol 2002; Jabbour J et al., Ann Surg Oncol 2007*) However, the role of LN coverage in sentinel LN Bx–or LND– pts is controversial.
What is the evidence for concurrent CRT after surgery for MCC?	Data on concurrent CRT for MCC are **limited.** Phase II trials have shown that CRT is tolerable (*Poulsen MG et al., IJROBP 2006*), but no trials have established superior efficacy over RT alone.
What is the historical LF rate after surgery alone and with adj RT?	Historical rates are **45%–75%** with surgery alone and **15%–25%** with adj RT.
Estimate the 3-yr OS for MCC by informal staging.	3-yr OS by informal staging: <u>Stage I (localized)</u>: 70%–80% <u>Stage II (LN+)</u>: 50%–60% <u>Stage III (DM)</u>: 30%
After recurrence, can Merkel cell be retreated?	Yes. Multimodality surgery +/– RT +/– chemo is recommended, with improved survival over single modality for recurrent Dz. (*Eng TY et al., IJROBP 2004*)

▶ TOXICITY

What specific follow-up studies do MCC pts require?

Frequent CXR imaging, consideration of serum neuron-specific enolase testing for recurrence, and total skin exam for life (high rates of 2nd skin cancers)

What follow-up intervals are recommended by the NCCN for MCC?

NCCN recommended follow-up schedule: H&P and clinically indicated imaging q3–6mos for 2 yrs, and q6–12mos thereafter.

86 Nonmelanoma Cutaneous Ear Cancer

Updated by Eva N. Christensen

▶ BACKGROUND

What staging system is used for cancer of the ear?

The **AJCC 7th edition (2011) for nonmelanoma skin cancer staging system** is used for ear cancer (refer to Chapter 84).

▶ WORKUP/STAGING

What is the general workup for tumors of the inner ear?

Tumor of the inner ear workup: H&P, otoscopy, LN exam, CT/MRI, tissue Bx, and audiometry

What structures constitute the outer and inner components of the ear?

Outer ear: pinna (auricle), external auditory canal, tympanic membrane, and middle ear
Inner ear: temporal bone (mastoid bone of bony and membranous labyrinth)

What is the lymphatic drainage of the ear?

The ear drains to the **parotid, retroauricular, and cervical nodes.**

What are the most common cancer histologies of the outer vs. the inner ear?	<u>Pinna</u>: basal cell carcinoma <u>Rest (canal, middle ear, mastoid)</u>: squamous cell carcinoma (SCC) (85%)
What % of pts with ear cancer present with nodal mets?	<15%
What anatomic site in addition to the ear has been added as a high-risk subsite per the 7th AJCC edition?	Hair-bearing lip
Why is a tumor of the ear considered a high-risk feature per the 7th edition AJCC?	Increased LR and potential for metastatic spread
What are all of the high-risk features for the primary tumor staging (T)?	DOI >2 mm, Clark level ≥IV, +PNI, poorly differentiated or undifferentiated, primary site ear or non-hair-bearing lip

▶ TREATMENT/PROGNOSIS

What is the general Tx paradigm for a pt with ear cancer?	Surgery or definitive RT (surgery preferred for cartilage invasion)
What features of the primary tumor merit consideration of elective LN irradiation?	Elective LN irradiation is considered for **large tumors (>4 cm) and deep invasion of underlying structures (i.e., cartilage).**
How should SCC of the mastoid be treated?	SCC of the mastoid Tx: mastoidectomy or temporal bone resection → PORT
How are tumors of the pinna treated?	Electrons or orthovoltage RT (1-cm margin for <1-cm tumors; 2–3-cm margin for larger tumors)
How should tumors of the external auditory canal be treated?	Include in the Tx volume the entire external auditory canal and temporal bone with 2–3-cm margins, and include ipsi regional nodes (pre-/postauricular, level II); these tumors should be treated to **60–70 Gy.**
How should the RT doses be modified based on tumor size?	Conventional fx of 1.8–2 Gy: <u>Small thin lesions</u> <1.5 cm: 50 Gy <u>Larger tumors</u>: 55 Gy <u>Min cartilage/bone involvement</u>: 60 Gy <u>Cartilage/bone involvement</u>: 66 Gy
When should higher-energy electrons be used for ear lesions?	Higher-energy electrons should be used for **large, deep, unresectable tumors** (to cover the deepest extent).

What simple technique can reduce heterogeneity and reduce inner dose in a pt being treated with electrons?	Per *Morrison WH et al.* (*IJROBP 1995*), place pt in true lat position, and use water bolus to account for inhomogeneity when treating external ear.

 TOXICITY

What is the max dose allowed in order to minimize the likelihood of osteoradionecrosis?	Osteoradionecrosis can be minimized by keeping bone doses to **<70 Gy** (~10% rate for doses >65 Gy).
What are some complications in the Tx of the ear with RT?	RT complications include **osteo- or cartilage necrosis, hearing loss, chronic otitis, and xerostomia.**
Data from Canadian series (*Hayter C, IJROBP 1996; Silva P et al., IJROBP 2000*) suggest what Tx feature was associated with increased necrosis risk?	Large fx size; to prevent necrosis, doses <4 Gy daily should be used.

Part XIV Palliative

87 Brain Metastases

Updated by Jason D. Kehrer and Bronwyn R. Stall

▶ BACKGROUND

What is the most common intracranial tumor?	**Brain met** is the most common intracranial tumor (outnumber primary brain tumors 8:1).
What is the annual incidence of brain mets in the U.S.?	**170,000–200,000 cases/yr** of brain mets in the U.S., with development in up to 30% of pts with systemic cancer
Why is the incidence of brain mets increasing?	The incidence is increasing due to advancements in systemic therapy (improved extracranial control) with limited penetration of the blood–brain barrier in conjunction with increased utilization of MRI/ surveillance imaging.
What cancers are associated with hemorrhagic brain mets?	Hemorrhagic brain mets is associated with **melanoma, renal cell carcinoma, and choriocarcinoma.**
What do the terms *solitary* and *single brain met* connote?	A solitary brain met is **only 1 brain lesion and the only site of Dz.** A single brain met is **only 1 brain lesion in addition to other sites of met Dz.**
What cancers are most likely to metastasize to the brain?	Cancers associated with brain mets: lung (40%–50%), breast (15%), melanoma (10%)
In what % of pts are brain mets the 1st manifestation of Dz?	5%–20% of pts present with brain mets from an unknown primary. Pts presenting with brain mets without a prior Dx of cancer most often have a **lung primary.**
Should Bx or resection be recommended if a new Dx of brain mets is suspected?	**Yes.** Bx should be considered in pts with a new Dx of brain mets as 11% of pts (6/54) enrolled in the 1st Patchell trial were found to have a primary brain tumor (3 pts) or inflammatory/infectious process (3 pts) despite MRI or CT findings consistent with metastatic Dz. (*Patchell R et al., NEJM 1990*)

What is the more common type of brain mets: single or multiple?	Most pts have **multiple** brain mets rather than a single lesion, with increased detection of small, multifocal lesions on MRI typically not appreciated on CT.
How do pts with brain mets present?	Presentation of pts with brain mets: Sx of ↑ ICP (HA, n/v), weakness, change in sensation, mental status changes, and seizure
What is carcinomatous meningitis?	Carcinomatous meningitis is a clinical syndrome caused by leptomeningeal met with widespread involvement of the cerebral cortex. The Dx is associated with a poor prognosis.
Where do most brain mets occur?	Most brain mets arise in the **gray/white matter junction** due to hematogenous dissemination with narrowing of blood vessels. (*Delattre J et al., Arch Neurol 1988*)
Are most brain mets infra- or supratentorial?	The majority of brain mets are **supratentorial.**
What is the distribution of brain mets within the brain?	The distribution of brain mets correlates with relative weight and blood flow: Cerebral hemispheres: 80% Cerebellum: 15% Brainstem: 5% (*Delattre J et al., Arch Neurol 1988*)
What is the overall median time from initial cancer Dx to development of brain mets?	The median overall time from initial cancer Dx to development of brain mets is **1 yr.**
Do most pts with brain mets die from their CNS Dz?	**No.** ~30%–50% of pts with brain mets die from their CNS Dz.

▶ **WORKUP/STAGING**

Describe the workup of a brain met.	Brain met workup: H&P focus on characterization of any neurologic Sx, evaluation for infectious causes (fever, CBC), careful neurologic exam, MRI brain +/– gadolinium, assessment for status of extracranial Dz, determination of Karnofsky performance status (KPS), and neurosurgery consult
What is the DDx for a new lesion in the brain?	Brain lesion DDx: mets, infection/abscess, hemorrhage, primary brain tumor, infarct, tumefactive demyelinating lesion, and RT necrosis
What imaging features are suggestive of brain mets?	Imaging features suggestive of brain mets include lesions at gray/white matter junction, multiple lesions, ring-enhancing lesions, and significant vasogenic edema

| What is triple-dose gadolinium, and why is it used? | Triple-dose gadolinium: **0.3 mmol/kg.** It is used **to increase the sensitivity of MRI.** |

▶ **TREATMENT/PROGNOSIS**

| Describe the RTOG recursive partitioning analysis (RPA) classes for brain mets. (*Gaspar L et al., IJROBP 1997*) | |

Class	KPS	Age	Disease
1	≥70	<65	Primary controlled, and no extracranial mets
2	≥70	**Either** age >65	**Or** primary uncontrolled
3	<70		

KPS, Karnofsky performance score.

| What is the MS time for RTOG RPA classes I, II, and III? | MS according to the RTOG brain met RPA:
 Class I: 7.2 mos
 Class II: 4.2 mos
 Class III: 2.3 mos |

| What is the Sperduto Index? | The Sperduto Index is a graded prognostic assessment based on age, KPS, # of brain mets, and the presence or absence of extracranial mets developed from an analysis of 1,960 pts in the RTOG database. Criteria is based on a point system:
 0 points: age >60 yrs, KPS <70, >3 brain mets, presence of extracranial mets
 0.5 points: age 50–59 yrs, KPS 70–80, 2 CNS mets
 1 point: age <50 yrs, KPS 90–100, 1 CNS met, no extracranial mets

 The sum of points predicts MS in mos:
 0–1 point: 2.6 mos
 1.5–2.5 points: 3.8 mos
 3 points: 6.9 mos
 3.5–4 points: 11 mos

 (*Sperduto P et al., IJROBP 2007*) |

| What is the Diagnosis Specific Graded Prognostic Assessment (DS-GPA)? | The DS-GPA is a graded prognostic assessment developed from a retrospective database of 4,259 eligible pts from 11 institutions with determination of significant prognostic factors based on the primary histology. (*Sperduto P et al., IJROBP 2010*) |

| What are the significant prognostic factors? | The significant prognostic factors vary by Dx:
 Non-small cell lung cancer (NSCLC)/small cell lung cancer: age, KPS, presence of extracranial mets and number of brain mets
 Renal cell/melanoma: KPS and the number of brain mets
 Breast/GI: KPS |

In pts with untreated brain mets, what is the MS?	MS of untreated brain mets is **1 mo.**
What Tx may be used for brain mets?	Brain met Tx: steroids, surgery, fractionated RT (WBRT), and SRS
In pts with brain mets treated with steroids alone, what is the MS?	MS in pts with brain mets treated with steroids alone is **2 mos.**
Are there randomized data to support improvement in pt survival or QOL with the addition of WBRT to best supportive care?	**No.** The ongoing MRC Quartz trial is a randomized, noninferiority phase III trial investigating the role of optimal supportive care (OSC) + WBRT (4 Gy × 5 fx) vs. OSC alone in pts with inoperable brain mets from NSCLC. The primary outcome measure is quality-adjusted life yrs.
How are steroids for brain mets typically prescribed?	Steroid dose for newly diagnosed brain mets: **4 mg dexamethasone q6hrs;** may give initial loading dose of 10 mg.
Why are steroids used for symptomatic brain mets?	In pts with symptomatic brain mets, **steroids reduce leakage from tumor vessels,** therefore decreasing edema and mass effect.
What pharmacologic Tx should always accompany steroid Tx?	When prescribing steroids, also provide **GI prophylaxis with a proton-pump inhibitor or H2 blocker.**
Should anticonvulsants be used prophylactically?	**No.** In accordance with guidelines from the American Academy of Neurology, pts with newly diagnosed brain tumors should not be started on prophylactic anticonvulsants. (*Glantz M et al., Neurology 2000*) The 2010 guidelines from the American Association of Neurological Surgeons/Congress of Neurological Surgeons do not recommend routine prophylactic use of anticonvulsants. (*Mikkelsen T et al., J Neurooncol 2010*)
Are there any randomized data on the dose for WBRT?	**Yes.** The RTOG conducted several RCTs from 1970–1995 of WBRT alone, assessing different fractionation schemes. The 1st 2 trials **(RTOG 6901 and 7361)** included >1,800 pts randomized to 40 Gy/20, 40 Gy/15, 30 Gy/15, 30 Gy/10, or 20 Gy/5. No significant difference was found in response rates, length of response, or OS. The MS in the 1st study was 4.1 mos and 3.4 mos in the 2nd. (*Borgelt B et al., IJROBP 1980*)
	2 ultrarapid fractionation schemes were also tested on these studies and reported separately; 10 Gy/1 **(RTOG 6901)** and 12 Gy/2 **(RTOG 7361)** in 26 and 33 pts, respectively. These schedules were associated with worse toxicity and time to neurologic progression than the standard fractionation. (*Borgelt B et al., IJROBP 1981*)

2 studies showed no MS advantage to giving a higher total dose. **RTOG 7606** randomized 255 pts to 30 Gy/10 vs. 50 Gy/20. MS was 4.1 and 3.9 mos, respectively. (*Kurtz J et al., IJROBP 1981*) **RTOG 9104** randomized 429 pts to 30 Gy/10 vs. 54.4/1.6 Gy bid. MS was 4.5 mos in both arms. (*Murray K et al., IJROBP 1997*)

What dose and fractionation schemes are considered standard for WBRT?

The most standard WBRT dose is **30 Gy/10.** Pts with a good KPS and longer life expectancy may be treated to 37.5 Gy/15, 40 Gy/20, or 50 Gy/20.

What % of brain met pts have Sx improvement with WBRT?

WBRT improves Sx from brain mets in **~60%** of cases.

What is the rate of CR to WBRT for brain mets?

~25% of pts have a CR to WBRT for brain mets.

What data support surgery + RT rather than Bx + RT for brain mets?

The 1ˢᵗ **Patchell study** for brain mets randomized 48 pts with 1 brain met and KPS ≥70 to surgery + WBRT vs. Bx + WBRT. WBRT in both arms was 36 Gy in 3 Gy/fx. Pts treated with surgery had a longer MS (40 wks vs. 15 wks, p <0.01), longer functional independence (38 wks vs. 8 wks), and ↓LR (20% vs. 52%, p <0.02). (*Patchell R et al., NEJM 1990*)

Did the Netherlands trial of WBRT +/− surgery support or refute the Patchell study?

The Noordijk study **supported** the findings of the 1ˢᵗ Patchell study. It randomized 63 pts to WBRT alone or surgery + WBRT. WBRT was 40 Gy in 2 Gy bid fx. Pts treated with surgery had improved MS (10 mos vs. 6 mos, p = 0.04) and longer functional independence (7.5 mos vs. 3.5 mos, p = 0.06). (*Noordijk E et at., IJROBP 1994*)

Does adj WBRT after surgical resection of a brain met improve OS?

No. Postop WBRT following resection of a brain met does not improve survival. In the 2ⁿᵈ Patchell study for brain mets, 95 pts following surgical resection of a single met were randomized to no further Tx or WBRT (50.4 Gy in 1.8 Gy/fx). WBRT decreased LR (10% vs. 46%), decreased the rate of any brain failure (18% vs. 70%), and decreased the rate of neurologic death (14% vs. 44%) but did not significantly change MS (48 wks vs. 43 wks). (*Patchell R et al., JAMA 1998*)

Why did the investigators choose a nonstandard WBRT dose?

The dose and fractionation schedule were chosen to achieve 90% microscopic Dz control probability.

What are the indications for surgical resection?

Single lesion amenable to resection, controlled or absent extracranial Dz, **KPS >70, age <60 yo, life expectancy >2 mos, need for immediate relief of neurologic symptoms secondary to mass effect, need to establish a tissue Dx.**

Are there any current randomized studies that support the role of adjuvant WBRT?

Yes. EORTC 22952 enrolled 359 pts with 1–3 brain mets s/p surgery or SRS randomized to no further Tx vs. WBRT (30 Gy in 3 Gy/fx). Adjuvant WBRT reduced the 2-yr relapse rate both at initial sites (surgery: 59% to 27%; SRS: 31% to 19%) and new sites (surgery: 42% to 23%; SRS: 48% to 33%) with decreased rates of death secondary to intracranial progression (44% vs. 28%) **without** improvement in the duration of functional independence or OS. Pts randomized to observation were more likely to require salvage therapy (51% vs. 16%). (*Kocher M et al., JCO 2010*)

What is the rationale for SRS in the Tx of brain mets?

Spherical/pseudospherical target, generally noninfiltrative lesions (<3–4 cm) located along the gray–white junction (noneloquent regions), ability to deliver a higher dose than can be achieved with WBRT alone (improved LC), Tx of unresectable lesions.

What was the 1st RCT study of WBRT +/− an SRS boost?

The 1st RCT of WBRT +/− an SRS boost was conducted at the **University of Pittsburgh.** 27 pts with KPS ≥70 and 2–4 mets ≤2.5 cm that were at least 5 mm from the chiasm were randomized to WBRT (30 Gy/12 fx) +/− a 16-Gy boost. The trial closed early b/c of significant difference in brain control. The SRS arm had a longer time to LF (36 mos vs. 6 mos, $p = 0.0005$) and longer time to any brain failure (34 mos vs. 5 mos, $p = 0.002$) but no difference in OS (11 mos vs. 7.5 mos, $p = 0.11$). (*Kondziolka D et al., IJROBP 1999*)

According to RTOG 9508, which pts had a survival advantage with the addition of an SRS boost to WBRT?

RTOG 9508 randomized 331 pts with 1–3 brain mets to WBRT + SRS boost vs. WBRT alone. WBRT on both arms was 37.5 Gy in 2.5 Gy/fx. The SRS boost dose was dependent on size in accordance with RTOG 9005. On univariate analysis, the addition of SRS improved the MS for pts with a single brain met (6.5 mos vs. 4.9 mos, $p = 0.39$). On subgroup multivariate analysis (MVA), RPA class I pts had improved survival with the SRS boost, as did pts with a lung cancer primary. (*Andrews D et al., Lancet 2004*)

What is the main determinant in selecting the Rx dose for SRS Tx of a brain mets?

The SRS Rx dose for a brain met is determined by **size** in accordance with the results of **RTOG 9005,** a dose escalation study: 24 Gy if <2-cm diameter, 18 Gy if 2–3 cm, and 15 Gy if 3–4 cm. (*Shaw H et al., IJROBP 1996*)

In the RTOG SRS dose escalation study, did pts rcv WBRT?

Yes. In **RTOG 9005,** an SRS dose escalation study, 64% of pts had recurrent brain mets (median prior dose of fractionated radiation 30 Gy) while 36% of pts had recurrent primary brain tumors (median initial dose of 60 Gy).

What retrospective data support the omission of upfront WBRT in pts treated with SRS for brain mets?

Sneed et al. compiled a database from 10 U.S. institutions to assess the effect of omitting upfront WBRT in pts treated with SRS for brain mets. 983 pts were analyzed and excluded pts treated with surgery (159 pts) and pts with a >1-mo interval between WBRT and SRS (179 pts). Of 569 evaluable pts, 268 had SRS alone and 301 had upfront WBRT + SRS. When adjusted for RPA class, there was no difference in survival. 37% of pts Tx with SRS alone rcvd salvage therapy (median 5.7 mos) vs. 7% of pts Tx with RS + WBRT (median 8.0 mos). No local control data were provided. (*IJROBP 2002*)

What data argue against omission of WBRT following SRS alone?

Regine et al. retrospectively analyzed 36 pts Tx with planned observation following SRS alone (median dose 20 Gy). With a MS of 9 mos, brain tumor recurrence occurred in 47% (17/16 pts) with 71% symptomatic at the time of recurrence and 59% with a neurologic deficit. (*IJROBP 2002*)

According to randomized data, what is the effect of delaying WBRT after SRS for pts with 1–4 brain mets?

JROSG99–1 showed that the omission of WBRT after SRS for 1–4 brain mets does not affect survival but increases the risk of intracranial relapse (46% with SRS + WBRT vs. 76.4% with SRS alone) and thus increases the need for salvage Tx. (*Aoyama H et al., JAMA 2006*)

What was the 1st randomized trial to assess the effect of delaying WBRT after SRS?

The 1st trial to assess the effect of delaying WBRT after SRS was **JROSG99–1.** 132 pts with 1–4 mets were randomized to SRS or WBRT + SRS. The SRS dose was based on size (lesions ≤2 cm to 22–25 Gy; lesions >2 cm to 18–20 Gy) and randomization (30% SRS dose reduction for pts on the WBRT arm). The WBRT dose was 30 Gy in 10 fx. (*Aoyama H et al., JAMA 2006*)

What prospective data support the omission of WBRT in pts treated with SRS alone?

Chang EL et al. randomized 58 pts with 1–3 brain mets (57% single) with KPS ≥70 to SRS alone vs. SRS + WBRT (30 Gy in 2.5 Gy/fx). SRS + WBRT resulted in a significant decline in 4-mo recall (24% vs. 52%) and median OS (15 mos vs. 6 mos) as compared to SRS alone. Pts treated with SRS + WBRT experience improved 1-yr LC (100% vs. 67%) and 1-yr distant brain control (73% vs. 44%) with SRS alone patients requiring more frequent salvage therapy. (*Lancet 2009*)

What are some criticisms of the trial?

Utilization of a single neurocognitive metric to assess learning and memory (HTLV-R) at a single time point (4 mos post-Tx); decreased survival in the SRS + WBRT group despite 100% 1-yr LC and improved neurologic DFS (73% vs. 27%); incomplete accrual (stopped early due to worse cognitive outcomes in the WBRT + SRS arm).

Are any ongoing protocols investigating the role of SRS +/– WBRT?

Yes. RTOG 0671 is an RCT of pts with 1–3 cerebral metastases treated with SRS randomized to WBRT. The trial is open to accrual with a primary endpoint of OS.

Are there any data on SRS dosing with planned WBRT?

Yes. Retrospective data from the **University of Kentucky** showed that optimal control of brain mets ≤2 cm was achieved with SRS of 20 Gy + WBRT. Pts treated with >20 Gy SRS + WBRT had higher rates of grade 3–4 neurotoxicity. (*Shehata M et al., IJROBP 2004*)

Are there any data comparing surgery + WBRT with SRS alone?

Yes. Retrospective data from **Germany** comparing RPA class I–II pts with 1–2 brain mets treated either with surgery + WBRT or SRS alone suggests that SRS is as effective. Of 206 pts treated from 1994–2006, 94 pts had SRS alone (18–25 Gy), and 112 pts had resection + WBRT (30 Gy/10 or 40 Gy/20). At 12 mos, there was no difference in OS (~50% in both groups), LC, or brain control. There was no difference according to the RPA group. (*Rades D et al., Cancer 2007*)

What is the role for hypofractionated stereotactic radiotherapy (hfSRT)?

Large metastases (>3 cm) and irregular shaped lesions correlate with inferior outcomes and result in increased toxicity with SRS. *Martens B et al.* retrospectively analyzed therapeutic results in 75 pts with 108 intracranial mets (48% rcvd primary hfSRT while 52% were treated following prior WBRT) with a variety of dose concepts (primary hsFRT: 5 Gy × 6–7 fx and 6 Gy × 5 fx; recurrent hsFRT 4 Gy × 7–10 fx and 5 Gy × 5–6 fx). A cumulative EQD2 (equivalent dose 2 Gy) of ≥35 Gy resulted in improved LC with acceptable toxicity. (*Cancer 2012*)

Can pts treated with WBRT for brain mets be reirradiated?

Yes. *Wong WW et al.* reported on a series of 86 pts Tx with reirradiation (median dose 20 Gy) due to progressive brain mets (median initial dose 30 Gy). 70% experienced neurologic improvement (24% complete resolution; 47% partial resolution). (*IJROBP 1996*)

What dose should be used for reirradiation after WBRT for brain mets?

The optimal dose for reirradiation after WBRT is **unknown.** 20 Gy in 10 fx is often used.

How are the fields arranged for WBRT?

WBRT is delivered using opposed lat fields; a post gantry tilt of 3–5 degrees is used to avoid divergence into the eyes; and multileaf collimation or custom blocks are used to ensure adequate coverage of the cribriform plate, temporal lobe, and brainstem while protecting the eyes, nasal cavity, and oral cavity. The inf border is generally set at C1-2.

Should surgery be used for recurrent tumors?	**Yes.** Retrospective data from MDACC have suggested that reoperation for recurrent brain mets can prolong survival and improve QOL. Multivariate analysis revealed several negative prognostic factors: presence of systemic Dz, KPS <70, short time to recurrence (<4 mos), age ≥40 yrs, and breast and melanoma primaries. (*Bindal R et al., J Neurosurg 1995*)
What is the advantage of tumor bed radiosurgery after brain met resection?	Retrospective data from the University of Sherbrooke in Canada have suggested that SRS to the tumor bed following resection for brain mets achieves LC rates that are comparable to WBRT but does not impact the development of remote brain mets. 40 pts underwent resection → SRS at a median of 4 wks postresection. 73% achieved LC, and 54% developed new brain mets. (*Mathieu D et al., Neurosurgery 2008*)
Are any prospective trials investigating the role of SRS vs. WBRT for resected metastatic brain Dz?	**Yes,** RTOG 1270 is an RCT open to accrual investigating the role of postoperative SRS boost to the surgical cavity vs. adjuvant WBRT following surgical resection of intracranial mets.
Are professional guidelines available to provide Tx recommendations for pts with newly diagnosed brain mets?	Yes, ASTRO published an evidence-based guideline of Tx recommendations dependent on the goal of Tx (survival, local control, distant brain control, and neurocognitive function) and estimated prognosis. (*PRO 2012*)

▶ TOXICITY

What are potential acute toxicities of WBRT?	Potential WBRT acute toxicities: alopecia, fatigue, HA, n/v, ototoxicity
What are potential long-term toxicities of WBRT?	Potential WBRT chronic toxicities: thinned hair, decline in short-term memory, altered executive function, leukoencephalopathy, brain atrophy, normal pressure hydrocephalus, RT necrosis
What is the relationship between WBRT-induced brain mets shrinkage and neurocognitive function?	WBRT-induced brain met shrinkage correlates with improved neurocognitive function. This was demonstrated in an analysis of 208 pts with brain mets randomized to WBRT alone on a phase III trial of WBRT +/– motexafin gadolinium. Pts with a good response (>45% tumor volume reduction at 2 mos) to WBRT had a longer time to decline in neurocognitive function. (*Li J et al., JCO 2007*)

What is the reported risk of severe dementia with WBRT?

DeAngelis L et al. reported an 11% (5 pts) risk of radiation-induced dementia in long-term brain mets survivors (>12 mos) based on a retrospective review of 47 pts Tx with WBRT. 3 pts were treated with nonstandard fractionation, 1 pt rcvd concurrent adriamycin, and 1 pt rcvd 30 Gy in 3 Gy/fx with a radiosensitizer. Of 15 pts Tx with **<3 Gy/fx without systemic therapy, 0 developed severe dementia or neurocognitive symptoms.** (*Neurosurgery 1989*)

What is the most important determinant of neurocognitive function?

The most important determinant is brain tumor control/delay of intracranial progression.

What other factors contribute to neurocognitive decline?

Anticonvulsants, benzodiazepines, opioids, chemo, surgical intervention (craniotomy), and systemic progression of Dz

What daily fx size in WBRT is associated with RT necrosis?

WBRT administered in fx sizes **>3 Gy/day** are associated with RT necrosis. (*DeAngelis L et al., Neurology 1989*)

Name the potential acute toxicities of SRS for brain mets.

Potential acute toxicities of SRS for brain mets: HA, nausea, dizziness/vertigo, seizure

What is the risk of symptomatic RT necrosis after SRS for brain mets?

There is an ~5% risk of symptomatic RT necrosis secondary to SRS for brain mets. This is usually treated with steroids but may require surgery or bevacizumab for refractory cases.

What are the dose limits to critical structures with SRS?

Brainstem 12.5 Gy, optic chiasm or optic nerves 10 Gy, other cranial nerves 12 Gy

88 Bone Metastases

Updated by Delnora L. Erickson and Bronwyn R. Stall

▶ BACKGROUND

What are the top 3 sites of metastatic Dz?

Top 3 sites of metastatic Dz:
1. Lung
2. Liver
3. Bone

What is the route of spread of cancer cells to the bone?

Most bone mets arise from **hematogenous** spread of cancer cells.

What part of the skeleton is more commonly affected by bone mets: axial or appendicular?

Bone mets more commonly affect the **axial** rather than the appendicular skeleton.

What part of the spine is most commonly affected by bone mets?

The **thoracic** spine is the most common site of bone mets. (*Bartels RH et al., CA Cancer J 2008*)

What 5 tumors are known to stimulate osteoclast activity?

Tumors known to stimulate osteoclast activity:
1. Breast
2. Prostate
3. Lung
4. Renal
5. Thyroid

In decreasing order, what 5 tumors carry the highest risk of bone mets?

Top 5 tumors with regard to the risk of bone mets (in decreasing order):
1. Prostate
2. Breast
3. Kidney
4. Thyroid
5. Lung

What is the most common presenting Sx of bone mets?

Most pts with bone mets present with **pain.**

▶ WORKUP/STAGING

What is the workup for bone mets?

Bone met workup: H&P, characterization of pain, assessment of fracture risk, assessment for weight-bearing bone, orthopedic consult as necessary, plain films, and bone scan

What imaging test is 1st line in evaluating bone mets?

Initial imaging of asymptomatic bone mets usually involves a **bone scan** (skeletal scintigraphy). If symptomatic, directed plain films and bone scan as well as subsequent clinically directed CT and/or MRI may be beneficial.

When may plain films be useful when evaluating bone mets?

In the setting of **bone pain with a positive bone scan,** plain films may show an impending fracture or a pathologic fracture.

What cancer is associated with mixed lytic and sclerotic lesions?

Breast cancer is associated with mixed sclerotic and lytic lesions.

What cancers are associated with primarily blastic lesions?

Tumors with predominantly blastic lesions:
1. Prostate
2. Small cell lung cancer
3. Hodgkin lymphoma

What cancers are associated with primarily lytic lesions?

Tumors with predominantly lytic lesions:
1. Renal cell
2. Melanoma
3. Multiple myeloma
4. Thyroid
5. Non–small cell lung cancer
6. Non-Hodgkin lymphoma

What imaging test can help to differentiate degenerative Dz from mets?

CT and/or MRI can help to distinguish between degenerative Dz and bone mets.

When cord compression is suspected, what imaging is indicated?

MRI of the entire spine is indicated if cord compression is suspected.

What scoring system predicts for pathologic fracture?

The **Mirels scoring system** is a weighted system based on a retrospective review that predicts the risk of pathologic fracture through metastatic lesions in long bones. Score ranges from 4–12. A score <7 can be treated with RT alone, while a score ≥8 requires internal fixation prior to RT. (*Mirels H et al., Clin Ortho Res 1989*)

What are the components of the Mirels scoring system?

Score	Pain	Location	Cortical Destruction	Appearance
1	Mild	Upper limb	<1/3	Blastic
2	Moderate	Lower limb	1/3–2/3	Mixed
3	Severe	Peritrochanteric	>2/3	Lytic

(*Mirels H et al., Clin Ortho Res 1989*)

What 2 risk factors predict for pathologic fracture of the femur?

Factors predicting for pathologic fracture of the femur:
1. Axial cortical involvement >30 mm
2. Circumferential cortical involvement >50%

(*Van der Linden Y et al., J Bone Joint Surg Br 2004*)

▶ TREATMENT/PROGNOSIS

Name 6 Tx for bone mets.

Bone met Tx:
1. Chemo
2. Radionuclides
3. Local EBRT
4. Endocrine therapy
5. NSAIDs
6. Narcotics

What supportive measures can be used for pts with painful bone mets?

Supportive care for bone mets may include orthopedic braces such as **thoracolumbosacral orthosis, canes, walkers, and wheelchairs.**

What interventional procedures can decrease pain from cancer-associated vertebral body collapse (i.e., compression fracture)?

Kyphoplasty and vertebroplasty are procedures performed by interventional radiologists that can address pain from vertebral body collapse. They are often performed in conjunction with EBRT.

What is the difference between kyphoplasty and vertebroplasty?

Vertebroplasty utilizes fluoroscopic guidance to inject bone cement (methyl methacrylate) into the collapsed vertebral body. In **kyphoplasty,** an inflatable bone tamp is inserted to restore the height of the vertebral body, creating a cavity that can be filled with bone cement.

According to the ASTRO Guidelines for Palliative RT for bone mets, what factors favor the inclusion of surgical decompression in addition to EBRT for spinal cord compression?

1. Solitary site of tumor progression
2. Absence of visceral or brain mets
3. Spinal instability
4. Age <65 yrs
5. Karnofsky performance score (KPS) ≥70
6. Projected survival >3 mos
7. Slow progression of neurologic symptoms

8. Maintained ambulation
9. Nonambulatory for <48 hrs
10. Relatively radioresistant tumor (i.e., melanoma)
11. Site of origin suggesting relatively indolent course (i.e., prostate, breast, kidney)
12. Previous EBRT failed

(*Lutz S et al., IJROBP 2011*)

In what cancers may chemo eradicate bone mets?

Chemo can cure bone mets from **lymphomas and germ cell tumors.**

What is the chief action of bisphosphonates? Name 2.

Bisphosphonates **inhibit osteoclast activity. Pamidronate and zoledronic acid** are 2 common bisphosphonates.

What is denosumab (XGEVA)?

Denosumab is a fully human monoclonal antibody that targets receptor activator of nuclear factor-kappa beta ligand (**RANKL**), thereby inhibiting maturation of osteoclasts.

What are the American Society for Clinical Oncology (ASCO) 2011 guidelines for bone-modifying agents (BMAs) in the Tx of bone mets from breast cancer?

ASCO 2011 guidelines state that either bisphosphonates (pamidronate or zoledronic acid) should be administered **q3–4wks** or denosumab should be administered **q4wks** to breast cancer pts with evidence of bone metastases. BMAs are adjunctive therapy, not recommended for 1st-line therapy and should be used concurrently for pain relief with analgesics, chemo, RT, and/or hormonal therapy. (*Van Poznack C et al., JCO 2011*)

Name 4 radionuclides used to treat bone mets.

Radionuclides available in the U.S. for Tx of bone mets:
1. Strontium-89
2. Samarium-153
3. Phosphorus-32
4. Radium-223 (currently for prostate cancer only)

For each of these radionuclides, name the method of decay, half-life, average particle energy per decay, and particle range.

	Sr-89	Sm-153	P-32	Ra-223
Decay method	β emission to Y-89	β and γ emission	β emission to S-32	α emission
Half-life	50.6 days	1.9 days	14.3 days	11.4 days
Avg decay energy	0.58 MeV	0.22 MeV	0.69 MeV	27.4 MeV
Range	7 mm	4 mm	8.5 mm	<0.1 mm

Describe the clinical implications of the differences in physical properties between strontium-89, samarium-153, phosphorus-32, and radium-223.

1. Both strontium-89 and phosphorus-32 emit β particles with higher energy than those of samarium-153, causing deeper tissue penetration. Though these higher-energy β particles may have a therapeutic benefit, they can also cause greater marrow toxicity.
2. The half-life of samarium-153 is much shorter than that of strontium-89. Thus, the planned RT dose from samarium-153 is delivered more quickly, leading to faster time to pain relief in many published trials.
3. Radium-223 emits high-energy α particles, which have high linear energy transfer inducing double-stranded DNA breaks, but a short range resulting in very limited toxic effects on adjacent healthy tissues.

Why is phosphorus-32 seldom used for bone mets?

Phosphorus-32 was the 1st radionuclide to be used for bone mets, but it has **greater hematologic toxicity** compared with the other radionuclides available in the U.S.

When should radionuclides be considered?

Radionuclides should be considered in pts with **adequate blood counts and multifocal painful bone mets** imaged on bone scan.

What are some contraindications to radionuclides for bone pain?

Contraindications for using radionuclides for bone pain:
1. Myelosuppression
2. Impaired renal function
3. Pregnancy
4. Cord compression
5. Nerve root compression
6. Impending pathologic fracture
7. Extensive soft tissue component

What randomized data support the use of samarium-153?

A **double-blind placebo controlled study** of samarium-153 supports its use. 118 pts with symptomatic bone mets were randomized to low-dose samarium-153 (0.5 mCi/kg), high-dose samarium-153 (1 mCi/kg), or placebo. Pts receiving high-dose samarium-153 had significant improvement in pain during the 1st 4 wks per pt and medical evaluation. Relief persisted until at least wk 16 in 43% of pts. There was a significant reduction in the pain score and analgesic use only in pts receiving the high dose. (*Serafini A et al., JCO 1998*)

What randomized data supports the use of radium-223?

ALSYMPCA is a multi-institution **double-blind placebo controlled study** of radium-223 that showed an **overall survival benefit** for pts with castrate-resistant metastatic prostate cancer (14.9 mos vs. 11.3 mos, p <0.001). Pts were randomized 2:1 to 6 IV injections of radium-223 (dose 50 kBq per kg) q4 weeks vs. placebo injections on the same schedule. The trial was stopped early due to OS benefit on planned interim analysis. (*Parker C et al., NEJM 2013*)

What RTOG study originally reported no difference in bone pain relief between different fractionation schemes?

RTOG 7402 randomized 759 pts. Those with solitary bone mets were randomized to 40.5 Gy (2.7 Gy × 15) vs. 20 Gy (4 Gy × 5). Pts with multiple mets were randomized to 30 Gy (3 Gy × 10), 15 Gy (3 Gy × 5), 20 Gy (4 Gy × 5), or 25 Gy (5 Gy × 5). The initial report revealed that 90% of pts had some pain relief, and 54% had eventual CR of pain. There was no difference between regimens. (*Tong D et al., Cancer 1982*) Reanalysis showed that a higher # of fx correlated with CR of pain, suggesting that a more protracted course was more effective. The analysis was based only on physician assessment of pain. (*Blitzer P et al., Cancer 1985*)

Which pts are generally excluded from RCTs of different fractionations for bone-met RT?

RCTs assessing different fractionation schemes for the Tx of bone mets have generally excluded **pts with cord compression and pathologic fracture.**

Did the study by the Bone Pain Trial Working Party support single- or multi-fx Tx of bone mets?

The Bone Pain Trial Working Party supported **single-fx** Tx. The study (UK/NZ) randomized 765 pts with painful bone mets to 8 Gy × 1 vs. a protracted regimen (2 Gy × 5 or 3 Gy × 10). Pain relief was evaluated for up to 1 yr post-Tx by the use of a validated pt questionnaire. There was no difference in pain control between the arms. Re-Tx was twice as common with single-fx Tx (23% vs. 10%), though this may have been due to a greater willingness to re-treat pts who rcvd only 8 Gy × 1. (*No author, Radiother Oncol 1999*)

Did the Dutch Bone Metastasis Study support single- or multi-fx Tx of bone mets?

The Dutch Bone Metastasis Study supported **single-fx** Tx. 1,171 pts were randomized to 8 Gy × 1 fx vs. 4 Gy × 6 fx. Pain relief was evaluated for up to 2 yrs post-Tx by the use of a validated pt questionnaire. No difference was seen with respect to pain relief. However, re-Tx was more common in the single-fx arm (25% vs. 7%). (*Steenland E et al., Radiother Oncol 1999*) Reanalysis suggested that the higher rate of re-Tx in the single-fx arm may be related to a greater willingness to re-Tx pts who rcvd only 8 Gy × 1 fx. (*Van der Linden YM et al., IJROBP 2004*)

Did RTOG 9714 support single- or multi-fx Tx of bone mets?

RTOG 9714 supported **single-fx Tx.** The study randomized 898 pts with breast or prostate cancer to 8 Gy × 1 fx vs. 3 Gy × 10 fx. There was no difference in complete pain relief (15% vs. 18%) or partial pain relief (50% vs. 48%), but there was increased acute toxicity in the 3 Gy × 10 arm (10% vs. 17%). The re-Tx rate was significantly greater in the 8 Gy × 1 arm. (*Hartsell W et al., JNCI 2005*)

What were the results of the *Chow et al.* meta-analysis of trials comparing single- vs. multi-fx Tx of bone mets?

In this meta-analysis of trials comparing single- vs. multi-fx Tx of bone mets, no significant differences between fractionation schemes with respect to pain control were shown. However, re-Tx was more common with single-fx Tx. (*Chow et al., JCO 2007*)

What study supported use of hemibody irradiation (HBI) after focal RT for bone mets?

RTOG 8206 randomized pts treated with focal RT to HBI (8 Gy) vs. no further Tx. HBI increased the time to progression as well as the time to re-Tx. (*Poulter C et al., IJROBP 1992*)

What are the published response rates of RT for palliation of symptomatic bone mets irrespective of the fractionation scheme?

The published response rates of RT for palliation of symptomatic bone mets are **60%–80%.**

What is the benefit of PORT after orthopedic stabilization?

PORT following orthopedic stabilization of impending or pathologic fracture decreases the need for 2nd surgery (2% vs. 15%) and increases the rate of regaining normal function (53% vs. 11.5%) as compared with surgery alone. (*Townsend P et al., JCO 1994*)

What data support the use of SRS for spinal mets?

Prospective nonrandomized data from the **University of Pittsburgh** support the use of SRS for spinal mets. 500 cases were treated with CyberKnife to a median dose of 20 Gy. SRS improved pain in 86% of cases (defined as a 3-point improvement on a 10-point pain scale). The majority of pts had prior Tx; however, in the 65 cases treated with SRS as the primary modality, the LC was 90%. (*Gerstzen P et al., Spine 2007*)

What is the MS of pts with metastatic cancer who present for palliative RT?

Risk factors: (1) nonbreast primary, (2) sites of mets other than bone, (3) KPS ≤60.

# of risk factors	MS
0–1	~60 wks
2	~25 wks
3	~10 wks

(*Chow E et al., JCO 2008*)

▶ TOXICITY

What are the expected acute and late RT toxicities associated with Tx of bone mets?	Potential toxicities from focal RT for bone mets: Acute: skin irritation Late: fibrosis, nerve damage, fracture, lymphedema
What is the main toxicity of radionuclide Tx?	Radionuclide Tx can cause **significant myelosuppression.**

89 Cord Compression

Updated by Jason D. Kehrer and Bronwyn R. Stall

▶ BACKGROUND

What % of cancer pts develop cord compression?	**5%–10%** of cancer pts develop cord compression.
What is the median survival in pts with cord compression?	Median survival in pts with cord compression is ~3 mos (dependent on Hx of primary, extent of visceral/osseous met, degree of motor dysfunction, and performance status)
What is the most important prognostic factor?	Pre-Tx ambulatory status directly influences functional outcome and survival.
What are 3 routes of metastatic spread to the spine?	Routes of metastatic spread to the spine: hematogenous, direct extension, and CSF. (*Abeloff MD et al., Abeloff's Clin Oncol. 4th ed. 2008*)
What malignancies commonly cause cord compression?	Lung, breast, and prostate each account for 15%–20% of cases, whereas renal cell, lymphoma, and multiple myeloma each account for 5%–10% of cases of cord compression.
What is the most common site of origin?	Cord compression origin: epidural (extradural) in 95% > leptomeningeal (intradural extramedullary) in 4%–5% > intramedullary in 0.5%–1%
How do pts with cord compression present?	Presenting Sx of cord compression: back pain, radicular pain, weakness, sensory deficits, bowel/bladder dysfunction, and paralysis

What is the most common presenting Sx of cord compression?	The most common Sx of cord compression is **back pain** present in 90%–95% of pts (often precedes neurologic Sx > 2 mos).
Describe the presentation of cauda equina syndrome?	Presenting Sx of cauda equina syndrome: pain, lower extremity weakness, sensory disturbance ("saddle anesthesia"), and autonomic dysfunction including urinary retention and fecal incontinence
What is the pathophysiology of cord compression?	Gradual progression results in epidural venous congestion, vasogenic edema, and demyelination (potentially reversible) while rapid progression results in disruption of arterial blood resulting in ischemia and cord infarction (irreversible)
What part of the vertebra is most commonly involved by metastatic Dz?	Metastatic Dz typically involves the **vertebral body** rather than the posterior elements. Compression originates directly from the vertebrae (85%–90%) or via neural foramina extension (5%–10%)
What part of the spine is most often involved in cord compression?	The **thoracic** spine (70%) is most commonly affected by cord compression > lumbosacral (20%) > cervical (10%).

▶ WORKUP/STAGING

Describe the workup of cord compression.	Cord compression workup: H&P with careful attention to complete neurologic exam to include DRE, evaluation of sensation to determine level of the lesion, assessment of pain, prior cancer management to include prior RT, assessment of bowel/bladder function, and screening MRI spine
Why is a screening MRI of the spine ordered to evaluate cord compression?	Pts with suspected cord compression should be evaluated with a screening MRI of the spine b/c **multilevel involvement is not uncommon.**
Is a gadolinium-enhanced MRI necessary to evaluate cord compression?	No, it is not required to diagnose epidural compression. Contrast improves identification of leptomeningeal and intramedullary mets.
Why is CT useful in evaluating cord compression?	CT evaluation of spinal cord compression **helps to delineate osseous structures,** including retropulsed fragments, and **aids in surgical planning.**

▶ TREATMENT/PROGNOSIS

What modalities are used to treat spinal cord compression?	Modalities used to treat spinal cord compression: steroids, surgery, and RT

What is the initial management of cord compression?

For initial management of cord compression, start dexamethasone (include GI prophylaxis with proton-pump inhibitor or H2 blocker) and consult neurosurgery or orthopedics, depending on the institution, to assess spine stability.

What initial bolus dose of dexamethasone should be used in cord compression?

For newly diagnosed cord compression, a loading dose of 10 mg IV is generally given → 4 mg orally q6hrs. *Vecht CJ et al.* randomized 37 pts to 10 mg IV vs. 100 mg IV, both → 16 mg daily in divided oral doses. There was no difference in pain control, rate of ambulation, or bladder function. (*Neurology 1989*)

Historically, what type of surgery was used to treat spinal cord compression?

Historically, **laminectomy** was used to treat spinal cord compression. However, this was abandoned b/c it can lead to instability, and improved surgical stabilization techniques have allowed for anterior decompressive approaches.

What pts with cord compression are appropriate for decompressive surgery?

Pts with MRI evidence of cord compression in a single area and a life expectancy >3 mos who do not have radiosensitive tumors (lymphomas, leukemias, germ cell tumors, multiple myeloma) may be good candidates for decompressive surgery → RT. (*Patchell R et al., Lancet 2005*)

What are further indications for surgery?

Spinal instability and/or bony retropulsion, previous RT, Dz progression despite RT, unknown primary tumor (therapeutic and diagnostic), paraplegia <48 hrs

What was the trial design and outcome of the Patchell study of decompressive surgery for cord compression?

The Patchell cord compression trial was a multi-institutional RCT of 101 pts with MRI-confirmed spinal cord compression restricted to a single area with >3-mo life expectancy. Exclusion criteria included being paraplegic >48 hrs, radiosensitive tumors, Hx of prior cord compression, and other pre-existing neurologic conditions. Pts were randomized to decompressive surgery + RT vs. RT alone. RT was 30 Gy/10 delivered to the lesion + 1 vertebral body above and below. Surgery was tailored to the individual lesion to provide circumferential decompression and stabilization as needed (anterior corpectomy for 60% of cases involving only the vertebral body). The study was stopped at interim analysis. Surgery significantly improved the ambulatory rate (84% vs. 57%), duration of ambulatory status (122 days vs. 13 days), and survival (122 days vs. 100 days). Pts nonambulatory prior to Tx were more likely to walk after surgery (62% vs. 19%). (*Patchell R et al., Lancet 2005*)

What are some criticisms of the Patchell data?

RT alone results were worse than historical prospective controls, small sample size, 18 pts in the RT alone group had an "unstable" spine, surgery provides immediate decompression in pts with rapid onset of Sx (delayed response with RT).

Can surgery be delayed following RT?

Due to a decline in neurologic function (nonambulatory), 10 pts in the radiation group (20%) underwent surgery; 3 regained the ability to walk (30%) with results inferior to surgery upfront

Is SBRT utilized for primary Tx of cord compression?

No, direct tumor contact with the spinal cord (epidural compression within 3 mm) and/or spinal instability are contraindications.

What pts with cord compression should be treated with RT alone?

Cord compression pts treated with RT alone: life expectancy <3 mos, no spinal instability or bony compression, multilevel involvement and radiosensitive tumor

Does the interval between development of motor deficits and RT predict response?

Yes, a longer time interval results in **improved** functional outcome. A retrospective review of 96 pts demonstrated improved function in 86% of pts when motor Sx were present >14 days. In contrast, only 10% improved when Sx were present <7 days. (*Rades D et al., IJROBP 1999*)

How are conventional RT fields arranged to treat the cervical, thoracic, and lumbar spine?

Field arrangement for cord compression:
  Cervical: opposed lats
  Thoracic: AP/PA or PA alone, respecting cord
    tolerance
  Lumbar: AP/PA

Encompass the lesion + 1–2 vertebral levels above and below.

Are there data to support the use of hypofractionation for cord compression?

Marranzano et al. enrolled 300 pts with metastatic spinal cord compression and short life expectancy (≤6 mos) randomized to short-course (8 Gy × 2 fx, 1-wk apart) or split-course (5 Gy × 3 fx, 4-day rest, and then 3 Gy × 5 fx). No significant difference was observed between the 2 schedules with median follow-up of 33 mos (response, duration of response, survival or toxicity). (*JCO 2005*) A follow-up trial randomized 327 pts to 8 Gy × 2 fx (1 wk apart) vs. 8 Gy × 1 fx without a difference in outcome. No myelopathy was registered with a median follow-up of 31 mos. (*Radiother Oncol 2009*)

Is reirradiation possible with recurrent cord compression?

Rades et al. reviewed the outcome of 124 pts with in-field recurrence (69% ambulatory) with improvement in 36% and stable motor function in 50% with reirradiation. No radiation myelopathy was observed at a median follow-up of 11 mos with cumulative biological effective dose ≤120 Gy_2 in 92%. (*Cancer 2008*)

What are potential acute toxicities of RT for cord compression?	Potential toxicities of RT for cord compression: odynophagia, globus, esophagitis, nausea, diarrhea, myelosuppression, rare spinal cord injury

90 Superior Vena Cava Syndrome

Updated by Delnora L. Erickson and Bronwyn R. Stall

▶ **BACKGROUND**

What vessels form the SVC?	The **right and left brachiocephalic veins** join to form the SVC.
What is SVC syndrome?	SVC syndrome is extrinsic or intrinsic obstruction of blood flow through the SVC, leading to proximal congestion.
Describe the course of the SVC.	The SVC begins at the **sternal angle,** extends inferiorly along the right lat side of the ascending aorta, and inserts into the right atrium.
What predisposes the SVC to compression?	The SVC is a thin-walled vessel with relatively low intravascular pressure and is therefore susceptible to compression by **surrounding rigid structures** including enlarged LNs and the trachea, sternum, pulmonary artery, and right main stem bronchus.
What vessels form the collateral system of the SVC?	The collateral system of SVC is formed by the azygos, mammary, vertebral, lat thoracic, paraspinous, and esophageal vessels.
What vessels join to form the azygos vein?	The **right subcostal and right ascending lumbar veins** coalesce to form the azygos vein.

What is the most common cause of SVC syndrome?

Malignancy is the most common cause of SVC syndrome accounting for ~60% of cases. Malignancy previously accounted for 90% of cases, but with increased use of implantable intravenous devices (i.e., central venous catheters, pacemaker leads), this has decreased. (*McCurdy M et al., Crit Care Med 2012*)

Name 5 benign causes of SVC syndrome.

Benign causes of SVC syndrome:
1. Catheter-induced thrombosis
2. Chronic mediastinitis
3. Retrosternal goiter
4. CHF
5. Aortic aneurysm

Name 6 cancers most commonly associated with SVC syndrome, in decreasing order of incidence.

Cancers associated with SVC syndrome:
1. Non–small cell lung cancer (NSCLC): 50%
2. Small cell lung cancer (SCLC): 22%
3. Lymphoma: 12%
4. Mets: 9%
5. Germ cell tumors: 3%
6. Thymoma: 2%

(*Wilson L et al., NEJM 2007*)

Are NSCLC or SCLC pts more likely to develop SVC syndrome?

SCLC pts are more likely to develop SVC syndrome than NSCLC pts b/c of their propensity toward rapid growth in central airways.

What is the most common cause of SVC syndrome in pts <50 yo?

In pts <50 yo, the most common cause of SVC syndrome is **lymphoma.**

Which types of NHL are associated with SVC syndrome?

NHL types associated with SVC syndrome:
1. Diffuse large B-cell lymphoma
2. Lymphoblastic lymphoma
3. Primary mediastinal B-cell lymphoma with sclerosis

What is the typical duration of Sx prior to presentation with SVC syndrome?

Pts with SVC syndrome may have Sx over days to wks but usually present **within 1 mo of onset.**

Do most pts presenting with SVC syndrome have a prior cancer Dx?

No. Most pts presenting with SVC syndrome do not have a prior cancer Dx.

Why is SVC syndrome considered an emergency?

SVC syndrome **may cause airway obstruction and cerebral edema;** however, severe Sx are uncommon, and life-threatening Sx are rare.

What are the common presenting Sx of SVC syndrome?

Presenting Sx of SVC syndrome:
1. Face and neck swelling
2. Upper extremity swelling
3. Cough/stridor
4. Dyspnea
5. Dilated chest veins

(*Rice T et al., Medicine 2006*)

What is the most common Sx of SVC syndrome?	The most common Sx of SVC syndrome is **facial swelling.**
What physical exam findings are associated with SVC syndrome?	Signs of SVC syndrome: plethora, facial edema, jugular venous distension, and visible collateral venous drainage on the ant chest

▶ **WORKUP/STAGING**

Describe the workup of SVC syndrome.	SVC syndrome workup: H&P, assessment of respiratory status, CXR and/or CT chest with contrast (best to visualize the extent of blockage), determination of the best Bx route if Dx is unknown, labs (AFP, LDH, β-HCG), and BM aspirate and Bx
Name 5 ways to obtain tissue Dx for SVC syndrome.	Methods to obtain tissue Dx in SVC syndrome: 1. Sputum cytology 2. Bx of palpable LNs 3. Bronchoscopy 4. Mediastinoscopy 5. Video-assisted thorascopic surgery
What is usually seen on CXR in SVC syndrome?	CXR findings in SVC syndrome include a widened mediastinum and the presence of a mass near the SVC.
What CT finding is closely associated with SVC syndrome?	The **presence of collateral vessels** is a CT finding that closely relates to SVC syndrome.
Why should RT not be given prior to a histologic Dx in SVC syndrome?	RT **may obscure the histologic Dx** and should be deferred until diagnostic Bx is obtained in SVC syndrome. However, empiric Tx may be considered in the setting of airway obstruction or cerebral edema.

▶ **TREATMENT/PROGNOSIS**

What is the 1st step in Tx of SVC syndrome?	The 1st step in treating SVC syndrome is to **establish a pathologic Dx,** which will determine further interventions.
What Tx may be used for SVC syndrome?	SVC syndrome Tx: RT, chemo, surgery, and stents
What supportive measures can be taken to manage SVC syndrome?	Elevation of head of bed and supplemental oxygen. Diuretics can be used for cerebral edema. (*McCurdy M et al., Crit Care Med 2012*)
What is the role of steroids in SVC syndrome?	Steroids are **frequently used** in SVC syndrome, but there are limited data to support their use except in lymphoma and thymoma.

In which malignant causes of SVC syndrome is chemo 1ˢᵗ-line Tx?

Chemo is the Tx of choice in SVC syndrome caused by **lymphoma, germ cell tumors, and SCLC.**

What is the most rapid way to manage SVC thrombosis?

The most rapid method to manage SVC thrombosis is by **intraluminal stenting.**

What Tx should be considered if a pt with SVC syndrome presents with thrombosis?

Use **anticoagulation therapy** for pts with SVC syndrome presenting with thrombosis unless contraindications are present.

Which pts with SVC syndrome require emergent Tx?

SVC syndrome pts with central airway compromise, severe laryngeal edema, or coma secondary to cerebral edema require emergent Tx.

What fractionation is used to emergently treat SVC syndrome?

Fractionation for emergent SVC Tx is **2.5–4 Gy × 3 fx.** There are conflicting retrospective data on the benefit of hypofractionation.

When treating SVC syndrome, what should the RT fields encompass?

RT fields for SVC syndrome include encompassing gross Dz and adjacent nodal tissue while respecting normal tissue toxicity, esp the lungs and heart.

What should guide the total RT dose used for SVC syndrome?

The total RT dose for SVC syndrome depends on the **underlying histology** (i.e., lung cancers are treated to ≥60 Gy, while lymphomas are treated to 35–45 Gy).

Does SVC syndrome portend a bad prognosis?

No. The prognosis in SVC syndrome depends on the underlying cause rather than the presence of the syndrome itself. Median survival is about 6 mos for cancer-induced SVC syndrome. However, based on etiology, many will survive longer or even be cured.

What is the overall symptomatic response to RT in SVC syndrome?

The overall response rate to RT for SVC syndrome is **~60%.**

Over what approximate timeline can pts expect symptom relief from RT?

Normally, response time to RT is **7–15 days,** but in some cases, relief may be experienced as soon as 72 hours. (*Wan J et al., Emerg Med Clin N Am 2009*)

Does RT for SVC syndrome restore normal flow in the SVC?

No. RT for SVC syndrome does not generally restore normal vascular flow despite improving Sx.

What non-Tx event likely contributes to symptomatic improvement in SVC syndrome?

The **development of collateral vessels** largely contributes to Sx improvement in SVC syndrome.

What is the Tx if RT or chemo are not effective?

Vascular stents are recommended, with angioplasty 1ˢᵗ if the lumen needs to be expanded.

TOXICITY

What are potential acute toxicities of emergent RT for SVC syndrome?

Potential acute toxicities of emergent RT for SVC syndrome: fatigue, skin irritation, cough, esophagitis

What are potential subacute and chronic toxicities of RT for SVC syndrome?

Potential subacute and chronic toxicities of RT for SVC syndrome: RT pneumonitis, pericarditis, pulmonary fibrosis, esophageal stenosis

Part XV Benign Disease

91 Heterotopic Ossification Prophylaxis

Updated by Jing Zeng and Michael J. Swartz

▶ BACKGROUND

What is heterotopic ossification (HO)?

HO refers to **abnl bone formation outside the skeleton.** It often appears after trauma or surgery in periarticular soft tissue and is commonly associated with injury to the hip.

What are common Sx of HO?

In HO, **functional impairment** such as joint stiffness is the most common Sx. **Pain** can also occur, beginning as early as a few days after surgery.

What is the etiology of HO?

The etiology of HO is not completely understood. It is assumed that pluri potent mesenchymal cells present in periarticular soft tissue and develop into osteoblastic stem cells, which then produce bone.

What are the highest risk factors for developing HO?

Pts who already have ipsi or contralat HO carry the greatest risk of developing further HO. Their risk is 80%–100%. Pts with osteophytes at the femoral head and socket, acetabular fractures, ankylosing spondylitis, and other hyperostosis conditions of the skeleton also carry a high risk for HO. This condition is more common in males than in females.

▶ WORKUP/STAGING

How soon after surgery can radiologic evidence of HO be detected?

Radiologic evidence of HO can be detected **2–6 wks** after surgery as calcified structures with blurred contours on x-ray. Bone scans typically show increased uptake in the soft tissues adjacent to the hip and can detect HO several days before it becomes apparent on plain film.

593

What is the most common staging system used for HO?	The most common staging system used for HO was developed by *Brooker et al.*

Grade 1: bone islands in soft tissue around hip

Grade 2: exophytes in pelvis or proximal end of femur with at least 1 cm between opposing bone surfaces

Grade 3: exophytes in pelvis or proximal end of femur with <1 cm between opposing bone surfaces

Grade 4: bony ankylosis between proximal femur and pelvis

Grades 3–4 are considered clinically relevant even if there is no pain or impaired mobility.

▶ TREATMENT/PROGNOSIS

What is the role of surgery in the Tx of HO?

Clinically relevant HO should be surgically removed. The risk of subsequent recurrence may be lower if the ectopic bone is removed after it has reached maturity. At the time of surgery, prophylaxis against future HO should be taken.

Other than RT, are there any other effective methods for prophylaxis against HO?

For prophylaxis against HO, **indomethacin and ibuprofen** (prostaglandin synthesis inhibitors) have been shown to decrease the incidence of HO compared to placebo. (*Fransen M et al., Cochrane Database Syst Rev 2004*)

What should be the RT dose and fractionation for prophylaxis against HO?

There have been multiple randomized trials and retrospective series on the RT dose and fractionation for prophylaxis against HO:

Sylvester J et al. (*IJROBP 1988*) compared 20 Gy × 10 fx vs. 10 Gy × 5 fx, and *Pellegrini V et al.* (*J Bone Joint Surg Am 1992*) looked at 8 Gy × 1 fx vs. 10 Gy × 5 fx. There were no significant differences between those doses and fractionation schemes. More recent studies looked at using lower doses.

Healy W et al. (*J Bone Joint Surg Am 1995*) compared 7 Gy × 1 fx against 5.5 Gy and concluded that 5.5 Gy is not a sufficient dose.

Padgett D et al. (*J Arthroplasty 2003*) looked at 5 Gy × 2 fx or 10 Gy × 5 fx. There was a trend toward increased HO of any grade in the 5-Gy group.

What is the efficacy of preop RT for HO prophylaxis compared with PORT? What are the advantages and disadvantages of preop RT vs. PORT?

In 1 study, preop RT at 7–8 Gy × 1 fx gave the same rates of prophylaxis as the same dose given PORT. (*Gregoritch S et al., IJROBP 1994*) Preop RT decreases pt discomfort associated with transport and positioning for RT but is often not feasible due to scheduling issues.

How soon should PORT be given after surgery for prophylaxis against HO?

PORT prophylaxis against HO should be given **no later than 4 days and ideally within 3 days** of surgery. (*Seegenschmiedt M et al., IJROBP 2001*)

What is the timeframe for giving preop RT for HO prophylaxis?

The randomized trial comparing preop RT vs. PORT for HO prophylaxis using 7–8 Gy × 1 fx (*Gregoritch S et al., IJROBP 1994*) gave preop RT within 4 hrs of surgery. Other nonrandomized series have suggested that preop RT can be given as early as 8 hrs preop without a significant decrease in efficacy. (*Seegenschmiedt M et al., IJROBP 2001*)

Are there randomized trials comparing RT against indomethacin in HO prophylaxis?

Yes. Burd T et al. (*J Bone Joint Surg Am 2001*) randomized 166 pts to rcv either indomethacin or RT postoperatively for HO prophylaxis. Grades 3–4 HO occurred in 14% of the indomethacin group as compared with 7% of the RT group, but the results were not SS ($p = 0.22$).

A meta-analysis by **Pakos E et al.** (*IJROBP 2004*) looked at 7 randomized trials comparing RT vs. NSAIDs. They concluded that RT postop >6 Gy tended to be more effective than NSAIDs in preventing Brooker grade 3 or 4 HO, but the absolute difference was only 1.2%.

What is the typical RT field for HO prophylaxis?

The RT fields for HO prophylaxis typically includes the usual area at risk for HO. When treating the hip for HO prophylaxis, the cranial border is usually 3 cm above the acetabulum and inferiorly includes two-thirds of the shaft of the implant. Field size is usually around 14 × 14 cm. The prosthesis may be blocked from RT if a cementless fixation is used, but observational data suggest that this blocking strategy is associated with higher rates of subsequent HO.

▶ TOXICITY

What are the rates of increased wound-healing complications after RT for HO prophylaxis?

RT for HO prophylaxis has not been associated with an increased incidence of wound-healing complications.

Is there an increased risk of nonfixation of cementless implants after RT for HO prophylaxis?

No. There is not an increased risk of nonfixation of cementless implants after RT for HO prophylaxis based on multiple studies. (*Seegenschmiedt M et al., IJROBP 2001*) Animal studies have shown a transient decrease in force required to remove an implant after RT, but this difference resolved by wk 3 (*Konski A et al., IJROBP 1990*).

What is the rate of RT-induced tumor after RT for HO prophylaxis?	There is 1 case report of a RT-induced tumor after RT for HO prophylaxis. (*Farris M et al., Radiat Oncol 2012*) The rarity is thought to be the effect of both low doses of RT as well as an older pt population. As RT is employed for younger pts, this concern is worth considering.

92 Keloids

Updated by Jing Zeng and Michael J. Swartz

▶ BACKGROUND

What is a keloid?	A keloid is a **benign fibroproliferative growth** resulting from a connective tissue response to a variety of proposed factors such as surgery, burns, trauma, inflammation, foreign body reactions, endocrine dysfunction, and occasional spontaneous occurrence.
Is there a racial predilection for keloid formation?	**Yes. People of African descent** are more likely to be predisposed to keloid formation than other ethnic groups. Any skin insult (piercings, lacerations, infected skin lesions, surgery) can cause keloid formation in predisposed individuals. Less commonly, lesions can occur de novo.
Name 3 common locations for keloids.	Keloids most commonly affect areas of increased skin tension such as the ears, neck, jaw, presternal chest, shoulders, and upper back.
Name 3 Sx commonly associated with keloids.	Keloids can be asymptomatic but often are pruritic, tender to palpation, or occasionally cause pain.

▶ WORKUP/STAGING

What is the difference between a keloid and a hypertrophic scar?	Hypertrophic scars may initially appear similar to keloids but do not extend beyond the margins of the scar. Keloids are more infiltrative and can cause a local reaction such as pain and inflammation. Hypertrophic scars are much less likely to recur after resection.

▶ **TREATMENT/PROGNOSIS**

What are the indications for RT in keloid Tx?

The indications for RT in keloid Tx include demonstrated recurrence after resection, marginal or incomplete resection, an unfavorable location, or a larger lesion.

Within what timeframe should RT be given postop after keloid resection?

PORT for keloids should be initiated **within 24 hrs** after resection.

What is the typical target RT volume for keloid Tx?

The typical target RT volume for keloid Tx is **scar + a 1-cm safety margin.**

What is the typical RT dose and fractionation for keloids?

The typical RT dose and fractionation for keloids is **12–16 Gy in 3–4 fx.** Single doses of 7.5–10 Gy are also effective. (*Ragoowansi R et al., Plast Reconstr Surg 2003*) Some series suggest that a dose of at least 9 Gy is required to maximize the benefit from RT. (*Lo T et al., Radiother Oncol 1990; Doornbos J et al., IJROBP 1990*) Another series from Pittsburgh suggests that doses of at least 5–6 Gy per fx for 3 fx may be needed for 90%–95% control for earlobe keloids and 7–8 Gy per fx for 3 fx may be needed for similar control at other sites. (*Flickinger J, IJROBP 2011*)

What RT modalities can be used in the Tx of keloids?

For RT Tx of keloids, the most common modalities are **lower megavoltage electrons, kilovoltage photons, or brachytherapy.**

Name 7 Tx options for keloids other than surgery and RT.

Tx options for keloids other than surgery and RT include steroid injections, pressure earrings, silicone gel sheeting, cryosurgery, laser therapy, imiquimod, and injections of fluorouracil or verapamil.

What is the recurrence rate for keloids after PORT?

The recurrence rate for keloids after PORT is typically **10%–35%.** This can vary depending on the size, location, extent of excision, etiology, and other factors.

Is there any randomized data comparing surgery + RT against surgery + steroid injection?

Yes. A prospective randomized trial conducted by *Sclafani A et al.* looked at a series of 31 pts, comparing PORT vs. intralesional steroid injection. The recurrence rate after surgery + RT was 12.5%; the recurrence rate after surgery + steroid injection was 33%. (*Dermatol Surg 1996*)

For unresectable keloids, what is the efficacy of using RT alone?

Malaker K et al. looked at 86 keloids in 64 pts treated with RT alone. 97% had significant regression 18 mos after completing radiotherapy. 63% of the pts surveyed were very happy with the outcome of their Tx. (*Clin Oncol 2004*)

TOXICITY

What are the most common side effects after RT for keloids?

The most common side effects of RT for keloids are **hyperpigmentation, pruritus, and erythema.**

Is there a risk of radiation-induced malignancy after treatment for keloid?

There are a few anecdotal reports in the medical literature of malignant tumors developing in association with radiotherapy for keloid formation, but this outcome is extremely rare. Caution is warranted and risks should be discussed when considering radiotherapy for keloids in the very young and in particular for lesions involving the chest or breast tissue in young females. (*Botwood N et al., Br J Radiol 1999*)

Normal Tissue Constraint Guidelines

The radiation dose constraints below are meant to serve as a guide only and may not be applicable to all clinical scenarios. Most doses are derived from randomized studies or consensus guidelines and we have attempted to provide the sources for these recommendations. Please refer to the individual pediatric chapters for dose constraints in the pediatric population as these can vary greatly from protocol to protocol and tend to be particularly site and age dependent.

What are the recommended dose constraints for the following organs and clinical scenarios?	
Organ	*Constraints*
CNS (1.8–2.0 Gy/fx)	
Spinal cord	**max 50 Gy** (full cord cross-section); tolerance increases by 25% 6 mos after 1st course (for reirradiation) (QUANTEC); for hyperfractionation (1.5 Gy bid up to 45 Gy for small cell lung cancer), dose ≤41 Gy (RTOG 0538)
Brain	**max 72 Gy** (partial brain); avoid >2 Gy/fx or hyperfractionation (QUANTEC)
Chiasm/optic nerves	**max 55 Gy** (QUANTEC)
Brainstem	**entire brainstem <54 Gy, V59 Gy <1–10 cc** (QUANTEC)
Eyes (globe)	**mean <35 Gy** (RTOG 0225), **max 54 Gy** (RTOG 0615)
Lens	**max 7 Gy** (RTOG 0539)
Retina	**max 50 Gy** (RTOG 0539)
Lacrimal gland	**max 40 Gy** (Parsons)
Inner ear/cochlea	**mean ≤45 Gy** (consider constraining to ≤35 Gy with concurrent cisplatin) (QUANTEC)
Pituitary gland	**max 45 Gy** (for panhypopituitarism, lower for GH deficiency) (LENT)
Cauda equina	**max 60 Gy** (LENT)

What are the recommended dose constraints for the following organs and clinical scenarios? *(Continued)*

Organ	Constraints
CNS (single fraction)	
Spinal cord	**max 13 Gy** (if 3 fxs, max 20 Gy) (QUANTEC)
CNS (single fraction)	
Brain	**V12 Gy <5–10 cc** (QUANTEC)
Chiasm/optic nerves	**max 10 Gy** (QUANTEC)
Brainstem	**max 12.5 Gy** (QUANTEC)
Sacral plexus	**V18 <0.035 cc, V14.4 <5 cc** (RTOG 0631)
	V16 <0.035 cc, V14 <5 cc (RTOG 0631)
H&N (1.8–2.0 Gy/fx)	
Parotid gland(s)	**mean <25 Gy** (both glands) or **mean <20 Gy** (1 gland) (QUANTEC)
Submandibular gland(s)	**mean <35 Gy** (QUANTEC)
Larynx	**mean ≤44 Gy, V50 ≤27%, max 63–66 Gy** (when risk of tumor involvement is limited) (QUANTEC)
TMJ/mandible	**max 70 Gy** (if not possible, then V75 <1 cc) (RTOG 0615)
Oral cavity	nonoral cavity cancer: **mean <30 Gy,** avoid hot spots >60 Gy (RTOG 0920) oral cavity cancer: **mean <50 Gy,** V55 <1 cc, max 65 Gy (RTOG 0920)
Esophagus (cervical)	**V45 <33%** (RTOG 0920)
Pharyngeal constrictors	**mean <50 Gy** (QUANTEC)
Thyroid	**mean <30 Gy** for hypothyroidism (Monnier)
Thoracic (1.8–2.0 Gy/fx)	
Brachial plexus	**max 66 Gy, V60 <5%** (RTOG 0619)
Lung (combined lung for lung cancer treatment)	**mean <20–23 Gy, V20 <30%–35%** (QUANTEC)
Lung (ipsilateral lung for breast cancer treatment)	**V20 <15%, V10 <35%, V5 <50%** (RTOG 1005)
Single lung (after pneumonectomy)	**V5 <60%, V20 <4%–10%, MLD <8 Gy** (QUANTEC)
Bronchial tree	**max 80 Gy** (QUANTEC)
Heart (lung cancer treatment)	**V40 ≤80%; V45 ≤60%; V60 ≤30%; mean ≤35 Gy** (NCCN 2014)
Heart (breast cancer treatment)	**V25 <10%** (QUANTEC) **V20 <5%, V10 <30%, mean <4 Gy** (RTOG 1005)

What are the recommended dose constraints for the following organs and clinical scenarios? *(Continued)*	
Organ	**Constraints**
Esophagus	**V50 <32%** (Maguire), **V60 <33%** (LENT), mean <34 Gy (QUANTEC)
Thoracic (hypofractionation)	Total recommended cumulative dose by the number of fractions per NCCN 2014 (based on constraints used in RTOG 0618, 0813, 0915). Note: the max dose limits refer to volumes >0.035 cc (~3 mm³).
Spinal cord	1 fraction: 14 Gy 3 fractions: 18 Gy (6 Gy/fx) 4 fractions: 26 Gy (6.5 Gy/fx) 5 fractions: 30 Gy (6 Gy/fx)
Esophagus	1 fraction: 15.4 Gy 3 fractions: 30 Gy (10 Gy/fx) 4 fractions: 30 Gy (7.5 Gy/fx) 5 fractions: 32.5 Gy (6.5 Gy/fx)
Brachial plexus	1 fraction: 17.5 Gy 3 fractions: 21 Gy (7 Gy/fx) 4 fractions: 27.2 Gy (6.8 Gy/fx) 5 fractions: 30 Gy (6 Gy/fx)
Heart/pericardium	1 fraction: 22 Gy 3 fractions: 30 Gy (10 Gy/fx) 4 fractions: 34 Gy (8.5 Gy/fx) 5 fractions: 35 Gy (7 Gy/fx)
Great vessels	1 fraction: 37 Gy 3 fractions: 39 Gy (13 Gy/fx) 4 fractions: 49 Gy (12.25 Gy/fx) 5 fractions: 55 Gy (11 Gy/fx)
Trachea/large bronchus	1 fraction: 20.2 Gy 3 fractions: 30 Gy (10 Gy/fx) 4 fractions: 34.8 Gy (8.7 Gy/fx) 5 fractions: 32.5 Gy (6.5 Gy/fx)
Rib	1 fraction: 30 Gy 3 fractions: 30 Gy (10 Gy/fx) 4 fractions: 30 Gy (7.5 Gy/fx) 5 fractions: 32.5 Gy (6.5 Gy/fx)
Skin	1 fraction: 26 Gy 3 fractions: 30 Gy (10 Gy/fx) 4 fractions: 36 Gy (9 Gy/fx) 5 fractions: 40 Gy (8 Gy/fx)
Stomach	1 fraction: 12.4 Gy 3 fractions: 27 Gy (9 Gy/fx) 4 fractions: 30 Gy (7.5 Gy/fx) 5 fractions: 35 Gy (7 Gy/fx)

What are the recommended dose constraints for the following organs and clinical scenarios? *(Continued)*

Organ	Constraints
GI (1.8–2.0 Gy/fx)	
Stomach	**TD 5/5 whole stomach: 45 Gy** (QUANTEC)
Small bowel	**V45 <195 cc** (QUANTEC) **V15 <275 cc,** individual loops, with chemo (Banerjee) **V15 <830 cc,** peritoneal space, with chemo (Banerjee)
Liver (metastatic disease)	**mean liver <32 Gy** (liver = normal liver minus gross disease) (QUANTEC)
Liver (primary liver cancer)	**mean liver <28 Gy** (liver = normal liver minus gross disease) (QUANTEC)
Colon	**45 Gy, max dose 55 Gy** (LENT)
Kidney (bilateral)	**mean <18 Gy, V28 <20%, V23 <30%, V20 <32%, V12 <55%.** If mean kidney dose to 1 kidney >18 Gy, then constrain remaining kidney to V6 <30%. (QUANTEC)
GI (single fraction)	Dose constraints per RTOG 0631
Duodenum	**V16 <0.035 cc, V11.2 <5 cc**
Kidney (cortex)	**V8.4 <200 cc**
Kidney (hilum)	**V10.6 <66%**
Colon	**V14.3 <20 cc, V18.4 <0.035 cc**
Jejunum/ileum	**V15.4 <0.035 cc, V11.9 <5 cc**
Stomach	**V16 <0.035 cc, V11.2 <10 cc**
Rectum	**V18.4 <0.035 cc, V14.3 <20 cc**
GU (1.8–2.0 Gy/fx)	
Femoral heads	**V50 <5%** (RTOG GU Consensus)
Rectum	**V75 <15%, V70 <20%, V65 <25%, V60 <35%, V50 <50%** (QUANTEC)
Bladder	**V80 <15%, V75 <25%, V70 <35%, V65 <50%** (QUANTEC)
Testis	**V3 <50%** (RTOG 0630)
Penile bulb	**mean dose to 95% of the volume <50 Gy. D70 ≤70 Gy, D50 ≤50 Gy** (QUANTEC)

What are the recommended dose constraints for the following organs and clinical scenarios? *(Continued)*

Organ	*Constraints*
GU (LDR prostate brachytherapy)	
Urethra	urethral volume receiving a % of prescribed dose **(UV5) <150%, (UV30) <125%,** difficult to achieve in small (<20 cc) prostates (ABS 2012)
Rectum	volume of rectum receiving 100% of prescribed dose **(RV100) <1 cc** on day 1; **<1.3 cc** on day 30 (ABS 2012)
GYN	
Bladder point (cervical brachytherapy)	**max 80 Gy** (LDR equivalent dose) (ABS 2000)
Rectal point (cervical brachytherapy)	**max 75 Gy** (LDR equivalent dose) (ABS 2000)
Proximal vagina (mucosa) (cervical brachytherapy)	**max 120 Gy** (LDR equivalent dose) (Hintz)
Distal vagina (mucosa) (cervical brachytherapy)	**max 98 Gy** (LDR equivalent dose) (Hintz)

Sources: **ABS 2000:** American Brachytherapy Society consensus statement for HDR brachytherapy for cervical cancer (Nag S et al., *IJROBP* 1;48(1):201–211, 2000); **ABS 2012:** American Brachytherapy Society consensus statement for transrectal US-guided permanent prostate brachytherapy (Davis BJ et al., *Brachytherapy* 11:6–19, 2012); **Banerjee:** Small bowel dose parameters predicting grade ≥3 acute toxicity in rectal cancer patients treated with neoadjuvant chemoradiation: an independent validation study comparing peritoneal space vs small bowel loop contouring techniques (Banerjee R et al., *IJROBP* 1:85(5), 2013); **LENT:** Late Effects of Normal Tissues (LENT) Consensus Conference (*IJROBP* 31:5, 1995); **Hintz:** Radiation tolerance of the vaginal mucosa (Hintz BL et al., *IJROBP* 6(6): 711–716, 1980); **Maguire:** Clinical and dosimetric predictors of radiation-induced esophageal toxicity (Maguire PD et al., *IJROBP* 45:97–103, 1999); **Monnier:** Late effects of ionizing radiations on the thyroid gland (Monnier A, *Cancer Radiother* 1(6):717–731, 1997); **NCCN 2014:** www.nccn.org; **Parsons:** Response of the normal eye to high dose radiotherapy (Parsons JT et al., *Oncology* 10(6):837–847, 2006); **QUANTEC:** QUANTEC Consensus Guidelines (panel of experts, *IJROBP* 76(3), Suppl, 2010); **RTOG** protocols: www.rtog.org; **RTOG GU** consensus: RTOG GU Radiation oncology specialists reach consensus on pelvic lymph node volumes for high-risk prostate cancer (Lawton CA et al., *IJROBP* 74(2):383–387, 2009).

INDEX

Page numbers followed by "t" indicate table, and "f" indicate figure.

A

Abdominal mass of unclear etiology, 23
Abdominoperineal resection (APR), 357
Abiraterone, 392, 393
Acoustic neuromas (ANs), 124–128
Acral lentiginous, 546
ACTH-secreting adenoma, 107
Active surveillance, 370
Adamantinomatous craniopharyngioma, 68
Adenocarcinoma
    of cervix, 436
    cholangiocarcinoma, 334
    endometrial, 453
    esophagus, 298
    of gallbladder, 334
    gastric, 308
    NSCLC, 208, 209
    pancreatic, 316–327
    periampullary, 316–327
Adenoid cystic carcinoma, 174, 175
Adenomas
    pituitary, 113
    pleomorphic, 173
    villous, 341
Adenomatous polyposis coli (*APC*) tumor suppressor gene, 342
Adenopathy, painless, 484
Aggressive fibromatosis. *See* Desmoid tumors (DT)
AJCC (American Joint Committee on Cancer) staging
    anal cancer, 356
    bladder cancer, 402, 403
    bone tumors, 515, 518–519
    cervical cancer, 437
    cholangiocarcinoma, 336–338
    colorectal cancer, 343–344
    endometrial cancer, 454
    esophageal cancer, 299, 300
    gastric cancer, 310
    hepatocellular carcinoma, 329–330
    invasive breast cancer, 262

major salivary gland tumors, 176
maxillary tumors, 153
melanoma, 547–548
Merkel cell carcinoma, 561
mesothelioma, 252
nasopharyngeal cancer, 148
NSCLC, 212–213
ocular melanoma, 131
pancreatic adenocarcinoma, 320
papillary and follicular thyroid cancer, 193
penile cancer, 421
prostate cancer, 368–369
renal cell carcinoma, 431
soft tissue sarcoma, 528
squamous cell carcinoma, 555
testicular tumors, 410–411
urethral cancers, 427
Albinism, 554
Allogeneic transplants, 508–509. *See also* Transplant
Anal canal, 354
Anal cancer, 353–362
Anal verge, 354
Androgen deprivation therapy (ADT), 386, 389, 396
Androgen suppression (AS), 391, 392, 394
Ann Arbor staging system
    eye lymphomas, 137
    Hodgkin disease, 476–477
    for MALT lymphoma of GI tract, 492
    of non-Hodgkin lymphoma, 485–486
ANs. *See* Acoustic neuromas (ANs)
Ant compartment dissection, 203
Anterolateral neck dissection, 202
Antiandrogens (AAs), 392, 394
Antibiotics, in MALT lymphoma, 493
Anticoagulation therapy, 591
Ant neck dissection, 202
Arctan, 55
Argon plasma coagulation, 301
Arteriovenous malformation (AVMs), 120–123
Asbestos exposure, and mesothelioma, 250
ASCUS (Atypical Squamous Cells of Unknown Significance), 435
Askin tumor, 14

ASTRO criterion, 385
Astrocytoma
  central nervous system, 77
  juvenile pilocytic, 75
  pilocytic, 82, 83, 85–86
  spinal cord, 114, 116
  subependymal giant cell, 82
Audiometry, 125
  for acoustic neuromas, 125
Auricotemporal nerve, 159
Auriculotemporal nerve syndrome, 178
Autologous transplant, 508–509.
        See also Transplant
AVMs. *See* Arteriovenous malformation (AVMs)
Azygos vein, 588

B

Barrett esophagus, 300
Basal cell carcinoma (BCC), 553–559
  background, 553–555
  toxicity, 558–559
  treatment/prognosis, 556–558
  workup/staging, 555
BCC. *See* Basal cell carcinoma (BCC)
bcl-2, 136
Beam spoilers, 510
Beckwith-Wiedemann syndrome, 21
Benign lip lesions, 159
Benign prostatic hypertrophy (BPH), 363
β_2-microglobulin, 499
Biliary cancer, 334–340
Birbeck granules, 45
Bisphosphonates
  in bone metastases, 580
  in multiple myeloma, 501
Bladder cancer, 400–408
  and urethral cancer, 425
Bleomycin, 70, 419
Blueberry muffin sign, 32
Bone metastases, 577–584
  background, 577
  toxicity, 584
  treatment/prognosis, 579–583
  workup/staging, 578–579
Bone-modifying agents (BMAs), 580
Bone scan, 578
Borrmann classification, of gastric cancer, 308
Bowen disease, 420, 555
Brachiocephalic veins, 588
Brachytherapy, for prostate cancer, 395–400
Brain metastases, 567–575
  multiple, 568

  single, 567
  solitary, 567
Brainstem gliomas (BSGs), 74–76
BRCA1, 258
BRCA2, 258, 317
Breast cancer, 257–264, 578
  background, 257–261
  breast MRIs and, 259–260
  ductal carcinoma in situ, 264–271
  early-stage, 272–283
    background, 272–273
    treatment/prognosis, 275–283
    workup/staging, 273–275
  lobular carcinoma in situ, 264–271
  locally advanced, 283–295
    background, 283–284
    follow-up/toxicity, 294–295
    treatment/prognosis, 284–293
    workup/staging, 284
  in pregnancy, 283
  screening for, 259
  tissue microarray classification system, 260
  toxicity, 263–264
  workup/staging, 261–263
Breast reconstruction, 293
Broca motor area, 80
Bronchial neuroendocrine tumor, 233–243
BSGs. *See* Brainstem gliomas (BSGs)
Buccal mucosa cancer, 156, 160
Bulbomembranous urethra, 426
Bulky mediastinal disease, 476

C

CA125, 446
Carboplatin, 237
Carcinomatous meningitis, 568
Cauda equina syndrome, 585
CD20, 136
CD133, 79
CD207 (langerin), 45
CD1a, 45
CEA, 345
Central nervous system (CNS) tumors, 77–81
  lymphoma, 96–103
Cerebellopontine angle (CPA), 124
Cerebellum, 71
Cervical cancer, 435–444
Chang staging system, for MB, 50
Chest radiograph (CXR), Wilms tumor, 23
Child-Pugh score, 330
Chlamydia psittaci, 137
Cholangiocarcinoma (CC). *See* Biliary cancer